# Infectious Diseases

## Focus on Clinical Diagnosis

Edited by

### HARAGOPAL THADEPALLI, M.D.

Chief, Division of Infectious Diseases
Martin Luther King, Jr. General Hospital;
Associate Professor of Medicine
Charles R. Drew Postgraduate School of Medicine
University of Southern California School of Medicine
Los Angeles, California

 Medical Examination Publishing Co., Inc.
an Excerpta Medica company

969 Stewart Avenue • Garden City, New York 11530

**SIMULTANEOUSLY PUBLISHED IN:**

| | | |
|---|---|---|
| Brazil | : | GUANABARA KOOGAN<br>Rio de Janeiro, Brazil |
| Europe | : | HANS HUBER PUBLISHERS<br>Bern, Switzerland |
| Mexico,<br>Central America,<br>and South America<br>(except Brazil) | : | EDITORIAL EL MANUAL MODERNO<br>Mexico City, Mexico |
| South and East Asia | : | TOPPAN COMPANY (S) Pte. Ltd.<br>Singapore |

# Preface

This book is written for all practicing physicians and emphasizes such common diseases as tuberculosis, typhoid fever, amoebiasis and other parasitic diseases, as well as those diseases not commonly encountered. We have intentionally deleted therapy unless it was imperative.

Unfortunately, no two patients are alike; each patient is a unique jigsaw puzzle, a pattern to be assembled with a keen sense of coordination. One ought to know what one is treating; there is no such thing as a textbook case. It is important to gather together facts and pieces of information at the bedside and boil down the data to a certain limited number of probabilities. Every investigation done thereafter should lead one step closer to the diagnosis; if not, it is a wasted effort. This book will help to confirm the diagnosis when clinically suspected and to assess the relative value, advantages and disadvantages of each test as compared with previous tests done for the same disease.

I am grateful to my undergraduate and postgraduate teachers in India for their emphasis on bedside teaching and diagnosis. I am immensely grateful to my teachers in the United States who taught me the skills of the actual practice of medicine, and who inculcated the technique of synthesizing the clinical and laboratory medicine into an art of diagnosis.

I have greatly benefited from the preparation of this book and have learned a great deal during the several hundreds of hours I spent reviewing the literature.

I am very grateful to my co-authors for their enthusiastic support and for the many hours of valuable time they spent in the preparation of this manuscript.

Haragopal Thadepalli

# Contributors

**LARRY J. BARAFF, M.D.,** Assistant Professor of Pediatrics, University of California at Los Angeles, School of Medicine, Los Angeles, California

**HANS E. EINSTEIN, M.D., F.A.C.P., F.C.C.P.,** Clinical Professor of Medicine, University of Southern California School of Medicine, Los Angeles, California

**A. PAUL KELLY, M.D.,** Associate Professor of Medicine; Chief, Division of Dermatology, Charles R. Drew Postgraduate School of Medicine, Los Angeles, California

**TOM MADHAVAN, M.D., F.A.C.P.,** Staff Physician, Division of Infectious Diseases, Henry Ford Hospital; Clinical Assistant Professor of Internal Medicine, University of Michigan Medical School, Ann Arbor, Michigan

**GARY OVERTURF, M.D.,** Assistant Professor of Pediatrics, University of Southern California; Director, Communicable Diseases Unit, Los Angeles County General Hospital, Los Angeles, California

**FRANK A. SALEM, M.D.,** Associate Professor of Pathology, Charles R. Drew Postgraduate School of Medicine, Los Angeles, California

**LOUIS D. SARAVOLATZ, M.D.,** Fellow in Infectious Diseases, Henry Ford Hospital, Ann Arbor, Michigan

**TOSHIYUKI TANAKA, M.D.,** Assistant Professor of Radiology, Charles R. Drew Postgraduate School of Medicine, Los Angeles, California

**HARAGOPAL THADEPALLI, M.D.,** Chief, Division of Infectious Diseases, Martin Luther King, Jr. General Hospital; Associate Professor of Medicine, Charles R. Drew Postgraduate School of Medicine, University of Southern California School of Medicine, Los Angeles, California

**DAVID D. ULMER, M.D.,** Professor of Medicine, Charles R. Drew Postgraduate School of Medicine, University of Southern California School of Medicine; Chairman, Department of Medicine, Martin Luther King, Jr. General Hospital, Los Angeles, California

**LALIT H. VORA, M.D.,** Assistant Professor of Radiology, Charles R. Drew Postgraduate School of Medicine, University of California at Los Angeles, Los Angeles, California

**DAVID W. WEBB, M.D.,** Fellow in Infectious Diseases, Charles R. Drew Postgraduate School of Medicine, Los Angeles, California

**CAROLINE H. YEAGER, M.D.,** Assistant Professor of Radiology, Charles R. Drew Postgraduate School of Medicine, Los Angeles, California

# Contents

Contents (cont'd)

## D.  HEART

## E.  GENITOURINARY INFECTIONS

## F.  SKIN AND SOFT TISSUE INFECTIONS

## G.  BONE AND JOINT INFECTIONS

## H.  INFECTIONS OF THE LYMPHATIC SYSTEM

### I. DISTURBANCES IN BODY TEMPERATURE

### J. PARASITIC INFECTIONS

### K. RICKETTSIA

### L. VIRAL INFECTIONS

Contents (cont'd)

## M.  MISCELLANEOUS CATEGORIES

## N.  DIAGNOSTIC PROCEDURES

To

Carmen, Fernando, and Harini

# Acknowledgments

We are greatly indebted to Mrs. Lois E. Pickering for her dedication and innumerable hours spent on the preparation of this manuscript, through to the last stages of completion. Page after page she struggled to decipher the hieroglyphics of my handwriting and that of my co-authors; patiently she typed and retyped, read and reread until this book was found to be pleasing and presentable to the publisher before the deadline.

We are grateful to Dr. Neville C.W. Smith, our staff physician in radiology, for contributing many of the roentgenograms depicted in this book.

We would like to thank Mr. George W. Sanders, supervisor of the Drew Medical Illustration Department; Mr. William F. Hixon, medical photographer; and Mrs. Jane Sakai, graphic artist for contributing their time toward the illustration of this book.

We are immensely grateful to Medical Examination Publishing Company and Mr. Howard Granat for giving us the opportunity to prepare this book.

**The Authors**

## notice

The editor(s) and/or author(s) and the publisher of this book have made every effort to ensure that all therapeutic modalities that are recommended are in accordance with accepted standards at the time of publication.

The drugs specified within this book may not have specific approval by the Food and Drug Administration in regard to the indications and dosages that are recommended by the editor(s) and/or author(s). The manufacturer's package insert is the best source of current prescribing information.

# SECTION A: GASTROINTESTINAL INFECTIONS

## 1: SALMONELLOSIS, TYPHOID FEVER AND ENTERITIS
by H. Thadepalli

### DEFINITION

Typhoid fever is caused by the obligatory human pathogen, Salmonella typhi. Enteric fevers are caused by a number of different Salmonella serotypes. The enteritis is an acute infection, resulting from ingestion of contaminated food containing Salmonella organisms. Salmonella of any species can produce a syndrome clinically indistinguishable from typhoid fever, salmonellosis, enteritis or food poisoning. With the exception of food poisoning caused by Salmonella toxins, diarrhea is not the pronounced feature of these diseases. Unlike most other diarrheas, Salmonella infections are systemic infections.

### EPIDEMIOLOGY

Salmonellosis occurs in all parts of the world, and it can affect all age groups, more frequently those who are younger than thirty years of age. It has no special sex predilection. In the United States, nearly 400 cases of Salmonella typhi infection are reported per year.

### SYMPTOMS AND SIGNS

Typhoid fever, contrary to general belief, starts with symptoms of upper respiratory tract infection, such as cough (60%) or epistaxis (10%),[1] following which patients develop stepladder-type fever; 99° to 100°/101°F. for the first three to five days, increasing to 104° to 105°F. during the second week. Because of the respiratory type of onset, it can be mistaken for bronchitis. A daily fluctuation in temperature is generally within 1° to 2°F. An occasional patient may have fever of abrupt onset with a chilly sensation, but classic "rigors" are rare. Two-thirds of the patients do not have diarrhea.

In most instances, typhoid fever begins as an undiagnosed fever. During the second week of fever, the clinical symptoms may be more serious. The patient may then have cloudy consciousness or delirium. During the second week, the characteristic "rose spots" may appear in 60% to 70%. They are faint, salmon-colored macules of 2 to 4 mm. in size and blanch on pressure, usually less than fifteen in number. They appear on the abdomen or the lateral portions of the trunk. Other areas of the body may be involved, but this is rare. Typhoid organisms can be isolated from these lesions. These spots can be marked as they appear so as to recognize the new spots as they appear.

Several modes of onset of this disease have been recognized. Typhoid fever, at onset, may be mistaken for meningitis, pneumonia, appendicitis, nephritis, cholecystitis, hepatitis, acute diarrhea, intra-abdominal abscess, endocarditis, or tuberculosis.

MENINGITIS-TYPE: The patient is usually confused or has other mental symptoms, such as delirium or coma, and may have neck stiffness. Occasionally, the spinal fluid may show slightly increased protein and lymphocytosis. The spinal fluid is almost always sterile. Frank meningitis, due to S. typhi, is rare.

PNEUMONIA TYPE: Sputum cultures are usually negative, but may occasionally be positive.

INTRA-ABDOMINAL ABSCESS, CHOLECYSTITIS TYPES: These may not be distinguished without a stool culture.

TUBERCULOSIS: Typhoid fever can be mistaken for miliary tuberculosis at the onset. Sputum examination for acid-fast organisms, blood cultures and stool cultures, obtained as a part of the work-up for fever of undetermined origin, reveal the diagnosis.

BACTERIAL ENDOCARDITIS: The diagnosis becomes obvious after the blood culture results, for endocarditis due to Salmonella organism is rare. Anemia and heart murmur, with lung infiltrates, fever and splenomegaly, may occur in both conditions.

DIARRHEA: This might occur at the onset in 30% as the so-called "illness of infection".

During the third week, a dull, disoriented state of muttering delirium may set in. The abdomen becomes tumid, along with the onset of the so-called "pea soup" diarrhea. The illness lyses during the fourth week.

## PHYSICAL SIGNS

Prominent signs of typhoid fever include fever ranging from 100° to 106°F. , with little fluctuation during the day, associated with chills and sweats in the evening hours, but no rigors.

The patient may have bradycardia (Table 1, Fig. 1) with disproportionately slower pulse rate than body temperature. Relative bradycardia is not a constant feature, but when present, is a valuable clinical clue.

The spleen may not be palpable during the first three to four days of illness, but characteristically, there is subcostal tenderness. The spleen becomes readily palpable at the end of the first week, and in most instances, it is palpable during the second week. The spleen is soft and tender, and felt one or two inches below the costal margin.

Right iliac fossa tenderness may be present in 25% to 30% of the patients, but the rebound tenderness is not as severe as in acute appendicitis.

## COMPLICATIONS

Hemorrhage and perforation are the most frequent complications associated with typhoid fever, occurring in 10% to 20% during the second or the third week of typhoid fever. Other less frequent complications are: relapses, myocarditis, osteomyelitis, arthritis, lymphadenitis, acute cholecystitis and rarely thrombosis and Zenker's degeneration of the muscle of the anterior wall of the abdomen.[2]

## LABORATORY FEATURES

Pancytopenia is common with typhoid fever, probably secondary marrow suppression due to endotoxin. The leukocyte counts may be 2,000 to 5,000/cu. mm. It is rare to find any eosinophilia in a well-developed case of typhoid fever.[2] As a general rule, in typhoid fever, the inflammatory response is a mononuclear, but not polymorphonuclear, response. The lesions produced in the intestine are dominated by mononuclear cells. Extra-abdominal infections may cause polymorphonuclear leukocytosis. Polymorphonuclear leukocytosis in typhoid fever, therefore, calls for clinical re-evaluation for such complications

## TABLE 1: NORMAL PULSE - TEMPERATURE CHART

| PULSE : | 50 | 60 | 70 | 80 | 90 | 100 | 110 | 120 | 130 | 140 |
|---|---|---|---|---|---|---|---|---|---|---|
| TEMP $^0$F.: | 96 | 97 | 98 | 99 | 100 | 101 | 102 | 103 | 104 | 105 |
| TEMP $^0$C.: | 35.6 | 36.1 | 36.7 | 37.2 | 37.8 | 38.3 | 38.9 | 39.4 | 40.0 | 40.6 |

The pulse rate in untreated and uncomplicated enteric fever is, as a rule, 30 to 40 beats per minute slower than as indicated above. For example, a patient with 103$^0$F. (39.4$^0$C.) may have a pulse rate of 90 or lower, instead of 120 per minute.

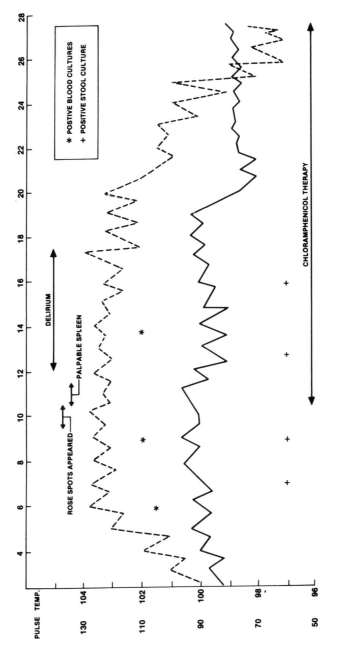

FIG. 1: Typhoid fever with graph of pulse rate.

as intestinal perforation or abscess of the liver or spleen. The serum transaminases, including SGOT and SGPT may be elevated. A small percentage of patients may develop reversible jaundice. The urinalysis may show 1 to 2+ protein with or without casts.

## DIAGNOSIS

Salmonella typhosa is an aerobic, gram-negative, motile organism belonging to the Enterobacteriaceae group. It does not ferment lactose and produces hydrogen sulfide, but no free gas. S. typhi characteristically possesses the Vi antigen. S. typhi belongs to group D, although there are other organisms classified under this group.

BLOOD CULTURE: Blood cultures are usually positive during the first week of illness. Contrary to the usual belief, blood cultures may be positive during the second and third week as well. It is a fallacy to think that the greater the amount of blood collected, the greater will be the yield. On the contrary, as small as 1 to 2 cc. of blood in 5 to 10 ml. of broth may give better results. The addition of substances such as bile and liquoid (sodium polyanethol sulphonate) to the medium may help to counteract the bactericidal action of the blood. The dilution factor may be even more important in patients receiving antibiotics. The average percentage of positive blood culture is from 10% to 50% during the first week. The chances decrease, somewhat, during the second and third weeks of illness.

CULTURE OF FECES: Nearly one-half of the patients with typhoid fever will have positive cultures of feces during the first week. Fecal cultures should, therefore, be obtained on the very first day of admission in all cases of suspected enteric fever. Subsequently, the number of organisms increases in the stool. In spite of antibiotic administration, fecal cultures may remain positive in nearly 50% of the patients during the third and fourth weeks. The overall yield by stool culture is around 90%. Rectal swabs are not satisfactory for culturing S. typhi, therefore, rectal swabs, alone, should not be used for the diagnosis of enteric fever.

URINE CULTURES: These are positive in one-fourth to one-third of all cases. Typhoid bacilluria is temporary, but in carriers, it may be prolonged. Quantitative urine cultures are not required to demonstrate the organism. Even one colony in urine is just as pathognomonic as one million organisms/ml. of urine.

CULTURE OF BILE: S. typhi are found in great concentrations in the bile. Bile can be obtained by duodenal intubation or by string-capsule technique. The latter involves a string capsule swallowed by the patient at night. The nylon thread is pulled up in the morning. The tip of the nylon thread, which is frequently bile-stained, is cut and dropped into a broth for culture of the organisms. The string-capsule technique was reported to yield positive cultures in one-third of the cases of enteric fever.

WIDAL TEST: S. typhi has both H or flagellar antigen, and O or somatic. They may be increased in recent infections. A four-fold increase in their titer, or a single O antigen titer in excess of 1:60 or more in a case with a clinical picture of typhoid fever, is a presumptive evidence of that disease. In acute infection, the O antigen may rise without a corresponding rise in H antigen titers. Antimicrobial therapy may interfere with the Widal test. Both O and H antigens might be increased in cases of recent vaccination. The vaccine contains the antigens of paratyphi A, paratyphi B and S. typhi. The paratyphi A is a rare infection; hence, a positive Widal test with increased titers for paratyphi A should mean that the accompanying increase in titers for S. typhi is due to vaccination, but not due to recent exposure to S. typhi.

A titer of 1:40 for O and H antibodies during the first week of fever in non-endemic areas should also suggest typhoid fever. They should be repeated within four days to demonstrate the rise in titer, generally considered diagnostic. Such titers are of no diagnostic value in patients from the endemic areas. The Widal reaction should not be relied upon for diagnosis. Every effort should be made to culture the organism from the blood, stool or urine before antibiotic therapy.

VIRULENT ANTIGEN (Vi antigen): This is possessed by S. typhi and S. dublin, both group D, and S. hirschfeldii (S. paratyphi C) of group C (1) of Salmonella species. A group D Salmonella organism containing the virulent antigen could be either S. typhi or S. dublin. S. dublin does not have the group "d-H" antigen.

CEREBROSPINAL FLUID: This is rarely (0.3% to 0.5%) positive on culture.

LACTOSE-FERMENTING SALMONELLA: Most Salmonella organisms do not ferment lactose. In one study, 86 (15.6%) of the 552 Salmonella cultures fermented lactose. This had been isolated from dried milk products.[3] Lactose-positive Salmonella typhimurium is endemic to Sao Paulo, Brazil,[4] isolated from stool cultures of infants under one year of age. They suggested a simple procedure for detecting lactose-positive Salmonella mixed with ordinary lactose-positive E. coli. It consists of picking twelve successive colonies and inoculating them in a peptone iron agar. Hydrogen sulfide production becomes apparent even if only one colony of Salmonella was picked. The true incidence of lactose-positive Salmonella remains unknown, because most laboratories do not look for them.

ILEAL PERFORATIONS: Intestinal perforations comprise nearly two-thirds of all the common complications associated with typhoid fever. The average mortality of ileal perforation is around 25%. The typhoid bacilli and its toxins may cause extensive necrosis of the Peyer's patches and ulceration, but cicatrization is rare. There is no relationship between the severity of clinical illness, degree of ulceration, and the chances of perforation. Abdominal distention with pain and tenderness, associated with guarding, fever and vomiting, is the symptom complex of typhoid ileal perforation. Antibiotic therapy may mask these symptoms. It is also difficult to detect among patients with protracted illness. The bowel sounds may be present in nearly two-thirds of the patients with perforation. A sudden decrease in the hemoglobin, with leukocytosis, hypotension and/or demonstration of free air under the diaphragm, suggests perforation. Perforations which occur while on medical therapy are twice as grave as typhoid perforations without therapy, because the former may go undetected for a period due to lack of symptoms. [5]

S. DUBLIN: This, as mentioned, also has Vi antigen. It is an infrequent isolate east of the Rocky Mountains. Nearly 80% of these cases reported in the U.S. are from the state of California. Most of them are of bovine origin, indicating the host specificity of S. dublin for cattle. Drinking raw milk, a recent fad among the naturalists, may be a frequent cause of S. dublin infection among humans.

## PROGNOSIS

The prognosis of typhoid fever is good in more than 95% of the cases if the diagnosis is suspected early enough and treated with appropriate antimicrobial agents. Chloramphenicol, ampicillin and sulphamethoxazole-trimethoprim are some of the recommended agents.

## THE CARRIER STATE

Regardless of the vehicle, the ultimate source of typhoid fever is invariably the human carrier. Food is the common vehicle of infection. All patients with typhoid fever should be periodically examined for the possible development of carrier state. Most patients with typhoid fever are free of the organisms within a period of three months. One who excretes S. typhi for more than one year is called a carrier. Approximately 3% of the patients become carriers. The carrier state was reported as 1 in 1,000 in Hong Kong and 1 in 100,000 in the United Kingdom. The carrier may be asymptomatic or may suffer periodic gastrointestinal illnesses, cholecystitis or recurrent urinary tract infections. Most carriers are females between ages 30 to 50.

The fecal carrier can be detected by stool cultures, duodenal intubation, bile culture or by the string-capsule test mentioned earlier. Carrier state can be eliminated in 90% by cholecystectomy combined with antimicrobial therapy. Urinary carriers are rare. Most urinary carriers are men between ages 30 to 50. All urinary carriers should be examined for the underlying urinary tract abnormality, either an anatomical defect or the development of renal stones. The underlying diseases should be treated to eliminate the carrier state. Schistosoma hematobium infections may predispose to the development of S. typhi carriers.

## ENTERIC FEVERS (PARATYPHOID)

For clinical purposes, the distinction between typhoid and paratyphoid serves no useful purpose, although such distinction is necessary for therapeutic purposes. The diagnosis is based upon the isolation of the causative organism and identification. Generally, if the organism identified is a Salmonella, but not S. typhi, and if the patient is asymptomatic, supportive therapy is all that is necessary. But if the patient is seriously ill or is too young or too old, he should be treated with antibiotics.

## SALMONELLOSIS

### EPIDEMIOLOGY

The mean, national annual incidence for the entire seven-year period (1968-1974) in the United States was 11.8 cases/100,000 population;[6] highest from Hawaii (76.6/100,000) and the lowest from Nebraska (2.2/100,000). Salmonella typhimurium is the most frequent, accounting for 26.5% of all isolates. Less common isolates were S. enteritidis, S. newport, S. heidelberg, S. infantis, and S. saint-paul. S. agona is reportedly imported in contaminated Peruvian fish meal. Approximately 280,000 cases per year of salmonellosis occurred in the United States during 1970 and 1971 due to pet turtles. Importing uncertified turtles or turtle eggs to the United States is now prohibited. After this, nearly two-thirds of the so-called certified turtles were later found to harbor Salmonella organisms. [7] Infections due to S. dublin associated with dairy products were discussed earlier.

## SYMPTOMS

Enteritis begins within eight to forty-eight hours after the ingestion of contaminated food or drink. [8] The onset is abrupt, associated with fever, body pains, headaches and generalized lethargy. A banquet or a family picnic is the usual starting point. Meat was the main contamination source in nearly one-half of the cases. It can be transmitted from person to person by hospital personnel. The infection is caused by the elaboration of enterotoxin. This disease is severe among children and young adults.

## PREDISPOSING CAUSES

The predisposing causes are subtotal gastrectomy, previous antibiotic therapy, and severe underlying debilitating illness. The fever may vary (99⁰ to 104⁰F.). Vomiting and diarrhea are common. The diarrhea may be severe enough to lead to dehydration requiring fluid replacement therapy. Untreated illness lasts for a week, and treated illness sometimes lasts longer. The peripheral cell counts are usually within normal limits. Blood cultures are of no value in the diagnosis of enteritis. Stool culture is a primary source for the organisms present in nearly all patients.

## DIFFERENTIAL

Salmonella enteritis resembles shigellosis. The stools in salmonellosis are usually watery in nature, rarely blood-stained. Vomiting is not a feature of shigellosis. Other disorders to be distinguished from Salmonella enteritis are Clostridium welchii enteritis, E. coli diarrhea and acute staphylococcal food poisoning. These conditions can be differentiated by positive stool cultures for Salmonella group of organisms.

Fecal smears examined for leukocytes may be of value in differentiating between Shigella dysentery and Salmonella enteritis.

Stool culture for C. perfringens, in counts of more than 1 x
$10^5$ organisms/gram of stool, is diagnostic of food-borne disease due to C. perfringens. Similarly, demonstration of more
than 1 x $10^6$ organisms/gram of stool of Staphylococcus aureus
is diagnostic of staphylococcal food poisoning (see pages 39,41).
Other diseases to be excluded are post-vagotomy diarrhea,
cholera, E. coli diarrhea, carcinoid syndrome, medullary carcinoma of the thyroid and Zollinger-Ellison syndrome.

COLONIC INVOLVEMENT: Involvement of the large bowel is a
fairly common feature of human salmonellosis and may, perhaps,
play an important role in the causation of diarrhea. In one study,
21 of 23 inpatients with acute Salmonella infection had active
colitis.[9] One who presents with bloody diarrhea, and has Salmonella in his stool, may be suffering from either acute ulcerative colitis with incidental Salmonella infection or Salmonella
enteritis. In such cases, one cannot distinguish these two syndromes with confidence.[10] Ulcerative colitis may either predispose or be associated with Salmonella infections.

Antibiotic therapy in acute salmonellosis may increase the duration of excretion of the organisms, thereby increasing its
chances of spread and the potential development of antibiotic
resistance.

ARIZONA HINSHAWII: A. hinshawii resembles Salmonella serologically and biochemically. Like Salmonella, it possesses H
and O antigens and produces hydrogen sulfide. Arizona ferments
lactose, unlike most Salmonella, but does not ferment tartrate
or dulcitol. Infections caused by A. hinshawii resemble the
spectrum of clinical syndromes seen with Salmonella infections.[11] It occurs mostly among patients with other serious underlying illnesses, such as Hodgkin's disease, renal transplant
recipients, mentally retarded patients, and those with sickle
cell disease. Arizona is of the group of Enterobacteriaceae. A.
hinshawii may be cultured from the stools, blood, sputum or
transtracheal aspirate. Most antimicrobial agents effective
against Salmonella are also effective against Arizona. The final
outcome is generally dependent upon the underlying host factors.

## REFERENCES

1. Christie, A. B. : Typhoid and Paratyphoid Fevers. Infectious
   Diseases: Epidemiology and Clinical Practice. Livingstone,
   Ltd. , London, 1969, pp. 54-121.

2. Boyd, W.: Typhoid Fever, Diseases of the Intestine. Pathology for the Physician, 7th Edition. Lea & Febiger, Philadelphia, 1965, pp. 414-421.

3. Blackburn, B. O., Ellis, E. M.: Lactose-fermenting Salmonella from dried milk products. Appl. Micro. 26:672, 1973.

4. Falcao, D. P., et al: Unusual Enterobacteriaceae - lactose-positive Salmonella typhimurium which is endemic in Sao Paulo, Brazil. Clin. Microbiol. 2:349, 1975.

5. Archampong, E. Q.: Typhoid ileal perforation: Why such mortalities? Br. J. Surg. 63:317, 1976.

6. Ryder, R. W., et al: Salmonellosis in the United States, 1968-1974. J. Inf. Dis. 133:483, 1976.

7. Polk, L. D.: Salmonellosis in children from pet turtles certified Salmonella-free. Clin. Pediatrics 13:719, 1974.

8. Overturf, G., Mathies, A. W., Jr.: Salmonellosis. Communicable and Infectious Diseases, 18th Edition, Ch. 59, (Eds.) Top, F. H., Wehrle, P. F., C. V. Mosby Co., St. Louis, 1976, pp. 598-611.

9. Mandal, B. K., Mani, V.: Colonic involvement in salmonellosis. Lancet 1:887, 1976.

10. Lindeman, R. J., et al: Ulcerative colitis and intestinal salmonellosis. Am. J. Med. Sci. 254:855, 1967.

11. Johnson, R., et al: Arizona hinshawii infections: New cases, antimicrobial sensitivities and literature review. Ann. Int. Med. 85:587, 1976.

## 2: SHIGELLA DYSENTERY
by H. Thadepalli

Shigella dysentery is a disease of the tropics and subtropics, prevalent during the rainy season and for a short period thereafter. [1] Overcrowding and poor sanitation are the two most prominent predisposing causes, assuming epidemic proportion during wars and in mental asylums. It has an incubation period of a few hours to seven days. It is a disease of the large intestine. Low-grade fevers are common, but fevers above 104°F. are rare except in Shigella shigae infections. Excruciating pain in the rectum, due to tenesmus, is very common with Shigella dysentery. It is a disease of low mortality, but among the hospitalized patients, the death toll may vary from 1% to 20% of the affected. The onset may be either insidious or fulminating. Vomiting may occur to start with, but rarely persists. The spleen is rarely palpable. The abdomen is difficult to palpate during the early stages because of tenderness and rigidity.

### STOOL EXAMINATION

The initial evacuations may be viscid mucus and blood-stained, resembling "red currant jelly". [2] It may change to a fulminating form of dysentery, with mucus mingled with large amounts of altered blood, resembling "meat washings". Shigella dysentery may at times be very alarming and highly pyrexial with a great degree of prostration in the patients passing large clots of blood in watery stools, resembling "tomato soup". The stools, in general, are small (a few teaspoonfuls), passed nearly twelve to eighteen times per day. An unfortunate victim may have a single protracted bowel movement, leaving the victim "glued to the commode". On the second day of illness, the stools are less hemorrhagic, but more purulent. On the third and fourth days, less blood and pus is passed, but the stools are more greenish, due to bile pigments.

Fecal smears should be stained with Wright's stain and examined for leukocytes. Sheets of polymorphonuclear cells are very common with Shigella dysentery, which is in contra-distinction to mononuclear cells found in typhoid fever. Polymorphs constitute 90% of the total cells in the stool. Macrophages of size 20 to 30 microns, containing vacuoles, are seen sometimes even ingested with red blood cells. They may be mistaken for E. histolytica. The macrophages are non-motile.

Shiga's bacillus dysentery may be abrupt and fulminating in onset, beginning with chills and rigors associated with vomiting, headache, and a quick rise in body temperature to 104°F. (40°C.), followed shortly thereafter with severe purging, and the stools quickly assume the dysenteric character. The abdomen may be soft or acutely tender; the stools may become liquidy or watery, as in cholera. On occasion, the patient might develop disseminated intravascular coagulation or circulatory failure within a few hours to a few days. The fatalities associated with Shiga bacillus are high.

Shigella sonnei is a common Shigella infection in the United States. [3] S. sonnei attacks are often mild and associated with dysentery or diarrhea. Fever is usually low-grade, and the stools are seldom more than twelve per day. A significant number of patients may have associated respiratory tract symptoms.

Other associated features of Shigella infections are: peripheral neuritis, conjunctivitis, measles-like rash, non-pyogenic arthritis and urethritis resembling Reiter's syndrome. Other complications, such as unilateral or bilateral parotitis, may also occur. Intussusception is one of the catastrophic problems associated with Shigella dysentery among children. Liver abscesses, splenic abscesses, enlargement of the spleen, peritonitis, perforation and intestinal hemorrhage are rare complications.

Blood cultures are useless to diagnose Shigella dysentery.

Stool cultures are diagnostic. The best specimen is one with blood and mucus in the stool.

## ISOLATION OF THE ORGANISMS

Stool cultures should be done on three to four successive occasions to increase the yield. Table 2 describes the characteristic biochemical differentiating features of Shigella from other enteropathogenic organisms. Table 3 depicts the biochemical characteristics of four classical strains of Shigella.

Dysentery is caused by Shigella shigae (Shiga's bacillus) Shigella flexneri, Shigella sonnei and Shigella boydii. Nearly 80% of isolates in the United States are S. sonnei. S. flexneri is the next most common. Shiga bacillus infections are rare in the United States. Shiga's bacillus is prevalent in Asia, Africa and South America.

TABLE 2: BIOCHEMICAL DIFFERENTIATION OF SHIGELLA AND SALMONELLA FROM OTHER ENTEROBACTERIACEAE

| Reaction | E. coli | Shigella* | Salmonella | Arizona | Edwardsiella | Alkalescens dispar |
|---|---|---|---|---|---|---|
| Gas from glucose | + | + | + | + | + | + |
| Lactose | + | - | - | +- | - | - |
| Sucrose | +- | - | - | · - | - | +- |
| Mannitol | + | +- | + | + | - | + |
| Sorbitol | + | +- | - | d | + | - |
| Arabinose | + | +- | + | + | - | - |
| Indole | + | - or + | - | - | + | + |

(cont'd)

(Table 2 cont'd)

| Reaction | E. coli | Shigella* | Salmonella | Arizona | Edwardsiella | Alkalescens dispar |
|---|---|---|---|---|---|---|
| Hydrogen sulfide | - | - | + | + | + | - |
| Simmon's citrate | - | - | +(1) | - | - | - |
| Lysine decarboxylase | - | - | +(2) | + | - | + |

* : See Table 3 for detailed speciation.
d : Different biochemical types.
(1): S. typhi and paratyphi A are citrate-negative. S. cholera suis is delayed positive.
(2): S. paratyphi is lysine-negative.

TABLE 3: DISTINGUISHING CHARACTERISTICS OF THE
SHIGELLA (S.) SPECIES

| Reaction | S. dysenteriae | S. flexneri | S. boydii | S. sonnei |
|----------|----------------|-------------|-----------|-----------|
| Lactose  | -  | -  | -  | (+) |
| Mannitol | -  | +  | +  | +   |
| Sucrose  | -  | -  | -  | (+) |
| Dulcitol | d  | -  | d  | -   |
| Xylose   | -  | -  | d  | -   |
| Ornithine| -  | -  | -  | +   |
| Arginine | -  | -  | -  | d   |

d : Character inconsistent
(+): Slow reaction

Spinal fluid examination, even among patients with convulsions, is almost always negative. Nearly 20% to 30% of spinal fluid specimens may show pleocytosis with an increased protein, but normal glucose, level.

## DIFFERENTIAL DIAGNOSIS

The fecal smears in dysentery due to Salmonella contain mononuclear cells. See Table 36, page 534 for differentiation between bacillary and amoebic dysentery. E. coli dysentery may resemble shigellosis, which can be distinguished by stool cultures. The cholera stools are watery and seldom contain red blood corpuscles or pus cells. Tenesmus seldom occurs in cholera. Ulcerative colitis may be indistinguishable from shigellosis. An occasional patient with ulcerative colitis may develop Shigella dysentery. Staphylococcal food poisoning and Clostridium perfringens food poisoning are usually conspicuous by vomiting. Vomiting is a mild and early feature in shigellosis.

CARRIERS: With or without long-term therapy, the Shigella carrier state may occasionally exist for a year or more.[4] Therapeutic responses are excellent among the Shigella carriers. Lomotil (diphenoxylate hydrochloride with atropine) may retard the intestinal motility and thereby increase the duration of bacillary excretion.[5]

Bacillary dysentery may be associated with parasitic infections, notably E. histolytica or Giardia lamblia. Shigella dysentery is also found along with virus diseases, such as measles or polio.

## REFERENCES

1.  Bevenson, A. S. (Ed.): Control of Communicable Diseases in Man, 12th Edition. Amer. Pub. Health Association, Washington, D. C., 1975, pp. 285-288.

2.  Manson-Bahr, P. H.: Bacillary Dysentery. Manson's Tropical Diseases, 16th Edition. Balliere, Tindall & Cassell, London, pp. 406-422, 1966.

3.  Gangarosa, E.: Shigellosis. Communicable and Infectious Diseases, 18th Edition, (Eds.) Top, F. H., Wehrle, P. F. C. V. Mosby Co., St. Louis, 1976, pp. 616-622.

4.  Levine, M. M., et al: Long-term Shigella - carrier state. New Eng. J. Med. 288:1169, 1973.

5.  Dupont, H. L., Hornick, R. B.: Adverse effect of Lomotil therapy in shigellosis. J. A. M. A. 226:1525, 1973.

## 3: TRAVELERS' DIARRHEA
## by H. Thadepalli

Travelers' diarrhea is characterized by the onset of watery diarrhea, sometimes up to ten to twenty episodes a day, within ten days of arrival to a new country. It is frequently accompanied by such symptoms as abdominal cramps, nausea, anorexia, vomiting, malaise, chills and fever, and may last for one to five days. It is generally a self-limiting illness, and exceptions may last for a week. It affects both sexes and all age groups.

Recent investigations implicate Escherichia coli as the etiologic agent.[1,2] Both enteropathogenic and non-enteropathogenic E. coli types, those that liberate heat-labile, or heat-stable toxins, were isolated from the stools of patients with travelers' diarrhea. Toxigenic E. coli may cause cholera-like profuse watery diarrhea, and invasive strains may cause dysentery, akin to the dysenteries caused by Shigella, Salmonella and Entamoeba histolytica.

There is no correlation between serotyping, toxigenicity, enteropathogenicity, mucosal adherence and actual clinical illness. Serotyping E. coli is of little diagnostic value. Not all travelers develop diarrhea. Some may have immunity. The Guatemalan or East Indian traveler to Mexico has less chance of developing travelers' diarrhea than the North American or Canadian visiting Mexico.

### DIAGNOSIS

Extensive diagnostic procedures are not recommended for routine purposes. To be certain of the presence or absence of enteropathogenic strain, one may have to examine at least ten different colonies from each stool specimen. An examination of fresh stool specimens should be made for isolation of E. coli, in addition to Salmonella, Shigella and Vibrio parahaemolyticus group of organisms. In travelers' diarrhea, one may have more than one pathogen in the stool.

### REFERENCES

1. Gorbach, S. L. , et al: Travelers' diarrhea and toxigenic Escherichia coli. New Eng. J. Med. 292:933, 1975.

2. Merson, M. H. , et al: Travelers' diarrhea in Mexico. New. Eng. J. Med 294:1229, 1976.

4: CHOLERA
by H. Thadepalli

The most appropriate descriptive name for cholera is "vanthi-bedi", which in my mother tongue, Telugu, means vomiting and diarrhea. Most cases occur during December and January in Dacca (Bangladesh) and during June and July in Calcutta (India).

Cholera starts like any ordinary case of diarrhea. After the initial purgation of the feces from the colon, the stool becomes clear and watery, compared to "rice water" stools. The preliminary looseness of stools is known as premonitory diarrhea or cholerine, or mild form of diarrhea (green color stool). During this period, the patient may be somewhat depressed in spirits and develop lethargy.

True cholera then heralds with profuse watery stools without pain, but occasionally, abdominal discomfort. The first fecal stools are malodorous, but the watery diarrhea is odorless or may have fishy odor. The amount of water lost can be so profuse that a patient might lose as much water as his own body weight in three days. In cholera, vomiting frequently follows the onset of diarrhea. It is profuse and occurs without nausea. Muscle cramps develop secondary to severe water loss. At this stage, the patient may develop peripheral circulatory failure and collapse.

Consequent to the loss of body water, the soft parts of the body shrink; cheeks fall in, the nose becomes pinched and thin, eyeballs sunken deep; and the skin over the fingers shrivels like "washer-womens' hands".[1] Those who have not seen washer-womens' hands may compare it with the hands of one who has been swimming in the sea for several hours.

The body temperature may be normal or subnormal, occasionally going down to 94°F. The rectal temperature, however, may be normal or increased to 101° to 105°F. (38.3° to 40.6°C.). The patient is restless with a hoarse, low-pitched voice, unrecordable blood pressure, and may soon pass into a comatose state. Coma occurs secondary to dehydration, acidosis and renal failure.

Varying stages and degrees of the disease might manifest in an epidemic. Not all patients affected with cholera require hospitalization. Only 1 of 100 patients are sick enough to be hospitalized. In a non-endemic area where the population has no resistance to cholera, 25% to 50% of those affected may be hospitalized. The fatality rates are nearly 50% without proper medical care. With proper fluid replacement, the mortality today is less than 1%.

Poverty, insanitation, malnutrition and previous history of gastrectomy, vagotomy or pyloroplasty are some of the predisposing causes for cholera. The chief source of infection is the human species.

The first sign of recovery is marked by the passage of a few ounces of turbid high-colored urine, followed by profuse diuresis, which strongly resembles the recovery stage of acute glomerulonephritis. Hyperpyrexia is a rare, but fatal, complication. Not all cholera victims have profuse diarrhea prior to death.

## COMPLICATIONS

Dehydration may dry up the lacrimal secretion, leaving the eyeballs vulnerable to ulceration of the cornea. An occasional patient may go into coma with eyes half open (coma vigil), and the cornea may ulcerate and slough, leading to scar formation at the lower limbus of the cornea.[1] Cataracts might develop during dehydration and may go unnoticed for several months. Severe dehydration may cause hemoconcentration and gangrene of the tips of the fingers or the toes, or the entire genitalia. [1]

## BACTERIOLOGY

Cholera is caused by Vibrio (V.) cholerae, a gram-negative comma-shaped, self-propelling, flagellated aerobic organism that grows well on thiosulfate-citrate-bile-salt agar (TCBS). V. cholerae, the classic strain, is endemic to the Gangetic and Brahmaputra delta areas in India and Bangladesh. Biotype El Tor strain has been endemic to Indonesia during the last decade. This strain has traveled to several parts of Asia, Africa and Southern Europe. Cholera is rare in the United States. A single case was reported in 1973. Nevertheless, a physician practicing in the U.S. should be familiar with this disease. West Africa was free of cholera during the 20th century until 1970, when a devastating epidemic of more than 150,000 cases occurred with 20,000 deaths. [2,3]

The organism, as the name Vibrio implies, is a motile bacillus which can be seen readily in the stool and vomitus of the patient.

These organisms are usually present in $1 \times 10^{10}$/ml. concentration in these specimens. The first stool may contain a mixture of organisms, but the characteristic rice water stool predominantly contains V. cholerae. They can also be seen under phase-contrast or dark field microscopy and diagnosed within hours. The serotypic diagnosis can also be established within hours by sero-agglutination techniques.

There are three serotypes in biotype El Tor, i.e., Inaba, Ogawa and Hikojima. Vibrio can also be detected by its scintillating rotating movements in hanging-drop preparations. Vibrio may also be stained by carbol fuchsin. Rectal swabs may be obtained for culture. El Tor strains are hemolytic, but the classical strain of cholera is non-hemolytic.

The El Tor disease has now virtually replaced the classic strain of cholera in Calcutta. Carrier state has been described. It may be found in bile. See Table 4 for the differences between the classic and the El Tor strain of cholera.

TABLE 4: DIFFERENTIATION OF VIBRIO CHOLERAE
CLASSIC STRAIN FROM EL TOR

| CHARACTER | CLASSIC STRAIN | EL TOR |
|---|---|---|
| Hemolysis of sheep red blood cells | --- | + or - |
| Chicken erythrocyte agglutination (slide test) | --- | + |
| 50 I. U. polymyxin B disc test | Susceptible | Resistant |
| Susceptibility to Group IV cholera phage | Susceptible | Not Susceptible |

Vibrio cholerae seldom penetrates through the intestinal mucosa. The disease is essentially caused by its toxin.

### DIFFERENTIAL DIAGNOSIS

E. coli may produce clinical symptoms indistinguishable from Vibrio cholerae. The differentiation from these diseases should be based on actual culture techniques and, in the endemic areas, exclusion of V. cholerae as the agent. Rarely, either bacillary dysentery or amoebic dysentery produce such a profuse diarrhea. Fecal leukocytes are absent in cholera stools, but they are usually present in bacillary and amoebic dysentery. In addition, tenesmus, the outstanding feature of bacillary dysentery, is characteristically absent in cholera. Abdominal pain (in contrast to discomfort) is absent in cholera and is usually present in other forms of bacterial and parasitic dysenteries. Acute salmonellosis can be differentiated by the presence of fecal leukocytes and stool cultures. Staphylococcal food poisoning may resemble cholera. Gram's stain of the vomitus may show gram-positive cocci in staphylococcal food poisoning and gram-negative rods in cholera. True cholera may be hard to differentiate from mushroom poisoning. History of a common food source is available in mushroom poisoning. Violent and distressing vomiting precedes diarrhea in most cases of food poisoning. Diarrhea precedes vomiting in cholera. Both abdominal pain and offensive stools are absent in cholera. The differentiating features between food poisoning and cholera are listed in Table 5. The choleraic form of subtertian malaria may simulate cholera, but blood smears would settle the diagnosis. Acute arsenic or antimony poisoning may be indistinguishable from acute cholera. Acute arsenic poisoning may go undetected in endemic areas when there is an outbreak of an acute cholera. Arsenic poisoning can be diagnosed by estimating arsenic content of the vomitus and stool, in addition to hair and nail levels of arsenic. Pancreatic cholera, due to non-islet cell pancreatic adenoma, resembles cholera. Vomiting is not a feature of acute pancreatic cholera.

TABLE 5: DIFFERENTIAL DIAGNOSIS OF FOOD POISONING FROM CHOLERA

| SYMPTOMS AND SIGNS | FOOD POISONING | CHOLERA |
|---|---|---|
| Nausea and retching | Common | Rare |
| Vomiting | Violent and distressing, never watery (contains food) and precedes diarrhea | Follows diarrhea, watery and projectile |
| Tenesmus | Present | Absent |
| Stools | Liquid, fecal and offensive | Watery and copious |
| Urine output | Never decreased | Decreased |

## REFERENCES

1.  Manson-Bahr, P.: Cholera. Manson's Tropical Diseases. Balliere, Tindall & Cassell, London, 1966, pp. 389-405.

2.  Goodgame, R. W., Greenough, W. B.: Cholera in Africa: A message for the West. Ann. Int. Med. 82:101, 1975.

3.  Isaacson, M., et al: The recent cholera outbreak in the South African gold mining industry. S. A. Med. J. 48:2557, 1974.

5: CLOSTRIDIUM PERFRINGENS FOOD POISONING
by H. Thadepalli

Clostridium perfringens is one of the leading causes of food
poisoning in the United States. The vehicle may be cooked meat
or poultry products that are inadequately refrigerated and re-
heated to serve. It occurs among groups attending picnics or
parties, and occasionally in improperly maintained restaurants.

Nausea, vomiting, abdominal cramps and diarrhea, with or
without fever, are present. The onset is explosive and comes
eight to twelve hours after the ingestion of food, beginning with
nausea, vomiting and abdominal cramps. Fever and chills are
not common features of C. perfringens food poisoning. The
entire episode may terminate from a few hours to twenty-four
hours. It is rarely fatal.

C. perfringens is an anaerobic bacteria. Type A strain causes
this disease. The disease, itself, is produced by an enterotoxin.
Type F strains produce enteritis necroticans. C. perfringens
is present in two to six per cent of stools among normal population.

DIAGNOSIS

Diagnosis is established by culturing large numbers of these
organisms from the stool specimens of the victims and also
from the food vehicle. Organisms isolated from the food and
the victim should be of the same type. Types A, C, and D are
implicated in the causation of this disease. C. perfringens
toxin may also be demonstrated in the stool and the serum of
the victims.

THE AGENT

Clostridium perfringens are gram-positive, anaerobic, sporebearing bacilli; some are heat-tolerant and some intolerant.
Most infections reported from the United Kingdom are due to
heat-tolerant strains, and most outbreaks in the United States are
caused by heat-intolerant strains. All of these strains produce an
alpha toxin at the time of their germination from the spores.
The alpha toxin and the spores are resistant to cooking at
$100^{o}C.$ for one to three hours. Neuraminidase production is
characteristic of pathogenic strains. Laboratory identification
is based upon the anaerobicity of the organism, production of
alpha toxin (licithinase), hemolysis and opalescence on human

serum (Nagler's reaction on the egg-yolk media). These are some of the identification features for <u>Clostridium perfringens.</u>

## DIFFERENTIAL DIAGNOSIS

It should be differentiated from <u>Bacillus cereus</u> food poisoning. B. cereus food poisoning is characterized by nausea and vomiting, with or without diarrhea, occurring one to six hours following ingestion of a meal. <u>B. cereus</u> infection may be acquired from vegetable sources, such as cereals and fried rice. Diagnosis is established by the demonstration of at least $1 \times 10^5$ organisms/gram of stool and also from the food sample.

## REFERENCES

1. McClung, L. S.: Human food poisoning due to growth of <u>Clostridium perfringens</u> (C. welchii) in freshly cooked chicken: Preliminary note. J. Bacteriol. 50:229, 1945.

2. Nakamura, M.: <u>Clostridium perfringens</u> food poisoning. Ann. Review of Microbiol. 24:359, 1970.

3. Loewenstein, M. S.: Epidemiology of <u>Clostridium perfringens</u> food poisoning. New Eng. J. Med. 286:1026, 1972.

4. Hobbs, B. C.: <u>Clostridium welchii</u> and <u>Bacillus cereus</u> infection and intoxication. Postgrad. Med. J. 50:597, 1976.

5. Mortimer, P. R., McCann, G.: Food poisoning episodes associated with <u>Bacillus cereus</u> in fried rice. Lancet 1:1043, 1974.

## 6: STAPHYLOCOCCAL FOOD POISONING
### by H. Thadepalli

Food poisoning is caused by enterotoxin produced by Staphylococcus (S. ) aureus. It starts with nausea, vomiting and diarrhea, without fever, after the ingestion of contaminated foods.
Recovery is rapid and fatalities are rare. It is usually abrupt
in onset, often violent, but of brief duration. Diagnosis is established by epidemiologic evidence and the demonstration of
enterotoxin and/or coagulase-positive Staphylococcus aureus
in significant numbers (1 x $10^6$/gram) in the food, vomitus or
stool.

Staphylococcus aureus is a gram-positive aerobic coccus which
occurs in grape-like clusters and grows well in 10% salt solution. It coagulates citrated rabbit and human plasma, referred
to as coagulase-positive reaction. Several outbreaks in the
United States were produced by phage-group III organisms. They
produce type A or type D enterotoxin. S. aureus may be isolated
from the nose, throat, feces or any other skin surface from
normal, healthy persons. Epidemiologic search may lead to
the fingers of cooks as the most likely source.

An outbreak which involved 142 passengers, all Japanese soft
drink dealers on a chartered trip, on close search, led to a
cook who had ulcerating lesions in the hand. [2,3] Coagulase-
positive S. aureus phage 53 and 83AA (group III) was isolated
from the leftover ham samples, and from the ulcerating lesions
on the hands of the cook who prepared the food. In this outbreak,
nearly one-half of the passengers had fever, one-sixth of them
developed bloody diarrhea, and only two became critically ill,
of which one developed shock and anuria and the other developed
temporary cerebral ischemia with hemiparesis, but both recovered from the illness completely. The remaining persons
recovered within a period of a few hours.

Staphylococcal food poisoning can occasionally be fatal. In one
outbreak, four persons developed staphylococcal food poisoning
three to four hours after the consumption of a "cold plate" lunch
served at a restaurant. [1] One patient with rheumatoid arthritis,
on steroids, became ill three hours and forty-five minutes after
the consumption of the cold plate; within five hours and fifteen
minutes, he became unresponsive to external stimuli and died.
In this outbreak, once again, phage 83A/85 (group III) was isolated from the ham plate and also from the hands of the chief
cook who prepared the ham.

## REFERENCES

1. Currier, R. W. , II, et al: Fatal staphylococcal food poisoning. South. Med. J. 66:703, 1973.

2. Effersoe, P. , Kjerulf, K. : Clinical aspects of outbreak of staphylococcal food poisoning during air travel. Lancet 2:599, 1975.

3. Eisenberg, M. S. , et al: Staphylococcal food poisoning aboard a commercial aircraft. Lancet 2:595, 1975.

7: VIBRIO PARAHAEMOLYTICUS INFECTIONS
by H. Thadepalli

Vibrio (V.) parahaemolyticus infection is acquired by consumption of incompletely cooked seafood, such as shell fish, dried sardines, and sushi (raw fish), the most popular food in Japan. It is characterized by an abrupt onset of diarrhea, beginning ten to sixteen hours after the consumption of infected food, lasting for one day at best and at worst, for five days. The clinical symptoms reported from thirteen outbreaks of V. parahaemolyticus food poisoning are summarized in Table 6. Sigmoidoscopic examination might show ulceration of the colon. The fecal leukocyte count may be 10,000 cells/cu. ml., mostly polymorphs. Dysentery is rare with this infection. This disease is rarely fatal (mortality is 0.05% in Japan).

V. parahaemolyticus infections are reported from Japan, the United Kingdom,[1] the United States,[2] India, Indonesia, Panama, and several other countries. Nearly 60% of cases of diarrhea in Japan are due to V. parahaemolyticus infections. It occurs in summer, because V. parahaemolyticus, which is at the bottom of the marine mud during winter, surfaces during summer.[3]

TABLE 6: CLINICAL MANIFESTATIONS IN VIBRIO
PARAHAEMOLYTICUS INFECTIONS*

| SYMPTOMS | APPROXIMATE % OF FREQUENCY |
|---|---|
| Diarrhea | 98 |
| Abdominal Cramps | 82 |
| Nausea | 71 |
| Vomiting | 52 |
| Headache | 42 |
| Fever | 27 |
| Chills | 24 |

* Modified from Barker, W. H., Jr.[2]

CARRIER: Healthy carriers are uncommon. Seven per cent of sushi cooks in Japan harbor this organism.

BACTERIOLOGY

V. parahaemolyticus is a motile, halophilic, non-sporing facultatively anaerobic, gram-negative bacillus. The haemolytic strains are pathogenic to man, and the non-haemolytic strains are not. The organisms that produce haemolysin are called "Kanagawa-positive", and the organisms that do not are called "Kanagawa-negative". Most strains found in sea fish are Kanagawa-negative, whereas most strains recovered from human infections are Kanagawa-positive. The Kanagawa-negative strains usually do not transform to Kanagawa-positive strains even on ingestion of $1 \times 10^9$ organisms/ml. These organisms can be recognized in the TCBS media (thiosulfate-citrate-bile salts-sucrose agar) or mannitol salt agar. They are gelatinase-positive, oxidase-positive, and lactose-negative organisms. They need salt for growth (8% to 10% sodium chloride). They grow better at 43°C. than at 37°C. The incubation period is usually 12 to 24 hours.

## DIFFERENTIAL DIAGNOSIS

CHOLERA: Sudden onset of abdominal pain and diarrhea, when it occurs in localized epidemic form, may cause V. parahaemolyticus infection to be confused with cholera. Clinically, these two diseases are indistinguishable. V. parahaemolyticus can be identified and differentiated from Vibrio cholerae by agglutination reaction and also by the affinity of V. parahaemolyticus to salt.

E. COLI DIARRHEA: This diarrhea resembles the V. parahaemolyticus food poisoning. History of ingestion of raw seafood, especially sushi, should be inquired about in such cases. Isolation of a non-lactose-fermenting, halophilic organism should establish the diagnosis.

Salmonella and Shigella infections may cause similar symptoms. Fecal leukocytes will be found in all three diseases. Splenomegaly is not a feature of V. parahaemolyticus infection. Differentiation is based upon culture results.

## REFERENCES

1. Barrow, G. I., Miller, D. C.: Vibrio parahaemolyticus: A potential pathogen from marine sources in Britain. Lancet 1:485, 1972.

2. Barker, W. H., Jr.: Vibrio parahaemolyticus outbreaks in the United States. Lancet 1:551, 1974.

3. Kaneko, T., Colwell, R. R.: Ecology of Vibrio parahaemolyticus in Chesapeake Bay. J. Bacteriol. 113:24, 1973.

8: YERSINIA ENTEROCOLITICA
by H. Thadepalli

## PRESENTING FEATURES

Fever and diarrhea are the outstanding symptoms of this disease. Nausea, vomiting, headache, arthritis, conjunctivitis, and abdominal pain may occur in 20% to 50% of the patients. Yersiniasis may be mistaken for acute appendicitis in nearly one-fifth of the patients when it involves the ileocolic lymph nodes. A small number (6%) might have ocular symptoms, such as iritis.

Arthritis (non-suppurative) occurs in one-third of the Yersinia infections, often involving the fingers, knees, and ankles, or the sacro-iliac region. It may last for one to twenty weeks. [1]

Abdominal lymphadenitis and thoracic lymphadenitis may also occur in one-third of the patients.

Septicemia and abscesses of the liver, lung and spleen caused by Yersinia enterocolitica are reported, but rare.

Yersinia (Y.) enterocolitica is more prevalent among women than men, and occurs more frequently (88%) among the young, ten to fifteen years old.

Skin changes, such as erythema multiforme and erythema figuratum, [2] may be found in one-third of the patients, mostly women. Cultures of these sites are invariably negative.

Y. enterocolitica infections are reported from Norway, Finland, Sweden, South Africa, Belgium, Japan, United States and Canada. It is believed to be acquired by fecal-oral contamination, although a zoonotic spread has been suspected. [3] Pigs, hares, chinchillas, dogs, cattle, bush babies, oysters, ocelots, sheep and mink are reported to be the carriers of Y. enterocolitica. In adult volunteers, $3.5 \times 10^9$ organisms/ml. were required to cause disease.

## LABORATORY DATA

Leukocytosis, greater than 10,000 cells/cu. mm may be present in one-half of the patients. Sedimentation rate may be increased. SGOT, SGPT and alkaline phosphatase are usually within normal limits.

The synovial fluids sample is frequently sterile. The synovial fluid may have 400 to 60,000 leukocytes/cu. mm, predominantly polymorphonuclear cells.

Stool culture is the most common positive source. Y. enterocolitica is not a normal flora.

Roentgenogram of the joints and chest is usually negative. Hilar lymphadenopathy may be noted in the chest x-rays resembling sarcoidosis.

The disease is commonly caused by serotypes 3, 5 and 8. Serum antibody titers of 1 in 160 or more are considered to be an evidence of infection.

Y. enterocolitica grows well on routine culture media. The problem is not that of identification, but of cognizance. It is a non-lactose fermentor, which does not produce hydrogen sulfide. It is dextrose-positive, dulcitol-, citrate-, lysine- and phenylalanine-negative. It splits urea and is motile at 22°C., but not at 37°C.

Yersinia enterocolitica is a disease with extremely low mortality.

## REFERENCES

1. Alvoren, P., Sievers, K., Alro, K.: Arthritis associated with Yersinia enterocolitica infection. Acta. Rheum. Scand. 15:232, 1969.

2. Niermik, M., Hannuksela, M., Salo, O. P.: Skin lesions in human yersiniosis. Brit. J. Derm. 94:155, 1976.

3. Zen-Yoji, H., et al: Isolation of Yersinia enterocolitica and Yersinia pseudotuberculosis from swine, cattle and rats at an abbatoir. Japan J. Microbiol. 18 (1):103, 1974.

## 9: ADULT NECROTIZING ENTEROCOLITIS
### by H. Thadepalli

Adult necrotizing enterocolitis is a disease of sudden onset, associated with abdominal distention, diarrhea, abdominal discomfort or cramps, dehydration, and fever. Severe toxicity associated with hypotension may occur either during the illness or at the end stage of this disease.

The exact cause of this disease is unknown. However, various drugs, antibiotics, vasopressor agents and bacterial toxins have been implicated. Staphylococcus aureus and Clostridium perfringens are associated with this disease, but have not been proven as the causative agents. Unrecognized, it runs a fulminating course, complicated by perforations, peritonitis, septicemia, shock, and death.

### ROENTGENOGRAM OF THE ABDOMEN

The diagnosis of necrotizing enterocolitis may be characterized by simple, but massive, dilation of the large bowel, local or generalized ileus, variable mucosal edema and loss of haustra.[1,3,4] Demonstration of air in the intramural area, submucosal, or subserosal areas, and air in the portal system or pneumoperitoneum with or without edema of the bowel, should suggest the diagnosis of necrotizing enterocolitis.

On celiotomy, the large bowel is either greenish or bluish in color, with or without gangrene, but the serosa is intact with extensive ulceration in the mucosa. Resection of the colon is the treatment of choice when the diagnosis is established.[1] Such decisions are often made after celiotomy.

### DIFFERENTIAL

Acute necrotizing enterocolitis should be differentiated from acute bacterial dysentery, salmonellosis, acute amoebic dysentery, ischemic colitis, and acute ulcerative colitis. Fecal leukocytes are found in all these situations when there are ulcerations on the mucosa of the colon. The enteropathogenic E. coli may produce similar disease, but it lasts for about three to four days. Certain other bacterial infections, such as Yersinia enterocolitica and Vibrio parahaemolyticus infections also need differentiation by appropriate culture techniques. The diagnosis of necrotizing enterocolitis should not be made, and celiotomy deferred, until the bacterial cultures of the stool have been reported as negative, and several stools and sig-moidoscopic examinations for parasites are negative. When facilities are available, a specimen of serum should also be tested by hemagglutination test for E. histolytica.

Profuse watery diarrhea associated with shedding of mucous membranes in a patient who was previously on a macrolide antibiotic, such as lincomycin, clindamycin or erythromycin, should make one suspect the possibility of pseudomembranous colitis. [2] Demonstration of Salmonella or Shigella organisms by culture would make the diagnosis specific for those bacterial agents.

Demonstration of gas in the portal or renal system, or demon-stration of gas in the wall of the large bowel with an acute gas-eous dilation of the large bowel, suggests the possibility of necrotizing enterocolitis. I saw such a picture in a diabetic woman with severe E. coli cystitis. Since the treatment of choice for necrotizing enterocolitis is total colectomy, every attempt should be made to rule out all treatable causes before celiotomy.

## REFERENCES

1. Rosen, I. B. , Cooter, M. B. , Ruderman, R. L. : Necro-tizing enterocolitis. Surgery, Gynecol. & Obstet. 137:645, 1973.

2. Schapiro, R. L. , Newman, A. : Acute enterocolitis. A com-plication of antibiotic therapy. Radiology 108:263, 1973.

3. Tully, T. E. , Feinberg, S. B. : Those other types of entero-colitis. J. Roentgenol. Rad. Ther. and Nuc. Med. 121:291, 1974.

4. Siegel, R. L. , et al: Early diagnosis of necrotizing entero-colitis. Am. J. Roentgenol. 127:629, 1976.

## 10: PSEUDOMEMBRANOUS COLITIS
by H. Thadepalli

Pseudomembranous colitis is a state of protracted diarrhea secondary to extensive ulceration of the colon, associated with pseudomembrane formation (membrane formed by cellular debris rather than by mucous membrane).

Pseudomembranous colitis may be caused by a variety of drugs, [1] most notably antibiotics, such as clindamycin, lincomycin, ampicillin, amoxycillin, cephalosporins, tetracycline, erythromycin, oral penicillin, gentamicin, neomycin, vancomycin and sulfamethoxazole-trimethoprim. It may be worsened by Lomotil (diphenoxylate hydrochloride). Clindamycin has received a great deal of attention in this respect. [2] In my experience with nearly 500 patients treated with clindamycin, as well as the prospective studies done by others, pseudomembranous colitis was rarely seen. [3] Clindamycin in this respect appears to have been more sinned against than sinning. The manufacturers of this drug refer to this complication as occurring in one of 100,000 treatment courses. Administration of Lomotil and concomitant clindamycin may worsen the attack. Clostridium difficile was suspected to be an etiologic agent in antibiotic-associated pseudomembranous colitis. [5]

The diarrhea may be of abrupt or insidious onset with yellowish-greenish or watery stool, much mucus, and occasionally, blood, and rarely, frank bloody diarrhea (5 to 24 stools per day). Abdominal discomfort is more common than pain, but no tenderness may be present. Occasionally, abdominal pain may be severe enough to warrant a clinical suspicion of bowel perforation.

Rectal examination may give a nodular feeling in the anterior surface of the rectum in one-fifth of the patients. The mucus on the examining finger should be examined microscopically, and may reveal numerous pus cells, frequently loaded with red blood cells.

The peripheral blood cell count might be increased to 11,000 to 70,000/cu. mm/l. The leukocytes may show toxic granulation The hemoglobin content and the protein albumin content may also be decreased secondary to diarrhea. The serum potassium levels may also be lowered.

Stool cultures are often unrewarding. Sophisticated anaerobic culture techniques, laborious search, and speciation yielded C. difficile or C. sordellii. Utilization of a selective medium may improve the chances for isolation of this organism.[6]

## DIAGNOSIS

A plain film of the abdomen may show the small bowel as being normal, but the large bowel may show gaseous distention with "giant thumb printing" in all areas of the colon. [4]

Barium enema examination may show serrations of the colonic margins, with wide haustral folds, but no bowel shortening. Irregularities due to mucosal protrusions into the barium column may be seen.

The rectal biopsy might show epithelial gland tubules filled with mucus, polymorphonuclear leukocytes and desquamated epithelial cells, which coalesce and form the pseudomembrane.

## DIFFERENTIAL

Pseudomembranous colitis should be distinguished from bacterial and acute amoebic dysentery and acute ulcerative colitis associated with or without toxic megacolon. Proctosigmoidoscopic examination in pseudomembranous colitis reveals the characteristic appearance of edema of the mucous membrane, associated with erythema, granularity and multiple areas of pseudomembrane formation which, on dislodging, might show no active bleeding underneath. The mucosal biopsy in pseudomembranous colitis shows polymorphonuclear infiltration and pseudomembrane formation. The diagnosis of bacterial dysentery is established by stool culture results; acute amoebic colitis by demonstration of amoebae. But amoebae may be seen only half of the time in acute amoebic dysentery. The mucous membrane between the ulcers in amoebic colitis, however, is normal.

## REFERENCES

1. Slagle, G. W., Boggs, W.: Drug-induced pseudomembranous colitis: A new etiologic agent. Dis. Colon and Rectum 19:253, 1976.

2. Tedesco, F. J., Barton, R. W., Alpers, D. H.: Clindamycin-associated colitis: A prospective study. Ann. Int. Med. 81:429, 1974.

3. Swartzberg, J. D. , Maresca, R. M. , Remington, J. E. : Gastrointestinal side effects associated with clindamycin. Arch. of Int. Med. 135:876, 1976.

4. Stanley, R. J. , et al: Plain film findings in severe pseudomembranous colitis. Radiology 118:7, 1976.

5. Bartlett, J. G. , et al: Antibiotic-associated pseudomembranous colitis due to toxin-producing clostridia. New Eng. J. Med. 298:531-534, 1978.

6. George, W. L. , Sutter, V. L. , Citron, D. , Finegold, S. M. : Selective and differential medium for isolation of Clostridium difficile. J. Clin. Microbiol. 9:214, 1979.

## 11: PRIMARY OR SPONTANEOUS PERITONITIS
by H. Thadepalli

Spontaneous peritonitis is a non-tuberculous bacterial infection of the peritoneum that develops in the absence of any evidence of direct extension from abdominal organs.[1] Spontaneous peritonitis is not a common disease, but if it is missed, it is fatal.

### AGE AND PREDISPOSING CAUSES

Spontaneous peritonitis, in adults, may occur during the third or fourth decade of life; usually in association with ascites due to cirrhosis of the liver, or occasionally, in association with the nephrotic syndrome.[1,3] Frequently, no predisposing cause is present; when present, it might be an intestinal erosion, salpingitis, renal abscess or an ischemic small or large bowel. Laennec's cirrhosis of the liver is, by far, the most common predisposing cause of spontaneous peritonitis.

### CLINICAL FEATURES

The relative prevalence of physical signs and laboratory features are listed in Fig. 2. Fever, abdominal pain, and impending hepatic coma are the three outstanding features of spontaneous bacterial peritonitis. A patient diagnosed to have cirrhosis of the liver with ascites, who shows signs of decreased mentation, abdominal tenderness, loss of weight, or develops jaundice, with or without fever, should be investigated for possible spontaneous peritonitis. The bowel sounds may be hypoactive or absent (60% to 70%). Hypotension (50% to 60%) might occur, sometimes in association with coma. The presence of free fluid in the abdomen is a sine qua non for spontaneous peritonitis.

### DIAGNOSIS

BACTERIOLOGY: Both blood and ascitic fluid specimens should be routinely cultured for both aerobic and anaerobic bacteria. Spontaneous peritonitis is predominantly caused by gram-negative aerobic and facultative bacteria. Escherichia (E.) coli is the most common cause. (Klebsiella and Pseudomonas are less frequent). Pneumococcus is the second most common and anaerobic bacteria are perhaps the third. In most instances, spontaneous peritonitis is monobacterial, but occasionally, it may be a polymicrobial infection. Blood cultures are positive in 75% mostly due to an organism that may also be found in peritoneal fluid cultures.

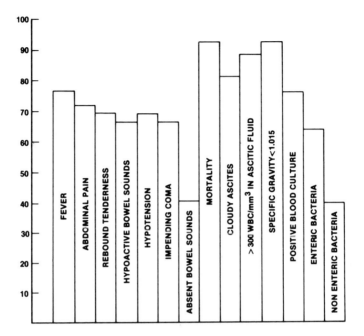

FIG. 2: Relative prevalence of physical signs and the laboratory features in spontaneous bacterial peritonitis.

Paracentesis of the abdomen should be routinely performed in
all suspected cases of spontaneous peritonitis. I prefer to tap
through the midline (linea alba), midpoint between the symphysis
pubis and the umbilicus. The patient should have the urinary bladder completely emptied before this procedure is done. If necessary, catheterization should be done to empty the bladder.
All sterile techniques should be adhered to while doing paracentesis. Diagnostic paracentesis may be done with an 18-gauge
needle attached to a 30-cc. or 50-cc. syringe. Rapid paracentesis with a trocar and cannula is unnecessary and should be
avoided.

The ascitic fluid may be straw-colored in nearly 10% or totally
purulent in 90%. The aspirate should be processed for specific
gravity, protein analysis, leukocyte count, and aerobic and anaerobic cultures. Microscopic examination (gram's stain of the smears
of the sediment) may demonstrate bacteria of morphotype similar
to bacteria cultured from ascitic fluid in nearly one half of the
patients. The specific gravity of the ascitic fluid may range from

1.014 to 1.024, with a total protein of 1 to 3 grams/100 ml.
High protein ascites may occur in uncomplicated hepatic cirrhosis subjected to repeated diagnostic paracentesis. [2] The
total leukocyte count of the fluid may be unreliable. [4] A high
leukocyte count does not always suggest peritonitis, and counts
of less than 300 do not exclude this disease. The only reliable
evidence of peritonitis is the positive peritoneal fluid culture,
but not its color, protein content or the leukocyte count.

Lysozyme content of peritoneal fluid was studied in cases of
peritonitis. It was found to be increased to 10 mcg/ml. when
infected. It is probably derived from the white cells by the action of bacterial endotoxin.

Laboratory features include leukocytosis in nearly 50% with a shift
to the left, anemia, sudden drop of hematocrit, elevated serum bilirubin in 90% and occasionally elevated alkaline phosphatase.
None of these findings are characteristic of bacterial peritonitis.

In my experience, of 175 cases of intra-abdominal infections
diagnosed during a four-year period, eleven patients had spontaneous peritonitis. Eight were monobacterial and three were
polymicrobial infections. Only three patients had pneumococcal
peritonitis, two had coccidioidomycosis peritonitis, and the
remaining were due to E. coli, Clostridium (C.) perfringens,
C. innocuum, C. sordellii, C. capitovale, Klebsiella, Enterobacter, Staphylococcus aureus and Streptococci. Eight of these
patients had cirrhosis of the liver and had no obvious source
of infection. Five patients had positive blood cultures (Pneumococcus, 2; Clostridia, 2; Streptococcus, 1). Ten patients,
when promptly diagnosed and treated, improved, but one patient in whom the diagnosis was delayed, and who was treated
with inappropriate antibiotics, died.

## DIFFERENTIAL DIAGNOSIS

The protein content of peritoneal fluid may be increased in tuberculous peritonitis, nephrosis, constrictive pericarditis and
occasionally, in polyserositis. It is around 2.9 G/100 ml. or
higher in pancreatic ascitis[6] and 0.5 to 1.5 G/100 ml. in cirrhosis.

Recurrent ascites may result from peritoneal dialysis due to
a sudden fall in the serum albumin level. Usually, the fall
of serum protein to 2.5 grams per 100 cc. is reversible,
and peritoneal dialysis need not be suspended for this reason. [7]

Gas-producing bacteria, such as Clostridium, might occasionally cause pneumoperitoneum. Gaseous peritonitis, in my experience, was always found in association with a defect in the colon either due to cancer, diverticulitis or perforation.

CANDIDA PERITONITIS: It is usually secondary to peritoneal dialysis, gastrointestinal surgery, or perforation of an abdominal viscus.[8] It is usually limited to the abdomen, but in moribund patients, blood cultures might be positive.

TUBERCULOUS PERITONITIS: Tuberculous peritonitis is generally indolent and clinically indistinguishable from other bacterial peritonitis. The hallmarks of this disease are abdominal pain, fever, exudative ascites and occasionally, abdominal mass. In developing countries, tuberculous peritonitis is more frequent among young females than among the elderly.[9,10] Abdominal enlargement is an inconstant feature of tuberculous peritonitis, present in only 50% of cases. Tuberculous peritonitis is associated with fluid in the peritoneum (wet peritonitis), or it may be adhesive or dry (plastic peritonitis). Wet peritonitis is more common than the dry. The laboratory findings in tuberculous peritonitis are similar to that of spontaneous peritonitis, except the liver enzymes SGOT, SGPT and the bilirubin levels may be normal. Table 7 summarizes the differences between tuberculous and spontaneous peritonitis.

Tuberculous peritonitis is diagnosed by peritoneoscopy (Fig. 3), peritoneal biopsy, or exploratory celiotomy. Demonstration of caseating granulomas in a peritoneal mass confirms the diagnosis of tuberculosis. The specific gravity in tuberculous peritonitis is higher than that of spontaneous peritonitis. It is around 1.024 in tuberculous peritonitis, with a range of 1.015 to 1.033. The protein content of ascitic fluid in tuberculous peritonitis is high in spite of low serum protein. See Table 14, page 158 for further details.

Positive sputum smears are rare in abdominal tuberculosis.

Intravenous pyleography may show evidence of urinary tract tuberculosis. Hysterosalpingograms may reveal irregularity of the intimal layers of the salpinx, suggesting tuberculosis. Endometrial biopsies are of immense value in the diagnosis of early genital and abdominal tuberculosis. Today, the mortality of tuberculous peritonitis is still around 10%.

TABLE 7: DIFFERENTIAL DIAGNOSIS OF SPONTANEOUS PERITONITIS FROM TUBERCULOSIS

| DIFFERENTIAL FEATURE | SPONTANEOUS PERITONITIS | TUBERCULOUS PERITONITIS |
|---|---|---|
| Usual age | >30 | <30 |
| Sex | both sexes | predominantly female |
| Association with cirrhosis of liver | 80% | may or may not |
| Ascites | must | may or may not |
| Palpable mass in abdomen | unusual | 40% |
| Serum bilirubin | usually elevated | usually normal |
| Serum SGOT, SGPT | elevated | normal, unless complicated by miliary tuberculosis |
| Positive blood cultures | 50% | may or may not |
| ASCITES FLUID ANALYSIS: | | |
| Color | turbid or purulent | straw-colored |
| Cell count* | 80% polymorphs | 60% lymphocytes |
| Protein | less than 2 G./100 ml. | $\geqslant$2 G./100 (4 G./100 ml.) |
| Gram stain | positive | negative |

*WBC count is of no value in differential diagnosis.

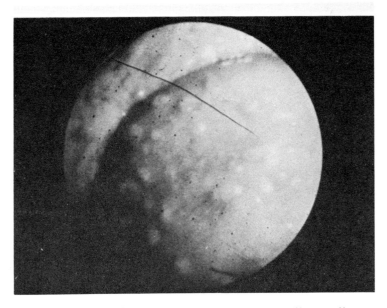

FIG. 3: Tuberculous peritonitis, seen through the peritoneo-
scope, showing multiple, small nodular granulomas.

Guinea pig inoculations of ascitic fluid may not always be successful. Appropriate therapy should be promptly instituted
after obtaining a peritoneal biopsy while still waiting for the
peritoneal fluid culture results.

## REFERENCES

1.  Conn, H. O. , Fessel, J. M. : Spontaneous bacteria peri-
    tonitis in cirrhosis. Variations on a theme. Medicine 50:
    161, 1971.

2.  Sampliner, R. E. , Iber, F. L. : High protein ascites in pa-
    tients with uncomplicated hepatic cirrhosis. Am. J. Med.
    Sci. 267:275, 1974.

3.  Curry, N. , McCallum, R. W. , Guth, P. H. : Spontaneous
    peritonitis in cirrhotic ascites. A decade of experience.
    Digest. Dis. 19:685, 1974.

4.  Kline, M. M. , McCallum, R. W. , Guth, P. H. : The clini-
    cal value of ascites fluid culture and leukocyte count studies
    in alcoholic cirrhosis. Gastroenterol. 70:408, 1976.

5. Wardle, F. N. : Simple method for detection of infection of peritoneum during dialysis. Brit. Med. J. 1:518,1973.

6. Smith, R. B. , et al: Pancreatic ascites. Ann. Surg. 177: 538, 1973.

7. Rodriguez, H. J. , et al: Recurrent ascites following peritoneal dialysis: A new syndrome? Arch. Int. Med. 134: 283, 1974.

8. Bayer, A. S. , et al: Candida peritonitis: Report of 22 cases and review of the English literature. Amer. J. Med. 61:832, 1976.

9. Barhannesh, F. , et al: Tuberculous peritonitis: Prospective study of 32 cases in Iran. Ann. Int. Med. 76:567, 1972.

10. Novis, B. H. , Banks, S. , Marks, I. N. : Gastrointestinal and peritoneal tuberculosis. S. A. Med. J. 47:365, 1973.

## 12: SUBPHRENIC ABSCESS
by H. Thadepalli

### GENERAL CONSIDERATIONS

Right-sided pleural effusion, right-lower-lobe consolidation or collapse, or abscess in the right lower lobe of the lung in any patient, requires exclusion of subdiaphragmatic abscess as a possibility. [1]

Subphrenic abscess, by definition, means either a mere collection of pus right underneath the diaphragm or within the substance of the liver or spleen. The liver is attached to the posterior surface of the abdomen. The liver divides the subphrenic region into suprahepatic, hepatic and the infrahepatic compartments. The falciform ligament divides the suprahepatic space into the right and the left compartments.

The subphrenic abscesses are more frequent on the right than on the left. The subphrenic abscess may be bilateral in 3% to 4%. Hematogenous liver abscesses are often located in the bare area on the posterior surface of the liver. Bacterial liver abscess is frequently within the liver substance. If the abscess is located on the posterosuperior aspect of the liver, it is more frequently amoebic, rather than bacterial, in origin.

### AGE AND SEX

It is a disease of the adult in the fourth or fifth decade of life and preponderantly (70%) a disease of the male. [2]

### ETIOLOGY

The subphrenic abscess, in 90% of the cases, is secondary to infections, injury or perforation of the appendix, colon, stomach or duodenum. [3,4] A small number arise from the hepatobiliary system.

### SYMPTOMS AND SIGNS

The most frequent symptoms are fever, associated with abdominal pain and tenderness, chest pain or shoulder pain with leukocytosis. An occasional patient may have no specific complaint other than being just "sick", "no pep", "run down". Anorexia is common. The peripheral cell counts may be normal. Only 25% are diagnosed by clinical examination alone.

Roentgenographic examination improves the diagnostic yield up to 50% to 90%. Of the subdiaphragmatic abscess patients, nearly 10% die undiagnosed.

The physical signs of subdiaphragmatic abscess are schematically represented in Fig. 4. In most instances, one or more, or even none of these features, may be present. The old adage "pus somewhere, pus nowhere - pus under the diaphragm" is a helpful tip in the diagnosis of subdiaphragmatic abscess.

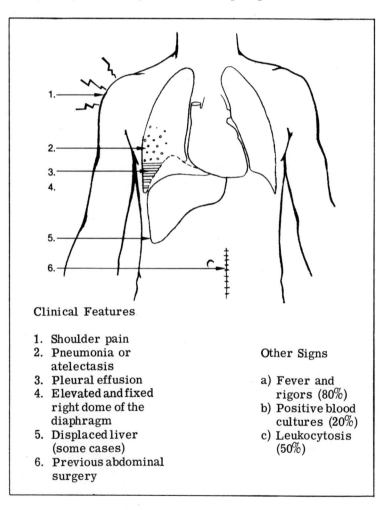

Clinical Features

1. Shoulder pain
2. Pneumonia or atelectasis
3. Pleural effusion
4. Elevated and fixed right dome of the diaphragm
5. Displaced liver (some cases)
6. Previous abdominal surgery

Other Signs

a) Fever and rigors (80%)
b) Positive blood cultures (20%)
c) Leukocytosis (50%)

FIG. 4: Subdiaphragmatic abscess.

Clear-cut distinction between the subdiaphragmatic abscess and the liver abscess may at times be difficult in spite of extensive scintigraphic and ultrasonic procedures. Many a time I erred both ways. In a great majority of cases, such a distinction, preoperatively, is of academic interest and, at best, an intellectual gamble. What is more important is the distinction between the metastatic subdiaphragmatic or liver abscess from the primary abscess elsewhere in the abdomen, by thorough investigation. The investigations should include:

1) a roentgenogram of the chest
2) Ga-67 scan
3) liver-lung scan
4) Tc-99 liver-spleen scan
5) ultrasound of the right-upper quadrant of the abdomen
6) fluoroscopic visualization of the immobile right leaflet of the diaphragm
7) $CO_2$ insufflation to visualize the subdiaphragmatic space
8) angiography of the liver
9) other miscellaneous studies to exclude primary focus of infection elsewhere, such as:
   (a) appendix
   (b) diverticulitis
   (c) perirectal abscess
   (d) gastric or duodenal perforation
10) abdominal abscess other than subdiaphragmatic abscess:
   (a) perirectal
   (b) pancreatic
   (c) prostate

The radiologic, scintigraphic and ultrasonic procedures used in the diagnosis of intra-abdominal abscess are discussed separately (see Chapter 13).

REFERENCES

1. Ariel, I. M. , Kazarian, K. K. (Eds. ): Classification, Diagnosis and Treatment of Subphrenic Abscess. Diagnosis and Treatment of Abdominal Abscess. Williams and Wilkins Co. , Baltimore, 1971.

2. Ochsner, A. , DeBakey, M. E. : Subphrenic abscess. Collective review and analysis of 3,608 collected and personal cases. Surg. Gynec. Obstet. 66:426, 1938.

3.  Harley, H. R. S.: Subphrenic abscess with particular reference to the spread of infection. Ann. Roy. Coll. Surg. Eng. 17:201, 1955.

4.  Magilligan, D. J.: Suprahepatic abscess. Arch. Surg. 96: 14, 1968.

## 13: ABDOMINAL ABSCESS: GENERAL DIAGNOSTIC CONSIDERATIONS
by H. Thadepalli

The abdomen is a magic box. It may have many surprises in store. Intelligent collection of data base and a keen and dexterous physical examination may avert such surprises.

### CLINICAL FEATURES

Abdominal pain, fever with or without chills or rigors and leukocytosis are the important early clues to the diagnosis of abdominal abscess. Vomiting, diarrhea or constipation and abdominal distention are delayed features.

PAIN: Pain or discomfort is a relatively constant feature. Acute abdominal abscess more frequently causes pain, but chronic infection may cause no more than "discomfort", not amounting to pain. Pain radiates, but "discomfort" does not.

When there is irritation of the area supplied by the fourth and the fifth cervical nerves (such as the diaphragm, gallbladder, surface of the right and left lobes of the liver, spleen and upper pole of the left kidney), the pain may radiate to the tip of the right or left shoulder and to the interscapular area. Pain around the navel is a symptom of appendicitis, typhlitis, perityphlitis, rupture, or infection of the Meckel's diverticulum or oophoritis, but is rarely due to an acute salpingitis or tuboovarian abscess. This sign is of no value in children, for they tend to point towards the umbilicus as the source of pain, regardless of where it is.

Pain radiating to the back is commonly due to an infection or irritation of the posterior wall of the abdomen, such as pancreatic abscess, perforating duodenal ulcer, gastric ulcer, metastasis to the pancreatic lymph node as a result of cancer, and occasionally, due to involvement of the kidney.

Pain radiating to the tip of the penis or into the testes suggests renal colic, either due to stones or infection.

FEVER: Hectic fevers were common in the pre-antibiotic era. Fever is still an outstanding feature of abdominal abscess. It may often be irregular and low-grade in the morning, spiking to as high as 103°F. in the evening; usually reaching the peak at midnight. Hyperpyrexia (>106°F) is rare. The body temperature is higher than normal (99°-100°F), unless interrupted by antipyretics.

CHILLS AND RIGORS: A chill is a "cold" sensation when several blankets are drawn to keep oneself warm, in spite of one having above normal temperature. A rigor is an intense "teeth chattering" and limb-shaking chill. They are common with all suppurative infections. Unless complicated, they are infrequent in typhoid fever and tuberculosis.

LEUKOCYTOSIS: Leukocytosis might occur, often up to 12,000 to 15,000/cu. mm. In some, it may go up to 20,000 to 30,000/cu. mm. Counts higher than 40,000 are rare. Highest leukocyte counts may be obtained late in the evening, or early in the morning. Frequently, there is a shift to the left. The eosinophil count is lowered (0 to 2%). Eosinophil counts higher than 5% may suggest an associated allergic manifestation or parasitic infection.

PHYSICAL SIGNS: Most patients have very few physical signs. Local guarding and tenderness, a palpably enlarged and tender intra-abdominal organ, when present, may lead to the diagnosis. Right intercostal fullness and tenderness may suggest subdiaphragmatic and/or liver abscess.

The reader should refer to certain books of physical signs for details on all types of intra-abdominal abscess. [1]

Four additional sites should be routinely included with the abdominal examination. They are, (1) pupillary light reflexes, (2) spine, (3) testis and (4) rectal and pelvic examination. Light reflexes are lost (Argyll-Robertson pupil) in tabes dorsalis, which may manifest as an acute abdominal catastrophe mistaken for either visceral perforation or appendicitis. The tuberculous cold abscess of the spine may be mistaken for other pyogenic abscesses. The intra-abdominal testes may become malignant or undergo torsion, and present as an abdominal problem which may be diagnosed by their absence from the scrotum. Similarly, a strangulated hernia can be mistaken for gram-negative sepsis and shock, if one fails to examine the scrotum.

The importance of rectal and pelvic examinations needs no special emphasis. Their value in the diagnosis of appendicitis, prostatic abscess, or pelvic abscess are well known. The following case history illustrates an example:

A 36-year-old male with fever and chills, and abdominal pains, was examined. On physical examination, he had a temperature of 104°F. and appeared very toxemic, but was otherwise unremarkable. Urinalysis revealed many pus cells, but the cultures were negative. He was treated, as an outpatient, with Azo Gantrisin for the presumed urinary tract infection. Three days later, the abdominal pain worsened, necessitating hospitalization. Rectal examination was tender and "very painful; hence, it was not pursued". He was then treated with an intravenous cephalosporin. Five days later, he developed septic shock and was placed on a vasopressor agent. Routine physical examination at this time again revealed no septic focus. The rectal examination was then repeated in spite of pain, when an extremely tender bulge was felt in the anterior wall of the rectum. He was then diagnosed to have an abscess of the prostate, which was incised and drained per rectum, following which he showed rapid and steady improvement.

## DIAGNOSIS

BACTERIOLOGY OF INTRA-ABDOMINAL AND PELVIC ABSCESS: Anaerobic bacteria predominate and are often the exclusive flora in intra-abdominal abscess. The chief isolates are Peptostreptococci, Peptococci, Bacteroides and Clostridia.[2] Bacteroides fragilis, a bacterium resistant to the commonly used antibiotics, such as penicillin, cephalothin, tetracycline, and gentamicin, may occur in 20% to 30% of the patients. The foul smell of the intra-abdominal pus is due to the production of short-chain, volatile fatty acids produced by the anaerobes. These fatty acid products yield valuable clues to the rapid diagnosis of anaerobic infection by direct gas-liquid chromatography Effective anti-anaerobic antibiotics frequently eliminate the anaerobes from the site of infection. Persistence of anaerobes at the site of infection, while on effective anti-anaerobic therapy, may suggest an underlying, surgically correctable disorder, such as enteric fistula. Such patients may need barium contrast examination of upper and/or lower bowel to exclude internal fistulae.

RADIOLOGY: An intra-abdominal abscess may manifest as a soft tissue density displacing the bowel. On occasion, it may be seen as an extra-luminal gas with branching linear shadows.[3] Gas shadows are of no value in recently operated patients. Elevation of the diaphragm, generalized ileus or scoliosis with concavity towards the side of the lesion, are additional diagnostic clues. Intrathoracic changes may include basilar pneumonia, pleural effusion or occasionally, segmental atelectasis.

Routine films should include the supine, upright and both de-cubitus positions to look for the air fluid levels, if any. Con-trast studies, such as pneumoperitoneum or barium (upper or lower intestinal) series may help in further localization of the abscess. In a sick patient, one may favor the barium series in scintigraphy and ultrasonography. The clinician should share his observations with the radiologist to help arrive at a more accurate diagnosis.

Lesser sac (pseudocyst) abscess may be diagnosed by the an-terior displacement of the stomach and downward displacement of the colon. Abscess of the left lobe of the liver may also show similar signs, but it displaces the stomach, not only anteriorly, but also medially. The pelvic abscess might present as a mere homogenous density. If there is free fluid in the pelvis, on prone position, it may disappear altogether. The pelvic abscess may displace the urinary bladder and the sigmoid colon. Massive tubo-ovarian abscess might displace the small bowel shadows upwards as it rises into the abdominal cavity.

Pneumatosis intestinalis might occasionally be mistaken for intra-abdominal abscess. It may be diagnosed by the linear and parallel lucent gas shadows within the wall of the bowel. The barium series may characteristically show circular gas shadows along the bowel wall.

The presence of subcutaneous gas shadows in a closed abdom-inal surgical wound may imply wound infection and abdominal wall abscess.[4] Gas shadows in the gallbladder area in the right-upper quadrant are characteristic of emphysematous cholecys-titis, usually caused by Clostridium perfringens. Such a com-plication is more frequent in elderly diabetics (Fig. 5).

THE SCANS:

Gallium scan: Gallium citrate (Ga-67) accumulates at the site of inflammatory and malignant lesions. In one study of 36 pa-tients with suspected infections, 25% had positive scans,[5] and negative patients with infection had no evidence of abscess for-mation. Both false-positive and false-negative scans do occur, although they are infrequent. Gallium scans are traditionally obtained after 24 or 48-hour intervals; often, however, suffi-cient information can be obtained by scanning at 6 hours.[6] In pyogenic liver abscess, the Ga-67 uptake is increased. The amoebic liver abscess may show a negative uptake at the site of infection, surrounded by a ring of increased accumulation of Ga-67.[7]

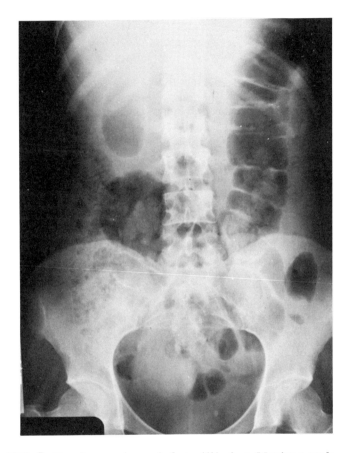

FIG. 5: Emphysematous cholecystitis in a Mexican male
due to Clostridium perfringens infection. He
also had diabetes mellitus.

The gallium scan, by itself, is a non-specific test. It is of limited value in infections around the large bowel, urinary bladder and the kidneys, for gallium is normally excreted by these organs. Catharsis, enemas and bladder drainage may somewhat prevent this problem, but a patient with an acute infection may not tolerate such drastic procedures. False-negative scans may occur due to antiobiotic therapy.

Selective labeling of leukocytes with Ga-67 may be promising in the localization of abdominal infections.

Lung-liver scan: Several isotope combinations may be used in the lung-liver scan. The lung-liver scan is helpful in delin-eating a subdiaphragmatic abscess seen as a radionuclide "gap" or "cold area" between the lung and the liver scans. I-131-macroaggregated human serum albumin and Tc-99 sulfides are used for this procedure. The accuracy of diag-nosis of subdiaphragmatic abscess by this method is nearly 80%. It is a relatively simple and a safe procedure to do, and, therefore, is of immense value in the diagnosis of subdiaphrag-matic abscess. A subdiaphragmatic abscess, at times, may be difficult to distinguish from a liver abscess.

Tc-99 colloid liver scan: This scan may show liver abscesses of 2 cm. in size or more. Abscesses of smaller size do occur with septicemia and they are missed by all scintigraphic pro-cedures.

Tc-99 and Ga-67 scans: Decreased uptake of Tc-99 and in-creased uptake of Ga-67 at a site within the liver suggest pyo-genic liver abscess. Both Ga-67 and Tc-99 uptake are de-creased in the amoebic liver abscess. The scans may be done at two separate sittings or simultaneously by the subtraction technique. [8] The subtraction technique is based on simultane-ous differential concentration of two different radiopharmaceu-ticals. This technique is useful in the diagnosis of infections of the upper abdomen. In one study by subtraction technique, 13 of 15 patients with abscesses located in the upper abdomen were correctly diagnosed. [9] They have used Ga-67 for the localiza-tion of the lesion, and Tc-99m labeled human albumin and Tc-99 sulfur colloid for subtraction.

The expected diagnostic yield of liver scans when liver abscess is clinically suspected is nearly 80%, but, when the liver scans are routinely ordered without clinical suspicion, the diagnostic yield is infinitely small. A normal scan does not exonerate the liver as the site of infection (remember that it is positive only in 80%, and 20% are missed). The diagnostic yield of routine scans of any part of the body, as a part of routine fever work-up, is expensive and terribly discouraging, not to mention the needless exposure to radiation and, therefore, it should be condemned.

ULTRASOUND: The ultrasound, with a frequency of 2.25 million cycles per second, is being used to localize the lesion and differentiate between solid and cystic lesions. Ga-67 scans cannot differentiate between cystic and solid inflammatory lesions. The ultrasound can detect lesions that are 3 cm. or more. Of 102 patients suspected of having a postoperative abdominal abscess, there were no (0%) false-positive results and 2% false-negative results.[10] Avoidance of false-positives is the most important aspect of ultrasound, for it avoids needless laparotomy. False-negatives may occur when the abscesses are posteriorly located. It may be avoided by ultrasound examination from the back. Ultrasound examination may be done prior to scintiscans, when one suspects postoperative intra-abdominal abscess.

Unlike scans, the ultrasonic examination requires very little patient cooperation. It is non-invasive; not contraindicated in pregnancy; does not need catharsis; can be done at any time; and it differentiates the solid from the cystic lesions with precise anatomic localization. Therefore, ultrasound examination is an extremely useful procedure in the diagnosis of intra-abdominal abscess. A negative ultrasonic examination of the liver nearly always excludes liver abscess that is 3 cm. or more.[11]

When the site of infection is not known, searching for an abscess with the transducer is laborious and discomforting to the patient; therefore, the gallium scans are preferred. The ultrasound examination does not differentiate between an abscess and a non-inflammatory cyst.

Ultrasonically guided needles have been used for the aspiration of the abscesses when surgery is not feasible.[12] Extension of infection is a potential risk associated with this procedure. We have used the ultrasound to locate and determine the size and volume of the amoebic liver abscesses, and, having measured the distance from a mark placed on the skin to the center of the abscess, the pus was aspirated at the bedside through a single large-bore needle. (This is not always necessary.)

ANGIOGRAPHY: Super selective catheterization of small blood vessels by percutaneous angiography, with image-intensified fluoroscopy, has improved the diagnostic accuracy. Angiography can help differentiate an abscess from a tumor. Most liver abscesses can be diagnosed by scans and ultrasound. An occasional afebrile patient may need angiography to exclude malignancy. Displacement of the arteries around an avascular defect, with a thin halo of hyperemic stain, may be noted in liver abscess. [13] An angiogram can accurately differentiate the subdiaphragmatic abscess from the intrahepatic abscess. A long-standing granulomatous infection, such as actinomycosis, may show hypervascular parenchyma with stretching of the intrahepatic arteries. Pancreatic cysts or pseudocysts may cause marked displacement of the blood vessels, although the mass, by itself, may be avascular. Angiography can also be used to differentiate pancreatitis from a pseudocyst. Splenic abscess may be diagnosed by the displacement of the intraparenchymal blood vessels. In one series of 76 cases of pancreatic disease studied by angiography, inflammatory disease of the pancreas was differentiated from carcinoma, with confidence, in nearly 85% of the cases. [14]

Angiography should not be used as a routine. It is contraindicated in bleeding disorders. Even in expert hands, serious complications might occur in 0.5% to 1% of the patients.

## REFERENCES

1.  Ariel, I. M. , Kazarian, K. K. : Diagnosis and Treatment of Abdominal Abscesses. Williams & Wilkins Co. , Baltimore, 1971.

2.  Gorbach, S. L. , Thadepalli, H. , Norsen, J. : Anaerobic Microorganisms in Intra-abdominal Infections, Ch. XXXII. Anaerobic Bacteria: Role in Disease, (Eds. ) Balows, A. , et al. Charles C Thomas, Springfield, 1975.

3.  Meyers, M. A. , Whalen, J. P. : Radiologic Aspects of Intra-abdominal Abscess. Diagnosis and Treatment of Abdominal Abscesses. Williams & Wilkins Co. , Baltimore, 1971.

4.  Nelson, J. A. , Coggs, G. C. : Occult infections of abdominal incision as seen on lateral chest roentgenogram. Amer. J. Roentgenol. Rad. Ther. Nuc. Med. CXVII: 846, 1973.

5.  Kumar, B. , Coleman, E. , Anderson, P. O. : Gallium citrate Ga-67 imaging in patients with suspected inflammatory process. Arch. Surg. 110:1237, 1975.

6.  Hopkins, G. B. , Kan, M. , Mende, C. W. : Early Ga-67 scintigraphy for the localization of abdominal abscesses. J. Nuc. Med. 16:990, 1975.

7.  Miyamoto, A. T. , Thadepalli, H. , Mishkin, F. S. : Gallium images of amoebic liver abscesses. New. Eng. J. Med. 291:1363, 1975.

8.  Beihn, R. M. , Damron, J. R. , Hafner, T. : Subtraction technique for the detection of subphrenic abscesses using Ga-67 and Tc-99m. J. Nuc. Med. 15:371, 1974.

9.  Damron, J. R. , Beihn, R. M. , DeLand, F. H. : Detection of upper abdominal abscesses by radionuclide imaging. Radiology 120:131, 1976.

10. Makland, N. F. , Doust, B. D. , Baum, J. K. : Ultrasonic diagnosis of postoperative intra-abdominal abscess. Radiology 113:417, 1974.

11. Doust, B. D. , Doust, V. L. : Ultrasonic diagnosis of abdominal abscess. Digestive Diseases 21:569, 1976.

12. Smith, E. H. , Bartrum, R. J. : Ultrasonically guided percutaneous aspiration of abscesses. Amer. J. Roentgenol. Rad. Ther. Nuc. Med. 122:308, 1974.

13. Pollard, J. J. , Nebesar, R. A. : Abdominal angiography. New. Eng. J. Med. 275:1035-42, 1093-99, 1148-51, 1968.

14. Goldstein, H. M. , Neiman, H. L. , Bookstein, J. J. : Angiographic evaluation of pancreatic disease. Radiology 112: 275, 1974.

14:  BACTERIAL ABSCESS OF THE LIVER
by H. Thadepalli

Liver abscess may be amoebic or bacterial. In my experience, one has been just as frequent as the other. Most of my patients with amoebic liver abscess were born outside of the United States. It is important to distinguish these two entities because surgical drainage is unnecessary for amoebic liver abscess, whereas it is mandatory for bacterial liver abscess.

The primary focus of infection for bacterial liver abscess is the appendix or colon or the biliary tract.[1-4] The symptoms and signs are that of an intra-abdominal abscess. The liver may or may not be palpable. The intrathoracic complications secondary to liver abscess include pleural effusion, pneumonia, atelectasis or lung abscess.

## LABORATORY FEATURES

Polymorphonuclear leukocytosis (10,000 to 50,000/cu. mm.) might occur along with iron-deficiency anemia. The sedimentation rate is always raised. Alkaline phosphatase is usually elevated. Serum albumin may be decreased with increased gamma globulin. Vitamin $B_{12}$ may be raised (greater than 2,000 pg/ml.) because of liver tissue destruction in bacterial liver abscess, and malignancy (see Chapters 13 and 71).

MICROBIOLOGY OF BACTERIAL LIVER ABSCESS: Surgically drained pus from the liver should be cultured for aerobes and anaerobes as well. It should be collected in bottles or tubes previously filled with oxygen-free carbon dioxide (see Chapter 19). Suboptimal techniques are the common causes of "sterile pus" reports. The pus is rarely sterile. Anaerobic or microaerophilic cocci are the most common causes of bacterial liver abscess. Other anaerobes are less frequent. The most common aerobic isolates are Escherichia (E.) coli, and Streptococcus viridans, found in 20% to 35%, often in mixture with anaerobic bacteria.

BLOOD CULTURES: Blood cultures are positive in 25% to 40% of the cases.[2] Streptococci and E. coli are the most frequent isolates. Positive blood cultures, on occasion, might be the only available clue to the underlying infection. Therefore, a positive blood culture in a febrile patient with abdominal pain needs exclusion of intra-abdominal abscess. Blood cultures are rarely positive in amoebic liver abscess. Amoebic liver abscess may occasionally be contaminated with bacteria. Of twenty-four consecutive cases of amoebic liver abscesses that I witnessed during the recent three-year period, pus was cultured for both aerobic and anaerobic bacteria in every case. Two specimens (8%) had bacteria on gram's stain and culture, but in neither instance were blood cultures positive. [5]

## AMOEBIC LIVER ABSCESS VS. PYOGENIC LIVER ABSCESS

Amoebic and pyogenic liver abscess may be clinically indistinguishable. I found the following criteria to be useful in their differentiation: Amoebic liver abscess is the most likely, if the patient is an immigrant from Latin American countries, Africa or Asia, or has history of recent travel to these parts of the world. The exception to this rule was one American-born black male who had spent five years in the California State Penitentiary. He was hospitalized ten days after his release on parole. He was admitted with right-sided pleural effusion and pneumonia, initially mistaken by the house officers for Mycoplasma pneumonia, and was treated with tetracycline with some clinical improvement. Six weeks after discharge, the liver abscess was discovered by scintiscan, by which time he had developed a hepatobronchial fistula with pseudohemoptysis (expectoration of an anchovy-sauce-colored sputum). The diagnosis was confirmed by increased hemagglutination inhibition titers and Gallium-67 scan. Anchovy-sauce-colored pus was later aspirated from the liver. When a contrast medium was injected into the liver after aspiration, he coughed up radiopaque material (see Fig. 104, page 542).

Indirect hemagglutination (IHA) test is the most sensitive of all diagnostic tests thus far available for amoebic liver abscess. A positive IHA test in a patient with clinical signs of liver abscess is diagnostic of amoebic liver abscess.

## PROGNOSIS

The overall mortality of bacterial abscess improved from 80% in 1955-1957 to 28% in 1965-1969 and the diagnostic accuracy improved from 20% to 78%. The mortality of undrained bacterial liver abscess is still close to 100%. Surgical drainage is the treatment of choice for bacterial liver abscess. [3] Neither surgery nor antibiotics, one exclusive of the other, are effective. Whereas the surgical techniques have remained unchanged, early diagnosis by scintiscan methods and the use of modern potent antibiotics should be credited for the improved mortality in liver abscess. However, hasty antibiotic therapy may suppress the clinical signs and thereby delay the much required surgical drainage. It is a major cause of death due to liver abscess today.

## REFERENCES

1. Barbour, G. L. , Juniper, K. : A clinical comparison of amoebic and pyogenic abscess of the liver in sixty-six patients. Am. J. Med. 53:323, 1972.

2. Sabbaj, J. , Sutter, V. L. , Finegold, S. M. : Anaerobic pyogenic liver abscess. Ann. Int. Med. 77:629, 1972.

3. Lazarchick, J. , et al: Pyogenic liver abscess. Mayo Clinc. Proc. 48:349, 1973.

4. Altmeier, W. A. : Liver Abscess: The Etiologic Role of Anaerobic Bacteria. Anaerobic Bacteria: Role in Disease, (Eds. ) Balows, A. , et al. Charles C Thomas, Springfield, 1975.

5. Mandal, A. K. , Thadepalli, M. : Surgical Aspects of Amoebiasis and Diagnostic Clues. Amer. Surgeon 44: 564-570, 1978.

## 15: BORRELIOSIS
by H. Thadepalli

Borreliosis is a form of relapsing fever caused by Borrelia, a corkscrew-shaped organism belonging to Spirochaetales, classified as shown in Table 8.

## CLINICAL FEATURES

The clinical features of the louse-borne relapsing fever caused by B. recurrentis are indistinguishable from the tick-borne relapsing fever caused by B. duttonii. The incubation period is two to ten days. Men are more frequently affected than women. Most patients are young - the average age is less than twenty-five to fifty.

1) Periods of continuous fever lasting for two to seven days, punctuated by afebrile intervals lasting for seven to ten days, are characteristic of relapsing fever. The febrile period may end with drenching sweats and diarrhea; occasionally, the temperature may drop to $95^{0}$ to $97^{0}$F.

2) Cough due to bronchitis may be present during the first two weeks in 15% to 20%. [1]

3) Petechiae or rose-colored spots of 5 to 7 mm. in size may appear (in 25% to 30% of patients)[1] on the neck and shoulder girdle.

4) Conjunctivitis and iritis may be noticed in 20%.

5) Splenomegaly (50% to 75%).

6) Abdominal pains and generalized muscle aches may occur.

7) Epistaxis or uterine hemorrhage may result from disseminated intravascular coagulation.

8) Delirium, cranial palsies and peripheral neuritis are infrequent (10% to 15%).

9) Jaundice (10% to 15%) is a frequent feature in India. Vomiting is common, and the liver may be enlarged (17%).

TABLE 8: CLASSIFICATION OF SPIROCHAETALES

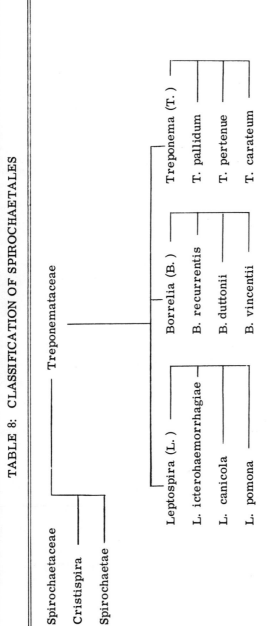

Spirochaetaceae — Treponemataceae

Cristispira

Spirochaetae

Leptospira (L. )

L. icterohaemorrhagiae

L. canicola

L. pomona

Borrelia (B. )

B. recurrentis

B. duttonii

B. vincentii

Treponema (T. )

T. pallidum

T. pertenue

T. carateum

Spirochaetaceae are not human pathogens, but all other species of Treponemataceae listed above can cause disease in man.

10) Proteinuria is infrequent.

11) Leukocytosis (15,000 to 30,000/cu. mm. ) frequently occurs during the febrile paroxysms.

12) The erythrocytic sedimentation rate is often increased (40 to 70 mm. /hour. )

## THE PATHOGEN

Borrelia (B.) recurrentis is transmitted by the body louse (Pediculus humanus) while it sucks the blood of man, when it may be accidentally killed by the host. It is not a transovarially transmitted disease, such as B. duttonii infection, to be mentioned later. It may occur in epidemic form. B. recurrentis infection is rare in the United States. It is a disease of famine and wars, prevalent during the winter months and propagated by the unhygienic conditions that prevail in several parts of the world. Man is the only known host for this organism.

Borrelia (B. ) duttonii and other Borrelia species are transmitted by the tick called Ornithodoros, which causes sporadic outbreaks of relapsing fevers. It occurs in all parts of the world. The tick transmits the organism during the act of biting, by discharging its coxal fluid either simultaneously or soon after the blood meal. Many varieties of rodents host this organism. The contagion, unlike B. recurrentis, mentioned earlier, is transmitted transovarially in the tick. Table 9 summarizes the epidemic and endemic relapsing fevers.

## DIAGNOSIS

1) Peripheral blood smears: Both thick and thin blood smears should be obtained at the height of the fever ($102^\circ$F. or more), stained with Leishman's [2] or Giemsa's stain and examined for the characteristic corkscrew-shaped organisms. Thick smears should be dehemoglobinized before further examination. Borrelia organisms may be found in the blood smears of nearly 70% of the patients. Often the blood smears are negative when the patient becomes afebrile.

2) Direct examination: Mix one drop of blood with one drop of sodium citrate, and place it under a cover slip on a slide and examine under 400X for the helical rotation and twisting movements of Borrelia.

TABLE 9: DIFFERENTIATING FEATURES OF EPIDEMIC AND ENDEMIC RELAPSING FEVERS

| CHARACTER | EPIDEMIC | ENDEMIC |
|---|---|---|
| 1. Bacteria | B. recurrentis | B. duttonii and other B. species |
| 2. Transmitted by | Louse (Pediculus humanus) | Tick (Ornithodoros) |
| 3. Unaffected countries | U. S. A. | New Zealand and Australia |
| 4. Transovarial spread in the vector | No | Yes |
| 5. Mode of infection | By intimate contact with louse-infected population | Acquired in the caves, at rodent burrows in mountainous countries where tick infections occur |
| 6. Route of infection by blood meal | Crushed lice through the abraded skin | The tick discharges coxal fluid at the site |
| 7. Animal host | Man | Mostly rodents |
| 8. Number of relapses | 2 to 4 | 5 to 11 |

3) Animal inoculation: Inject 0.1 ml. to 0.2 ml. of 1:1 dilution of blood with sodium citrate, either subcutaneously or intra-peritoneally into a 21-day-old Swiss mouse. Three to four days later, begin examining the tail blood smears for a period of at least fourteen days for bacteria. These smears may be stained with Leishman's or Giemsa's stain or by silver impregnation technique. The animal inoculation may be positive in nearly 90% of the patients.

4) Cerebrospinal fluid (CSF): The CSF pressure may be in-creased with either mononuclear or polymorphonuclear leu-kocytosis; 950/cu. mm. (750 to 2,200); protein - 97% (56 to 160). The spirochaetes may be found in the CSF of nearly 12% of the patients.

5) VDRL: False-positive blood VDRL may occur in nearly one-half of the patients, but the CSF VDRL is rarely pos-itive.

6) Complement-fixation test: This is a useful diagnostic tool in obscure cases. The antigen is derived from a suspension of spirochaetes.

7) Proteus OXK agglutinins: Proteus OXK agglutinins, used as a diagnostic tool for tsutsugamushi fever, may be pos-itive in more than 90% of the cases of borreliosis at 1:40 or more. Nearly 30% of the louse-borne Borrelia infections have high titers of 1:100 or more. However, one-third of the patients with tick-borne typhus have low titers of 1:40 or less.

8) Borrelia immobilization test: This is positive in most in-stances during the first four to six weeks of the disease. The test is similar to Treponema pallidum immobilization test.

9) Borreliolysin: This is produced during the early phase of the disease, especially during the crisis of the first attack. Addition of the patient's serum, obtained at this time, lyses the Borrelia organisms obtained from the stock cultures.

## DIFFERENTIAL DIAGNOSIS

Borreliosis may be mistaken for:

1) Malaria, which is diagnosed by blood smears.

2) Acute abdominal catastrophe, such as perforation and acute appendicitis. It is because of the infection of the spleen, which is an infrequent complication of borreliosis.

3) Dengue fever.

4) Typhus diagnosed by Weil-Felix reaction.

5) Yellow fever.

6) Hemorrhagic smallpox or chickenpox can be established by skin biopsy.

7) Leptospirosis. Borrelia are rarely found in the urine, whereas the Leptospira are frequently found.

Dengue fever, typhus, and yellow fever can be excluded by the demonstration of the spirochaetes in the blood.

## TREATMENT

Tetracyclines are the drugs of choice. The response to penicillin is slow. Tetracycline, 250 mg., may be administered every six hours for five days. Relapses are rare after tetracycline therapy, but adverse effects like Jarisch-Herxheimer type of reaction can occur during therapy. It begins (prodromal phase) one hour after the first dose with rigors and chills, associated with fever above 102°F. Severe respiratory alkalosis may occur at this stage. Six to eight hours later, it is followed by the "flush phase", when the fever may increase or drop to subnormal, accompanied by the fall of blood pressure. Fibrinolysis (DIC) can also occur, and fibrin degradation products may be found in the blood during this stage. Eight to twelve hours later, the recovery phase (defervescence) ensues.

## REFERENCES

1. Southern, P. M., Sanford, J. P.: Relapsing fever. A clinical and microbiologic review. Medicine 48:129, 1969.

2. Johnson, R. (Ed.): The Biology of Parasitic Spirochetes. Academic Press, New York, 1976.

16: INFECTIONS OF THE PANCREAS
by H. Thadepalli

Pancreatic infections might manifest as:

1) pancreatitis
2) pancreatic ascites
3) pseudocyst of the pancreas
4) pancreatic abscess

Pancreatitis in the United States is essentially a disease of the alcoholic and, therefore, its associated infections are those peculiar to alcoholics. The duodenum is normally sterile, but it may be colonized with gram-negative aerobic bacilli in the alcoholic. Hence, the infections associated with acute pancreatitis are usually due to the enteric gram-negative bacilli. In spite of aggressive therapy, the mortality associated with acute pancreatitis is around 10% to 12%. Shock is a sign of fatal prognosis in acute pancreatitis, but if the patient survives, there is a tendency to develop pancreatic abscess.

## PANCREATITIS

Abdominal pain, nausea and vomiting are the constant signs of pancreatitis, and they occur in 90% of the cases of pancreatitis. [1] Fever and chills are inconstant features and they occur in only 10%. Serum amylases in pancreatitis are always elevated. Abdominal tenderness is present in nearly all the patients. Abdominal distension and decreased bowel sounds occur in nearly one-half of the patients. Leukocytosis might be present in 60%. The chest films may reveal pleural effusion on one or both sides, with or without atelectasis. The flat plate of the abdomen alone is usually unrewarding.

BACTERIOLOGY: Only 4% to 10% of pancreatitis patients have positive blood cultures. The most frequent isolates in acute pancreatitis are Klebsiella-Enterobacter group of organisms.

RADIOLOGY: Some of the bizarre clinical signs and symptoms of pancreatitis and its radiological features can be explained if one understands the relationship of the pancreas to various anatomic fascial planes in the abdomen. [2] Extravasation of the enzymes in pancreatitis follow certain set anatomic planes, as shown in Fig. 6.

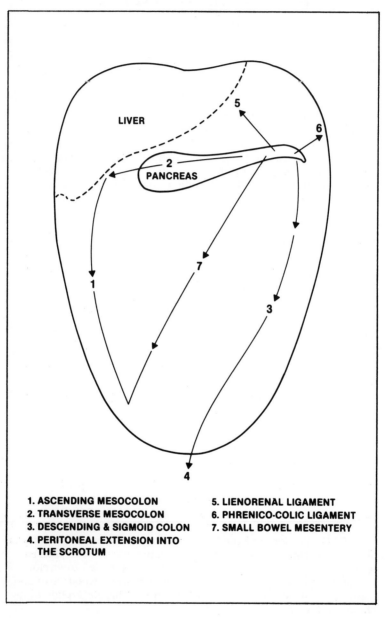

FIG. 6: Dissemination of pancreatic enzymes by anatomical planes.

## DIAGNOSIS

Hyperamylasemia is usually present in acute pancreatitis. Amylases might also be elevated in other situations. Hyperamylasemia might occur following surgery of the upper gastrointestinal or biliary tract. [3] In patients with acute pancreatitis, the amylase/creatinine clearance ratio may increase significantly, [4] whereas it is unaltered or normal in others.

Several signs of pulmonary involvement occur secondary to acute pancreatitis. They may be mistaken for bronchopneumonia and lobar pneumonia gram-negative sepsis. At times, they are also mistaken for a severe degree of hypoxia, which may occur due to acute pancreatitis, but is largely reversible. [5] Acute pancreatitis may also cause pleural effusion of either right and/or left side, and ascites. A positive blood culture in association with these symptoms needs exclusion of the possible underlying pancreatic abscess.

Diabetes mellitus may occur secondary to acute pancreatitis or the associated gram-negative sepsis. Bacterial infection, by itself, may cause diabetes mellitus, due to: (1) stimulation of pancreatic alpha cell function and liberation of glucagon[6] or, (2) insufficient production of insulin secondary to generalized pancreatic inflammation.

The value of antibiotics in the treatment of acute pancreatitis is controversial. They are administered to prevent infection and also to arrest abscess formation. In a prospective controlled double-blind study, ampicillin failed to substantiate this prediction. [7]

## PANCREATIC ABSCESS

A diagnosis not thought of is seldom made. The clinical signs and symptoms, the radiological clues of pancreatic abscess are subtle. If one is not aware of this condition as a possibility, it is missed. When untreated, pancreatic abscess may give rise to severe and dramatic complications and death. [8,9]

## CLINICAL FEATURES

Persistent fever, abdominal ileus and tenderness are common. Clinical deterioration of a patient one to four weeks after the initial improvement, following an attack of pancreatitis, should be suspected as a possible sign of pancreatic abscess.

Fevers ($100°$ to $102°$F. ) are common. Leukocytosis, above 15,000/cu. mm. is frequent. The serum amylases may or may not be elevated; occasionally, hypoalbuminemia and increased alkaline phosphatase may occur.

A distinct fullness or a palpable mass in the epigastrium may or may not be present. The abscess may be located in the head, body or tail of the pancreas; or around or behind it; or occasionally, in the lesser sac. It may extend into the paracolic gutter down to the pelvis or into the scrotal sac, as outlined in Fig. 6.

Certain clinical features of pancreatitis are summarized in Table 10.

TABLE 10: SIGNS, SYMPTOMS AND CLINICAL FEATURES OF PANCREATIC ABSCESS (Among 121 Cases)[8,9,10]

| SYMPTOMS: | | INVESTIGATIONS: | |
|---|---|---|---|
| Abdominal pain | 97% | Leukocytosis ( >10, 000) | 91% |
| Fever | 82.3% | Pulmonary abnormalities, i.e. , x-rays and lung function tests | 67% |
| Nausea and vomiting | 67% | | |
| History of pancreatitis | 94% | | |
| History of gallbladder disease | 35% | | |
| Diarrhea | 10% | | |
| SIGNS: | | MORTALITY: | |
| Upper abdominal tenderness | 85% | Mortality without surgery | 98% |
| Mass in upper abdomen | 43% | Mortality in spite of surgery | 26% |
| Shock | 16% | | |

The important diagnostic factors of pancreatic abscess are:

1) awareness of the possibility
2) acute pancreatitis and hypovolemic shock preceding that event

3) persistent fever associated with leukocytosis for more than two weeks following an attack of pancreatitis
4) palpable mass in the epigastrium with tenderness
5) a barium meal x-ray examination of the stomach or duodenum showing a displacement or deformity of these structures due to an extrinsic mass
6) toxicity is absent in pancreatic cyst and pancreatic ascites, but it is invariable in all cases of pancreatic abscess.

The diagnosis may not be obvious until surgically explored.

As mentioned earlier, death may occur from septicemia, renal failure, and electrolyte imbalance. The mortality rate among those operated on is around 26% and 98% among the non-operated. In spite of appropriate antibiotic therapy, the postoperative course of these patients is extremely stormy.

BACTERIOLOGY (Table 11): In one study, 13 of the 32 patients (41%) had more than one type of bacteria. Staphylococcus aureus, Escherichia coli, Streptococci, Proteus, Enterobacter, Klebsiella and Pseudomonas are the most frequent. The presence of anaerobic bacteria, although generally suspected, is infrequently reported with pancreatic abscess. Eighty to ninety-five per cent of cases are culture-positive and about fifteen to twenty per cent are sterile.

TABLE 11: BACTERIOLOGY OF PANCREATIC ABSCESS
(From 121 Cases)[8,9,10]

|  | Approximate Per cent |
| --- | --- |
| Number of patients with positive pus cultures | 85 |
| No growth | 15 |
| Polymicrobial infection | 40 |
| Escherichia coli | 30 |
| Staphylococcus aureus | 25 |
| Klebsiella | 20 |
| Enterococcus | 20 |
| Proteus | 15 |
| Pseudomonas | 10 |
| Aerobacter aerogenes | 5 |

RADIOLOGY: Displacement of intra-abdominal viscera may be demonstrated by barium examination of the upper gastrointestinal series. A small number may show gas within the abscess cavity. The presence of retroperitoneal gas, or "soap-bubble appearance", is pathognomonic of pancreatic abscess or abscess of the lesser sac. A routine chest roentgenogram may show elevation of the right or left leaflet of the diaphragm. Fluoroscopy may reveal decreased motion of the diaphragm.

## DIFFERENTIAL DIAGNOSIS

Pancreatic abscess is a diagnosis made by the process of systematic exclusion of other diagnoses. Abdominal pain and fever, associated with or without a positive blood culture should first suggest an intra-abdominal infection. Exclusion of liver abscess, subdiaphragmatic abscess and an abscess of the spleen may be made on the basis of clinical examination and gallium scans. The usefulness of gallium scans in the diagnosis of pancreatic abscess is not well established.

ABSCESS OF THE LESSER SAC:  Theoretically, the pancreatic abscess may have to be distinguished from the non-pancreatic abscess of the lesser sac. The latter may be preceded by a bout of acute pancreatitis, due to perforation of the stomach or the duodenum.

NON-PANCREATIC LESSER SAC ABSCESS:  This abscess should also be diagnosed promptly and drained within a period of three weeks, because a delay in diagnosis for more than eighteen days is associated with 75% mortality.[11]

The differential diagnoses of pancreatic lesions are listed in Table 12. I have diagnosed pancreatic abscess ante mortem or postmortem among 6 of 180 cases (3.3%) of miscellaneous intra-abdominal and pelvic abscesses. All six patients gave history of pancreatitis and alcoholism or upper gastrointestinal surgery. Four patients were diagnosed to have pancreatic abscess ante mortem and were successfully treated, following surgical drainage, with antibiotics to cover both anaerobic and aerobic bacteria. In two patients, the diagnosis was made at autopsy. Anaerobic bacteria were found in three of four abscesses diagnosed ante mortem, and both cases at autopsy.

## PSEUDOCYST OF THE PANCREAS

Pseudocyst of the pancreas might occur as a complication of subacute or chronic pancreatitis. By this time, the serum amylase may have returned to normal levels, and the patient is relatively asymptomatic. Pancreatic pseudocyst can be diagnosed by both clinical and radiological means.

## TABLE 12: DIFFERENTIAL DIAGNOSIS OF PANCREATIC LESIONS

| | PANCREATITIS | PANCREATIC PSEUDOCYST | PANCREATIC ABSCESS | NON-PANCREATIC ABSCESS OF THE LESSER SAC |
|---|---|---|---|---|
| Fever | 99° to 101°F. | normal | usually 102°F. or above | usually 102°F. or above |
| History of pancreatitis | yes | yes | yes | not necessarily present |
| History of perforation and ulcer disease | maybe | maybe | maybe | usually present |
| Serum amylase | increased | may be normal | may be normal | normal or increased |
| Stool guaiac | may be positive | may be positive | may be positive | usually positive |
| Clinical toxicity (graded 0 to 4+) | 0 to 4+ | 0 to 2+ | 3 to 4+ | 1 to 3+ |
| X-ray: "Soap bubble" appearance in lateral view of abdomen | no | no | may be seen | may be seen |

Table 12 (Cont'd)

|  | PANCREATITIS | PANCREATIC PSEUDOCYST | PANCREATIC ABSCESS | NON-PANCREATIC ABSCESS OF THE LESSER SAC |
|---|---|---|---|---|
| **X-ray:** |  |  |  |  |
| Ultrasound | usually negative | usually positive | may be positive | usually positive |
| Mass seen by plain x-ray | no | usually seen | may be seen | usually seen |
| Displacement of an adjacent organ as seen by barium examination | no | may be displaced | may be displaced | usually displaced |
| Blood cultures | + − | always negative | + − | + − |

Abdominal pain and vomiting associated with previous history of gastrointestinal bleeding (ulcer disease), with or without elevated serum amylases associated with the palpable mass, should suggest the possibility of pancreatic pseudocyst.[12] Infected pancreatic pseudocyst and pancreatic abscess are preoperatively indistinguishable.

The radiological signs of pseudocyst of the pancreas usually consist of a demonstrable mass in the retroinfragastric, retrogastric or anterior gastric area. This mass may push the colon down or may show a "cutoff" sign of the colon and/or the duodenum.

Angiograms of the pancreas are extremely useful in the diagnosis of pancreatic abscess, but their use in the diagnosis of pseudocyst is limited.

A ruptured or a rupturing pseudocyst is neither palpable nor radiologically demonstrable.

Ultrasonic scanning may be useful in the demonstration of space-occupying lesions of the pancreas. By ultrasonic scanning of the abdomen, a cross-section of views of the organs, including the pancreas, can be seen, and lesions may be demonstrated, provided they are at least one inch in diameter. They may be outlined on an oscilloscope screen. When they are outlined, a guided puncture can be performed with a special ultrasonic transducer, which has a central canal through which an ultrasonically guided needle may be introduced. This procedure has been used, not only for verification of ultrasonic diagnosis, but also for definitive therapy and for decompression in cases of threatening rupture.

Despite the refined roentgenographic, endoscopic and isotopic techniques, the diagnosis of pancreatic lesions is still a problem in many instances.

REFERENCES

1. Olsen, H.: Pancreatitis: A prospective clinical evaluation of 100 cases and review of literature. Amer. J. Digest. Dis. 19:1077, 1974.

2. Myers, M. A., Evans, J. A.: Effects of pancreatitis of the small bowel and colon, spread along mesenteric planes. Am. J. Roentgen. Rad. Ther. and Nuc. Med. CXIX:151, 1973.

3. Miller, S. F., Whitaker, J. R., Snyder, R. D.: Incidence of elevated serum amylase levels and pancreatitis after abdominal surgery. Amer. J. Surg. 125:535, 1973.

4. Warshaw, A. L., Fuller, A. F., Jr.: Specificity of increased renal clearance of amylase in diagnosis of acute pancreatitis. New Eng. J. Med. 292:325, 1975.

5. Ranson, J. H. C., et al: Respiratory complications in acute pancreatitis. Ann. Surg. 179:557, 1974.

6. Rocha, D. M., et al: Abnormal pancreatic alpha cell function in bacterial infections. New Eng. J. Med. 288:700, 1973.

7. Finch, W. T., Sawyers, J. L., Schenker, S.: A prospective study to determine the efficacy of antibiotics in acute pancreatitis. Ann. Surg. 183:667, 1976.

8. Kune, G. A., King, R.: The late complications of acute pancreatitis, pancreatic swelling, cyst and abscess. Med. J. Aust. 1:1241, 1973.

9. Miller, T. A., et al: Pancreatic abscess. Arch. Surg. 108:545, 1974.

10. Altmeier, W. A., Alexander, J. W.: Pancreatic abscess: A study of 32 cases. Arch. Surg. 87:96, 1963.

11. Wilson, S. E., Gordon, H. E., Passaro, E., Jr.: Non-pancreatic abscess of the lesser sac. Amer. J. Surg. 126:235, 1973.

12. Komaki, S., Clark, J. M.: Pancreatic pseudocyst: A review of 17 cases with emphasis on radiologic findings. Am. J. Roentgen. Rad. Ther. and Nuc. Med. 122:385, 1974.

SECTION B: RESPIRATORY INFECTIONS

17: PNEUMONIA: DIAGNOSTIC TECHNIQUES
by David W. Webb

Pneumonia is the most common cause of death due to infection.
Despite its prevalence, it is one of the most frequently misdiagnosed conditions. Appropriate diagnostic studies are therefore crucial to establish its etiology. This chapter deals with
the bacterial pneumonias. Tuberculosis (see Chapter 23) and
the viral pneumonias are discussed elsewhere.

DIFFERENTIATION OF PNEUMONIA FROM MALIGNANCY

Cough and fever are the two common symptoms for both conditions. Physical examination and the roentgenogram of the
chest together are preliminary for differentiating pleuropulmonary infections from carcinoma. Often, carcinoma of the
lung may present with a picture clinically indistinguishable
from bacterial pneumonia. Carcinoma and pneumonia may coexist; therefore, diagnosis of one does not exclude the other.
Recent onset of cough lasting for more than four weeks' duration
and weight loss should lead one to suspect tuberculosis or cancer.
Low-grade fevers are not uncommon with malignancy, but chills
and rigors often spell bacterial infection. Final diagnosis rests
on the exfoliative cytology of either expectorated sputum or
bronchoscopy specimen. Carcinoma should be suspected in all
cases of pneumonia that fail to respond to an adequate course
of appropriate antibiotics. Ordinarily, the chest roentgenogram of pneumococcal pneumonia clears within a month.[1]
Further delay in its resolution warrants bronchoscopy to exclude malignancy.

DIFFERENTIATION OF PNEUMONIA FROM EMBOLISM

Pulmonary embolism, with or without pulmonary infarction,
can be confused with bacterial pneumonia. A pulmonary infarct
can be secondarily infected. Pleuritic pain, dyspnea, low-grade
fever, cough with hemoptysis and leukocytosis may be present
with both infection and infarction. A pulmonary embolus may
show a wedge-shaped infiltrate on x-ray, or could be altogether
normal. High fever, rigors and productive cough with purulent
sputum are rare with infarction, unless secondarily infected.

91

Signs of phlebitis, such as calf pain and tenderness with a palpable cord or a positive Homan's sign, in our experience, are more frequently absent than present in cases of pulmonary infarction. Hypoxemia can occur with both. The characteristic EKG findings, such as tachycardia, right axis deviation, partial or complete right bundle branch block, or an S I, Q III, T III pattern may occur in pulmonary embolism.

Perfusion and ventilation lung scan may help to differentiate infection from infarction.[2] A perfusion scan is done by intravenous injection of I-131 tagged albumin or Tc-99m. It demonstrates the areas of the lung perfused by blood. Areas of decreased uptake represent areas with decreased blood flow. The perfusion defects are nonspecific; seen in cases other than pulmonary embolism, i.e., emphysema, carcinoma, and infection. Specificity is enhanced by also performing a ventilation scan with xenon-133. The patient inhales this gas. It normally shows up in areas of good ventilation in the lungs. When both tests are combined, two patterns emerge; the first is pulmonary vascular disease (pulmonary embolism), wherein the involved area shows decreased perfusion with normal ventilation, and the second is parenchymal disease (infection or tumor), wherein the affected area reveals normal perfusion with decreased ventilation. Parenchymal lung disease can produce two patterns. In emphysema and bronchial obstruction, when the patient rebreathes the xenon, the affected segment slowly fills. In pneumonia and carcinoma, there is no later uptake after the xenon is rebreathed. Ventilation/perfusion scans have their limitations; some cases of embolism will show no ventilation defects, and some may show both ventilation and perfusion defects, especially when an infiltrate is present.

A gallium-67 scan may be helpful in separating embolism from infection.[3] Normally, the lung takes up very little Ga-67, generally less than the soft tissue of the shoulder. Increased uptake of gallium should make one suspect infection or neoplasma.[42] Absence of such an increase on the face of a roentgenographic evidence of inflammation suggests pulmonary embolism as the likely cause.

Pulmonary angiography may be done to confirm the diagnosis of pulmonary embolism. Injection of contrast material into the pulmonary artery is made via a catheter inserted in the femoral vein.[4] A filling defect in one of the branches of the pulmonary artery will be seen on serial roentgenograms in cases of pulmonary embolism; but is absent in

cases of bacterial pneumonia. An abrupt 'cutoff' of one of these
vessels is considered pathognomonic of pulmonary embolism,
but it is seen infrequently. False-negative results are known,
but false-positive results are not common.

## ATELECTASIS AND PNEUMONIA

Atelectasis may mimic pneumonia. Infection can occur in the
collapsed segment. In cases of pneumonia, the bronchus may
be occluded due to mucus plugs and secondary atelectasis will
follow. Therefore, the differentiation of atelectasis from pneumonia is not always clear-cut. Atelectasis, along with pneumonia, can cause cough, fever and a pulmonary infiltrate.
Purulent sputum, high fevers and rigors suggest infectious
complications. Atelectasis can be diagnosed by the "plate-like"
infiltrates seen in the chest roentgenogram, associated with
or without a shift of the mediastinum, which is pulled toward
the collapsed segment. The gallium scan is normal in cases
of uncomplicated atelectasis. When atelectasis persists in
spite of vigorous physiotherapy, bronchoscopy should be performed to exclude malignancy. Visualization of the mucosal
plugs, and removal of them during bronchoscopy, may promptly relieve the collapsed segment. Associated infections should
be excluded by proper culture techniques.

## DIAGNOSTIC PROCEDURES

BLOOD CULTURES: Nearly 3% of all febrile patients, regardless of the nature of the infection, may have positive blood cultures.
Blood cultures are usually positive in 10% to 40% of the cases
of bacterial pneumonia. Demonstration of Streptococcus pneumoniae in the blood does not necessarily mean that it is the
cause of underlying pneumonia. Pneumococcal bacteremia can
occur in cases of tuberculosis or malignancy. Certain invasive
procedures, such as bronchoscopy, can also cause bacteremia.
Staphylococcal pneumonia is infrequent. If the blood culture
is positive for S. aureus, one should suspect endocarditis or
hospital-acquired infection. Bacteremia can occur in viral
pneumonia due to bacterial superinfection. Isolation of Bacteroides fragilis, anaerobic cocci and Enterococcus from the
blood, in cases of pneumonia, should lead one to suspect the
abdomen as the primary septic focus.

SPUTUM: Examination of the sputum for bacteria by Gram's
stain and culture often yields more misleading results. Nevertheless, it is a religiously performed ritual in all cases of

pneumonia. Diplococcus pneumoniae is a normal flora of the sputum, present in up to 35% of normal persons, [5] and is cultured only in 50% of the cases proven to have pneumococcal pneumonia. [6] Some believe that if the sputum has no epithelial cells and shows many polymorphs and intraleukocytic gram-positive diplococci, it is diagnostic of pneumococcal pneumonia. Demonstration of "intraleukocytic" diplococci is not pathognomonic of pneumococcal pneumonia. Gram's stain of the sputum, at its best, is just as (un) reliable as one's own clinical acumen. The only situation when a sputum Gram's stain can be considered to be of any value is when it contains only one morphotype, i.e., gram-positive cocci alone or gram-negative rods alone. Demonstration of more than one morphotype of bacteria in the sputum nullifies its diagnostic value.

Sputum examination is worthless for the diagnosis of anaerobic pneumonia, because anaerobes are normal flora of the mouth.

Gram-negative bacteria may be seen on Gram's stain of sputum in patients who do not have gram-negative pneumonia. Antimicrobial therapy, even for a short duration, can increase the prevalence of gram-negative bacilli in the sputum.

TRANSTRACHEAL ASPIRATION: Transtracheal aspiration (TTA) allows one to obtain uncontaminated sputum. It is indicated when:

1) anaerobic infection is suspected
2) the patient is unable to cough up an adequate sputum sample, and
3) the patient fails to respond to seemingly appropriate therapy

This procedure was found to be useful and reliable for the diagnosis of pneumonia. Demonstration of bacteria in the Gram's stain of a properly done TTA confirms the diagnosis of bacterial pneumonia. Pneumonia caused by the aerobes can be diagnosed with confidence within 24 hours and anaerobes within 48 hours after this procedure.

Transtracheal aspiration is safe provided certain precautions are taken. [7] It should not be attempted by the novice without guidance. It should not be done in the uncooperative patients, or in those with uncorrectable hypoxemia or bleeding tendencies. Routine clotting studies, such as platelet count, prothrombin time, and partial thromboplastin time should be obtained before this procedure is done.

Procedure: TTA is performed by extending the patient's neck over a pillow (Fig. 7) with the patient lying in the supine position. The area of the neck should be cleansed with an appropriate local antiseptic. Under local anesthesia, the cricothyroid membrane is first pierced by a 14 or 16-gauge needle with the bevelled edge of the needle extended caudad; a catheter is then threaded through the needle for nearly two to four inches down the trachea. The needle is then withdrawn with the catheter left within the trachea. Suction is then applied by a large 50 cc. syringe or a suction apparatus, and the sputum is collected into the syringe or a sterile container. If no sputum is obtained, 2 to 4 cc. of sterile saline may be injected into the trachea to stimulate cough. After a sample is obtained, the catheter is withdrawn, and gentle pressure is applied on the puncture site to prevent bleeding. The patient should remain in bed for several hours to minimize the risk of subcutaneous emphysema.

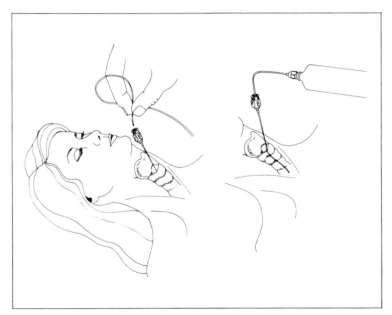

FIG. 7: Transtracheal aspiration.

Minimal subcutaneous emphysema is a common complication of TTA. Bleeding can be minimized if the cricothyroid membrane is punctured caudad, avoiding the blood vessels. [8] Streaks of blood in the sputum frequently occur; the patient should be cautioned not to be perturbed, for this is temporary. Serious bleeding, however, is rare if proper precautions are taken. Cardiac arrhythmias can occur in hypoxemic patients. [9] One's success with this procedure, like any other, depends on one's own experience.

Once the TTA sample is obtained, it should be promptly processed for culture of both aerobic and anaerobic bacteria. A Gram's stain and stain for acid-fast bacteria should be done routinely on all TTA specimens. It should be kept in mind that patients with chronic bronchitis may have colonization of their trachea by aerobic bacteria (particularly H. influenzae), and results of TTA culture in such patients must be interpreted in this light. [10]

Since the trachea or bronchial tree is normally sterile, isolation of any bacteria from a well done TTA should be interpreted as the most likely cause for the underlying lung infection. [11]

TRANSTHORACIC NEEDLE ASPIRATION AND BIOPSY: When TTA does not yield the diagnosis in cases of suspected lung infection, and the patient remains ill, one may resort to more invasive procedures, such as needle aspiration or biopsy of the lung. Often, in cases of pneumonia caused by unusual organisms, such as fungi and Pneumocystis carinii, these procedures are invaluable. [12] Needle aspiration of the lung is somewhat safer than percutaneous biopsy, but the latter has the advantage of securing tissue for histologic examination.

Both transthoracic needle aspiration and needle biopsy are done with the patient in the sitting position; following local anesthesia, direct puncture of the lung is made with the patient holding his breath in the expiratory position. A 20-gauge needle attached to a syringe is used for aspiration; a trephine biopsy cutting needle is used for biopsy. The precautions to be taken are the same as with transtracheal aspiration. In addition, severe hypoxemia and bullous lung disease are contraindications for this procedure. Immediate complications include pneumothorax and bleeding. These complications can occur in nearly 2% to 10% of patients undergoing needle aspiration; and up to 20% undergoing biopsy when done with a cutting needle. Most of these complications are of minor nature and they are often temporary and reversible.

BRONCHOSCOPY: Rigid or flexible fiberoptic bronchoscopy has become a useful tool in the diagnosis of certain types of pneumonia. The technique involves passing the instrument into the trachea and then down the bronchi. Fiberoptic bronchoscopy

has the advantage of visualizing fifth, and even sixth, order bronchi. [13] Peripheral lesions can be visualized and material obtained for culture. The technique is most useful in
certain cases of pneumonia caused by unusual organisms, such
as Mycobacterium tuberculosis and Pneumocystis carinii, which
are not normal flora of the mouth. It has no value in the diagnosis of common lung infections such as pneumococcal or Klebsiella pneumonia, and is also useless for the diagnosis of anaerobic lung infections, because these organisms are so often
part of the normal flora of the mouth. Secretions obtained by
bronchoscopy are invariably contaminated by mouth flora.
Furthermore, topical anesthetics used in bronchoscopy inhibit
bacterial growth, thus yielding falsely negative culture results. [14]

Bronchial brushing, via the bronchoscope, yields material suitable for staining and culture of unusual pathogens. [15] More
recently, transbronchial biopsy has been used as a means of
obtaining lung tissue for pathologic examination and culture. [16]
Transbronchial biopsy is done by a small forceps passed into
the lung via a flexible fiberoptic bronchoscope. In the hands of
the experienced, this procedure is considered safer than needle biopsy of the lung, but its overall safety awaits further
analysis. Bleeding can occur and coagulation parameters should
be assessed and corrected, if abnormal, before the procedure
is carried out.

LUNG BIOPSY: Open biopsy of the lung has the highest diagnostic yield, because a large sample of lung tissue can be obtained for histologic examination and cultures. This procedure
may be diagnostic when other less invasive means have failed. [17]
An open lung biopsy has become increasingly important in the
diagnosis of pneumonia in the immunosuppressed. Because a
host of highly fatal infections are known to be associated with
immunosuppression, either transthoracic needle aspiration or
open biopsy of the lung is resorted to when TTA does not yield
the diagnosis. Such procedures should only be done by those
experienced in such techniques.

## 18: SPECIFIC CAUSES OF PNEUMONIA
by David W. Webb


### PNEUMOCOCCAL PNEUMONIA

Streptococcus (Diplococcus) pneumoniae is the most common cause of bacterial pneumonia, accounting for at least 80% of the cases occurring in the community. The organism is a gram-positive lancet-shaped coccus, usually occurring in pairs. In adults, pneumonia is caused most frequently by serotypes 1, 3, 4, 7, 8 and 12. Type 3 is heavily encapsulated and causes a particularly virulent pneumonia with high fatality and a propensity to form a lung abscess. Between 5% and 35% of the healthy population are carriers of pneumococci, depending on the season, age of the patient, and whether or not children are present in the family. [5]

Carriage rates are highest in the winter, in young children and in adults with preschool children in the family. Carriage rates are highest for serotypes 3, 19 and 23. [18]

Pneumococcal pneumonia is more frequent during the winter months, and during the monsoon in India. Certain patients are predisposed to this illness, such as the malnourished, alcoholics, diabetics and those with sickle cell anemia, multiple myeloma, bronchogenic carcinoma, chronic obstructive lung disease, congestive heart failure, asplenia, or hypogamma-globulinemia. Pneumococcal pneumonia may follow an upper respiratory tract infection due to viruses.

Clinical features of pneumococcal pneumonia are not sufficiently distinctive to make the diagnosis; often the disease begins with one shaking chill, followed by fever and cough productive of rusty-colored sputum. Pleuritic chest pain is often present. Sometimes, pharyngitis or other symptoms of an upper respiratory tract infection have been present for several days before the initial rigor.

Physical examination reveals a febrile patient with tachypnea and tachycardia at rest. There may be splinting or decreased movement of the chest on the involved side. Physical examination of the chest usually reveals signs of consolidation (dullness to percussion, increased tactile and vocal fremitus). Wet rales and bronchovesicular breathing are usually heard over the involved segment. Decreased breath sounds over the involved area are one of the earliest signs of pneumonia. The

abdomen may show signs of an ileus, more infrequently, gastric atony as evidenced by a succussion splash. Herpes labi-
alis may be present. Mild icterus may be noted in some cases.

Laboratory values usually reveal a leukocytosis with a shift
of granulocytes to the left. Occasionally leukopenia will be
present. Leukopenia of less than 2,000/cu. mm. heralds a
poor prognosis. The erythrocyte sedimentation rate (ESR) is
elevated. Arterial blood gases may reveal hypoxemia with respiratory alkalosis and hypocapnia. Hyperbilirubinemia may
occur, but the remainder of the liver function tests are usually
normal.

The chest roentgenogram, in most cases, reveals lobar consolidation (Fig. 8). Commonly, one of the lower lobes is involved; but more than one lobe can occasionally be involved.
Early cavitation can occur in type 3 pneumococcal infections.
Pleural effusion is not common, but does occur in 10% of cases.
While the pneumococcus classically produces lobar pneumonia,
occasionally involvement of a single bronchopulmonary segment occurs, especially early during the course of illness. At
times, it may present as diffuse bronchopneumonia instead of
lobar pneumonia.

Sputum examination should be interpreted in the light of clinical and roentgenographic features. A fresh sample on Gram's
stain revealing the presence of a heavy concentration of polymorphs, suggests that the sample is from the lung. The presence of almost exclusively gram-positive, lancet-shaped diplococci, occurring both intra- and extracellularly, is highly
suggestive, but not necessarily diagnostic, of pneumococcal
pneumonia. When the diagnosis is in doubt, a TTA should be
performed (see page 95). Blood cultures should, of course,
be obtained in all cases prior to therapy. Once appropriate
cultures have been obtained, appropriate antibiotic therapy
should be started without waiting for the culture results. Because culture results may take a day or two, newer methods
have been developed for the presumptive identification of pneumococci. The "quellung" reaction occurs when pneumococci come
in contact with anticapsular serum; under the microscope, the
capsule of the organism becomes refractile. This reaction can
be applied directly to sputum. An air-dried smear of sputum
is covered with 0.01 ml. of omniserum (a commercially available pool of rabbit anticapsular serum) and examined immediately by microscope under oil immersion with the illumination
turned down. Pneumococci will appear refractile as the capsule
"swells". This procedure is more accurate than a Gram's stain

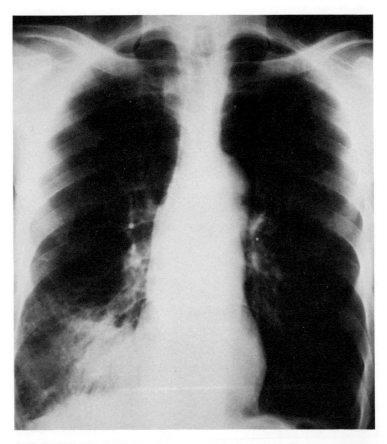

FIG. 8: Pneumococcal pneumonia. A 45-year-old alcoholic with cough and fever. Culture of transtracheal aspirate grew Streptococcus pneumoniae.

when compared to culture.[19] Counterimmunoelectrophoresis
(CIE) can also be used to rapidly detect pneumococci in sputum samples; this test may be useful in detecting pneumococci
in patients who have previously received antibiotics and whose
sputum cultures are negative.[20]

## COMPLICATIONS

In the penicillin era, certain complications of pneumococcal
pneumonia are rare. In desperately ill patients, these complications should be considered. Endocarditis may occur, usually affecting the aortic valve. It should be suspected when a
new murmur appears in the heart, particularly when it is a
murmur of aortic insufficiency. Meningitis can occur, and such
patients often have classical signs of meningitis (see Chapter 30).
However, in the elderly, meningitis should not be excluded on
the basis of absence of stiff neck. Some may show only changes
in mental status without obvious neck stiffness. Conversely,
some patients with pneumococcal pneumonia of the upper lobe
of the lung will have meningismus without meningitis. Diagnosis
of meningitis can only be made by examination and culture of
the cerebrospinal fluid (CSF). Lumbar puncture should be done
in all patients with meningeal signs or changes in mental status
disproportionate to the extent of pneumonia. Purulent pericarditis is, fortunately, rare, but is a rapidly fatal complication. It should be suspected when pericardial friction is heard.
Chest pain is often absent in such patients.

## TREATMENT

Treatment of pneumococcal pneumonia is best undertaken in a
hospital setting. Uncomplicated pneumonia can be treated with
penicillin G in a dose of 1.2 to 2.4 million units per day in divided doses. Initial treatment is best given intravenously. Complications, such as empyema, pericarditis, meningitis or endocarditis require much higher doses. A cephalosporin should
be used in patients allergic to penicillin, provided the allergic
reaction is not life-threatening. Erythromycin or clindamycin
can be used in those few patients with a history of serious reaction to penicillin. Treatment is usually continued for seven
to ten days.

## KLEBSIELLA PNEUMONIA

Klebsiella pneumoniae is an encapsulated gram-negative bacillus. Pneumonia is caused most frequently by serotypes 1 to 5.[21]

Higher serotypes are normal flora of the mouth in ten per cent of the population. Colonization is higher in patients with chronic obstructive lung disease. Probably less than one per cent of bacterial pneumonias are caused by this organism. They occur sporadically throughout the year.

Elderly patients or those with diabetes mellitus, alcoholism, chronic obstructive lung disease, renal failure, malignancy or renal disease are predisposed to this infection. Nosocomial infections are far more frequent with this organism than naturally acquired infections. It may spread within the hospitals by ventilatory equipment. At risk are those on assisted ventilation through tracheostomy or endotracheal tubes. The following description is pertinent to the naturally acquired Klebsiella pneumonia:

Signs of systemic toxicity are common with Klebsiella pneumonia. It often begins abruptly after a brief episode of an upper respiratory tract infection. High fever ($102^0$ to $105^0$ F. ), malaise and severe prostration are usually present, with multiple rigors. Productive cough with dyspnea is common. The sputum may be thick and tenacious or brick red due to blood, sometimes like currant jelly.

Physical examination may reveal cyanosis and signs of consolidation, usually of the upper lobe.

Laboratory values reveal leukocytosis with a shift to the left in most cases, although leukopenia is not rare. An anemia of the normochromic, normocytic type may be present. The sedimentation rate is elevated. Other laboratory values are unremarkable.

The chest roentgenogram may reveal an infiltrate, most often in an upper lobe (Fig. 9). When the upper lobe is involved, there may be downward displacement or "bulging" of the adjacent interlobar fissure. This sign is neither characteristic nor invariable for Klebsiella pneumonia. Associated pleural effusion may be present in about 15% of the cases. Necrosis and cavitation of the lung with abscess formation occurs frequently. Because of the destruction of the lung tissue and loss of volume, there may be a shift of the trachea to the involved side.

Sputum examination is the key to the diagnosis. It is often, although not invariably, thick and tenacious with a reddish-brown currant jelly appearance. Gram's stain often reveals many

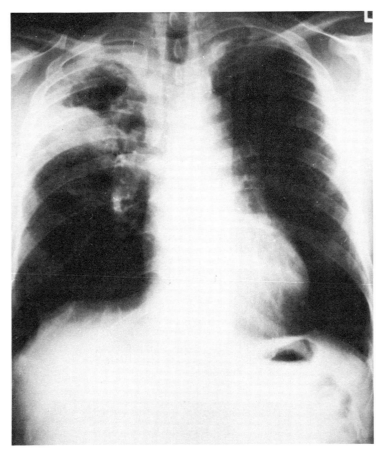

FIG. 9: Klebsiella pneumonia. A 45-year-old patient with juvenile diabetes mellitus, admitted with cough and fever. Culture of a transtracheal aspirate grew <u>Klebsiella pneumoniae</u>.

polymorphonuclear leukocytes and many gram-negative encapsulated bacilli. Most often, the smear predominantly, if
not exclusively, consists of these gram-negative bacilli. Culture of blood will reveal the organism in one-third of the cases.
Because many patients harbor Klebsiella in their oropharynx
(usually the higher serotypes), a TTA is usually required to
confirm the diagnosis. If Klebsiella are isolated from the TTA
specimen, or from blood cultures or both, the diagnosis is
certain.

In addition to the more usual acute form of the disease, a chronic
pneumonia due to K. pneumoniae has been described. Such patients present with symptoms spanning over several weeks,
and do not appear acutely toxic. Low-grade fever and cough are
the predominant symptoms. The chest roentgenogram may show
either a diffuse unilateral bronchopneumonia or a thin-walled
cavity. Most of these cases, in the past, were diagnosed on
the basis of sputum examination, which accounts for the large
number of cases of Klebsiella pneumoniae found in the literature.
Klebsiella pneumoniae has been rarely isolated from the TTA in
such cases. In most instances, in our experience, they had
several anaerobic bacteria in addition to Klebsiella, which is
often a bystander. The existence of such an entity as chronic
Klebsiella pneumoniae is questionable.

## TREATMENT

Klebsiella pneumoniae is usually sensitive to both the cephalosporins and the aminoglycosides (gentamicin, tobramycin, amikacin). Cephalosporins are preferable and may be used alone
in most cases; an aminoglycoside may be added in fulminant
cases. In vitro sensitivity testing must always be done,
as Klebsiella can be resistant to one or more of these antibiotics.

## STREPTOCOCCUS (S.) PYOGENES

S. pyogenes is a rare cause of bacterial pneumonia in the adult.
It may be primary or secondary. The secondary infection may
follow viral infections, such as influenza, rubella, rubeola or
varicella. [22] Primary infection usually occurs in military re-
cruits or other closed populations, but sporadic cases may occur as well. It may also occur following such infections as
tonsilitis, scarlet fever, or erysipelas.

It is usually of abrupt onset, with fever, shortness of breath,
chest pain, and cough productive of blood-streaked sputum.

Physical examination, in addition, may reveal cyanosis, pharyngitis in about half the cases, and rales on both sides of the chest. Signs of lobar consolidation are rare. Associated pleural effusions are frequent. Laboratory values reveal leukocytosis with shift to the left. The ESR is elevated.

The chest roentgenogram shows a patchy or diffuse bronchopneumonia with an interstitial pattern. It is often unilateral, but in some instances may be bilateral. Pleural effusion may be present.

Diagnosis is made by recovery of the organism from the sputum, blood or pleural fluid (if present). Because S. pyogenes may be harbored by about 10% of the population at any given time, the growth of S. pyogenes from expectorated sputum culture should be interpreted with caution. Precise diagnosis cannot be made without TTA. Streptococcal and staphylococcal pneumonia should always be suspected when signs of bacterial pneumonia complicate influenza or other viral infections.

## TREATMENT

S. pyogenes are uniformly sensitive to penicillin. The usual dose for pneumonia is four to six million units of penicillin G per day, given intravenously in divided doses. Therapy should be continued for at least two weeks.

## STAPHYLOCOCCUS AUREUS

Staphylococcus aureus causes about 10% of all bacterial pneumonia. Infection can be primary or secondary. During an epidemic of influenza and measles, secondary staphylococcal pneumonia is common. It may also follow other bacterial pneumonias. Certain patients with diabetes mellitus, connective tissue diseases, malignancy, or heroin or alcohol abuse are predisposed to staphylococcal pneumonia. Staphylococcal pneumonia most often affects infants and the elderly.

The clinical features vary with the type of infection. The mode of onset is usually abrupt with high fever, multiple chills, dyspnea, productive cough with purulent blood-tinged sputum and chest pain. Its course is fulminant, and the patient is acutely ill. Less frequently, the onset can be subacute; this commonly occurs in patients who had pneumonia due to septic embolism or bacteremia from a different source. Staphylococcal pneumonia in a heroin addict should suggest endocarditis of the tricuspid valve (Fig. 10). Staphylococcal bacteremia secondary to a boil, carbuncle or osteomyelitis can metastasize to the lung by the hematogenous route. Pleuritic chest pain, rather than cough, is more a prominent feature of such pneumonias.

Post-influenzal staphylococcal pneumonia often follows a fulminant course. Such patients may appear to be getting over an episode of influenza and seem entirely well for a day or two, when they develop a sudden onset of high fever, rigors and productive cough. When viral influenza pneumonia occurs as a complication of influenza, there is often no such disease-free interval between the two episodes.

## INVESTIGATIONS

Leukocytosis, with a shift to the left, and an elevated sedimentation rate, are common. In cases of overwhelming infection, leukopenia may occur. The chest roentgenogram may show diffuse nodular or "fluffy" infiltrates or lobar pneumonia, as in the case of infants and elderly patients. In infants, several pneumatoceles may characteristically appear either during the acute phase or during resolution. These are thin-walled cysts occurring in the interstitial tissue of the lungs. Several of these cavities may later coalesce during the illness and give rise to the so-called "vanishing lung" appearance. Pleural effusions are frequent. An interstitial bronchopneumonia, either unilateral or bilateral, may occur, especially when staphylococcal pneumonia occurs as a complication of viral influenza. Septic emboli early in the course often have the characteristic appearance of one or more round densities scattered throughout both lung fields; they may later appear as typical lobar or bronchopneumonia.

## DIAGNOSIS

Diagnosis can be suspected by the isolation of Staphylococcus aureus from the sputum. Blood cultures are often positive in cases of pneumonia due to a septic embolism from endocarditis. Gram's stain of the sputum usually reveals many polymorphonuclear leukocytes and gram-positive cocci in clumps. Diagnosis is established by isolating Staphylococcus aureus from a TTA sample. Because S. aureus is a normal flora of the mouth in 10% of healthy adults, sputum culture may be misleading.

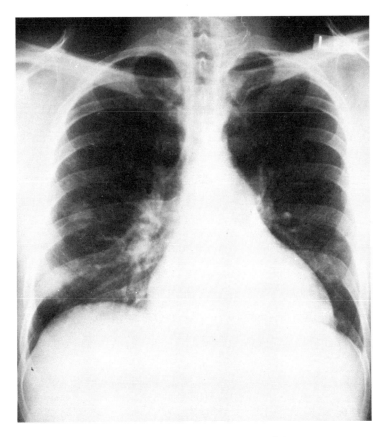

FIG. 10: Pneumonia due to septic emboli. A 24-year-old heroin addict admitted with chest pain, chills and fever. Blood cultures grew Staphylococcus aureus. He went on to develop a murmur consistent with tricuspid insufficiency. Note round densities in the right lung due to septic emboli.

## TREATMENT

Today, most Staphylococci are resistant to penicillin; therefore, treatment should be instituted with one of the semisynthetic penicillins (methicillin, oxacillin or nafcillin) or one of
the cephalosporins. The antibiotic should be given intravenously in full doses. If later sensitivity testing shows the organism
to be susceptible, penicillin G may be substituted. Treatment
should be continued for ten days in uncomplicated cases.

## GRAM-NEGATIVE PNEUMONIA (other than Klebsiella)

Besides Klebsiella, a variety of gram-negative bacteria are
responsible for pneumonia; Pseudomonas aeruginosa, Escherichia coli, Proteus and Serratia group of organisms are some
such examples. [23] At the outset, it is important to remember
that gram-negative pneumonia is an exceedingly rare disease
among the healthy population. Often, it is predisposed by diabetes
mellitus, congestive heart failure, chronic lung disease, alcoholism, malignancy, steroids or other immunosuppressive
drugs. Most notably, prior antibiotic therapy can shift the normal flora of the oropharynx toward predominantly gram-negative organisms. When debilitated patients aspirate these organisms, a gram-negative pneumonia results. Gram-negative
pneumonia today is the scourge of the hospitalized patient, unfortunately acquired through such life-saving devices as res-
pirators, tracheostomies and resuscitation equipment. Less
commonly, it can be secondary to bacteremia from a distant
septic focus, for instance, E. coli pneumonia secondary to
pyelonephritis, and Pseudomonas pneumonia, following skin
infections secondary to burns.

The clinical features of all gram-negative pneumonias are non-
specific. The patients are usually quite ill with fever, productive cough with purulent sputum, and pleuritic pain, often accompanied by respiratory distress. In patients with granulo-
cytopenia, the sputum may be thin because of the absence of
inflammatory response. Hemoptysis is rare. In patients with
pneumonia secondary to Serratia marcescens, there may be
pseudohemoptysis due to the presence of red pigment produced
by the organism itself.

## DIAGNOSIS

Leukocytosis may or may not be present. The findings on the
chest roentgenogram may vary from a mild patchy bronchopneumonia confined to a single lobe to an extensive bronchopneumonia affecting all lung fields. Microabscesses can be
seen occasionally with cavities greater than 1 cm in diameter.

A reliable diagnosis cannot be made from sputum cultures. Transtracheal aspiration is important to confirm the diagnosis. Nearly 16% of the healthy population harbor gram-negative bacilli as normal flora of the oropharynx, [24] and among hospitalized patients, this increases to about 50%. [25] It is for this reason that it is advisable to obtain blood culture and to perform a TTA when gram-negative pneumonia is suspected.

The most common clinical setting in the hospital for gram-negative pneumonia is the patient who is on a mechanical respirator and has either a tracheostomy or endotracheal tube in place. Such patients may colonize their entire respiratory tract with gram-negative bacteria. Tracheal aspiration in such case is unreliable because of contamination from the tracheal tubes. Diagnostic and therapeutic considerations in such cases are based on clinical grounds alone. Transient pulmonary infiltrates, due to atelectasis from "mucus plugs" of the bronchi, can also cause fever and leukocytosis and mislead one to use antibiotics. Bronchoscopy may be needed to dislodge these plugs and open up the obstructed segment of lung.

## TREATMENT

Treatment of gram-negative pneumonia will depend on the organism and in vitro sensitivity testing. An aminoglycoside (gentamicin, tobramycin or amikacin) is preferred therapy, pending identification of the organism. If the patient is immunosuppressed, carbenicillin or ticarcillin should be added to the regimen. Carbenicillin can be added to the aminoglycoside in cases of Pseudomonas pneumonia; pneumonia due to E. coli or Proteus can often be treated with carbenicillin, ampicillin, or a cephalosporin alone, depending on in vitro sensitivity results.

## MELIOIDOSIS

Melioidosis is a rare infection caused by Pseudomonas pseudomallei, a gram-negative bacillus. In southeast Asia, it occurs as a soil saprophyte, and the disease may occur in travelers to this area (particularly military personnel). The disease may have a long latent period and present many years after travel to an endemic area. [26] This emphasizes the need to ask the patient, "Where have you been?" Pseudomallei infection may occur either by inhalation, ingestion or through small breaks in the integrity of the skin.

Symptoms vary, depending on the severity and the spread of infection. Whereas inapparent infection is common at one end of the spectrum, a rapidly fatal septicemia may occur at the other. Localization of infection leads to pneumonia, osteomyelitis or abscess; in the U. S. , pneumonia is the most common manifestation of melioidosis.

The patient may present with fever, chills, weight loss and cough with productive blood-tinged sputum and pleuritic pain. Occasionally, it can take a fulminant course, but more typically, the presentation is either subacute or chronic.

Physical examination may reveal signs of consolidation of one or more lobes of the lungs; in addition to signs of generalized disseminated disease, such as draining sinuses, lymphadenopathy or hepatosplenomegaly.

### DIAGNOSIS

The white blood cell count may be up to 20,000/cu. mm., although it can be normal. The chest roentgenogram may show an infiltrate of an upper lobe of the lung (although any lobe may be involved). Cavitation often occurs. Empyema is uncommon but can occur. Melioidosis of the lung is often confused with tuberculosis or one of the fungal diseases; diagnosis depends on the clinical awareness of this entity and a carefully obtained travel history.

Once the diagnosis is suspected, it is confirmed by culture or serologic tests. Both sputum and blood should be cultured for the organism. P. pseudomallei can be grown on standard bacteriologic media. The most useful serologic test is the indirect hemagglutination (IHA) test; a titer of 1:40 is significant but may indicate old inapparent infection. A four-fold rise in titer is diagnostic of acute infection. A complement-fixation test (CFT) is also available; a titer of 1:8 indicates old or new infection. Both of these tests can cross react with Malleomyces mallei (the agent causing glanders).

### TREATMENT

Treatment of melioidosis is indicated if the organism is cultured, or if there is a four-fold rise in titer of the IHA or CFT. Therapy is a tetracycline supplemented with either a sulfonamide or chloramphenicol.

## HAEMOPHILUS INFLUENZAE

Although Haemophilus (H. ) influenzae pneumonia is rare in adults, it is more common than is generally recognized. H. influenzae is a gram-negative bacteria, a common pathogen in children between the ages of six months and five years. Among adults, alcoholics and patients with chronic obstructive pulmonary disease (COPD) are most at risk to develop H. influenzae pneumonia.

## CLINICAL FEATURES

Its features are non-specific. Fever, cough, dyspnea, and chills are the most common symptoms, in that order.[27] Leukocytosis and increased sedimentation rate may be present, but leukopenia may also be seen. The chest roentgenogram may reveal diffuse bronchopneumonia pattern in nearly three-fourths of the patients, and about one-fourth may show lobar consolidation. Pleural effusion is not common but may be present. Complications, such as empyema, abscess formation, or rarely, a meningitis secondary to bacteremia, may occur.

## DIAGNOSIS

Diagnosis of H. influenzae pneumonia may be difficult. Problems arise because patients with COPD often colonize their oropharynx and trachea with H. influenzae. Therefore, the isolation of H. influenzae from a sputum sample or even a TTA specimen does not necessarily mean that the pneumonia is caused by H. influenzae. Most H. influenzae strains which colonize the oropharynx and trachea of patients with COPD are unencapsulated and non-typable. Most of the strains producing actual pneumonia are encapsulated and belong to type B. Therefore, typing of the organism should be done. It can be done by a quellung reaction. If the organism is type B, it should be assumed to be pathogenic, although, on occasion, type B can be a mere commensal and contrarily, the non-typable H. influenzae strains can produce a pneumonia. When H. influenzae is isolated from a blood culture or pleural fluid sample, the diagnosis is more certain.

## TREATMENT

The treatment of choice is currently ampicillin, but because H. influenzae resistant to ampicillin have been isolated, antibiotic sensitivity testing must be done. Chloramphenicol may be used for strains resistant to ampicillin and in patients allergic to penicillin.

## MENINGOCOCCAL PNEUMONIA

Neisseria (N.) meningitidis rarely causes pneumonia without meningitis. Its true incidence is unknown. It can occur in young adults with recent history of viral influenza or adenovirus infection.

Meningococcal pneumonia has no distinctive features. Cough and fever are its usual presenting features, and in most instances, present symptoms for two to three weeks before the patient seeks medical help. It is rarely fulminant unless complicated by meningitis. Rash or arthritis, as seen with meningitis, does not occur with pneumonia. The chest roentgenogram may reveal a pattern of either lobar or bronchopneumonia.[28]

## DIAGNOSIS

Diagnosis should be made by TTA. If a Neisseria species is isolated, it should be tested by carbohydrate fermentation reactions to confirm the identification of N. meningitidis or one of the other Neisseria species, such as N. catarrhalis, which may normally be found in the mouth. The latter can also rarely cause pneumonia. If a Gram's stain of the TTA specimen shows many gram-negative diplococci, presumptive diagnosis of meningococcal or Veillonella pneumonia should be made.

## TREATMENT

Penicillin is the drug of choice. Dose is the same as for pneumococcal pneumonia, i.e., penicillin G, 1.2 to 2.4 million units I. V. daily in divided doses.

## PNEUMONIA DUE TO NOCARDIA

Of several species of Nocardia (N.) that are pathogenic to man, N. asteroides is the most common, although N. brasiliensis and N. caviae may also cause disease in man. Nocardia pneumonia is uncommon, but it must be recognized, for it requires therapy radically different from that of other common bacterial pneumonias.

N. asteroides is a true bacterium, not a fungus. It is an aerobic gram-positive bacillus that may also be acid-fast. Nocardia may produce a pneumonia, as well as other foci of infection. Most often, nocardiosis occurs in the compromised host.[29]

At special risk are those on immunosuppressive drugs and those with underlying malignancy or organ transplant (heart or kidney) recipients. Such predisposing conditions may not always be present.

## CLINICAL FEATURES

Most commonly, the symptoms are subacute. Fever, cough and pleuritic chest pain are common. Dyspnea is unusual. Sputum may be copious or scant, and it may be blood-tinged. The chest roentgenogram may show a unilateral or bilateral bronchopneumonia. More commonly, a nodular density is seen on chest film; occasionally multiple nodules are seen. The pneumonia may be necrotizing with single or multiple cavities. Bowing of the fissure may occur, which can be mistaken for Klebsiella pneumonia (see page 103). Pleural effusion or empyema may accompany the lung infection. Brain abscess can occur as a complication, or the infection may spread to the bone, skin, kidney, eye or liver. Such dissemination is more likely to occur in the immunosuppressed.

## DIAGNOSIS

Diagnosis is based on isolating the organisms from the involved site. In sputum, Nocardia on Gram's stain are indistinguishable from the normally present Actinomyces, therefore, Gram's stain is of no diagnostic value. Sputum should be examined with Ziehl-Neelsen stain in all suspected cases. Demonstration of acid-fast organisms should always be regarded as abnormal. Nocardia are only weakly acid-fast on Ziehl-Neelsen smear, and may be seen more readily if a weak decolorizing agent is used (1% aqueous sulfuric acid). Nocardia may be difficult to tell from Mycobacteria or Actinomyces. Mycobacteria does not branch as Nocardia does and tend to be more strongly acid-fast. Nocardia may be difficult to grow from sputum samples because of overgrowth of normal mouth flora. Nocardia is rarely a saprophyte of the respiratory tract and even less often a laboratory contaminant. Therefore, a culture that is positive for Nocardia must be presumed to be significant. [30] Blood culture is rarely positive for Nocardia but should be done in all cases; if positive, it suggests dissemination.[31] When multiple sputum cultures are negative for Nocardia, but the entity is strongly suspected, more invasive procedures should be considered. Such must be considered early in cases of immunosuppressed patients with pulmonary infiltrates. A transtracheal aspiration is useful in such patients. Paratracheal abscess due to Nocardia can occur as a complication. Definitive diagnosis may sometimes require lung biopsy, either through a bronchoscope, transthoracically, or by open lung biopsy.

## TREATMENT

Nocardia infections are curable if treated; therefore, every attempt to make the diagnosis should be done in patients suspected of having this infection. Treatment is a prolonged course of a sulfonamide, sulfamethoxazole-trimethoprim, clindamycin or doxycycline.

## 19: ANAEROBIC BACTERIAL INFECTIONS
### by David W. Webb

Anaerobic bacteria can cause lung infections either alone or in combination with aerobic bacteria. The most commonly involved anaerobic bacteria are Peptococci, Peptostreptococci, Fusobacteria, Bacteroides (B.) oralis, B. melaninogenicus and occasionally, B. fragilis, Eubacteria, Veillonella and Clostridia. Often, more than one organism is involved. Infections generally caused by anaerobic bacteria are aspiration pneumonia, lung abscess, necrotizing pneumonia and empyema. [32]

### ASPIRATION PNEUMONIA

Aspiration pneumonia often follows a state of compromised consciousness. Predisposing conditions include alcoholism, drug addiction, general anesthesia, central nervous system disease (such as seizures) and certain clinical states that cause prolonged vomiting. The bacteria that cause aspiration pneumonia are derived from aspiration or oropharyngeal contents. Normally, the anaerobic bacteria outnumber the aerobic bacteria by 10 to 1 in the oropharynx; it is therefore not surprising that such infections usually involve anaerobes, often in combination with aerobic bacteria. Dental infections are predominantly due to anaerobic bacteria; patients with dental abscess stand an increased risk of developing an anaerobic lung infection. Aspiration occurring in hospitalized patients involves anaerobes in only one-third of the cases; gram-negative aerobic bacteria are frequently seen in these infections. [33]

### CLINICAL FEATURES

Aspiration pneumonia can resemble other types of pneumonia. Perhaps the most important clue to the diagnosis of aspiration pneumonia is the clinical setting; it should always be suspected in patients with compromised state of consciousness as seen in alcoholics, drug overdose, seizures, or diabetic ketoacidosis. The presence of carious teeth or periodontal or gingival disease need not always occur; aspiration pneumonia due to anaerobes can occur even in edentulous patients.

The chest roentgenogram classically may show areas of consolidation in the posterior segment of the upper lobe and superior segment of the lower lobe; these are the dependent segments of the lung when the patient is in the recumbent position, the common position during unconscious state. If one aspirates in the sitting position, basal segments of the lower lobes are involved. When aspiration pneumonia is left untreated for a week or more, necrosis with cavity formation may occur. Aspiration pneumonia may develop into a lung abscess (Fig. 11). The gallium-67 scans often show increased uptake (Fig. 12) as in cases of malignancies.

## DIAGNOSIS

Diagnosis can only be made by performing a TTA to obtain material for anaerobic culture. Because the oropharynx normally contains anaerobic bacteria, expectorated sputum is not suitable for anaerobic culture. Specimens obtained by bronchoscopy are unsuitable, for oropharyngeal secretions frequently contaminate the bronchoscope while it is being passed down the trachea. Further, liquid xylocaine used for topical anesthesia is bacteriostatic; hence, the cultures may be falsely negative.[14] Some patients with COPD may normally harbor aerobic bacteria in their trachea (as determined by TTA samples) but colonization with anaerobic bacteria is rare.[10]

The Gram's stain of a TTA specimen in cases of aspiration pneumonia frequently shows polymorphonuclear leukocytes and mixed bacterial flora. Presence of more than one morphotype of bacteria on Gram's stain is characteristic of such infections, although at times only one organism may be seen. Because anaerobic culture techniques are time-consuming, treatment should be instituted based on the clinical suspicion and the Gram's stain results.

## TREATMENT

Treatment of aspiration pneumonia depends on the clinical setting. Community acquired aspiration pneumonia, not associated with B. fragilis responds to intravenous penicillin G, two to ten million units per day in divided doses.[34] Pneumonia associated with B. fragilis should be treated with clindamycin, carbenicillin, doxycycline or ticarcillin. Hospital acquired aspiration usually involves aerobic gram-negative bacilli as well as anaerobes. Therefore, an aminoglycoside (gentamicin, tobramycin or amikacin) should be used in combination with penicillin or alternatively, carbenicillin alone could be used in this situation; it is active against both anaerobic bacteria and aerobic gram-negative bacteria.[35]

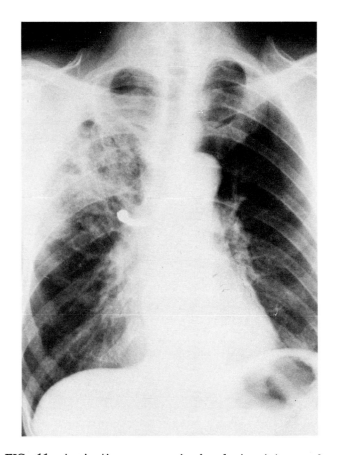

FIG. 11: Aspiration pneumonia developing into an abscess in the right upper lobe of the lung. Note
the highly radiopaque density due to partial den-
tures of the front teeth aspirated into the right
bronchus. Culture of the transtracheal aspirate
revealed a variety of anaerobic bacteria.

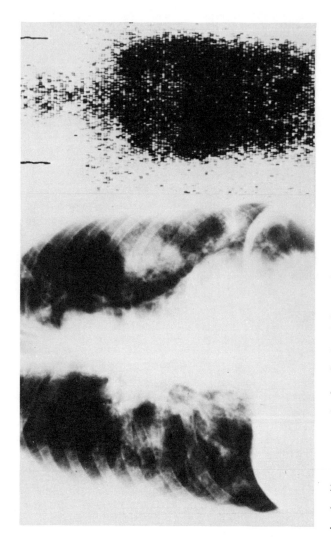

FIG. 12: Aspiration pneumonia developing into an abscess on the left side of the lung. Occasional infiltrates can be seen in the right lung as well as the left. Note the intense uptake of Ga-67 in the lung. Normally, Ga-67 uptake by the lung should not exceed that of the shoulder. Transtracheal aspiration revealed α-Streptococcus and Clostridium ramosum.

## NECROTIZING PNEUMONIA

Necrotizing pneumonia is often an anaerobic infection, characterized by destruction and cavitation of the lung, followed by suppuration and multiple abscess formation. It can be indolent and chronic, characterized by progressive weight loss and low-grade fever and unproductive cough, but it can be fulminant and associated with marked systemic toxicity and signs of acute pneumonia. Necrotizing pneumonia is first a radiologic and then a clinical diagnosis. The chest roentgenogram may show cavitation of the lung (with shaggy margins) often involving a single bronchopulmonary segment, progressing to involve an entire lobe. Roentgenographically, it resembles tuberculosis, fungal infections and resolving lobar pneumonia or cavitating carcinoma (Fig. 13). The diagnosis is established by the isolation of aerobic and/or anaerobic bacteria from a TTA specimen. Bronchoscopy is often required to exclude underlying malignancy.

### TREATMENT

Necrotizing pneumonia will respond to the same agents used for aspiration pneumonia but the roentgenographic improvement may take longer.

### LUNG ABSCESS

Anaerobic bacteria are important pathogens in lung abscess. The pathogens in lung abscess are in general the same as in aspiration pneumonia. Although certain aerobic bacteria such as Staphylococcus aureus, Klebsiella pneumoniae, Proteus, Escherichia coli, and Pseudomonas can produce lung abscess either by themselves or in combination with anaerobic bacteria. The predisposing causes are the same as aspiration pneumonia. In addition, lung abscess can be secondary to metastatic infection from an abscess elsewhere. In most instances, the lung abscess can be mistaken for other common pneumonias, because pneumonia precedes cavitation. Staphylococcal lung abscess can be secondary to staphylococcal endocarditis.

### CLINICAL FEATURES

Lung abscess may begin as an acute fulminating pneumonia, with a highly toxic course with fever ($102^{\circ}$ to $105^{\circ}$F.), cough with voluminous expectoration and even chest pain and physical signs of consolidation associated with severe prostration. The acute toxicity subsides on antimicrobial therapy and then assumes

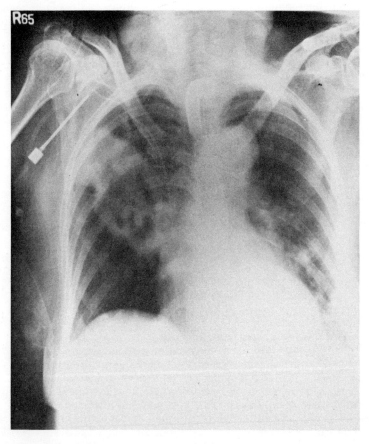

FIG. 13: Necrotizing pneumonia secondary to aspiration.

a somewhat subacute or chronic course. During this period, the patient continues to produce voluminous sputum with very offensive odor. This is the stage of gangrene of the lung.

Improperly and inadequately treated patients return with signs of cavitation and abscess formation with severe weight loss, and inanition.

The most characteristic roentgenographic feature of lung abscess is the "air fluid level." When the bronchus is occluded, the air is resorbed and the fluid level disappears, and one may see a circular density, or alternatively, one may cough out and empty the abscess, leaving behind only a cavity, when it is frequently mistaken for tuberculosis. (See Chapter 23) Fluid level in tubercular cavities almost always suggests other associated bacterial infections.

## DIAGNOSIS

The diagnosis is obvious on the chest roentgenogram, but the bacterial etiology can only be determined by transtracheal aspiration.

Tuberculosis, fungal infection (coccidioidomycosis, histoplasmosis and blactomycosis) or bronchogenic carcinoma can often present insidiously with weight loss and low-grade fever, with cavitation in the lung. The transtracheal aspirate should be examined for aerobic and anaerobic bacteria to confirm the diagnosis of bacterial lung abscess. The sputum coughed up after the transtracheal aspiration has greater diagnostic yield for cytology, and Mycobacteria and mycology cultures. We recommend bronchoscopy for all cases of lung abscess, more so if they do not respond to appropriate antimicrobial therapy within three to four weeks.

## TREATMENT

Lung abscess will respond to the same antibiotics used for aspiration pneumonia. Initial treatment should be parenteral. When systemic symptoms subside and the cavity begins to decrease in size, therapy may be switched to the oral route. Antibiotics should be continued until the cavity disappears or only a small, stable residual lesion remains. After three months, if treatment is effective, most cavities will have disappeared; resolution is slowest for large cavities and cavities of the right upper lobe.[36] Surgical resection is rarely required for bacterial lung abscess.

## EMPYEMA

Empyema is, simplistically, the presence of pus in the pleural space. Empyema may be caused by aerobic bacteria, anaerobic bacteria, or more commonly, a combination of both. Among the aerobic bacteria Staphylococcus aureus, Streptococcus pneumoniae, Streptococcus pyogenes, Streptococcus fecalis, Klebsiella pneumoniae, Pseudomonas, Proteus and E. coli are most frequent. The anaerobic bacteriology of empyema is similar to that of aspiration pneumonia. Parenchymal lung infection occurs first, in most cases with spread of the infection to the pleural space. A bronchopleural fistula may, at times, be present.

The predisposing causes are the same as the infections of the lung parenchyma; occasionally empyema can be secondary to intra-abdominal infection, such as a subdiaphragmatic, liver, or splenic abscess with or without rupture of pus across the diaphragm. Tuberculous and fungal infections of the lung may also be associated with empyema. It is to be emphasized that a thin, watery sympathetic parapneumonic pleural effusion may occur with any bacterial pneumonia.

## CLINICAL FEATURES

Chest pain with fever and cough are the presenting symptoms. The physical signs are those of pleural effusion. Diagnosis may not be often suspected unless a roentgenogram is obtained. However, when a patient diagnosed to have bacterial pneumonia shows unexplained worsening of clinical signs, leukocytosis, increased area of dullness over the chest to percussion disproportionate to the auscultatory evidence of pneumonia, empyema should be suspected and a roentgenogram of the chest should be obtained. Fluid in the pleural space may at times only be appreciated when a lateral decubitus film is taken and the fluid is seen to layer out. In cases of empyema secondary to an intra-abdominal process, the latter may be either clinically pronounced or silent. A careful abdominal examination is therefore imperative in all cases of empyema, especially when it is on the right side.

## DIAGNOSIS

This is established by thoracentesis. The empyema fluid has characteristics of an exudate in the pleural space. Empyema fluid is often thick, but in cases of pleural effusion secondary to infection by Streptococcus pneumoniae or Streptococcus pyogenes, the fluid is characteristically thin because of the production of proteolytic enzymes by these organisms. The pleural fluid in cases of empyema has the characteristics typical of that of an exudate. [37, 38] (See Table 16, page 177).

Gram's stain of the fluid should always be done, and it almost always shows bacteria (except tuberculous empyema). The fluid should be cultured for both aerobic and anaerobic bacteria, in addition to culturing for M. tuberculosis and fungi. Viruses do not cause empyema. In all cases of right-sided empyema the liver and the subdiaphragmatic space should always be examined by appropriate scintiscans or ultrasound.

ROENTGENOGRAPHY: A plain roentgenogram of the chest reveals evidence of pleural effusion, which should be verified by appropriate lateral decubitus films. Air fluid level in the pleural space indicates a prior attempt to aspirate the fluid, bronchopleural fistulae or an infection due to gas-producing organisms. A massive lung abscess can be mistaken for empyema; similarly, a small loculated empyema can be mistaken for a lung abscess. Distinction between the two, at times, can be difficult.

ULTRASOUND: Ultrasonography may have to be employed to delineate a loculated empyema. An ultrasonically guided needle can be used to obtain the fluid.

SCANS: Gallium-67 scan almost always shows increased uptake of Ga-67 in cases of empyema (Fig. 14). It can also be used to localize an associated intra-abdominal abscess, if any.

GAS LIQUID CHROMATOGRAPHY (GLC): GLC can be used to diagnose anaerobic empyema. Elution of multiple volatile fatty acids from the pus is characteristic of anaerobic infections.


THERAPY

It is to be emphasized that appropriate drainage of the pleural space with a chest tube is necessary in all cases of empyema. Antibiotic therapy should be directed against both aerobic and anaerobic microorganisms.

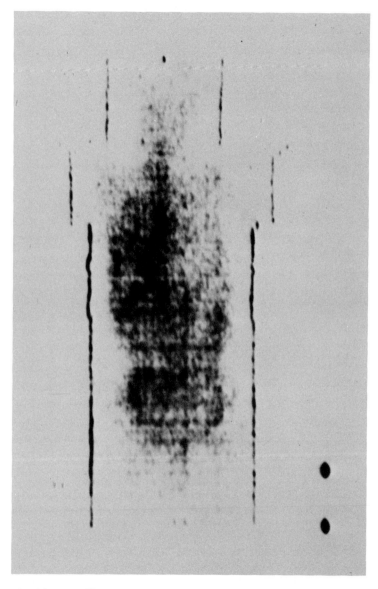

FIG. 14: Ga-67 scan in a case of empyema of the chest. Note the increased uptake of Ga-67 on the right side of the chest.

20: MYCOPLASMA PNEUMONIA
by David W. Webb

Mycoplasma pneumoniae is a true bacteria; it is, in fact, the smallest free-living organism. It lacks a cell wall and does not stain by the Gram's reaction. This organism may be associated with nearly one-third of all cases of pneumonia. Most commonly, children and young adults are affected, although it can affect any age group.

## CLINICAL FEATURES

It may present as bronchitis or pneumonia. The clinical symptoms are often suggestive of viral infection. Often, there is severe cough, fever and chills with malaise, headache, earaches and myalgias. Wheezing is common due to bronchiolitis, which can be mistaken for bronchial asthma.

Physical examination may reveal pharyngitis and a bullous myringitis, in addition to the features mentioned. The myringitis may be asymptomatic. Examination of the chest may reveal rales over the involved areas of the lung, but no definite signs of consolidation are present. Often the physical examination of the chest may be unrewarding. Mycoplasma pneumonia should always be suspected when bronchopneumonia develops in a young person, particularly when symptoms such as headache and myalgias are prominent.

Several complications have been associated with pneumonia caused by Mycoplasma. [39] Hemolytic anemia secondary to cold agglutinins may occur, but is rare. Hepatitis, arthralgias, aseptic meningitis, peripheral mononeuropathy, cerebellar ataxia, pericarditis, myocarditis and skin rashes (macular, petechial, morbilliform, erythema nodosum and urticaria) have all been reported in rare cases. The presence of any of these syndromes should indicate the need for doing appropriate studies to rule out Mycoplasma infection.

Laboratory tests may show an increase in the white blood cell count and sedimentation rate. Rarely is it associated with a normochromic normocytic anemia and reticulocytosis secondary to hemolysis.

The chest roentgenogram may show alveolo-bronchial infiltration involving one of the lower lobes. Often, the roentgenographic findings are out of proportion to the physical findings.

In one-third of the cases, the pneumonia is bilateral. Hilar adenopathy may be present, particularly in children (Fig. 15). Associated pleural effusions are not uncommon. They may be either unilateral or bilateral, but they are rarely massive.

## DIAGNOSIS

1) Sputum examination is not diagnostic - it is usually not purulent and only a moderate amount of polymorphonuclear leukocytes without bacteria are seen on Gram's stain.

2) A TTA is helpful only to detect bacterial causes that may occasionally coexist with Mycoplasma pneumoniae.

3) When facilities are available, Mycoplasma can be cultured from the sputum or throat washings.

4) Cold agglutinins appear in nearly one-half of the cases of Mycoplasma pneumonia. Cold agglutinins usually appear at the end of the first week and reach a peak at about four weeks. A titer of 1:40 is considered significant.

5) A screening test for cold agglutinins may be performed at the bedside. [40] To do this, 0.5 cc. of blood is placed in a citrated tube and placed in ice ($0°$ to $4°C$.) for about one minute. The tube is then examined for the presence of clumping of the red cells, indicating the presence of cold agglutinins. Unfortunately, cold agglutinins may also be present in such non-Mycoplasma infections as adenovirus pneumonia.

6) A complement-fixation test is available. Paired acute and convalescent serum should be obtained for this purpose, and a four-fold rise is considered diagnostic of Mycoplasma infection.

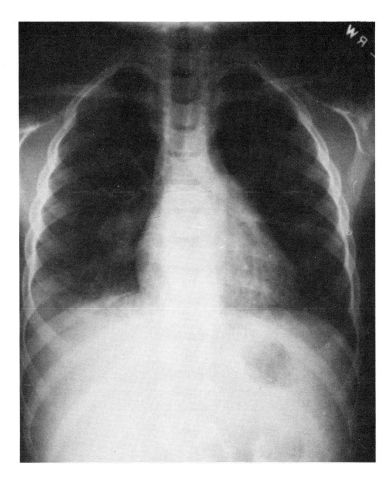

FIG. 15: Mycoplasma pneumonia. A 12-year-old boy with severe non-productive cough. Cold agglutinin titer was
positive at 1:256. Culture of pharynx grew Mycoplasma pneumoniae. Note hilar adenopathy and infiltrate on right.

## 21: PSITTACOSIS
by David W. Webb

Psittacosis (parrot fever) pneumonia is caused by an agent of the Chlamydia group, an obligate intracellular bacteria. The agent affects birds, such as parrots, parakeets, turkeys, chickens and ducks. Infected birds may have no symptoms, but are capable of infecting humans.

### CLINICAL FEATURES

Symptoms occur in about ten days after exposure to the infected birds. These include myalgias, headache, chills, fever and cough. Physical examination of the patient may show hepatomegaly. Splenomegaly may also occur, but lymphadenopathy is rare. The chest examination may reveal a few rales over the affected area of the lung. Patchy or diffuse interstitial bronchopneumonia may also be seen on x-ray. The sedimentation rate and white blood cell count are often normal.

### DIAGNOSIS

The sputum is not characteristic. It is usually scanty and not purulent. The organism cannot be seen on Gram's stain.

1) Culture: It can be grown by inoculation of chick embryo within one to three weeks. Giemsa-stained smears from yolk sacs show typical inclusions.

2) Serology: It can also be diagnosed by serologic methods. Complement-fixation titer - acute and convalescent serum should be obtained at least two weeks apart. A four-fold rise in the complement-fixation titer is diagnostic of psittacosis. If the acute phase titer is 1:16 or greater, a presumptive diagnosis may be made. [41]

### REFERENCES
(Chapters 17-21)

1. Jay, S. J., Johanson, W. G., Pierce, A. K.: The radiographic resolution of Streptococcus pneumoniae pneumonia. New Eng. J. Med. 293:798, 1975.

2. Moser, K. M., et al: Differentiation of pulmonary vascular from parenchymal diseases by ventilation/perfusion scintiphotography. Ann. Int. Med. 75:597, 1971.

3.  Niden, A. H. , et al:  $^{67}$Ga lung scan - An aid in the dif-
    ferential diagnosis of pulmonary embolism and pneumo-
    nitis. J. A. M. A.  237:1206, 1977.

4.  Grollman, J. H. , Gypes, M. T. , Helmer, E. :  Transfem-
    oral selective bilateral pulmonary artery seeking catheter.
    Radiology 96:202, 1970.

5.  Hendley, J. O. , et al:  Spread of Streptococcus pneumo-
    niae in families. I.  Carriage rates and distribution of types.
    J. Inf. Dis.  132:55, 1975.

6.  Barrett-Connor, E. :  The non-value of sputum culture in
    the diagnosis of pneumococcal pneumonia. Am. Rev. Res.
    Dis.  103:845, 1971.

7.  Hahn, H. H. , Beaty, H. N. :  Transtracheal aspiration in
    the evaluation of patients with pneumonia. Ann. Int. Med.
    72:183, 1970.

8.  Schillaci, R. F. , Iacovoni, V. E. , Conte, R. S. :  Trans-
    tracheal aspiration complicated by fatal endotracheal hem-
    orrhage. New Eng. J. Med. 295:488, 1976.

9.  Beaty, H. N. , Spencer, C. D. :  Complications of trans-
    tracheal aspiration. New Eng. J. Med.  286:304, 1972.

10. Jordan, G. W. , Wong, G. A. , Hoeprich, P. D. : Bacteri-
    ology of the lower respiratory tract. J. Inf. Dis.  134:428,
    1976.

11. Bartlett, J. G. :  Diagnostic accuracy of transtracheal as-
    piration. Bacteriologic studies. Am. Rev. Res. Dis. 115:
    777, 1977.

12. Brandt, P. D. , Blante, N. , Castellino, R. A. :  Needle di-
    agnosis of pneumonitis. Value in high-risk patients. J. A.
    M. A. 220:1578, 1972.

13. Khan, M. A. , Whitcomb, M. E. , Snider, G. L. :  Flexible
    fiberoptic bronchoscopy. Am. J. Med. 61:151, 1976.

14. Bartlett, J. G. , et al:  Should fiberoptic bronchoscopy as-
    pirates be cultured? Am. Rev. Res. Dis. 114:73, 1976.

15. Finley, R. , et al:  Bronchial brushing in the diagnosis of pul-
    monary disease in patients at risk for opportunistic infection.
    Am. Rev. Res. Dis. 109:379, 1974.

16. Feldman, N. T. , Pennington, J. E. : Pulmonary infiltrates and fever in patients with hematologic malignancy. Assessment of transbronchial biopsy. Am. J. Med. 52:581, 1977.

17. Greenman, R. L. , Goodall, P. T. , King, D. : Lung biopsy in immunocompromised hosts. Am. J. Med. 59:488, 1975.

18. Dowling, J. N. , Sheehe, P. R. , Feldman, H. A. : Pharyngeal pneumococcal acquisitions in "normal" families: A longitudinal study. J. Inf. Dis. 124:9, 1971.

19. Merrill, C. W. , et al: Rapid identification of pneumococci. Gram's stain vs. the quellung reaction. New Eng. J. Med. 288:510, 1973.

20. El-Refaie, M. , Dulake, C. : Counter-current immunoelectrophoresis for the diagnosis of pneumococcal chest infection. J. Clin. Path. 28:801, 1975.

21. Wilson, G. S. , Miles, A. : Topley and Wilson's Principles of Bacteriology and Immunity. Williams and Wilkins Co. , Baltimore, 1975.

22. Lerner, A. M. , Jankauskas, K. : The classic bacterial pneumonias. Disease-a-Month, February, 1975.

23. Pierce, A. K. , Sanford, J. P. : Aerobic gram-negative bacillary pneumonias. Am. Rev. Res. Dis. 110:647, 1974.

24. Rosenthal, S. , Tager, I. B. : Prevalence of gram-negative rods in the normal pharyngeal flora. Ann. Int. Med. 83: 355, 1975.

25. Johanson, W. G. , Pierce, A. K. , Sanford, J. P. : Changing pharyngeal bacterial flora of hospitalized patients. Emergence of gram-negative bacilli. New Eng. J. Med. 281: 1138, 1969.

26. Everett, E. D. , Nelson, R. A. : Pulmonary melioidosis. Am. Rev. Res. Dis. 112:331, 1975.

27. Levin, D. C. , et al: Bacteremic Hemophilus influenzae pneumonia in adults. Am. J. Med. 62:219, 1977.

28. Irwin, R. S. , Woelk, W. K. , Coudon, W. L. : Primary meningococcal pneumonia. Ann. Int. Med. 82:493, 1975.

29. Palmer, D. L. , Harvey, R. L. , Wheeler, J. K. : Diagnostic and therapeutic considerations in Nocardia asteroides infection. Medicine 53:391, 1974.

30. Williams, D. M. , Krick, J. A. , Remington, J. S. : Pulmonary infection in the compromised host. Part I. Am. Rev. Res. Dis. 114:359, 1976.

31. Roberts, G. D. , Brewer, N. S. , Hermans, P. E. : Diagnosis of nocardiosis by blood culture. Mayo Clin. Proc. 49:293, 1974.

32. Bartlett, J. G. , Finegold, S. M. : Anaerobic infections of the lung and pleural space. Am. Rev. Res. Dis. 110:56, 1974.

33. Lorber, B. , Swenson, R. M. : Bacteriology of aspiration pneumonia. A prospective study of community and hospital acquired cases. Ann. Int. Med. 81:329, 1974.

34. Bartlett, J. G. , Gorbach, S. L. : Treatment of aspiration pneumonia and primary lung abscess. J. A. M. A. 234:935, 1975.

35. Thadepalli, H. , Niden, A. H. , Huang, J. : Treatment of anaerobic pulmonary infections. Carbenicillin compared to clindamycin and gentamicin. Chest 69:743, 1976.

36. Weiss, W. : Cavity behavior in acute, primary non-specific lung abscess. Am. Rev. Res. Dis. 108:1273, 1973.

37. Light, R. W. , et al: Pleural effusions: The diagnostic separation of transudates and exudates. Ann. Int. Med. 77:507, 1972.

38. Potts, D. E. , Levin, D. C. , Sahn, S. A. : Pleural fluid pH in parapneumonic effusions. Chest 70:328, 1976.

39. Murray, H. W. , et al: The protean manifestations of Mycoplasma pneumoniae infections in adults. Am. J. Med. 58:229, 1975.

40. Griffin, J. P. : Rapid screening for cold agglutinins in pneumonia. Ann. Int. Med. 70:701, 1969.

41. Mufson, M. A. , Zollar, L. M. : Non-bacterial respiratory infections. Disease-a-Month, November, 1975.

42. Thadepalli, H., et al: Correlation of microbiologic findings and [67]Gallium scans in patients with pulmonary infections. Chest 72:442-448, 1977.

## 22: LEGIONNAIRES' DISEASE
### by Louis D. Saravolatz and Tom Madhavan

Legionnaires' disease is a respiratory illness caused by a previously unrecognized bacterium.  There have been several outbreaks of this disease, but it derived its name from an outbreak that occurred at the American Legion convention in July,
1976, in Philadelphia, resulting in 182 cases of pneumonia and
29 deaths.  The etiologic agent Legionella pneumophilia is a
pleomorphic bacillus 0.3-0.4 $\mu$m. wide and 2-3 $\mu$m. long,
although some may be as long as 50 $\mu$m.[1,2,3] Routine Gram's
stains are unsatisfactory, it takes Gimenez stain.  It belongs
to the family Legionellaceae, and 4 serotypes are described.
The source for this infection is uncertain, although respiratory
route is the suggested portal of entry.  Legionnaires' disease
has been reported from several parts of the world.

### CLINICAL FEATURES

It can occur at any age, although most patients are above forty,
and several were immunologically compromised.  Nosocomial
outbreaks have been described.

After an incubation period of two to ten days, patients develop
malaise, myalgias, headache, and productive cough.  Over the
next twenty-four to forty-eight hours, they complain of fever,
chills and rigors, while the cough becomes productive of small
amounts of non-purulent sputum.  Additional symptoms include
pleuritic chest pain (33%), abdominal pain, diarrhea and confusion or delirium (20%).   Early in the illness, the physical
examination may reveal fever (38°-40.6°C), and bilateral rales
without any definite evidence for consolidation.  As the illness
progresses, clinical evidence for consolidation later ensues.
The clinical course of a patient seen by us is shown in Fig. 16.

Patients often deteriorate during the first four to six days of
hospitalization; nearly one-fourth of them require assisted ventilation, and 10% may develop shock.   Renal failure unrelated
to hypotension may also occur with myoglobinuria, presumably
due to a bacterial toxin.  Transient liver failure can occur, which
may result in excessive blood levels of antibiotics (such as
erythromycin) metabolized by the liver.

Laboratory findings show leukocytosis (10,000 to 14,000 per cu.
mm.) with a shift to the left in nearly 60% of the patients.  Leukopenia is rare, but, when present, may suggest poor prognosis.
Proteinuria occurs in nearly 20% and microscopic hematuria

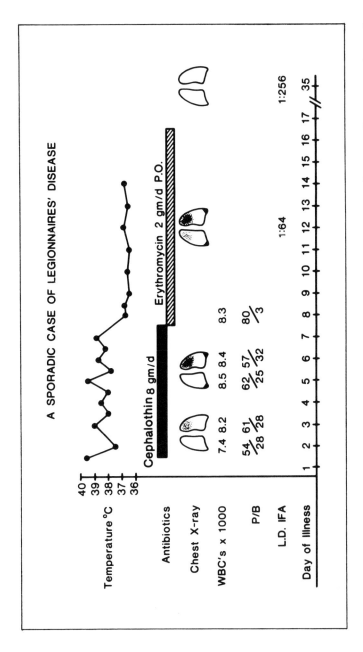

FIG. 16: Clinical course of Legionnaires' disease in one patient. Note the absence of response to cephalothin and the clinical improvement that ensued with erythromycin therapy.

in 10%.   Elevated glutamic oxalacetic transaminase, alkaline phosphatase and creatinine phosphokinase may also occur. Despite the state of mental confusion, the cerebrospinal fluid examinations are often normal.   Any patients with any three of the following criteria should be suspected to have this disease: 1) prodromal "viral" illness, 2) dry cough, confusion or diarrhea, 3) lymphopenia without marked neutrophilia and 4) hyponatraemia.

Nearly all patients with Legionnaires' disease have an abnormal chest roentgenogram showing interstitial infiltrates or consolidation but, in 10%, it can be normal. The infiltrates are bilateral in nearly 50% of the patients as shown in Fig. 17.   Effusions may be present and are minimal unless the patient was on corticosteroids.   Necrotizing pneumonia and abscess formation or empyema can also occur.   Like any other bacterial pneumonia, the roentgenographic resolution often lags behind clinical improvement by several days. For details, the reader should refer to one of the reviews on this disease.[5]

## DIAGNOSIS

Legionnaires' disease should be suspected mostly on clinical grounds.   Transtracheal aspiration is only occasionally helpful.

Three methods have been used to establish a diagnosis of Legionnaires' disease: 1) culture identification, 2) fluorescent antibody staining of tissue, and 3) serology.   Sputum cultures and blood cultures can also be positive. A special agar slant and broth with charcoal yeast agar is used for blood cultures.

CULTURE:  The most definitive method of establishing a diagnosis is to culture the Legionnaires' bacterium from the lung tissue or pleural fluid on Mueller-Hinton agar supplemented with 1% hemoglobin and 2% Iso-Vitalex.  It is later incubated under 5% $CO_2$ at 35°C for at least seven days.

Fluorescent antibody staining of the lung biopsy may provide a rapid diagnosis.  A conjugate prepared from hyperimmune rabbit antiserum was used to identify the organism from imprints of fresh lung tissue and in scrapings of formalin-fixed lung.  Other bacteria may also fluoresce due to certain natural antibodies in the serum of the immunized rabbit.   This technique is nonspecific; therefore, confirmation of the diagnosis by culture or an antibody titer rise is required for definitive diagnosis. Immunofluorescent staining of the sputum is a rapid and specific diagnostic test.

The histology shows inflammatory cellular exudate with both intracellular and extracellular organisms.

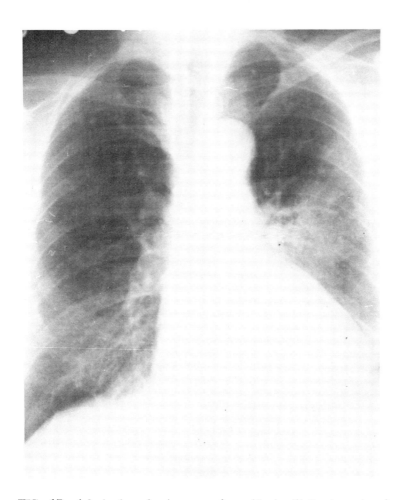

FIG. 17: Admission chest x-ray of a patient with Legionnaires'
disease.    Note the infiltrates in the left upper lobe
and the right and left lower lobes.

Usual stains, such as the Brown-Brenn modification of Gram's
stain, acid-fast and Giemsa stain, are not helpful.   The Kopo-
loff modification of the Gram's stain, or prolonged application
of the safranin counter stain for ten minutes, may reveal the
bacilli.    The most sensitive stain is the Dieterle silver stain
(Fig. 18); however, it lacks specificity, for it can stain spirochetes and coliforms as well.

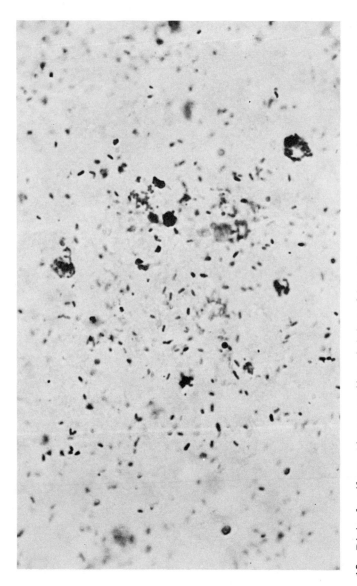

FIG. 18: Dieterle silver - impregnation staining of lung tissue obtained at open biopsy showing numerous, small, blunt bacilli (x 1430).

Legionnaires' disease antigen can also be diagnosed by enzyme-linked immunosorbent assay from clinical specimens such as urine and sputum. It is a rapid and specific test.

SEROLOGY: A set of acute and convalescent sera can be obtained 20-40 days apart, and if a patient with a negative or low titer shows a four-fold or greater rise in titer to 1:64 or higher by indirect fluorescent antibody, or a single antibody titer of 1:128 or greater, a diagnosis of Legionnaires' disease can be made.

## TREATMENT

The causative agent of this disease, L. pneumophilia, produces $\beta$-lactamase and therefore penicillins and cephalosporins are ineffective.

Clinical experience favors the use of erythromycin and tetracycline because they have the lowest case fatality ratio. It produces $\beta$-lactamase, an enzyme which develops penicillin. Failure rates were high with penicillin and cephalosporins. Despite favorable reports with oral erythromycin, parenteral erythromycin is recommended for severely ill patients. Adults should receive intravenous erythromycin in doses of 0.5-1.0 gm. every six hours, and children 15 mg./kg. every six hours. If they fail on erythromycin, rifampin may be added. Apparently rifampin alone may lead to the emergence of resistant strains. Treatment should continue for at least three weeks. Premature discontinuation may lead to relapse. Man to man transmission is rare and therefore, no isolation precautions are necessary.

## REFERENCES

1. Fraser, D.W., et al: Legionnaires' disease: Description of an epidemic of pneumonia. New Eng. J. Med. 297:1189, 1977.

2. McDade, G.E., et al: Legionnaires' disease: Isolation of a bacterium and demonstration of its role in other respiratory disease. New Eng. J. Med. 297:1197, 1977.

3. Chandler, F.W., et al: Demonstration of the agent of Legionnaires' disease in tissue. New Eng. J. Med. 297:1218, 1977.

4. Thornsberry, C., et al: In vitro activity of antimicrobial agents on Legionnaires' disease bacterium. Antimicrob. Agents and Chemother. 13:78, 1978.

5. International Symposium on Legionnaires' disease. Ann. Int. Med. 90(4):489-736, 1979.

## 23: TUBERCULOSIS
by H. Thadepalli

Tuberculosis is on the wane all over the world. But the active case rate in the urban ghettoes of the United States has remained unchanged during the past three decades. The new case rate for tuberculosis among children of the urban ghettoes in the U.S. is around 177/100,000, with 673 new converters per year. [1] Their major source of infection was their parents with undiagnosed or missed respiratory or urinary tract tuberculosis. Poverty, wherever it is, is a friend of tuberculosis. Among the professionals, the student nurses are the most vulnerable to tuberculosis, followed by pathologists, chefs and truck drivers. Diabetes mellitus and alcoholism are generally believed (although not proven) to be predisposing to tuberculosis.

With the advent of closing the sanatoriums, the diagnosis and treatment of tuberculosis in the U.S. is now the responsibility of the internist and the family practitioner. Currently, the attack rate of tuberculosis in the United States is between 14 and 16/100,000. In 1975, the highest attack rate was in Hawaii, 68.3/100,000, and the lowest was in Nebraska, 2.6/100,000. [2]

### DEMONSTRATION OF ACID-FAST BACILLI

The acid-fastness of mycobacteria can be demonstrated by the Ziehl-Neelsen procedures described below:

1)  Prepare a thin film of the specimen, air dry and heat fix. Do not do acid-fast smear examination on gastric fluid and urine. Acid-fast bacilli (AFB) are normally present at these sites.

    If the specimen is spinal fluid (CSF), centrifuge at high speed and place loopfuls or large drops of the supernatant (not the sediment) drop over drop on a slide, air dry and heat fix. Alternatively, the "pellicle" which forms on the top of CSF when left standing may be transferred onto a slide for staining. Gently heat fix.

    Flood the slide with carbolfuchsin (contains basic fuchsin with 90% of a 5% aqueous phenol solution).

    Heat the above smears in carbolfuchsin, warm to steaming, for a period of five minutes.

2) Rinse with water.
3) Decolorize with acid alcohol (1% hydrochloric acid and 70% ethanol) for ten to twenty minutes. Decolorize until the color no longer appears in the washings. One need not be concerned about over-decolorization. It rarely occurs. Rinse the slide with water for two to three minutes.
4) Counterstain with Loffler's methylene blue (methylene blue in alcohol, with potassium hydroxide and water) for fifteen seconds.
5) Rinse in tap water.
6) Dry in air.
7) Examine, using first a 4+ objective, and later with 100+ oil immersion and 10+ eyepiece.

The AFB stain red, and the background must be blue to recognize the acid-fast bacilli. A violet background, due to contamination of stain with gentian violet makes it impossible to detect AFB.

Kinyoun's stain is a cold stain; it requires no heating of the slide. The dye will penetrate the mycobacteria even without heat.

1) After heat-fixing, flood the slide with Kinyoun's carbolfuchsin and let stand for five minutes.
2) Decolorize with acid alcohol.
3) Counterstain with methylene blue.
4) Wash.

The acid-fastness of the organisms with Kinyoun's stain is similar to that of the Ziehl-Neelsen stain.

One's chances to recognize the AFB depend on one's experience. The sputum smears for AFB are positive in less than 43% of untreated cases of pulmonary tuberculosis.

False-positive (smear-positive but culture-negative) results are comparatively rare. [3] False-positive smears can result with partial treatments. A positive sputum smear for AFB strongly suggests pulmonary tuberculosis if that diagnosis was clinically suspected and roentgenographically suggestive.

False-negative smears (smear-negative but culture-positive) are common. They can occur in more than 50% of the patients. [4] Most sputa that are culture-negative are smear-negative as well.

As a rule, at least three or more AFB should be found on a smear to declare it as positive.

Niacin production is characteristic of Mycobacterium tuberculosis. The atypical mycobacteria are niacin-negative (see Table 15, page 163). Niacin-negative strains of M. tuberculosis may be found during long-term chemotherapy. [5]

## PRIMARY PULMONARY TUBERCULOSIS
### (Ghon's complex)

The Ghon's (primary) complex consists of an area of atelectasis or pneumonia in the right middle or lower lobes of the lungs, with mediastinal adenopathy of the corresponding side, seen on the chest roentgenogram. When infection occurs through the tonsillar bed, the cervical lymph nodes are enlarged. The Ghon's lesion is almost always quiescent. The Ghon's complex generally is a disease of children. But in the United States, it is now being increasingly found among adults, even in geriatric age groups of patients. The oldest patient I have seen with this lesion was 39 years old.

Under unfavorable circumstances, the lymph node breaks and discharges its contents into the adjacent bronchioles to produce progressive pneumonia. It is then called Ghon's progressive lesion, or progressive primary infection.

Ghon's complex, when it occurs in the adult, can be misleading. It can mimic malignancy by producing a middle lobe collapse. It may resemble staphylococcal pneumonia by producing bilateral "fluffy" infiltrates in the lungs. When the Ghon's lesion resolves, the lymph nodes become calcified. Measles, rubella, chickenpox and smallpox may occur coincidentally either with the Ghon's complex or miliary tuberculosis.

## LOWER LUNG FIELD (LLF) TUBERCULOSIS

Tuberculosis of the LLF is uncommon. When it affects the LLF, it involves (not as a rule) the upper portion of the lower lobe. LLF disease is more common during the third and fourth decades of life, and more frequent among women. [6] Fever, pneumonia, hemoptysis, or pleurisy are also more common with LLF tuberculosis.

Pregnancy, diabetes mellitus and alcoholism are some of the predisposing causes of LLF tuberculosis. It is often confused with bacterial or viral pneumonia. The sputum smears may be negative for AFB in LLF tuberculosis. On the other hand, transtracheal aspiration may reveal AFB. When cavities are found with a fluid level in such lesions, it suggests associated bacterial infections. On occasion, antibiotic treatment for the secondary infection is required before AFB may become manifest in the sputum or transtracheal aspiration. When a lower lobe pneumonia fails to improve on appropriate antibiotic therapy within a reasonable time, pulmonary tuberculosis should be suspected.

TRANSTRACHEAL ASPIRATION FOR THE DIAGNOSIS OF TUBERCULOSIS:  When pulmonary tuberculosis is suspected but sputa smears are negative, transtracheal aspiration (TTA) is an extremely valuable diagnostic procedure. In our hospital,[7] of 4,200 patients admitted over a period of three years, 126 were proven to have pulmonary tuberculosis, among which 35 or 28% had several induced sputa smears negative for AFB. On TTA, 31 of these 35 patients showed AFB in the TTA specimens. Interestingly, 18 of these 35 patients had associated bacterial infections due to aerobic and/or anaerobic bacteria. Tuberculin skin tests (PPD 5 TU) were negative in 14 of 35 sputum-negative patients (40%); 10 of 18 patients, or 56% with associated bacterial infections also had negative PPD skin tests. A smear and culture of TTA for tubercle bacilli are at times invaluable when pulmonary tuberculosis is suspected and sputa smears are negative for AFB.

Case report:  In an exceptional patient the diagnosis may still be missed in spite of such aggressive diagnostic procedures. For instance, one of my patients admitted for fever with minimal lung infiltrates initially had several sputa smears negative for AFB. No AFB were found in the smears of the aspirates obtained by TTA which were done on two separate occasions.  Furthermore, he had a negative skin reaction to intermediate strength PPD.  Two weeks later, he began to show a dense lesion in the lung.  He also appeared lethargic at this time.  Meningitis was suspected; therefore, a lumbar puncture (LP) was performed. The spinal fluid was unremarkable.  One week later, the LP was repeated when the spinal fluid showed lymphocytosis and elevated protein.  The patient died during the following week. Autopsy revealed tuberculosis of the lung (Fig. 19), tuberculoma of the brain and tuberculous meningitis.  Later the cultures of all sputa, TTA specimens and CSF were reported positive for M. tuberculosis.

In our study,[7] the sputa and the transtracheal aspirate smears were positive when there were at least 200 viable cells (colony forming units) per milliliter of the sample, which appears to be the critical minimum.  Transtracheal aspiration, by obviating the factor of salivary dilution, may increase the yield.

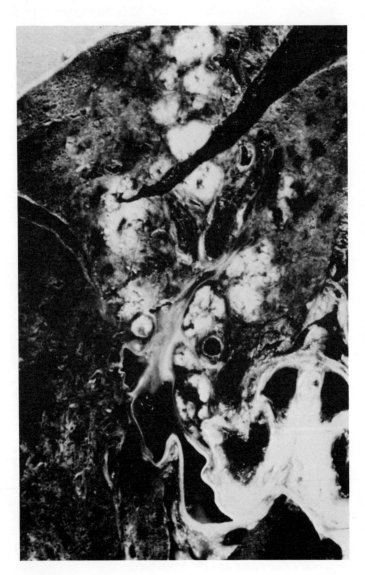

FIG. 19: Pulmonary tuberculosis; multiple parenchymal foci of white caseation are present.

## ASSOCIATED BACTERIAL INFECTIONS

Nearly one-half of the patients with associated bacterial infections due to aerobic or anaerobic bacteria have negative sputa for AFB. The tuberculin skin test may be unreliable in such patients. It is positive only in less than one-half of such patients. The associated bacterial infections can be due to aerobic and facultative bacteria or anaerobic bacteria alone, or more frequently due to the combination of both (Table 13). One-fifth of these patients may have bacteremia due to aerobic and anaerobic organisms. The septicemic patients are often admitted in acute respiratory distress. Pulmonary tuberculosis may present as an acute fulminating pneumonia or bronchopneumonia along with fever and leukocytosis because of the associated infection. The mortality among the septicemic patients is very high.

GALLIUM SCAN: The uptake of gallium is increased in most cases of sputum-positive pulmonary tuberculosis.[8] Increased uptake of gallium may also be found in cases of extrapulmonary tuberculosis. When the sputum smears are negative for AFB, the gallium scans of the lung are also usually negative. Therefore, it is of no value in the diagnosis of sputum-negative pulmonary tuberculosis.[9] Associated infections and carcinoma increase the gallium uptake. Gallium scans may be negative in tuberculous pleural effusions, and in most cases of miliary tuberculosis. Therefore, when sputa smears are negative for acid-fast bacilli (pending cultures), and pulmonary tuberculosis is suspected, increased uptake of gallium in the lung suggests bacterial infection or malignancy associated with pulmonary tuberculosis.

## BRONCHOGENIC CARCINOMA IN TUBERCULOUS PATIENTS

Bronchogenic carcinoma occurs in nearly one per cent of the patients with pulmonary tuberculosis.[10] Nowadays, there is a four fold increase in the incidence of lung cancer in tuberculosis patients, because tuberculosis is now occurring in the third and fourth decade of life. Therefore, all patients with pulmonary tuberculosis above age 35 must routinely have sputum cytologic studies.

Tuberculosis can mask the underlying cancer and often the unwary physician is reluctant to investigate further for another disease when he is lulled with the proven diagnosis of pulmonary tuberculosis. Clubbing of fingers is rare in tuberculosis.

TABLE 13:   BACTERIAL INFECTIONS OF THE LUNG
FOUND IN ASSOCIATION WITH SPUTUM-SMEAR-NEGATIVE
PULMONARY TUBERCULOSIS IN 25 PATIENTS

| AEROBIC AND FACULTATIVE BACTERIA | | ANAEROBIC BACTERIA | |
|---|---|---|---|
| Staphylococcus aureus* | 6 | Peptostreptococcus intermedius | 5 |
| Enterococcus* | 6 | Clostridium ramosum | 4 |
| Diplococcus pneumoniae | 4 | Clostridium perfringens* | 3 |
| Lactobacillus | 3 | Actinomyces naeslundii | 2 |
| Pseudomonas aeruginosa | 2 | Peptococcus magnus | 2 |
| β Hemolytic Streptococcus | 2 | Peptococcus constellatus | 2 |
| Citrobacter freundii | 1 | Diphtheroides (anaerobic) | 2 |
| ਠ Streptococcus not Group D | 1 | Actinobacillus | 1 |
| Streptococcus | 1 | Actinomyces israelii | 1 |
| α Hemolytic Streptococcus | 1 | Actinomyces viscosus | 1 |
| Nocardia asteroides | 1 | | |
| Neisseria species | 1 | | |
| Pseudomonas maltophilia | 1 | | |
| Proteus mirabilis | 1 | | |

*Also indicated from blood culture

Clubbing suggests associated bacterial infection, bronchiectasis, suppurative bronchiectasis or bronchogenic carcinoma. Unexplained anemia also should suggest the possible association with cancer. The mediastinal lymph nodes may be frequently involved in patients with scar carcinoma. Scar carcinoma on cytologic basis is indistinguishable from other forms of bronchogenic carcinoma. The prognosis of concurrent pulmonary tuberculosis and bronchogenic carcinoma is worse than either of them alone.

## MILIARY TUBERCULOSIS

Miliary tuberculosis is due to hematogenous dissemination. The size (miliary = millet) of the lesions is usually larger than that of a millet (2 mm. ). In spite of prompt chemotherapy, 20% to 30% of these patients die.

Loss of appetite, loss of weight, fever, cough and night sweats are by far the most predominant clinical features of miliary tuberculosis. One-fourth of them have shortness of breath and have pleuritic pain, and one-tenth of them may have meningitis. Mostly, it is a disease of the pediatric age group, and 7 to 8/1,000 cases of tuberculosis are of miliary onset. It is twice as frequent among men as women.

On physical examination, fever, rales and rhonchi may be present. The lungs are clear in one-half of the cases. The liver may be palpable in one-third, and the spleen may be palpable in about one-tenth of the patients. Nearly 10% are jaundiced. Miliary tuberculosis should be considered in a differential in all cases of fever of undetermined origin.

The predisposing causes for miliary tuberculosis are alcoholism, drug addiction, malnutrition, pregnancy, diabetes mellitus, previous gastrectomy, long-term steroid therapy, carcinoma and blood dyscrasias.

Chest radiograph may sooner or later show a miliary pattern. Most develop the classical radiologic signs of miliary tuberculosis within the first three to five days of hospitalization. The miliary tubercles as seen on the chest roentgenogram may appear as minute scattered radiopaque spots of size 2 to 3 mm. in diameter in multiple lung fields. Miliary tubercles during the first few days of its onset can be mistaken by the novice for increased vascular markings with an end-on appearance. When miliary tuberculosis is suspected, the radiograph should be examined more closely against a dim scattered light for miliary spots, with particular attention to the lower lung fields and the intercostal spaces. These spots can be missed if the radiograph is examined against the background of a bright light as is usually done.

Hilar adenopathy and cavitary lesions are rare with miliary tuberculosis. On occasion, the cavitary tuberculosis may disseminate in the form of miliary tuberculosis. Nearly 10% to 15% of the cases of miliary tuberculosis have pleural effusions, more frequently on the left side. Miliary tuberculosis can present as an acute adult respiratory distress syndrome. [11] In most instances, they have secondary bacterial infection. Miliary tuberculosis should, therefore, be considered in the differential diagnosis of adult respiratory distress syndrome.

Most patients with miliary tuberculosis are anemic. The leukocytes, however, may be normal, decreased or increased. Occasionally, miliary tuberculosis may be mistaken for leukemia, but the total white cell count seldom exceeds 50,000/cu. mm. Elevation of alkaline phosphatase might occur when the liver parenchyma is involved,[12] but the SGOT and SGPT are often within normal limits. The serum bilirubin levels are increased in a small number (10%).

Although the sputum smears are often negative, the cultures are usually positive in miliary tuberculosis. Gastric aspirates may be negative in two-thirds of them. The combined yield by culture of gastric contents and the sputum is close to 70%. Nearly 30% of the patients require other diagnostic procedures.

BRONCHIAL BRUSHINGS: Bronchial brushing involves passing, transnasally, a flexible polyethylene catheter under fluoroscopic control into the desired segment of the lung, then a nylon-tipped brush is advanced through the catheter onto the lesion. It is useful in nearly 20% of the cases of tuberculosis. Its value in the diagnosis of miliary tuberculosis is unknown.

GALLIUM SCANS: Gallium uptake is usually increased in cases of miliary tuberculosis. Gallium scan should be performed prior to transthoracic needle biopsy of the lung, for the latter procedure can falsely increase the uptake of gallium.

Transthoracic needle aspiration, or biopsy, is an extremely useful procedure for the diagnosis of miliary tuberculosis. When the diagnosis of miliary tuberculosis is uncertain because of negative sputum, and the transtracheal aspiration smears are negative, transthoracic needle aspiration and/or biopsy should be considered. It may reveal the evidence of granulomas and/or acid-fast bacilli (Figs. 20, 21).

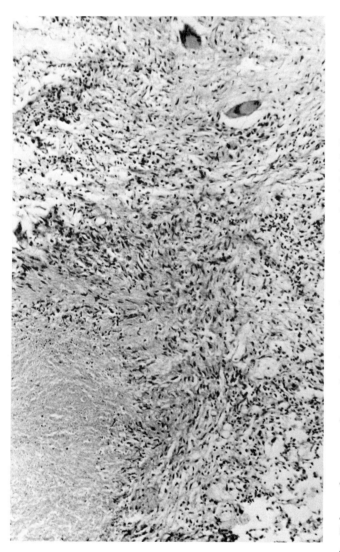

FIG. 20: Tuberculous granuloma showing granular caseous material in left upper part, surrounded by a mixture of inflammatory infiltrate formed of epithelioid cells, lymphocytes, histiocytes and multinucleated (Langerhan's) giant cells.

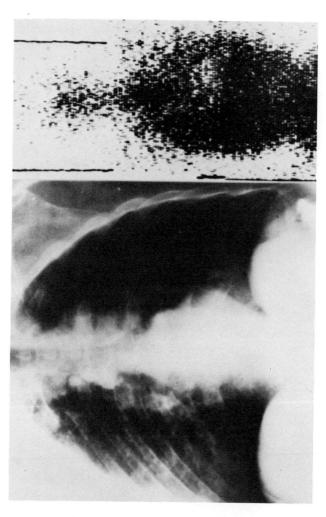

FIG. 21: A case of miliary tuberculosis with secondary infection due to Lactobacillus and Micrococcus, as evidenced by the positive culture from a transthoracic needle aspirate. Note the intense uptake of gallium in both lung fields (right) and the miliary pattern in the chest roentgenogram (left). (Reproduced with permission from Chest 72:442-448, 1977.)

The liver biopsy may show granulomas in nearly 30% of the cases of miliary tuberculosis. They are non-specific; nearly one-half of them reveal no organisms. Therefore, the relevance of a liver granuloma depends on the associated clinical evidence.

Scalene node biopsy should be considered when it is palpable or when the patient has cervical lymphadenopathy.

Pleural biopsy should be performed if there is pleural effusion, so that the fluid may be examined for acid-fast bacilli. At least two pieces of pleural biopsy should be obtained and submitted for histopathological examination.

Cerebrospinal fluid examination may reveal the acid-fast bacilli. Urine samples may be positive. When there is ascites, both ascitic fluid and the peritoneal biopsy should be examined for acid-fast bacilli. Peritoneal biopsy can be done either by suction or under direct visualization. Surgical exploration of the abdomen should be deferred in cases of miliary tuberculosis.

CERTAIN UNUSUAL FEATURES ASSOCIATED WITH MILIARY TUBERCULOSIS ARE:

1) alveolo-capillary block syndrome
2) disseminated intravascular coagulation
3) hyponatremia, with or without Addison's disease
4) inappropriate antidiuretic hormone (ADH) release syndrome. In this condition, the ADH content of the lung tissue is also high.

In spite of adequate and aggressive chemotherapy, the roentgenographic abnormalities in the lung noted in miliary tuberculosis may persist for two to three months.

SKIN TESTING (Mantoux test):   Administer 0.1 ml. of intermediate strength PPD (equivalent to 5TU Tween-80 stabilized) intradermally on the volar aspect of the forearm, previously cleansed with a local detergent. It is considered positive when the induration (not erythema) is of 10 mm. or more in diameter. It is in contrast to the mumps reaction, where erythema is important, but induration is not.

Skin testing may be done with the first strength, 1 TU PPD, Tween stabilized. In countries where tuberculosis is prevalent, the first strength PPD is more appropriate to use. When the first and the intermediate strengths are negative, the second strength of PPD (100 or 250 TU) may be employed. Second strength PPD should not be used routinely, because it can cause extensive reaction and even sloughing of the skin if the person is PPD positive. Further, it can yield excessively false-positive results by cross-reaction with atypical mycobacteria. PPD should be placed on both forearms at the same time. If the skin reactivity in one arm is less than 4 mm. even though it is 10 mm. or more on the other, it should be interpreted as negative. PPD conversion can be immediate (four to eight hours) in 2% of the patients. The skin reaction to PPD in 30% of the recent converters is temporary even without treatment. [14,15]

The PPD tablets (non-stabilized PPD) should not be used for skin testing because 25% of its potency is lost within 20 minutes of storage in the syringe and 80% of its potency may be lost in 24 hours. The clinician, therefore, must make sure that the PPD employed for testing is stabilized with Tween 80. Skin reactions measuring from 5 to 9 mm. are interpreted as "doubtful". I prefer not to use this term, for the skin test was done because tuberculosis is in doubt. Hence, a "doubtful" reaction contributes nothing more than what the clinician already knows. If second strength PPD is negative and tuberculosis is still suspected, it should be repeated before discharging the patient. Repeated skin testing can cause accelerated responses; the positive reaction can occur within a few hours to 24 hours, instead of the usual 48 hours.

False-negative skin tests can occur with overwhelming sepsis in elderly persons, Hodgkin's disease, sarcoidosis, steroid therapy, measles and other viral infections, and miliary tuberculosis. [13]

THE TINE TEST: The Tine test involves the application of a circular plastic disc, with four prongs previously immersed in old tuberculin of 5 TU strength. It is strongly pressed on the voral aspect of the forearm for one to two seconds and discarded. A 10 mm. induration, or the development of all four macules is read as a positive reaction. It is comparable to 5 TU PPD Mantoux (intermediate strength).

In countries and areas where the classic disease is uncommon, skin testing for atypical mycobacteria may also have to be done as follows: [16]

1) PPD-Y antigen from <u>Mycobacterium kansasii</u> to test for Runyon Group I organism (see Table 15, page 163)

2) PPD-G derived from <u>Mycobacterium intracellulare</u> to test for Runyon Group II organism

3) PPD-B antigen from Battey bacillus for Runyon Group III

The antigens for atypical mycobacteria should be placed on the forearm along with the intermediate strength PPD of M. tuberculosis (typical PPD). If the reaction to any or all of the PPD antigens for atypical mycobacteria are smaller than that for intermediate strength of typical PPD, it is unlikely that the tuberculin reaction is caused by atypical mycobacteria infection. If the reaction to the PPD antigens for atypical mycobacteria is larger than the typical PPD, it is likely that the sensitivity is caused by infection with atypical mycobacterium.[15]

## TUBERCULOSIS OF THE GASTROINTESTINAL TRACT

Although tuberculosis can affect any part of the gastrointestinal system, from the tongue to the anal canal, ileocecal tuberculosis is the most common. Abdominal lymph nodes are frequently involved. Involvement of other organs in the abdomen without ileocecal and lymph node involvement is rare. Tuberculous peritonitis is discussed in Chapter 11.

### CLINICAL FEATURES

Weight loss, abdominal pain and diarrhea are the most frequent symptoms. A palpable abdominal mass is present in one-fourth of the patients. Anemia, leukocytosis, elevated sedimentation rate and positive Mantoux test are usually present in more than one-half of the patients. Acid-fast bacilli are rarely found in sputum in cases of isolated gastrointestinal tuberculosis. It affects more men than women below the age of 40. Mostly it is a disease of the poor. Extra-intestinal manifestations are often absent. A palpable epigastric mass, loss of weight and abdominal pain associated with tenderness should make one think of omental or abdominal lymph node tuberculosis.

The erythrocytic sedimentation rate is often abnormal. Slight pain, tenderness with a mass, with concomitant radiologic findings suggestive of a mass in the right iliac fossa usually suggests ileocecal tuberculosis, amoeboma or colonic cancer.[17] If in doubt, one should give a therapeutic trial with

chemotherapy and anti-amoebic therapy prior to surgery. Ileocecal tuberculosis can be confused with Crohn's disease. Histological examination and guinea pig inoculation will establish
the differences. Malabsorption, protein-losing enteropathy, and
sprue-like syndrome, are some of the patterns of presentation
of intestinal tuberculosis. [18] Ileocecal tuberculosis is rare in
the United States and Canada. It is relatively common in India.
The colon, other than the cecum, is rarely involved with tuberculosis. [19] Pericolic abscess and subsequent fistula formation can occur with intestinal tuberculosis.

## DIAGNOSTIC TECHNIQUES

RADIOLOGY: Barium enema in gastrointestinal tuberculosis
may show five varieties of lesions: [18]

1) the hyperplastic type with the long segment of narrowing
   rigidity and loss of distensibility - the so-called pipe stem
   colon
2) the ulcerative type
3) the hyperplastic and ulcerative type
4) the carcinoma type
5) intussusception type

Most of these lesions are unifocal; multisegmental lesions are
rare. When these lesions are associated with ileocecal involvement, diagnosis of tuberculosis is more certain (Fig. 22). In
other conditions, diagnosis may not be clear.

## DIFFERENTIAL

Ileocecal tuberculosis should be differentiated from:

1) lymphogranuloma venereum
2) Schistosoma mansoni infections
3) actinomycosis, and
4) post-traumatic and post-radiation strictures
5) diverticular disease, and
6) endometriosis

Usually, the clinical history, as well as the laboratory and radiographic findings, help differentiate these disorders.

## TUBERCULOSIS OF THE URINARY TRACT

Tuberculosis of the urinary tract is generally a disease of the
young adult. [20] It may also be seen among the elderly. It affects
both sexes almost equally. Associated lung lesions are common,

although active disease is infrequent. Sputa smears may be positive for AFB in 15% to 30% of the cases.[21]

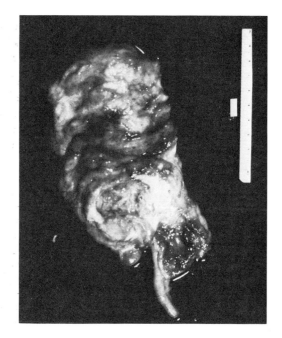

FIG. 22: Ileocecal tuberculosis. The cecum is contracted with fibrous adhesions and thick wall.

Renal tuberculosis is almost always secondary to a primary focus elsewhere, although it may not be readily apparent.

### CLINICAL FEATURES

1) sterile pyuria (60%)
2) painless hematuria (40%)
3) urinary frequency and loin pain (15% to 25%)
4) burning sensation at micturition, because of acid urea, may be present (15%)
5) fever is an inconstant feature (10%)
6) urgency, dribbling, painful micturition (10%)
7) perinephric abscesses are also infrequent (10%)
8) the sputum and urine cultures together are positive for Mycobacterium tuberculosis (90%)
9) culture-positive sputum (20% to 40%)
10) urine (80%) may be culture-positive

The first voided urine specimen is preferred over the 24-hour specimen collection. Isolation of other bacteria from urine cultures should not deter one's suspicion of urinary tract tuberculosis, because bacterial superinfections may occur. Other less frequent sources for culture are sperm, prostatic massage fluid, endometrium, cervical swabs, cervical biopsy and the fistulous tracts, if any.

OTHER INVESTIGATIONS: Intravenous pyelography is abnormal in nearly 70%. Skipped lesions are common with urinary tract tuberculosis. The kidney and bladder may be involved without involvement of the ureter.

SELECTIVE ANGIOGRAPHY: Tuberculosis can cause arteritis;[22] therefore, one may observe lack of blood supply, or absence of arteries on angiography. In pyelonephritis, however, one may find straightening of the arteries. Intravenous pyelography is not always helpful.

CYTOSCOPY: The urinary bladder is involved in more than 50% of the patients. It may show tubercles and ulcers. The ureterovesical junction is compared to a golf hole. Decreased bladder capacity, and therefore, frequency, can occur in advanced tuberculous cystitis. The bladder may shrink to such a small size that it may be compared with a thimble.

The urinary deposit, centrifuged or otherwise, should not be examined for acid-fast bacilli by smears. Innocent acid-fast bacilli, such as Mycobacterium smegmatis from the smegma contaminating the urine, may be mistaken for Mycobacterium tuberculosis.

TREATMENT

Almost all cases of genitourinary tuberculosis in the United States are now managed medically. Out of 800 cases reported in one study since 1958, none had nephrectomy. [20] This view, however, is not shared by the workers in the United Kingdom and India. They consider that the "putty kidney" or the "cement kidney" seen in the roentgenograms should be regarded as the storehouse of Mycobacteria, inaccessible to therapy, and therefore, should be surgically removed. [23] It is my opinion that if the patient is reliable, medical therapy alone must suffice. If not, surgery is an alternative.

ENDOMETRIAL TUBERCULOSIS

Endometrial tuberculosis is rare in North America. It has been found in only one per cent or two per cent of the cases of infertility. [24] In other parts of the world, the incidence is as high as ten per cent of all cases of infertility investigated. [25,26]

Lower abdominal pain, menstrual disorder, and abdominal swelling are the common complaints. The chest x-ray is often unremarkable. The diagnosis can be established by endometrial or endocervical curettage. This material should be submitted for histopathologic examination, microbiologic cultures and guinea pig inoculations. [27]

Hysterosalpingography may be abnormal in most instances. Multiple calcified lymph nodes, multiple constrictions in the salpinx, or an obstruction at the isthmus and ampulla, and decreased size of the endometrial cavity due to fibrosis, are some of its features (Fig. 23, also see Figs. 60 and 143, pages 324 and 788).

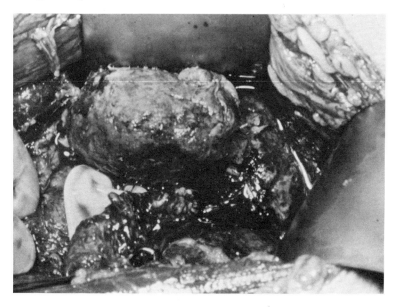

FIG. 23: Tuberculous salpingitis - at laparotomy, the fallopian tube is exposed, showing marked thickening and fibrous adhesions.

## TUBERCULOSIS OF THE TESTIS

Genital tuberculosis in men may present as a testicular mass which can be mistaken for a tumor. When far advanced, it can present with scrotal fistulae. Tuberculous orchitis is painful; syphilitic orchitis is painless. Acute epididymitis should be regarded as superfluous to tuberculous orchitis or secondary to urinary tract tuberculosis, and urine should be cultured for M. tuberculosis. Rectal examination should be done to examine for the enlargement of the prostate and seminal vesicles. They may be indurated and tender. These aforementioned signs may not be always present.

## TUBERCULOSIS OF THE BREAST

The breast is rarely involved in tuberculosis. It may present with a lump mistaken for cancer or sinuses discharging purulent material with or without accompanying pain.[26] Breast tuberculosis is often secondary to tuberculosis of the internal mammary lymph nodes.

## LARYNGEAL TUBERCULOSIS

Laryngeal tuberculosis is a rare but highly contagious disease. Less than two per cent with pulmonary tuberculosis may have laryngeal involvement. Tuberculosis of the larynx should be considered in the differential when a patient with a lung lesion has hoarseness of voice.[28] Other symptoms include cough, pharyngitis, dysphagia, pain in the ears and weight loss with or without fever, with or without otorrhea or hemoptysis. Syphilis, malignancy, Wagner's granulomatosis and polyarteritis nodosa should be considered in the differential diagnosis.

The sputum smears are almost always positive for acid-fast bacilli in upper respiratory tract tuberculosis, and the chest roentgenograms frequently are suggestive of pulmonary tuberculosis. Cervical lymphadenopathy although frequent with laryngeal carcinoma, is not a feature of laryngeal tuberculosis. The indirect laryngoscopy might reveal ulcerative lesions.[29] Laryngeal biopsy may show evidence of tuberculosis with acid-fast bacilli. On therapy, both clinical and roentgenographic improvement is expected within two to four weeks.

## TUBERCULOUS PLEURISY

Tuberculous pleurisy can occur at any age. Recently, its pre-valence has increased among the elderly. In India, it is still mostly a disease of the young adult. Although fever is an in-constant feature, the younger the patient, the more acute is the onset of illness. It may present with cough, chest pain, fever, night sweats, chilliness, dyspnea, weakness and weight loss. Chest pain may precede cough.[30]

Chest pain preceding non-productive cough and pleural effusion associated with normal white blood cell count is strongly sug-gestive of tuberculous pleurisy. If the skin test is positive, tuberculosis is the most likely diagnosis.

The skin reaction to intermediate strength PPD is negative in nearly one-third to one-half of the cases of pleural effusion. Most patients react to the second strength PPD. Lack of skin reactivity to the second strength one month following the onset of the illness, if the patient is not anergic, excludes the diag-nosis of tuberculosis.

The erythrocytic sedimentation rate is almost always high to start with, but tends to reverse on chemotherapy.

PLEURAL FLUID: The pleural fluid may be serosanguineous or clear. When secondarily infected, it turns purulent. The fluid may contain 1,000 to 6,000 or even up to 15,000 cells/cu. mm. Less than 400 cells would make the diagnosis of tuber-culous pleural effusion less likely. [32] It is predominantly poly-morphonuclear among those who are less than 35 years old, and predominantly lymphocytic among the older age group. The eosinophils are rare in tuberculous pleurisy. The protein con-tent is about 2.5 to 3 grams per 100 ml. The pleural fluid LDH is elevated in most cases. The glucose level is normal in two-thirds of the cases; decreased in one-third, and seldom below 10 to 20/100 ml. The pleural fluid glucose is not as diagnostic of infection as it is in the case of spinal fluid glucose in men-ingitis. See Table 14 for details on the characteristics of fluid in infection of the pleural space, meningitis, pericarditis, as-cites and arthritis.

Pleural biopsy is extremely valuable in the diagnosis of tuber-culous pleural effusion. At least two good pieces of pleura should be obtained at a given time. The diagnostic yield is pro-portionate to the number of bits biopsied.[31]

TABLE 14: COMPOSITION OF SEROUS EFFUSIONS IN TUBERCULOSIS INFECTION

| Diagnosis | Per cent of Occurrence | Naked Eye Examination | Approximate* Cell Count | G/100 Protein | Sugar | Comments and Cultures |
|---|---|---|---|---|---|---|
| Spinal fluid in meningitis | Nearly 10% | Turbid to cloudy; occasionally clear | 400 cells; 85% mononucleosis | > 50 mg | < 40 mg/100 | AFB may be found in the pellicle 20% to 30% of the time. Cultures are positive in nearly 80%. |
| Pleural effusion | < 10% | Straw-colored; occasionally turbid or sanguineous | Usually 1000 cells or more; WBC:10,000 (80% lymphocytes) | > 3 g | < 60 mg/ml | AFB may be found in centrifuged sediment, pellicle, standing or concentrate smear in 30-40%. |
| Ascitic fluid | < 10% | | 7500 cells;>75% mononuclear | > 3 g | | Rarely positive on direct smears, but cultures may be positive. |
| Pericardial effusion | < 15% | Occasionally hemorrhagic | | > 3 g | | Rarely positive on smear. Cultures are positive in nearly 50-60% of patients. |
| Arthritis fluid | | Turbid | 75,000 cells; 60% polymorphonuclear | | 0 to 10 | Rarely positive smears. Cultures are frequently positive. |

*Although mononuclear response is common, the initial response can be polymorphonuclear.

In cases of tuberculous effusion, pleural biopsies are positive in about 80% to 90%. Pleural fluid cultures are also positive in 75% to 80% of the cases. Gastric washings, alone, are positive in nearly a third of these cases.

## DIFFERENTIAL

It is often confused with pleural effusions secondary to bronchogenic carcinoma, cardiac failure, pulmonary embolism and acute autoimmune disorders. The skin reaction to PPD is of little help where tuberculosis is prevalent. The chest x-ray should be repeated after the pleural effusion is completely drained. It may help detect some of the parenchymal lesions. Bronchoscopy and cytologic examination of the pleural fluid will help in the diagnosis of malignancy. Occasionally, the malignancy may coexist with tuberculosis. LE and ANA antibody preparations are helpful in the diagnosis of autoimmune disorders. When in doubt, it is safer to treat for possible tuberculosis for six weeks, by which time culture results become available. When the cultures are negative and the patient shows no clinical improvement, antituberculosis therapy should be discontinued. In cases of pleural effusion, bronchogenic carcinoma should be suspected if no clinical and roentgenographic improvement occurs following a three-week course of effective antituberculosis therapy.

There is no need for the insertion of chest tubes or decortication in the management of uncomplicated tuberculous empyema. Effective antituberculosis chemotherapy is all that is required.

## REFERENCES

1.  Lee, M.W. , Adebonojo, F.O. : Tuberculosis among urban black children. Clin. Pediat. 15:1055, 1976.

2.  Morbidity & Mortality Weekly Reports: March 16, 1974, July 5, 1975 and July 16, 1976. Center for Disease Control, Atlanta.

3.  Burdash, N.M. , et al: Evaluation of the acid-fast smear. J. Clin. Micro. 4:190, 1976.

4.  Boyd, J.C. , Marr, J.J.: Decreasing reliability of acid-fast smear techniques for detection of tuberculosis. Ann. Int. Med. 82:489, 1975.

5.  Tsukamura, M.: Niacin negative Mycobacterium tuberculosis. Amer. Rev. Resp. Dis. 110:101, 1974.

6.  Chowdhury, J. R.: Observations on the disease pattern in lower lobe tuberculosis. J. Indian Med. Ass. 38:524, 1962.

7.  Thadepalli, H., Rambhatla, K., Niden, A. H.: Use of transtracheal aspiration for diagnosis of sputum smear negative tuberculosis: With special reference to associated infections. J. A. M. A. 238:1037-1040, 1977.

8.  Siemen, J. K., et al: Gallium-67 scintigraphy of pulmonary diseases as a complement to radiography. Radiology 118:371, 1976.

9.  Thadepalli, H., et al: Correlation of microbiologic and 67 Gallium scans in patients with pulmonary infections. Chest 72:442-448, 1977.

10. Gourin, A., Lyons, H.: Concurrent pulmonary tuberculosis and bronchogenic carcinoma. N. Y. State J. of Med. 174:2367, 1977.

11. Gelb, A. F., et al: Miliary tuberculosis. Amer. Rev. Resp. Dis. 108:1327, 1973.

12. Sahn, S. A., Neff, T. S.: Miliary tuberculosis. Am. J. Med. 56:495, 1974.

13. Holden, M., Dubin, M. R., Diamond, P. H.: Frequency of negative intermediate strength tuberculin sensitivity in patients with active tuberculosis. New Eng. J. of Med. 285:1506, 1971.

14. Ellenbogen, C.: Problems in interpreting tuberculin skin tests. When is a converter not a converter? A review. Military Medicine 138:276, 1973.

15. Rooney, J. J., Jr., et al: Further observations on tuberculin reactions in active tuberculosis. Amer. J. Med. 60: 517, 1976.

16. Chavalittamrong, B.: How to diagnose mycobacterial infections in children - An outline by principles. Clin. Pediat. 12:277, 1973.

17. Novis, B. H. , Bank, S. , Harks, I. N. : Gastrointestinal and peritoneal tuberculosis. S. A. Medical Journal 47:365, 1972.

18. Lewis, E. A. , Kolawale, T. M. : Tuberculous ileocolitis in Ibadan: A clinicoradiological review. Gut 13:646, 1972.

19. Mandal, B. K. , Schofield, P. F. : Abdominal tuberculosis in Britain. The Practitioner, 216:683, 1976.

20. Smith, A. M. , Lattimer, J. K. : Genitourinary tract involvement in children with tuberculosis. N. Y. State J. Med. 73:2325, 1973.

21. Levy, D. W. , et al: Pilot screening of cases of active pulmonary tuberculosis for evidence of renal or renal tract involvement. S. A. Med. J. 47:1687, 1973.

22. Peeters, F. L. M. : The renal angiogram in tuberculosis. Radiol. Clin. Biol. 42:488, 1973.

23. Ghoshal, S. K. , Sen, D. K. : A study of genitourinary tuberculosis in a Calcutta hospital. J. Indian M. A. 65:253, 1975.

24. Henderson, N. D. , Harkins, J. L. , Stitt, J. F. : Pelvic tuberculosis. Am. J. Obstet. & Gynec. 94:630, 1966.

25. Klein, T. A. , Richmond, J. A. , Mishell, D. R. : Pelvic tuberculosis. Obstet. & Gynec. 48:99, 1976.

26. Mukerjee, P. , Cohen, R. V. , Niden, A. H. : Tuberculosis of the breast. Amer. Rev. Resp. Dis. 104:661, 1971.

27. Hok, T. T. , Loew, L. K. , Chatim, A. : The isolation of tubercle bacilli from endocervical microcurettings of 100 consecutive infertile women. Arch. Gynak 208:143, 1969.

28. Rohwedder, J. J. : Upper respiratory tract tuberculosis. Ann. Int. Med. 80:208, 1974.

29. Travis, L. W. , Hybels, R. L. , Newman, M. H. : Tuberculosis of the larynx. The Laryngoscope LXXXVI:549, 1976.

30. Berger, H. W. , Mejia, E. : Tuberculous pleurisy. Chest 63:88, 1973.

31. Levine, H. , Szanto, P. B. , Cugell, D. W. : Tuberculous pleurisy: An acute illness. Arch. Int. Med. 122:329, 1968.

32. Benerjee, S. K. , Kundu, S. C. : Observations on tuberculous pleural effusion. J. Indian M. A. 61:427, 1973.

## 24: MYCOBACTERIOSES
by H. Thadepalli

### INFECTIONS CAUSED BY ATYPICAL MYCOBACTERIA

The atypical mycobacteria are ubiquitous in distribution (see Table 15 for classification of atypical mycobacteria). They are niacin-negative and grow more rapidly than Mycobacterium tuberculosis. Some of them produce pigment when exposed to light (photochromogen) and others produce pigment only in darkness (scotochromogen). [6]

TABLE 15: RUNYON'S CLASSIFICATION OF
ATYPICAL MYCOBACTERIA (M) [6]

| SKIN TEST ANTIGEN | GROUP | TYPE SPECIES |
|---|---|---|
| PPD-Y | I Photochromogen | M. kansasii<br>M. balnei<br>(marinum) |
| PPD-G | II Scotochromogen | M. scrofulaceum |
| PPD-B or<br>PPD-A | III Nonchromogen | M. intracellulare<br>(Battey bacillus)<br>M. avium<br>M. triviale |
| PPD-F | IV Rapid grower | M. fortuitum<br>M. smegmatis<br>M. phlei |

Other characteristics: Negative niacin test, absence of good cord formation, relatively rapid growth and ability to produce pigment, some in light (photochromogen) and some without light (scotochromogen).

### MYCOBACTERIUM (M.) KANSASII

Mycobacterium (M.) kansasii infections occur infrequently in the elderly and among those with other lung diseases, such as carcinoma of the lung, chronic obstructive pulmonary disease and multicavernous diseases of the lung. [1] Decreased host

resistance may also be a predisposing factor. M. intracellulare (Battey bacillus infection) and M. avium may also cause
lung infections.

The mycobacteriosis is clinically indistinguishable from the
typical pulmonary tuberculosis.[2] Mycobacteriosis, like classical tuberculosis, also causes cough and productive sputum
associated with low-grade fever, loss of weight and hemoptysis. The chest roentgenogram may show evidence of associated
lung disease. M. kansasii infection may occur sui generis or
in association with the M. tuberculosis. On occasion, M. kansasii might occur as a superinfection on the cavities of patients who were previously treated with antituberculosis chemotherapy for typical tuberculosis. [3]

## MYCOBACTERIUM INTRACELLULARE (Battey bacillus)

Battey bacillus infection is frequently found in association with
other lung diseases. In the United States, the Battey bacillus
infections are more frequent in the southeastern regions. The
water bubbles from the Atlantic Ocean were reported to dis-
perse a fine spray of multitudinous bacteria into the atmos-
phere; thus explaining this high incidence. Battey bacillus infections are generally indolent in onset and chronic in their
course. Disseminated disease is rare. It is the cause of death
in 11% of the patients infected with Battey bacillus.

## MYCOBACTERIUM MARINUM (balnei)

M. marinum is a water-loving organism. It is found in both
fresh and salt water. It is distinct from M. intracellulare,
which is found only in sea water. M. marinum is a parasite
of the fish and it causes swimming pool granulomas. It often
starts with an ulcer at the site of infection, followed by areas
of incrustation, which subsequently might coalesce to form a
granuloma (Fig. 24). [4] In general, these granulomas heal spontaneously. The fish tank granulomas frequently occur on the
fingers. These ulcers may sometimes start on the head, back,
neck, and, in general, over the cooler areas of the body. Associated regional lymphadenopathy is frequent.

## MYCOBACTERIUM SCROFULACEUM

M. scrofulaceum, as its name suggests, causes scrofular cervical lymphadenopathy. It is a disease of childhood, mostly
less than six years of age. It is often unilateral, with or without suppuration. They are occasionally calcified. These patients

do not usually respond to antituberculous chemotherapy or the clinical response is very slow. These patients usually have no history of previous exposure to tuberculosis.

## UNIDENTIFIED SPECIES

An unidentified species of mycobacteria which could not be cultured in the laboratory was reported to cause skin infections in the midwestern parts of the United States and Canada.[5] They started as reddish-purple papules on the leg, face or arm and rarely on the trunk, with or without associated regional lymphadenopathy. It occurs in fall and winter, with a peak incidence in the month of February. Microbiologically, it should be differentiated from other skin infections due to acid-fast organisms. The unidentified species are not cultivable. In this disease, unlike M. leprae infections, the skin sensations are intact. Mycobacterium fortuitum, marinum and intracellulare may also cause skin lesions, therefore, they must be distinguished from this unidentified species.

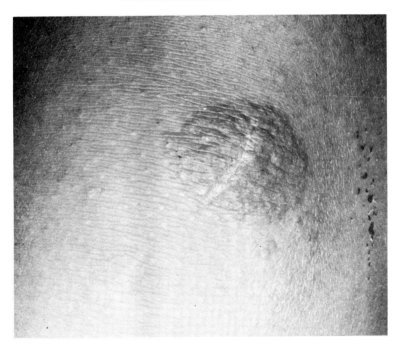

FIG. 24: A case of swimming pool granuloma on the elbow caused by M. marinum.

PPD skin test for mycobacterioses: See page 150 for details.

## REFERENCES

1. Lincoln, E. M. , Gilbert, L. A.: Diseases in children due to mycobacteria other than Mycobacterium tuberculosis. Amer. Rev. Resp. Dis. 105:683, 1972.

2. Wolinsky, E.: Non-tuberculous mycobacterial infections of man. Med. Clin. N. A. 58:639, 1974.

3. Owens, D. W.: General medical aspects of atypical mycobacteria. South. Med. J. 67:39, 1974.

4. Morbidity & Mortality Weekly Report: Atypical mycobacteria wound infections - North Carolina, Colorado: August 6, 1976. U. S. Dept. of Health, Education and Welfare Center for Disease Control, Atlanta.

5. Feldman, R. A. , Hershfield, E.: Mycobacterial skin infection by an unidentified species. A report of 29 patients. Ann. Int. Med. 80:445, 1974.

6. Runyon, E. H.: Classification of atypical mycobacteria. Med. Clin. N.A. 43:273, 1959.

25: ACTINOMYCES
by H. Thadepalli

## BACTERIOLOGY

Actinomyces is an anaerobic, gram-positive bacillus. It is a
normal flora of the mouth. There are five species of clinical
importance. In order of their prevalence, they are:[1]

1) Actinomyces (A.) israelii (95% are serotype 1)
2) Arachnia propionica (differs from Actinomyces by producing propionic acid)
3) A. naeslundii (clinical picture similar to A. israelii)
4) A. viscosus (facultative organism)
5) A. odontolyticus (rare cause of infections)

Arachnia propionica, as its name indicates, produces large
quantities of propionic acid; thus, it resembles Propionibacterium, a normal skin contaminant. The disease produced by A. propionica is indistinguishable from A. israelii.[2]

Not all Actinomyces branch like fungi; they may be bacillary,
colloid, filamentous or diphtheroid in appearance. Branching is difficult to demonstrate in clinical specimens. Contrary to general belief, most actinomycotic infections should
be diagnosed even in the absence of the typical sulphur granules. Arachnia propionica does not produce sulphur granules.

Actinomyces are not acid-fast organisms. Actinomyces is seldom a monobacterial infection; it is often a polymicrobial synergistic infection. Actinomyces may be found in association with
"other bacteria",[3] frequently a gram-negative coccobacillus,
appropriately called Actinobacillus actinomycetem-comitans,
and less frequently, anaerobic Streptococci, Staphylococci,
Bacteroides corrodens and even Clostridia. Some of these
"other bacteria" can prolong the clinical infection of Actinomyces long after it is eradicated. [4]

Actinomycotic infection is most often endogenous. Man-to-man
transmission is rare.

## CLINICAL FEATURES

Actinomyces can infect any organ in the body with the help of
other bacteria. Head and neck infections are the most frequent
(60%), followed by the chest (20%) and abdomen (20%). It can
affect any race, sex, age or occupation.

## BRAWNY INDURATION

Typically, actinomycotic infections are indolent and chronically suppurating, with areas of healing (fibrous tissue formation). When left untreated, they burrow out through the
skin with multiple discharging sinuses. Most actinomycotic
lesions have a characteristic "feel" to them on palpation.
They are slightly warm, but not hot; firm, but not hard.
There may be areas of softening and the lesion itself may
have indistinct margins - this is what is known as "brawny
induration". Every clinician needs to "feel" at least one
such lesion to recognize others when encountered. Once
appreciated, they have such a characteristic feel, whether
in the jaw, on the wall of the chest, abdomen or pelvis,
that they can be readily recognized.

## DENTAL INFECTIONS

Recurrent dental infections and trauma precede most actinomycotic infections of the jaw. Actinomycosis can cause the so-
called "gum boils", mastoid and maxillary sinus infections,
and frequently osteomyelitis of the mandible, the so-called
lumpy jaw (Fig. 25).[5] It may present with brawny induration, regional adenopathy and discharging sinuses.

Occasionally, Actinomyces can affect an isolated organ, like
the thyroid, tonsil, tongue or lip, but this is rare. One of my
patients, an elderly diabetic woman, had acute suppurative
thyroiditis and gaseous cellulitis caused by A. israelii and
"other bacteria" (Fig. 26).

## CHEST

Actinomycotic infection of the chest may present as a mere
cavity or a lung abscess, but more frequently as empyema.
History of trauma or dental extraction may be present. It is
only when the disease is far advanced that it presents with discharging sinuses on the chest wall. None of the actinomycotic
infections of the lung that I witnessed had sulphur granules. In
the sputum, they were diagnosed by transtracheal aspiration or
pus cultures.

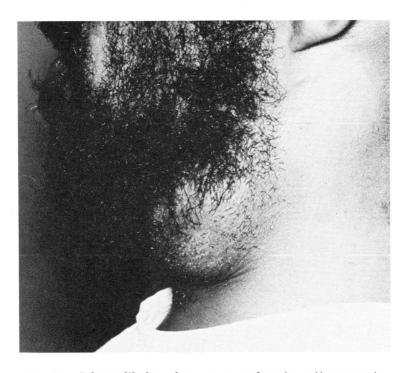

FIG. 25: Submandibular abscess secondary to actinomycosis. This patient had periodontal disease. The pus aspirated from the abscess yielded Actinomyces israelii and "other anaerobic bacteria".

At times, the ribs alone may be affected, but more frequently the rib involvement is due to empyema (Figs. 27, 28). Isolation of Actinomyces in pure culture is cumbersome and because of its association with "other bacteria" it can be hard to separate. Most actinomycotic infections of the lung are indistinguishable from the garden variety infections. Therefore, this organism should be sought for even if other bacteria are isolated. During the past six years, I encountered five patients with pulmonary tuberculosis that were later shown to have associated Actinomyces infections.

## ABDOMINAL

Chronic, recurrent, low abdominal pain with fever and progressive loss of weight, with anemia, with or without a palpable mass, and occasionally, discharging sinuses, are the

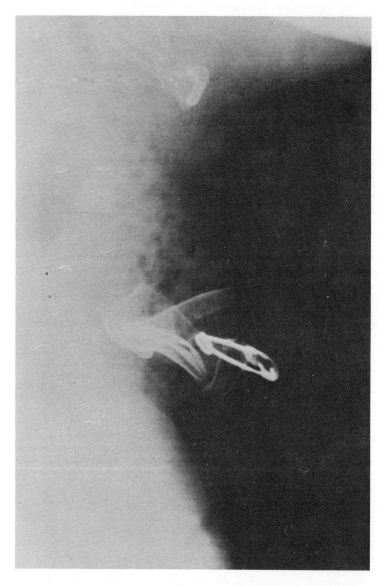

FIG. 26: Suppurative thyroiditis - a soft tissue roentgenogram of the neck following surgical drainage. Cultures yielded <u>Actinomyces israelli</u> and "other bacteria". Note the <u>gas bubbles</u>--no <u>Clostridia</u> were found.

features of abdominal actinomycosis. Often, there is history of abdominal trauma, appendicitis or appendicular perforation, diverticula of the colon or surgery of the large bowel.

Accidentally swallowed chicken bone or fish bone can perforate through the bowel wall or an ulcer and set up chronic peritonitis, later infected with Actinomyces. These bones have been recovered while draining the abdominal abscess.

The swelling due to Actinomyces infection can frequently present under the anterior wall, occasionally posteriorly. It may on occasion involve the lips, buttocks, scrotum, vertebrae, subdiaphragmatic space, pelvic or psoas muscle regions. Actinomyces can involve any solid organ in the abdomen, like liver, spleen, pancreas, kidney and others.

## PELVIC

Actinomyces is not usually found in the cervix. We isolated this organism in one out of 200 cervical specimens collected from 100 women (1%). Actinomycotic infections of the female genital tract are not common. The clinical picture is that of an intra-abdominal abscess. It more frequently involves the right lower quadrant than the left. Bilateral involvement is even less common.

History of appendicular infections or appendicular rupture, or criminal abortion are often present. In cases when such history is available, one should assume ascending infection as a possibility. More importantly, history of insertion of intrauterine contraceptive devices (IUCD) can cause endometritis and then predispose to actinomycotic infection. [6] Majzlin springs were frequently implicated with this complication, although any metallic IUCD can lead to actinomycotic infection. [7]

## DIAGNOSIS

HISTORY: Abdominal, pelvic or dental surgery, or insertion of IUCD or injury or surgery with a left-over foreign body, should lead one to suspect actinomycosis.

SULPHUR GRANULES: These are colonies of Actinomyces clumped together and when present, are the sine qua non of this infection. They are dull white or light brown in color, not yellow. They are translucent and refractive, of size 1 mm. x

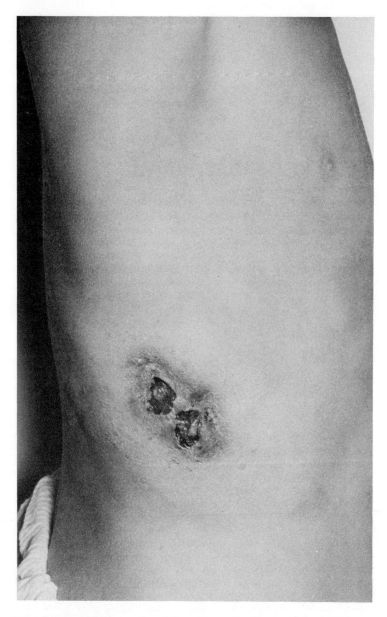

FIG. 27: Actinomycosis of the ribs with discharging sinuses on the right side of the chest.

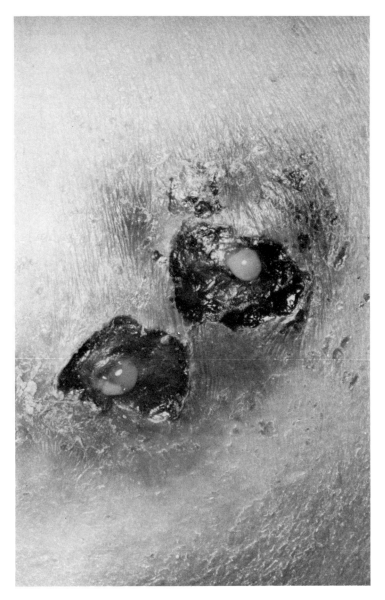

FIG. 28: Same as Fig. 27. Close-up showing drops of pus which showed sulphur granules; on culture, it yielded Actinomyces viscosus.

3 mm., irregular and roughly spherical. On Gram's stain, one may see gram-positive branching rods. Sulphur granules are not formed by A. viscosus.

RADIOLOGY: Appropriate roentgenographic examination should be performed to detect bone lesions, defects in the bowel (perforation, diverticula) and occasionally sinograms to detect the extent of infection. Ga-67 scans are almost always positive in actinomycotic infections. They are useful in most cases, except when the bowel is involved, as Ga-67 tends to concentrate the most in the bowel regardless of infection.

CHEST INFECTIONS: Actinomyces is a normal flora of the mouth; therefore, sputa examination and bronchoscopy specimens are worthless. The transtracheal aspirate and properly collected pus are the most reliable specimens.

BLOOD CULTURES: Blood cultures are rarely positive. In disseminated cases, Actinomyces or Actinobacillus may be isolated. Blood cultures should be collected in pre-reduced and anaerobically sterilized (PRAS) media.

FLUORESCENT ANTIBODY TECHNIQUE:    Can be used for identification of Actinomyces in the tissue specimens.

## TREATMENT

Penicillin or carbenicillin are the drugs of choice. In penicillin-allergic individuals, clindamycin or doxycycline can be used, to which it is susceptible.[8]  I have successfully used penicillin, carbenicillin, ticarcillin, doxycycline and clindamycin to treat this infection.

## REFERENCES

1.  George, L.K.: The Agents of Human Actinomycosis. Anaerobic Bacteria: Role in Disease (Eds.) Balows, A., DeHaan, R.M., Charles C Thomas, Springfield, 1974.

2.  Brock, D.W., et al: Actinomycosis caused by Arachnia propionica. A.J.C.P. 59:66, 1973.

3.  Holm, P.: Studies on the etiology of human actinomycosis. I. The "other bacteria" of actinomycosis and their importance. Acta. Path. et Microbiol. Scandinav. 27:736, 1950.

4.  Holm, P.: Studies on the etiology of human actinomycosis. II. Do the "other microbes" of actinomycosis possess virulence? Acta. Path. et Microbiol. Scandinav. 28:392, 1951.

5.  Gardiner, S.S.: Actinomycosis of the head and neck. Austr. New Zeal. J. Surg. 6:186, 1936.

6.  Dische, F. E. , et al: Tubo-ovarian actinomycosis associated with intrauterine contraceptive devices. J. Obstet. Gynecol. Brit. Commonwealth 81:724, 1974.

7.  Schiffer, M. A. , et al: Actinomycosis infections associated with intrauterine contraceptive devices. Obstet. & Gynecol. 45:67, 1975.

8.  Lerner, P. I.: Susceptibility of pathogenic actinomycetes to antimicrobial compounds. Antimicrob. Agents Chemother. 5:302, 1974.

## 26: PLEURAL EFFUSION
### by H. Thadepalli

Pleural effusion is a common diagnostic problem. The first step to diagnosis is to determine if the pleural fluid is a transudate or an exudate. Pleural effusion secondary to infection is exudative. Some diagnostic clues for an exudate (Table 16) are the following:

1) Specific gravity: Specific gravity (S.G.) is an unreliable test to differentiate exudate from a transudate. Most exudates have an S.G. greater than 1.016. Nearly 40% of tuberculous pleural effusions may have an S.G. lower than 1.016, and 10% of pleural fluids due to anasarca may have higher S.G. Pleural fluid protein concentration is more reliable than S.G.

2) Protein: Pleural fluid protein of 3 G. or higher suggests exudate. Only 10% to 15% of exudates have less than 3 G. of protein. Further, diuretic therapy can falsely increase the pleural fluid protein concentration. The pleural fluid and serum ratio is more reliable than the protein concentration in the pleural fluid.

3) Pleural fluid/serum ratio: In cases of exudate, this ratio is greater than 0.5. The diagnostic error by this method is less than 10%.

4) The pH: Most exudative effusions tend to be acidic in nature because of bacterial fermentation and cellular breakdown products. For the same reason, they also have lower $pO_2$ and higher $pCO_2$ values. A pH value of 7.30 or less is suggestive of an exudate that may require drainage with a chest tube.[1] Most benign effusions that may resolve without specific therapy tend to have a pH of greater than 7.30. Pleural fluid samples for analysis of pH should be collected with precautions similar to drawing arterial blood gases.

5) Leukocyte count:[2,3,4] The total white blood cell count in cases of exudative pleural effusion is usually greater than 1,000 cells. At least in 70%, the cell count is higher than 2,500 cells/cu. mm. Less than 10% of the transudates have more than 1,000 cells. Nevertheless, the pleural fluid (PF)/serum (SR) protein ratio of greater than 0.5 is a more reliable diagnostic clue of an exudate than total leukocyte count. Cell counts higher than 5,000 WBC/cu. mm. are diagnostic of infection.

TABLE 16: PLEURAL FLUID ANALYSIS

| CHARACTERISTIC | CUTOFF POINT | EXUDATE | TRANSUDATE |
|---|---|---|---|
| Specific gravity | 1.016 | Greater | Less |
| Protein | 3 gm. | Greater | Less |
| Pleural fluid/serum protein ratio | 0.5 | Greater | Less |
| pH | 7.30 | Less | Greater |
| Leukocyte count | 2,500/cu. mm. | Greater | Less |
| LDH | 250 to 350 | Greater | Less |
| LDH ratio - pleural fluid/serum | 0.5 to 0.6 | Greater | Less |
| Pleural fluid glucose | 50% of blood glucose | Less | Greater |
| Erythrocytes | 100,000/cu. mm. | Greater | Less |
| Hematocrit | 2% | Greater | Less |

When the lymphocytes predominate in the pleural fluid, they should be examined closely. They are lymphoblastic in cases of leukemia. The lymphocytes are mature in tuberculous pleurisy.

Differential cell count on occasion can also help to differentiate malignancy from tuberculosis. The mesothelial cells are less than 5% in tuberculosis; they are higher in malignancy.

6) Lactic dehydrogenase (LDH): In cases of exudate, the LDH levels are higher than 250 to 350 I.U. Like proteins, the pleural fluid/serum LDH ratio is often more reliable than absolute LDH concentration.[2]

7) LDH ratio: A ratio of pleural fluid/serum equal to or greater than 0.5 to 0.6 is highly suggestive of an exudate. If both protein ratio and LDH ratios are greater than 0.5, it is diagnostic of an exudate.

8) Erythrocytes and hematocrit: A bloody tap can be due to an exudative pleurisy; it does not mean infection. Even a leak of 2 ml. of blood into a liter of pleural fluid can look bloody. Less than 25% of transudates are bloody. It takes only 10,000 RBC/cu. mm. to give a blood appearance. Erythrocyte counts greater than 100,000/cu. mm., or the pleural fluid hematocrit greater than 2%, can be due to an exudative pleurisy, malignancy, trauma or pulmonary infarction.[5]

9) PF/serum amylase ratio: The PF/serum amylase ratio of greater than one can occur in cases of tumors.

10) Glucose: Simultaneous serum and pleural fluid glucose levels should be obtained. An absolute decrease of PF glucose to 40 mg.%, and PF/SR ratio less than 0.5, is suggestive of an exudative (inflammatory) pleurisy. Low glucose levels can also occur in malignancy and leukemia.

11) Gram's stain and acid-fast stain: Gram's stain and acid-fast stain are the most important steps that should be done routinely on all cases of pleural effusions. A positive Gram's stain of pleural fluid (when free of contamination) is diagnostic of infection. It should always be verified by culture. Acid-fast stains are often unrewarding.

12) Culture: All pleural fluid specimens should be submitted for both aerobic and anaerobic cultures. They should also be

routinely cultured for Mycobacterium tuberculosis and fungi
without regard to the initial appearance of the pleural fluid.
Viral cultures in general are of benefit only in retrospect.

13) Gas liquid chromatography: Gas liquid chromatography
(GLC) is useful to diagnose anaerobic empyema.[6] The test
can be done within 20 minutes. Elution of multiple volatile
fatty acids from the ether extracts of pleural fluid is diagnostic of anaerobic empyema.

14) Biopsy: It is a routine practice to obtain pleural biopsy in
all cases of pleural effusion whenever the fluid is aspirated.
Pleural biopsies can be dangerous in cases of empyema
because they can lead to rapidly spreading cellulitis. I recommend that thoracentesis be done first and the fluid analyzed for its nature. If it is an exudate, and if no bacteria
are seen in Gram's stain and none cultured within 48 hours,
and if the effusion still persists, then pleural biopsy should
be considered. Contrarily, if the fluid has the character
of an exudate and shows bacteria on Gram's stain or is positive
for culture within 48 hours, I do not recommend doing a biopsy,
insertion of a chest tube and drainage should be considered
instead.

## REFERENCES

1. Potts, D. E. , Levin, D. C. , Sahn, S. A. : Pleural fluid pH
   in parapneumonic effusions. Chest 70:328, 1976.

2. Chandrasekhar, A. J. , Buehler, J. H. : Diagnostic evaluation of pleural effusion. Geriatrics, 29:116, July, 1974.

3. Light, R. W. , Erozan, Y. S. , Ball, W. C. : Cells in pleural
   fluid. Arch. Int. Med. 132:844, 1973.

4. Dines, D. E. , Pierre, R. V. , Franzen, S. J. : The value of
   cells in pleural fluid in differential diagnosis. Mayo Clin.
   Proc. 80:571, 1975.

5. Light, R. W. , et al: Pleural effusions: The diagnostic separation of transudates and exudates. Ann. Int. Med. 77:507,
   1972.

6. Thadepalli, H. , Bartlett, J. G. , Gorbach, S. L. : Rapid
   diagnosis of anaerobic empyema by direct gas chromatography. Chest 68:428, 1975 (Abstract).

27: FUNGAL INFECTIONS OF THE LUNG
by Hans E. Einstein

## INTRODUCTION

Diagnostic accuracy in deep mycoses was, until recently, an intellectual exercise for many mycologists. Precise bacteriology did not become crucial until the antimicrobial era in the 1930s, so it was left to the 1950s to produce the great advances in diagnostic mycology. Again, the incentive was the beginning of effective anti-fungal therapy. Gradually, there has been a lessening of the average practitioner's lack of confidence in approaching these diseases; consequently, patient care has improved greatly. This is a fortunate development, for clearly the incidence of mycotic infections throughout the world is on the increase, with three-fold the incidence being reported from a number of centers since the beginning of the decade.

Basic differences from bacterial diseases need to be emphasized. Fungal infections are basically non-contagious and the soil is the reservoir for most of them. Free-living saprophytes become parasitic and pathogenic when the opportunity for inhalation usually, or implantation occasionally, presents itself. This has, in recent years, been facilitated by iatrogenic manipulations, such as immunosuppressive, cytotoxic or antimicrobial medications, organ transplantation, indwelling tubes and catheters and prosthetic devices.

Lengthened survival in serious disabling diseases, often with immunosuppression, as seen in malignancies, diabetes and collagen vascular diseases, and leukemia and lymphoma, is yet another major contributor to the emergence of opportunistic fungus infections.

In addition, the primary fungal pathogens are increasingly being seen out of their usual geographic habitats. World-wide travel and shipment of goods have made coccidioidomycosis, histoplasmosis and, most recently, blastomycosis a diagnostic concern for physicians everywhere. The latter diseases are the most common human infections, caused by the more than 200,000 specific fungi named in the mycological literature. Of these, over twenty species cause serious systemic disease and are the main concern of this chapter.

Deep mycoses are not rare diseases. [1,2] It has been estimated that over thirty million people in the United States have been infected by <u>Histoplasma capsulatum,</u> and the disease additionally has been reported from over fifty countries. Ten million people have been infected by and have recovered from coccidioidomycosis with another 100,000 or more joining the ranks annually. When one considers the above data of distribution and continued increase due to travel, disturbance of soil by housing, agriculture, mining, drilling, as well as the ever increasing breakdown of host defenses by administration of toxic agents and devices, it becomes apparent that fungus diseases will soon overshadow tuberculosis in their world-wide importance.

The clinical diagnosis of fungal infections, as with any disease, fundamentally must depend on the physician's index of suspicion. A vast area of diagnostic modalities is available; nevertheless, diagnoses are frequently missed or delayed. The setting in which the patient is seen is most important: Where has he lived and travelled? What exposures have there been? What are the underlying processes that may lead to disruption of normal symbiotic relationships, or alteration of intracellular biochemistry? What are the drugs that have been given, what procedures done? Once the possibility of fungal infection has been considered, an orderly diagnostic algorithm becomes possible in spite of the usual non-specific clinical appearance.

DEEP MYCOSIS OF THE LUNG - GENERAL CONSIDERATIONS

The pulmonary phase of the deep mycoses has many clinical similarities. An initial incubation period of from ten to twenty-one days usually culminates in a flu-like respiratory infection, the severity of which is thought to depend on the dose of the spore inoculum. A pneumonitis is usually present at this time, which tends to be basilar and frequently has a hilar component. While this primary infection is often asymptomatic, it leaves behind certain immunological diagnostic markers, which will be discussed for each mycosis separately. Culture identification is possible from the sputum during the primary phase, occasionally from the blood during fungemic phases (either early or late) from urine, sputum, pleural or spinal fluid, and occasionally by culture or histological examination of appropriate biopsy specimen from early or late lesions. While cultural or histopathological demonstration of the organism in exudate or tissue are the only definite methods of establishing a diagnosis, they have their pitfalls. Fungal cultures have certain risks to laboratory personnel. This is particularly true of coccidioidal and to a lesser extent, Histoplasma cultures. Histological examination also tends to mislead the inexperienced examiner because of the frequent deviation from the usual morphology on the part of many of the organisms. Thus, correlation between clinical, immunological, radiographic and histopathologic findings, confirmed, if possible, by cultural isolation becomes the diagnostic data base. In order to achieve this, proper collection of specimen and selection of tests is extremely important. Fortunately, chronic granulomatous fungal disease patients are usually not so desperately ill, when first seen, that a thorough diagnostic study cannot be carried out.

## COMMON DIAGNOSTIC FEATURES

RADIOGRAPHY: X-rays of the chest are generally abnormal at one stage of most of the deep mycoses. A pulmonary phase which usually is early in the disease is detectible only if the patient is symptomatic enough to present to the physician, which, as stated above, is frequently not the case. The roentgenographic appearance is never diagnostic per se; the mycoses resemble bacterial and Mycoplasma or viral diseases in their patterns; they can simulate tumors; they can and do resemble vascular lesions as well as pneumoconiosis, the various other pulmonary fibrotic syndromes and, of course, each other. Certain statements can, however, be made regarding their roentgenographic appearance.

Basically, the pulmonary lesion occurs at the portal of entry and is granulomatous with a hilar component frequently being present. A second hematogenous lesion can be seen later as part of the disseminated phase if it occurs. This is particularly true of coccidioidomycosis and blastomycosis. The primary granulomatous lesion can heal completely with or without calcification. The latter is almost universal in histoplasmosis, but much less common in coccidioidomycosis (12%). At other times, a granuloma may remain as a single or multiple so-called coin lesion or calcification. Cavitation can occur, especially in coccidioidomycosis and histoplasmosis. It must be emphasized that none of these patterns are particularly characteristic and again, only a high index of suspicion and consideration of all available clinical, epidemiological, microbiological and immunologic data can and will establish the diagnosis. Strontium lung scanning has recently been advocated as a way of rapidly and specifically identifying pulmonary aspergillosis.[3,4]

MICROBIOLOGICAL IDENTIFICATION: As with infectious
diseases in general, definite diagnosis depends on the isolation
of the organism or its demonstration in tissues or exudate.
Proper specimen collection is required for maximum information. Sputum is the most accessible; the traditional 24-hour
sputum is not appropriate to mycological examination due to
bacterial and saprophyte yeast overgrowth, especially in a hospital setting or from a sick patient. Fresh, single cough specimen collected after the morning hygiene, but before breakfast, is most suitable. Heated saline aerosol induction is
useful in patients without a productive cough. Daily samples
should be examined in a global fashion: bacteria including
Mycobacteria, cytology, mycology and, if indicated, the
physical and chemical characteristics should be determined.
The direct wet mount with potassium hydroxide should always be done (see page 219); frequently immediate diagnosis
can be made by the visualization of yeasts from pneumonic
lesion or mycelial clement from cavities. This is particularly useful with the sporangia of <u>Blastomyces dermatitidis</u>
and <u>Coccidioides immitis</u>. Cryptococcal elements can occasionally be seen with India ink preparations in sputum or
spinal fluid.

BRONCHOSCOPY: Bronchial and cavitary aspiration and brushings can be obtained either by transtracheal catheter or fiberoptic bronchoscope and sent to the laboratory after collection
in a Lukens tube. Biopsies can be performed transbronchially
or percutaneously by direct aspiration, high speed drill or with
special biopsy needles. Aspirates should again be sent to the
laboratory for total examination, as outlined previously as well
as the usual histological sectioning. Here, too, direct examination of the specimen by simple touching to a glass slide can
be rewarding. In the fixed section, special fungal stains are
mandatory, with the periodic Schiff, Hotchkiss-McManus and
the Grocott modification of the Gomori methenamine silver
stain having been proven the most useful. Surgically obtained
biopsy specimens should be handled in the same manner.

PLEURAL FLUID: Pleural fluid aspiration does not have a high
yield of culture identification; pleural biopsies by either the
Cope or Abbott techniques are very helpful, however, especially in coccidioidomycosis. [4] Handling of these specimens
must include all the parameters previously outlined. Pleural
fluid chemistries have not been particularly characteristic.
Pus from the pleura, from abscessed cavities, sinuses or fistulae is a rich source of material that generally is culturally
positive.

In addition to the direct visualization of organisms, the type
of cellular reaction can be fairly characteristic with an early
polymorphonuclear response, quickly replaced by a chronic
lymphocytic appearance with eosinophils occasionally predominating in both pleural and spinal fluids.

CEREBROSPINAL FLUID: Spinal fluid examination plays a
prominent part in the work-up of the patient with disseminated
mycotic disease. Coccidioides immitis, Cryptococcus neoformans and occasionally Histoplasma capsulatum can involve the
central nervous system and produce many puzzling clinical syndromes. The cellular response is polymorphonuclear in the
early stages but is soon replaced by a mononuclear predominance. Eosinophils have occasionally been seen in the spinal
fluid of coccidioidal meningitis; India ink staining can show
fungal elements in Cryptococcus neoformans infections. Cultural recovery of organisms is enhanced by constant draining
of cerebrospinal fluid. C. immitis will occasionally grow in
its own spinal fluid if left at room temperature for approximately one week. Spinal fluid in fungal meningitis does not usually
show significant chemical abnormalities. The colloidal gold
reactions are quite useful in coccidioidal infections, with a first
zone reaction being seen early and persisting throughout the
active infection.

BLOOD CULTURES: Blood cultures can be helpful, particularly in Candida species infection, also occasionally with
Cryptococcus neoformans and C. immitis. Skin lesions are a
rich source of diagnostic yield, both from direct swabs, cultures and biopsies. Bone marrow smear and culture are frequently positive in Histoplasma infections; occasionally, they
can be seen in the late pre-terminal disseminations of coccidioidomycosis, aspergillosis and cryptococcosis.

URINE CULTURES: Urine cultures yield Candida species,
Torulopsis glabrata, C. neoformans, C. immitis, H. capsulatum and occasionally B. dermatitidis. The interpretation
of a positive culture, especially for coccidioidomycosis[5] and
Candida, must be taken in the total context of the case and has,
at times, been over-interpreted. Prostatic secretions will
show yeast elements in from 10% to 15% of cases of blastomycosis and have been reported showing coccidioidal infections.

JOINT FLUID: Joint fluid and synovial biopsies are helpful in
synovitis and occasional osteomyelitis involving joints, particularly for sporotrichosis, blastomycosis and coccidioidomycosis.

CULTURES: In concluding the section on direct examination, brief mention should be made of special staining and culture procedures. Some of the stains have already been mentioned. In addition to the usual hematoxylin and eosin preparations, the Grocott modification of the Gomori methenamine silver stain is preferred, since it will highlight dead, as well as living, fungal cells. The modified, periodic acid Schiff, Hotchkiss-McManus and Gridley fungus stains are also useful. Sabouraud's dextrose-peptone medium remains the standard for culture growth, with chloramphenicol added for bacterial suppression, and cyclohexamide for inhibition of saprobic fungi. The former also tends to inhibit Nocardia, while the latter is toxic for C. neoformans and Candida species. A note of caution must be added here: The handling of fungal cultures requires extreme care, especially C. immitis and H. capsulatum. In the microscopic examination of organism and tissue, as well as direct examination of culture, colony characteristics should be noted. One should mainly look for budding yeasts or hyphal elements. Two to three micron sized yeasts with pseudohyphae suggest Candida albicans; intracellular yeasts of this size, surrounded by halo, are characteristic of H. capsulatum. The yeasts of both B. dermatitidis and C. neoformans are ten to fifteen microns in size, with single daughter buds. The attachment of these is broad in B. dermatitidis and rather hair-like in C. neoformans, where a thick capsule can also be seen. Coccidioidal spherules are recognized by the absence of budding and the large number of endospores.

Branching hyphae without budding are broad in appearance in Phycomycetes, somewhat more slender with septa in Aspergillus. The culture colonies also have certain characteristics which, however, usually require a mycologist for proper interpretation. Incubation with Sabouraud's is usually done at room temperature. Blood agar plates which should be inoculated simultaneously are incubated at 37°C. Growth occurs from two to fourteen days.

## IMMUNOLOGICAL PROCEDURES

The positive identification of fungal organisms in exudative tissue is frequently unachievable. Fortunately, a growing number of immunological procedures are available that can be performed on serum or spinal fluid. These, along with certain specific skin tests, give important epidemiological, diagnostic and, at times, prognostic information (Table 17).

TABLE 17: SEROLOGIC, IMMUNOLOGIC AND SKIN TESTS FOR THE PULMONARY MYCOSES

| DISEASE | TEST | VALUE |
|---|---|---|
| Aspergillosis | Skin | Helpful in allergic aspergillosis |
| | Agar gel double diffusion | Virtually diagnostic when positive in aspergilloma and allergic aspergillosis; no value in invasive aspergillosis |
| | Complement-fixation | Potential value in aspergilloma and allergic aspergillosis; patients with invasive disease are non-reactive |
| | Immunoelectrophoresis | Demonstrates antibody in patients with allergic aspergillosis, but not in those with invasive disease |
| Blastomycosis | Skin | None |
| | Agar gel double diffusion | If negative, is of no value; if positive, patient probably has blastomycosis |
| | Complement-fixation | If negative, is of no value; if positive in high or rising titer, patient probably has blastomycosis or another fungus infection |

| | Fluorescent antibody | Helpful in detection and identification of the fungus in cultures, clinical specimens and formalin-fixed tissues |
|---|---|---|
| Candidiasis | Skin | None |
| | Precipitating antibody | Positive reaction strongly suggestive of systemic candidosis |
| | Agglutinating antibody | Rising titers strongly suggestive of visceral candidosis; low titers found in normal persons and patients with superficial infections |
| | Fluorescent antibody | Useful in screening clinical specimens for some species, but not _Candida albicans_ |
| Coccidioidomycosis | Skin | Limited value (See text) |
| | Agar gel double diffusion (AGDD) | Negative reaction does not exclude coccidioidomycosis; positive reaction is virtually diagnostic; correlates with complement-fixation test |

Table 17 (cont'd)

| DISEASE | TEST | VALUE |
|---|---|---|
| | Complement-fixation (CF) | Negative reaction does not exclude diagnosis; positive reaction is strong presumptive evidence of coccidioidomy-cosis; cross reactions occur with his-toplasmosis; rising or falling titers are of prognostic value; useful in diagnosis of meningeal disease |
| | Tube precipitins (TP) | Useful for detection of early infections and relapse or spread of disease |
| | Latex particle agglutination (LPA) | Approximates tube precipitins in value |
| | Combination of AGDD and LPA tests | Reactive in 93% of cases, negative re-actions do not exclude; positive reactions are virtually diagnostic; false-positives occur |
| | Combination of CF and TP tests | Reactive in 83% of cases; negative re-actions do not exclude; positive reactions are virtually diagnostic; false-positives occur |

| | | |
|---|---|---|
| | Fluorescent antibody | Useful in detection and identification of fungi in cultures, clinical specimens and formalin-fixed tissues |
| Cryptococcosis | Latex agglutination | If negative, no value; if positive, virtually diagnostic; cross reacts with rheumatoid arthritis; titers are of prognostic value; useful in detecting cryptococcal meningitis |
| | Fluorescent antibody | Useful in detection and identification of fungi in cultures, clinical specimens and formalin-fixed tissues |
| Histoplasmosis | Skin | Useful in detecting recent infections in children; diagnostic value in adults is limited (see text for details) |
| | Complement-fixation (yeast form antigen) | If negative, does not rule out histoplasmosis but militates heavily against presence of chronic cavitary disease; less reliable with progressive disseminated forms; if positive in low titer, significance uncertain; if positive in high or |

Table 17 (cont'd)

| DISEASE | TEST | VALUE |
|---|---|---|
| | | rising titer, strong presumptive evidence of histoplasmosis or other fungal infection; titer fluctuations are of prognostic value |
| | Complement-fixation (mycelial form antigen) | Same general significance as yeast form complement-fixation; more likely to be elevated in chronic cavitary cases |
| | Histoplasmin latex agglutination | Unreliable in chronic cavitary cases, but useful in detecting acute primary infections |
| | Agar gel double diffusion | If positive, strong presumptive evidence of histoplasmosis; probably more specific than complement-fixation test, but cross reactions with blastomycosis and coccidioidomycosis may occur |
| | Fluorescent antibody | Useful to detect and identify this fungus in culture, clinical specimens and formalin-fixed tissues |

| | | |
|---|---|---|
| Paracoccidioidomycosis (South American blastomycosis) | Agar gel double diffusion | Highly specific; considered to be of both diagnostic and prognostic value |
| | Complement-fixation | A negative reaction militates heavily against the presence of paracoccidioidomycosis; positive reactions are virtually diagnostic; serial determinations are of prognostic value |
| Sporotrichosis | Agglutinating antibody | Promising diagnostic and prognostic value |
| | Agar gel double diffusion | Promising diagnostic and prognostic value |
| | Fluorescent antibody | Useful for detection and identification form of S. schenckii in clinical specimens and formalin-fixed tissues |

SKIN TESTS: While skin tests are the most commonly performed of these procedures, they are the least useful and the most over-interpreted. There is definite epidemiological value to skin testing in delineating an endemic area, establishing incidence and conversion rate, as well as a useful screening procedure for immunocompetence. However, in the diagnosis of a given clinical situation, skin tests are of very limited value;[0] only if the physician is able to witness a documented conversion of a recently negative skin test to positive, can a presumptive clinical diagnosis be entertained. Occasionally false-positive, and frequently false-negative skin tests confuse the diagnostic issues. Intercurrent disease, immunosuppression, age, infancy, along with technical factors involving both the manufacture and stability of material, as well as the technique of administration, make for much confusion. In addition, as in the case of Histoplasma, interference with future serologic procedures is produced by the injection intradermally of the skin test antigen.

## SKIN AND SEROLOGIC TESTS

INTRODUCTION: It must be emphasized again that the definitive diagnosis of fungus infection rests on identification of organisms in tissue or exudates, preferably by cultural means; morphologic recognition in smears, wet mounts and tissue sections are acceptable alternatives in experienced hands. Immunological methods, while never fully diagnostic, are frequently the most available and simplest way of arriving rapidly at a strongly presumptive diagnosis. As in all serological methods, it is particularly helpful if changing titers are encountered. Regarding skin tests, witnessing of a conversion from negative to positive by the clinician becomes strong presumptive evidence of recent infection. However, the greatest use of the skin test is as an epidemiological tool. There has been a trend in recent years as more skin tests become available to put too much diagnostic significance on either the presence or the absence of a positive reaction.[6] On the other hand, with greater understanding of the significance of cell-mediated immunity in the recovery from, and containment of, fungus infections, the skin test has recently assumed added significance as a marker of immunocompetence.

ASPERGILLOSIS: A skin test using Aspergillus (A.) fumigatus extracts is very useful in patients with allergic aspergillosis, producing the characteristic wheal and flare reaction, indicating type I and type III immunological response respectively in almost all cases. The Aspergillus fungus ball produces a positive skin test in less than one-fourth of the cases, with very little data being available of the use of the skin tests in invasive aspergillosis.

The immunological reactions in aspergillosis are of importance, since the diagnosis of any but the allergic form of the disease is difficult. Cultures are rarely positive even of bronchoscopy aspirates in aspergilloma cases. [7] On the other hand, direct examination and culture from sputum frequently gives positive results for Aspergillus that clinically may represent a false-positive. The fungi are found in the mouth of sputum of healthy patients, as well as those suffering from chronic bronchopulmonary suppuration, asthma or neoplasia. Aspergillosis can become a frequent colonizer in these situations without being a significant contributor to morbidity. Hence, immunologic tests that have recently been developed are most important. An agar gel double diffusion test is available for the demonstration of serum precipitins against aspergillosis species and has been found to be reliable. Precipitins are found in all patients with fungus ball and 70% of those with the allergic forms. False-positive tests can occur in controls: in a recent series, 39% of patients with pulmonary tuberculosis had a positive reaction. Nevertheless, strong presumption exists when precipitins are found in a patient. This test is of no value in invasive aspergillosis, nor are complement-fixation tests, immunoelectrophoresis or indirect fluorescence tests. [8]

BLASTOMYCOSIS: The previously available blastomycin skin testing material has been withdrawn from the market. Large numbers of false-positive, as well as false-negative, tests made it useless, both as a clinical and as an epidemiological tool. Research along these lines, however, is continuing, and hopefully another dermal antigen will soon be available. Recent work by Sarosi [9] suggests that this disease is more prevalent than suspected, and a good skin test is needed for epidemiological purposes.

The complement-fixation test for the yeast phase antigen of Blastomyces dermatitidis has been available for some years. However, there are many false-negative tests and thus a negative reaction does not exclude active disease. However, titers of 1:8 are quite indicative of active clinical disease; below this level, cross reactions have been seen with both Histoplasma and Coccidioides. This indicates the need for repeated samples in patients with low titers. More recently, the agar gel double diffusion test has come into use and shows greater specificity, with 70% reacting positively. A fluorescent antibody reagent has been developed and promises to be of help in demonstrating yeast forms and culture, as well as fresh preparations and in tissue.

CANDIDIASIS: Skin testing extract of <u>Candida albicans</u> has been commercially available for many years, producing an immediate reaction in one-third, and a delayed reaction in over half of normal people and, therefore, this method has no diagnostic value. It has been used for many years as a non-specific marker of cell-mediated immunity.

Candida precipitins are found only in patients with active, and probably invasive, systemic disease. Rising titers, therefore, or precipitins, are indicative of active disease.

See Chapter 28 for details on diagnosing Candidiasis.

COCCIDIOIDOMYCOSIS (Figs. 29-38): The coccidioidin skin test, made from the mycelial phase of the organism was developed by Smith[10] and has been in routine use for the past thirty years. It is a useful and reliable material. While it is probably the most specific of all the fungal skin tests, there are cross reactions with histoplasmosis, which occasionally cause clinical problems. The diagnostic value is limited by the considerations previously discussed, but recently, its use as an immunological marker has become important. The Mantoux technique is used with injection of one-tenth mg. of a 1:100 dilution usually. The reaction is read in 36 to 48 hours, and an area of induration of 5 mm. or more is considered a positive test. No stimulation of complement-fixing antibodies in the serum occurs. False-negative tests can be seen in patients with pulmonary cavities who are otherwise demonstrated to be immunocompetent.

Another skin test material developed by Stevens and Levine[11] is spherulin. As its name implies, it is derived from the parasitic phase of the organism. As might be expected, the yields have been considerably higher; well-controlled studies show 38% of patients reacting to spherulin without reacting to the standard coccidioidin.[11] The occasional cross reactions with histoplasmosis also occur. This material is commercially available and is recommended as the skin test material of first choice.

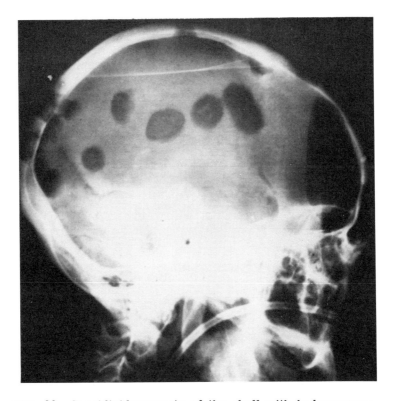

FIG. 29: Coccidioidomycosis of the skull with hydropneumo-
cephalus. Note the lytic lesion in the skull in a Negro
male. The holes were initially mistaken for burr
holes. The nodular swelling on the top of the calvarium is due to Omaya reservoir.

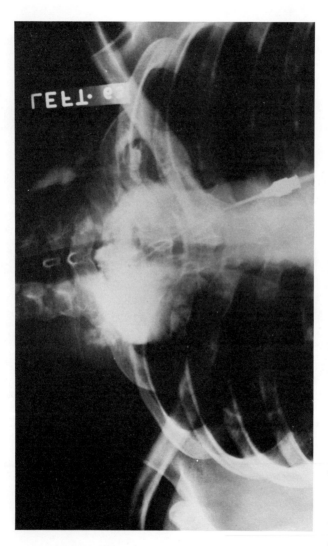

FIG. 30: A case of empyema necessitatis due to coccidioidomycotic infection of the lung. When a contrast material was injected into the abscess cavity on the chest wall, it escaped into the apices of both lungs and the root of the neck.

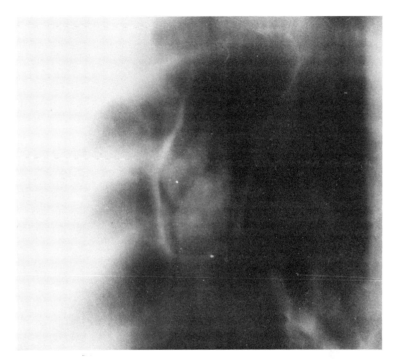

FIG. 31: The same patient as in Fig. 30, demonstrating a cavity with a "fungus ball" several months later, by which time the empyema healed. On lobectomy, he was found to have a fungus ball due to Coccidioides immitis. Further, Clostridium ramosum and Peptococcus were also isolated from the pus. (Figs. 31-34 are reproduced with kind permission from Thadepalli, H. , Rambuatla, K. , Salem, F. , Mandal, A.K. and Einstein, M. Pulmonary Mycetoma due to Coccidioides immitis. Chest 71: 429-430, 1977.)

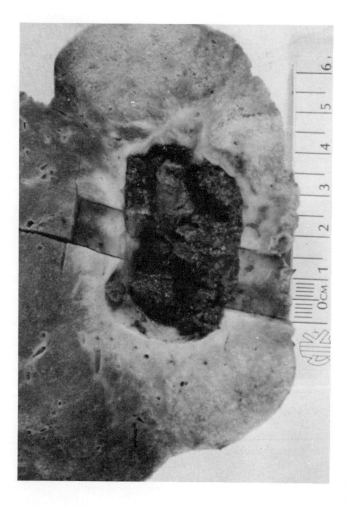

FIG. 32: Section of lung showing cavity lesion filled with pasty brown, grumous material (fungus ball). The surrounding lung parenchyma is indurated.

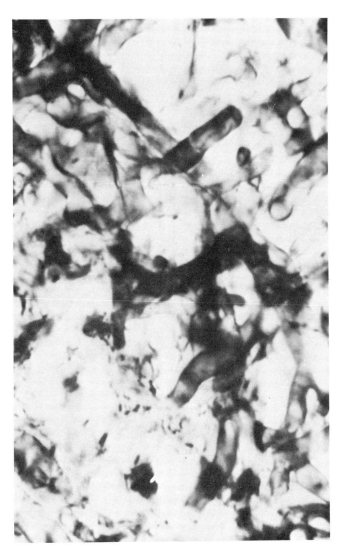

FIG. 33: Section of wall of cavity (shown in Fig. 32 and containing fungus ball) showing heavily and lightly stained hyphae with adjacent and superimposed microorganisms.

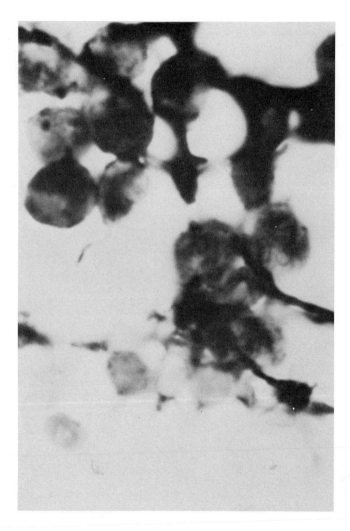

FIG. 34: Area adjacent to Fig. 33, showing spherules of coccidioidomycosis. Gomori methenamine silver stain.

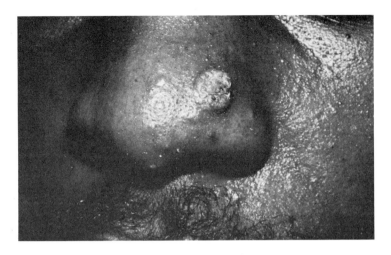

FIG. 35: Cutaneous coccidioidomycosis of tip of nose showing raised granular granulomatous ulceration of the skin.

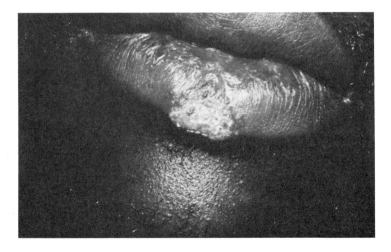

FIG. 36: Cutaneous coccidioidomycosis of lower lip showing raised granular granulomatous ulceration of the skin.

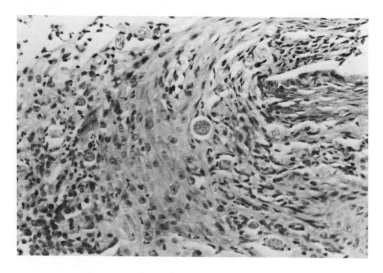

FIG. 37: Section of cutaneous lesion of coccidioidomycosis showing granulomatous inflammation and Coccidioides immitis spherules.

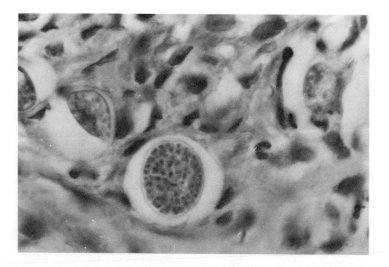

FIG. 38: Higher magnification showing the large, thick-walled spherules of Coccidioides immitis with endospores.

The coccidioidal complement-fixation and precipitin tests are the most generally available and best standardized of all the fungal serological procedures. They are performed by many public and commercial laboratories with good reliability and reproducibility. Precipitins are seen early in the disease within one to three weeks, but they do not stay very long and quantitatively have no prognostic significance. Their absence should never rule out the diagnosis of coccidioidomycosis. A tube precipitin test is commercially available as a rapid screening procedure for office and clinic use, but has the problem of considerable number of false-positive reactions. Complement-fixing antibodies appear somewhat later - usually two to four weeks after onset of clinical illness. This test is very reliable and is reproducible, using either coccidioidin or spherulin as the antigen. Quantitative titers are important and carry prognostic significance. Titers of 1:64 or above should raise suspicion that dissemination may be occurring, although a titer alone never makes the diagnosis of metapulmonary dissemination, since severe pneumonias can be seen with significantly elevated serum titers. [10] On the other hand, titers in the very high ranges of 1:264 and above almost always indicate involvement outside the thorax. Titers gradually come down over a period of months as the patient improves, but can persist in low dilutions much longer than the clinical illness. Relapses are marked occasionally by recurrence of precipitins and invariably by secondary or tertiary rises in the complement-fixing antibody level. False-negative serological titers are seen in some cases of cavitary pulmonary disease.

Complement-fixation titers should also be done on spinal fluid in suspected cases of meningitis; frequently, this is the only way of making the diagnosis, since positive cultures are obtained in not more than 20% of cases. A titer of any magnitude is important in the cerebrospinal fluid and usually indicates active meningitis. The only exceptions are the presence of paraspinous disease, which occasionally can give a low titer in the absence of meningitis. Also, recently, Pappagianis[12] has described the detection of serum antibodies in concentrated spinal fluids in patients with high serological titers, but no evidence of meningitis. This dilemma can occasionally be resolved by performing the colloidal gold test which, in coccidioidal meningitis, quite early shows a strong first zone reaction, whereas in the absence of meningitis, even when a low level of complement-fixation titer is present, the colloidal gold curve is flat. [13]

An agar gel double diffusion test has been developed by Huppert and Baily,[14] with a latex particle agglutination test as a corollary for a rapid detection of complement-fixing antibodies and precipitins respectively. Both of these are available and quite reliable in the case of the diffusion test, less so in the case of the particle agglutination test. However, using both tests in conjunction, a 93% accuracy can be obtained. These tests are useful, rapid screening procedures which, however, should always be followed by the conventional complement-fixation test. A counterimmunoelectrophoresis test of high specificity and quantitative value has recently been developed. [15]

Fluorescent antibody techniques are available for the study of Coccidioides immitis. However, the specificity of the procedure has not been fully satisfactory with cross reactions to both Histoplasma capsulatum and Blastomyces dermatitidis, as well as other fungi occurring. Manipulations of these procedures have increased specificity, and much work in this field is continuing.

CRYPTOCOCCOSIS (Figs 39-42): No commercially available skin test for cryptococcosis exists, nor does there appear to be one forthcoming. This will hopefully change, because this disease, like blastomycosis, undoubtedly is more prevalent than has been recognized, and a skin test would be a very useful epidemiological tool for studying its incidence, ecology and natural history.

Antigens have recently been developed for the study of the serological reaction of cryptococcosis. The indirect fluorescent antibody test is the most useful. A tube agglutination test for the detection of antigen is also available, as is a latex agglutination test. All three procedures should be performed, if possible. Some patients show antibody response, others show antigen reaction, and some both. A 95% agreement with cultural studies can be shown when all three tests are performed.

The latex agglutination test, while less specific, is the most sensitive. Rheumatoid arthritis has been the only major cross reactor in patients with rheumatoid factor in their serum. In its absence, a positive reaction is highly suggestive of the diagnosis of cryptococcosis. There is some prognostic value to this test also. Cerebrospinal fluid may show 71% positivity in cultural proven disease by the latex agglutination technique. The immunofluorescent antibody test is not positive in spinal fluid, but is 80% specific in non-meningeal disease with false-positive reactions occurring in patients with blastomycosis, histoplasmosis and other fungal infections. It may also simply reflect

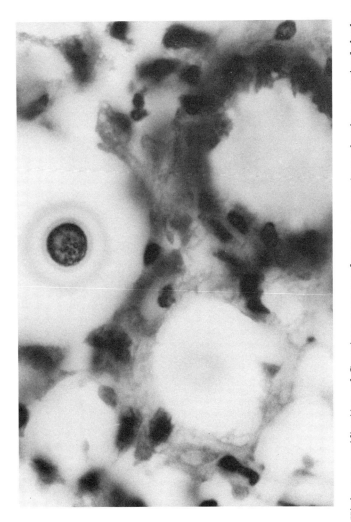

FIG. 39: Higher magnification of Cryptococcus neoformans organisms having a central dark portion and a prominent gelatinous capsule, creating a clear halo around the Cryptococcus.

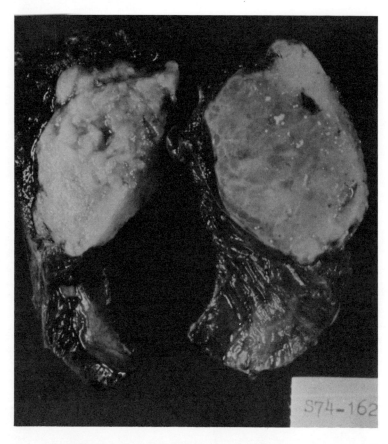

FIG. 40: Hemisectioned portion of a lung lobe showing a sub-
pleural "cryptococcoma" appearing as a well-defined,
solitary nodule having a granular, mucoid-cut surface.

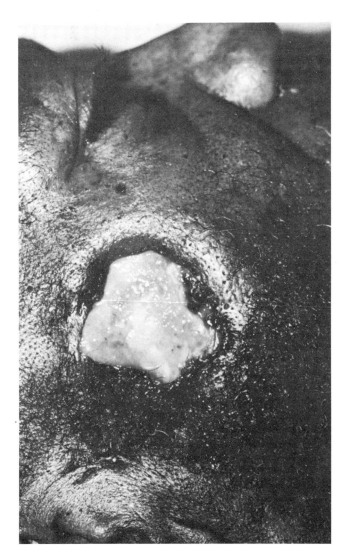

FIG. 41:  Cryptococcal skin ulcer in the region of the right parotid showing a gelatinous, necrotic base and elevated anterior margins.

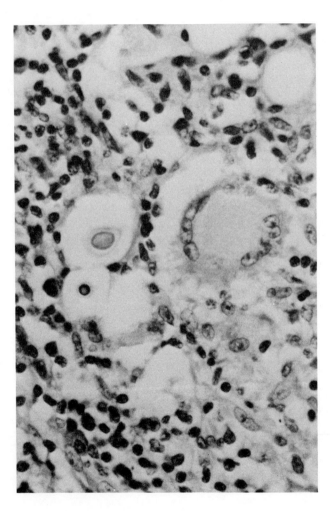

FIG. 42: Section of the same lung as Fig. 40 showing two organisms of Cryptococcus neoformans sur-rounded by a chronic granulomatous inflammation of lymphocytes, histiocytes and a multi-nucleated giant cell seen at the lower mid-part.

past cryptococcal infection and, therefore, evidence offered by
this test must be considered as presumptive only for clinically
active disease. Immunofluorescent techniques for tissue identification are available.

HISTOPLASMOSIS: The histoplasmin skin test has been widely
used for many years. It is virtually of no diagnostic value because of a high incidence of skin test reactivity, up to 90% of
people who have resided in an endemic area. Consequently, it
is of value only in such situations as pinpointing the nature of
pulmonary calcification in a tuberculin-negative individual, in
the identification of a pulmonary lesion in a recent casual visi-
tor to an endemic area and, again, during the witnessing of a
conversion, as discussed previously. There are false-positive
reactions in individuals previously infected with blastomycosis
and coccidioidomycosis, as well as to a wide variety of non-
pathogenic organisms. False-negative reactions are seen in the
majority of patients with progressive disseminated histoplasmosis. The stimulation of complement-fixing antibodies by the
skin test antigen needs to be re-emphasized at this point. The
skin test has some value in young children. Rising titers are of
significance prognostically, particularly since it has not been
reported that skin testing affects the yeast phase titer.

Complement-fixation tests are available with two antigens, the
mycelial and the yeast forms of Histoplasma capsulatum. [16]
The yeast phase is somewhat more sensitive.

In the acute primary form of the disease, yeast phase antigen
can be seen after an incubation period of two to three weeks.
The mycelial phase antibody develops somewhat later and titers
tend to be lower; the chronic cavitary form of histoplasmosis
develops higher mycelial phase titers, as might be expected.
Positive serological results have been observed in 97% of patients during the primary form and in all patients during the
chronic cavitary stage of the disease, when the sputum was culturally positive. When only histological confirmation is available, these figures are much lower. In progressive disseminated histoplasmosis, the complement-fixation reactions are
positive in only 60% to 80% of cases.

Positive titers are not usually considered diagnostic until they
reach a level of 1:16 or greater, since lower levels at times
represent false-positive values, or may represent an "immunological memory" of ancient infection. Again, rising titer is significant. However, occasionally, false-positive titers in 1:16
or above have been seen with coccidioidomycosis, blastomycosis,

cryptococcosis and other fungal infections, as well as in healthy people, patients with carcinoma and as a result of a histoplasmin skin test done previously. Twelve to twenty-seven per cent of patients show this type of reaction after skin testing, although usually in titers somewhat lower than 1:16. This is detected after fifteen days and may persist for as long as three months. Yeast phase titers also have occurred occasionally. The more virulent the skin test reaction, the higher the titer thus induced. For this reason, when histoplasmosis is suspected, blood should be drawn prior to performing the skin test. But even this precaution does not fully resolve the dilemma if the initial serology sample is obtained too early in the disease.

The level of complement-fixing titers in histoplasmosis, as in coccidioidomycosis, is significant, but very high titers have been seen without dissemination having occurred and, therefore, interpretation has to be based on careful clinical correlation. [17] If, after a period of months, the titer has leveled off at a certain point, usually 1:32 or above, without coming down after several months, a chronic, perhaps cavitary, pulmonary or extrapulmonary lesion should be suspected. As with coccidioidomycosis, recurrence of titer elevations suggests relapse or progression.

A histoplasmin latex agglutination test and an agar gel double diffusion test are available, although the latter is not yet being marketed commercially. These tests are indicative of primary acute infections, but have less value in the chronic, active or disseminated stages of the disease. The agar gel double diffusion tests, both the yeast and the mycelial phase antigen, are used and a double band is thus seen. The H band is the more specific, since it is less influenced by skin testing and tends to be positive in active, as well as progressive, disease. Immunofluorescence is used in the detection of H. capsulatum in culture and clinical specimen, as well as in tissue. It can also demonstrate antibodies in serum of the yeast form, but not as yet of the mycelial phase. As in coccidioidomycosis, counterimmunoelectrophoresis is simple, highly specific, and will undoubtedly have more application in the future.

PARACOCCIDIOIDOMYCOSIS: Skin tests with culture filtrates and polysaccharide fractions are being carried out by workers in South America, with reactivity approaching 100%. The material is not yet commercially available, and the diagnostic value has not been fully clarified.

An agar gel double diffusion precipitin test is available and highly specific. [18] The precipitins appear early in the disease, as they do with most fungal diseases, and can be found in the sera of virtually all patients. There is a quantitative relationship with the precipitin band being more intense in patients with severe disease and vice versa. Complement-fixing antibodies appear somewhat later and remain longer, and they are also positive in the vast majority of patients.

Localized disease produces low complement-fixation titers with disseminated lesions showing higher levels. Levels below 1:5 are considered not to indicate active disease and have been described as a "serologic scar". Titers of 1:10 or above are definitely indicative of activity. Recurrence of precipitins and complement-fixation titer rises suggests relapse. Fluorescent antibody techniques are available, but only through special laboratories.

SPOROTRICHOSIS: Sporotrichin, prepared from heat-killed yeast phase in a dilution of 1:1,000, is a very specific skin test, becoming positive as early as the first day after the appearance of skin lesions and remaining positive for long periods of time. This is not as yet commercially available, but promises to be useful.

Agglutination and immunodiffusion tests are available in sporotrichosis and appear to be of value, both diagnostically and prognostically. [19] Fluorescent antibody tests are developed for the tissue form of S. schenckii in exudate and cultures. They can also be used to stain the mycelial form.

PHYCOMYCOSIS (mucormycosis): Phycomycosis is a generally opportunistic infection caused by fungi of the class of Phycomycetes. The organisms are widespread and found in soil, manure, vegetables, wastes and elsewhere in nature. The infection is most commonly associated with diabetic acidosis, also with burns, malnourishment, leukemia, lymphoma and immunosuppression. The disease appears in various forms with the rhinocerebral form being the most common and serious. Pulmonary cases have also been seen. Entry is usually through the sinuses where orbital and paranasal disease is seen, as well as ulcers of the mouth and soft palate. From there, the fungus travels along nerve sheaths into the brain. This produces a rather characteristic clinical appearance of sinusitis, with purulent and bloody discharge from the nares, necrosis of the hard or soft palate with swelling of the bridge of the nose, facial paresis and ptosis. This is followed by localizing neurological

signs. The diagnosis is difficult to establish, since no serological procedures are available and sinusoidal, bronchial or
pulmonary biopsies are the only way of demonstrating it. [20]
The disease is rapidly progressive, and early and accurate
diagnosis depends on a high index of suspicion within the setting of the presentation of the case. The fungus shows characteristic broad non-septate hyphae, which are seen in tissue.

MYCETOMA: Mycetoma is a localized chronic deforming
swelling, usually of a foot or hand. Cutaneous and subcutaneous
tissue is involved with frequent sinus tracts. The common term
is madura foot. The lesion can be caused by a number of organisms, including several of the Actinomycetes. The most
common fungus causing this is Allescheria boydii, recently re-
named with the generic name, Petriellidium. [21] These are sap-
rophytic infections world-wide in their distribution. The organisms are found in the soil and can also be planned pathogens
which reside on vegetable debris and gain entrance through
abrasions into the skin. Non-dermatological cases have also
been reported, involving most frequently the lung. The diagnosis is most commonly made on direct examination of pus or
histologically. Culturally, a biopsy will usually grow the organisms also. There are no serological procedures of major
reliability, although recently, precipitin lines were established
in the sera of some patients, using gel diffusion techniques. This
will probably become more generally available and reliable in
the future. The cultural isolation is usually not difficult, since
the organism grows rapidly and shows a grossly characteristic
fluffy white aerial mycelium. The microscopic appearance shows
granules with septate hyphae on direct examination. The conidia
which are ovoid, light brown spores, occur at the ends of the
hyphae, singly or in groups of up to five. In tissue, differentiation between Petriellidium and Aspergillus species is difficult at times; the cultural differentiation becomes critical in
these cases.

## SUMMARY

A recent statement by the Committee on Fungus Diseases of the
American College of Chest Physicians regarding skin testing,
which is so commonly done by practicing physicians, yet has
such limited value, is appropriate at this time. [22] "The one
factor which exists needlessly and is most surely within the
power of the clinician to control, is the previously emphasized
adverse affect of the use of skin test antigens commercially
available; coccidioidin, histoplasmin and blastomycin. These
adverse affects include:

1) Falsely negative skin test reactions due to inert antigen
2) Falsely negative reactions due to cutaneous allergy in elderly patients, those with disseminated disease, those with complicating disorders such as measles and lack of reactivity resulting from unknown causes
3) Falsely positive reactions due to a general lack of specificity
4) Obscuring or altering the results of serological testing

"This criticism in no way denigrates the use of skin testing with certain preparations as an epidemiologic tool. The condemnation lies in skin testing as a hindrance to diagnosis and as a diversion from proper mycological studies of the ill patient".

With the ever-increasing array of immunological and cultural techniques, as well as improvement in histological staining, the diagnosis of fungal diseases is within the grasp of the average practitioner. At a time when the incidence of diseases is increasing, when more and more patients are being subjected to immunosuppression, as well as to increasingly invasive in-hospital procedures, fungus diseases will become, perhaps, more common ultimately than bacterial infections. World-wide travel contributes to this development. A detailed drug, procedure, hospitalization and travel history is a sine qua non for intelligent medical diagnosis. While the development of effective therapeutic agents has lagged far behind, we are beginning to see a broadening of a therapeutic approach, which hopefully will make accurate diagnosis of fungus diseases as mandatory for intelligent treatment, as has occurred in bacteriology. There exists now a need for accurate mycological diagnosis, and the tools are available.

## REFERENCES

1. Mycoses Surveillance, No. 3, Center for Disease Control, PSH, Dept. Health, Education and Welfare, Pub. No. (HSM) 72-8115, 1972.

2. Hammerman, K. J., Powell, K. E., Tosh, F. E.: The incidence of hospitalized cases of systemic mycotic infections. Sabouraudia 12:33, 1974.

3. Adiseshan, N. E., Oliver, W. A.: Strontium Lung Scans in the Diagnosis of Pulmonary Aspergillosis. Am. Rev. Resp. Dis. 108:441, 1973.

4. Lonky, S. A. , et al: Acute coccidioidal pleural effusion. Am. Rev. Resp. Dis. 114:681, 1976.

5. Patersen, E. A. , et al: Coccidioidouria: Clinical significance. Ann. Int. Med. 85:34, 1976.

6. Buechner, H. A. , et al: The current status of serologic, immunologic and skin tests in the diagnosis of pulmonary mycoses. Chest 63:259, 1973.

7. Young, R. C. , et al: Aspergillosis: The spectrum of the disease in 98 patients. Medicine 49:147, 1970.

8. Meyer, R. D. , et al: Aspergillosis complicating neoplastic disease. Am. J. Med. 54:6, 1973.

9. Sarosi, G. A. , et al: Clinical features of acute pulmonary blastomycosis. New. Eng. J. Med. 290:540, 1974.

10. Smith, C. E. , Saito, M. T. , Simons, S. A.: Pattern of 39,500 serologic tests in coccidioidomycosis. J. A. M. A. 160:546, 1956.

11. Stevens, D. A. , et al: Spherulin in clinical coccidioidomycosis. Chest 68:69, 1975.

12. Pappagianis, D. , Saito, M. T. , Van Hoosear, K. H.: Antibody in cerebrospinal fluid in non-meningitic coccidioidomycosis. Sabouraudia 10:173, 1972.

13. Einstein, H. E.: Coccidioidomycosis of the central nervous system. Advances in Neurology 6:101, 1974.

14. Huppert, M. , Baily, J. W.: The use of immunodiffusion tests in coccidioidomycosis. Amer. J. Clin. Path. 44: 364, 1965.

15. Aguilar-Torres, F. G. , et al: Counterimmunoelectrophoresis in the detection of antibodies against Coccidioides immitis. Ann. Int. Med. 85:740, 1976.

16. Kaufman, L.: Serology of systemic fungus diseases. Public Health Rep. 81:177, 1966.

17. Saslaw, S. , Prior, J. A.: The relationship of proved histoplasmosis to histoplasmin skin sensitivity in Ohio. Ohio State Med. J. 48:229, 1959.

18. Restrepo, A. , Greer, D. L. , Vasconcellos, M. : Para-coccidioidomycosis: A review. Rev. Med. Vet. Myc. 8:97, 1973.

19. Roberts, G. D. , Larsh, H. W. : The serologic diagnosis of extracutaneous sporotrichosis. Am. J. Clin. Path. 56: 597, 1971.

20. Brown, J. F. , Gottlieb, L. S. , McCormick, R. A. : Pul-monary and rhinocerebral mucormycosis. Arch. Int. Med. 137:936, 1977.

21. Lutwick, L. I. , et al: Visceral fungal infections due to Petriellidium boydii. Am. J. Med. 61:632, 1976.

22. Utz, J. P. , et al: The pulmonary mycoses: Diagnostic and therapeutic guidelines. Am. Coll. Chest Phys. Chicago, Ill. , 1976.

23. Conant, N. F. , et al: Manual of Clinical Mycology, 3rd Edition, W. B. Saunders, Philadelphia, 1971.

24. Emmons, C. W. , Binford, C. H. , Utz, J. P. : Medical Mycology, 3rd Edition, Lea & Febiger, Philadelphia, 1977.

25. Pan American Health Organization: Mycoses. Pan Ameri-can Health Organization, Washington, D. C. , 1975.

26. Rippon, J. W. : Medical Mycology: The Pathogenic Fungi and the Pathogenic Actinomycetes. W. B. Saunders, Phil-adelphia, 1974.

## 28: CANDIDIASIS
by H. Thadepalli

Candidiasis is caused by the fungus, Candida albicans. There are other species of Candida (C. ), namely, C. stellatoidea, C. parapsilosis, C. guilliermondi, C. krusei and C. tropicales. They may cause superficial or deep mycosis. The superficial mycotic lesions include mucocutaneous candidiasis.

## SKIN LESIONS

Systemic Candida infections may lead to macular, nodular lesions,[1] which are firm, raised nodules of size 0.5 to 1 cm. in diameter, hemorrhagic, and most of them are well-circumscribed and somewhat pinkish. Some of these lesions may appear maculopapular. In one study, 31% of 320 cases of skin infections were identified to be due to yeast organisms. [2] Other skin infections may include the intertriginous lesions that appear in the skin folds, under the breasts, in the groin, peri-anal areas and the axillae. These are maculopapular pruritic lesions. Paronychia can be caused by candidiasis, by infection of the nails. Occasionally, candidiasis can be generalized.

## THRUSH

Thrush is a condition of moniliasis of the mouth and tongue; occasionally, it may extend down into the esophagus and the rest of the gastrointestinal tract. It may present as multiple, patchy white lesions on the tongue; occasionally the entire papilla of the tongue may be denuded and appear like a rubbery tongue. Sometimes, there is hypertrophy of the papilla associated with glossitis, and if the patient is a heavy smoker, the tongue may appear black and hairy. Other mucosal involvements of Candida include perleche, which is an angular stomatitis secondary to riboflavin deficiency superinfected with Candida, and occasionally peri-anal infections.

The thrush syndrome may occasionally be caused by bacteria instead of moniliasis, especially in cases of patients who have had renal transplants. It can be caused by Staphylococcus, Streptococcus or Lactobacillus, occasionally coliforms. This condition may become worse, especially during the acute rejection phase of the transplanted kidney. Esophagitis may be diagnosed by endoscopy, wherein white, plaque-like areas may be seen in the mucosa of the esophagus, which can be scraped. Esophagoscopy should be performed in cases where there is a complaint of dysphagia with signs of moniliasis and positive serum Candida antibody titers of 1:160 or greater.[3]

## VULVOVAGINAL CANDIDIASIS

Candida is normal flora of 25% to 50% of women. Certain diseases, like diabetes, hypoparathyroidism, impaired host defense mechanisms, or patients who are on broad-spectrum antibiotics and those who are on oral contraceptives, tend to increasingly colonize with Candida. It may cause vulvovaginitis, with a white discharge, pruritis, symptoms mostly beginning before the onset of menses, occasionally associated with dyspareunia and dysuria. The diagnosis can be established by the physical examination and KOH preparations, Gram's stains, and Pap smears occasionally. The diagnostic yield for candidiasis by Pap smear is not very satisfactory. It may be positive in only 10% to 20% of the cases. Indirect immunofluorescence test has been used for the diagnosis of vaginal candidiasis, which was found to be unreliable. [4]

## DEEP MYCOSIS CAUSED BY CANDIDIASIS

Systemic candidiasis can occur in patients who are chronically ill, those who have had cardiac surgery or surgery on the gastrointestinal tract, renal transplant recipients, patients who have long-term intravenous catheters or hyperalimentation, prolonged antibiotic and broad-spectrum antibiotic therapy, immunosuppressive therapy, heroin addiction, patients who are on indwelling Foley's catheters, and those who are on long-term corticosteroid therapy. Systemic candidiasis may manifest as infection of the eye, bronchomoniliasis, pulmonary candidiasis, endocarditis, septicemia, meningitis, renal infection, peritonitis and, rarely, arthritis and osteomyelitis.

OCULAR CANDIDIASIS: The eye grounds must be examined in all patients who are suspected to be having deep mycosis. It is not unusual to see retinal involvement in patients who had chronic systemic candidiasis. Mostly, patients on systemic antibiotics with an indwelling intravenous catheter are prone to this complication. They may complain of blurring of vision, or spots before the eyes, occasionally pain around the eyes. A funduscopy examination may reveal focal glistening white mold-like lesions, seemingly on the surface of the retina, quite similar in appearance to the colony of Candida on the blood agar plate. [5] Occasionally, the lesions may appear in the intravitreous area. It may cause anterior uveitis, blepharitis, conjunctivitis and keratitis. Almost all species of Candida have been reported at one time or another causing ocular manifestations. [6, 7, 8] Ocular candidiasis is almost always secondary to systemic septicemia.

BRONCHOPULMONARY MONILIASIS: Bronchopulmonary moniliasis may manifest as bronchial moniliasis or pulmonary moniliasis. Bronchial moniliasis is an occupational disease of the tea tasters, referred to as "tea tasters cough" in Ceylon, Sri Lanka. Cough is the most distressing symptom of this disease. When it involves the lung, it may present with low-grade fever, cough and patchy infiltrates in the lung. Physical examination and the roentgenographic examination may be suggestive of bronchial pneumonia manifested with diffuse nodular densities on the pulmonary roentgenogram.

ENDOCARDITIS: See page 293.

SEPTICEMIA: The incidence of septicemia due to Candida is on the increase, mostly because of the predisposing factors that are already mentioned. There may be no clinical signs for the underlying septicemia other than ocular infiltrates. Yeast cells in the urine may be seen in systemic septicemia.

CANDIDIASIS OF THE URINARY TRACT: Candida albicans can involve the urinary tract frequently causing cystitis, secondary to chronic indwelling catheter associated with broad-spectrum antibiotic therapy. Torulopsis renal infection is often predisposed by diabetes mellitus, urinary tract obstruction or previous urological surgery. It may be associated with septicemia.

MENINGITIS: Meningitis is a rare manifestation of systemic candidiasis. The steroid therapy following neural surgery is the most frequent predisposing cause for Candida meningitis.

ARTHRITIS: This is a rare manifestation of Candida disease; it may follow transient Candida tropicales fungaemia. [9] Coccidioidomycosis is the most common fungal disease that affects the knee joint in North America, followed by blastomycosis, cryptococcosis and histoplasmosis.

OSTEOMYELITIS: This is also a rare disease, but it is peculiar to heroin addicts nowadays. [10] In a majority of cases in recent years, Candida osteomyelitis with hematogenous dissemination has been described in heroin addicts.

## DIAGNOSIS

BLOOD CULTURES: They are often positive in patients who have systemic candidiasis. Blood culture should be obtained in brain heart infusion broth with or without additional sucrose added. Higher recovery rate is reported when the culture bottles are vented. Biphasic medium, which contains brain heart infusion broth and brain heart infusion agar slant, apparently yields the best culture results. [11,12,13] Detection of fungaemia can be significantly improved with the use of biphasic medium.

BLOOD SMEARS: Examination of blood smears obtained from the catheter tip may be rewarding when blood cultures are negative or pending. It has been demonstrated that blastospores and pseudohyphae of Candida albicans can be seen from the blood from the CVP catheters. Smears of peripheral blood may also be a useful tool for the rapid diagnosis of systemic infections caused by both bacteria and fungi. [14,15]

SCRAPINGS: Scrapings and smears of the suspected lesions, and occasionally, biopsy specimens of the skin nodules, can be obtained for the detection of fungi by smears and cultures. Ten per cent KOH is added for the smears obtained from mucocutaneous lesions to eliminate most of the cells other than the Candida, which helps in delineating the Candida better. However, this has a disadvantage in vulvovaginal lesions, wherein Trichomonas vaginalis may be associated with it and may be destroyed by the KOH preparation.

GRAM'S STAINS: They may be done on these smears when the yeast organisms appear as ovoid bodies of size 2 to $5\mu$ with pseudohyphae, the diameter of which is about the same as the yeast organism.

ANIMAL INOCULATION: Rabbits may be injected with 1% saline suspension of the specimen and die within a period of four to five days with multiple abscesses in both kidneys. They can be examined for Candida organisms.

SEROLOGICAL TESTS FOR CANDIDIASIS: Precise diagnosis of Candida infection, is important, because amphotericin B, treatment for these infections, is toxic. The patient with invasive candidiasis may have no accessible tissue for examination. Most serological tests for candidiasis are based on the serotype A, Candida albicans, which is more common than serotype B.

To have a positive serological test for candidiasis, an antecedent antigenemia or antibodies must be present. Based upon these principles, various diagnostic procedures have been used.

a) Agar gel diffusion test (AGD): AGD may be positive in 85% of the cases of disseminated candidiasis. False-positive results can occur in 5%. A positive AGD and a positive counterimmunoelectrophoresis test, together, are diagnostic of deep-seated candidiasis. [16]

b) Counterimmunoelectrophoresis (CIE): CIE is positive in 90% of those patients with disseminated candidiasis. False-positive results can occur in less than 3%. A positive CIE test and the whole cell agglutination test, greater than 1:256 together, are diagnostic of candidiasis. A negative precipitin by CIE and whole cell agglutination test, antibody titer of less than 1:256, together, exclude the diagnosis of invasive candidiasis.[17,18]

c) Whole cell agglutination (AGGL) test: The test results vary from one laboratory to another. AGGL was found to be falsely positive in patients who had vulvovaginitis. False-positives occur in less than 15%. A titer of 1:80 or more is highly suggestive of invasive candidiasis. A negative AGGL test excludes the possibility of disseminated candidiasis.

d) Latex agglutination test (LAT): The false-positives and true-positives with this test are about the same as the AGGL test. The value of this test in the diagnosis of disseminated candidiasis has not been well established.

e) Mannan antigenemia: By hemagglutination inhibition assay, the surface antigen of the Candida, mannan, can be detected in cases of suspected disseminated candidiasis. A positive test is considered to be an early and a specific signal of invasive disease. Episodes of mannan antigenemia are followed by the production of anti-mannan antibodies. These antibodies can be detected in nearly one-third of the cases of invasive Candida infections, therefore, detection of mannan is specific for the diagnosis of invasive candidiasis.[19] The mannan antigen antibody test may not be positive in all cases of disseminated candidiasis. This test is not in common use. But, if proved reliable, this test may be useful. It becomes positive before the cultures becomes positive, thus signalling the physician to initiate proper and immediate therapy.

A positive CIE test and AGD test together indicate deep or disseminated candidiasis, whereas a negative AGGL test may exclude this disease.[20]

## REFERENCES

1. Bodey, G. I. , Luna, M. : Skin lesions associated with disseminated candidiasis. J. A. M. A. 229:1466, 1974.

2. Monohar, V. , Sirsi, M. , Ramananda Rao, G. : Yeasts in superficial mycosis. I. Incidence, isolation and characterization. Indian J. Med. Res. 63:261, 1975.

3. Baroukh, E. K. , et al: Candida esophagitis. Gastroenterology 71:715, 1976.

4. Warnock, D. W. , Hilton, A. L. : Value of the indirect immunofluorescence test in the diagnosis of vaginal candidiasis. Brit. J. Vener. Dis. 52:187, 1976.

5. Francois, J. , Rysselaere, M. : Oculomycoses. Charles C Thomas, Springfield, pp. 283-332, 1972.

6. Fishman, L. S. , et al: Hematogenous Candida endophthalmitis - A complication of candidemia. New Eng. J. Med. 286:675, 1972.

7. Edwards, J. E. , et al: Ocular manifestations of Candida septicemia: Review of seventy-six cases of hematogenous Candida endophthalmitis. Medicine 53:47, 1974.

8. Segal, E. , et al: Yeasts associated with ocular infections. Mycopathologia Mycologia Applicata 54:31, 1974.

9. Murray, H. W. , Fialk, M. A. , Roberts, R. B. : Candida arthritis. Am. J. Med. 60:587, 1976.

10. Edwards, J. E. , et al: Hematogenous Candida osteomyelitis. Am. J. Med. 59:89, 1975.

11. Roberts, G. D., Washington, J. A. II: Detection of fungi in blood cultures. J. Clin. Microbiol. 1:309, 1975.

12. Braunstein, H., Tomasulo, M.: A quantitative study of the growth of Candida albicans in vented and unvented blood culture bottles. J. Clin. Path. 66:87, 1976.

13. Roberts, G. D., Horstmeier, C. D., Ilstrup, D. M.: Evaluation of a hypertonic sucrose medium for the detection of fungi in blood cultures. J. Clin. Microbiol. 4:110, 1976.

14. Portnoy, J., et al: Candida blastospores and pseudohyphae in blood smears. New Eng. J. Med. 285:1010, 1971.

15. Parsons, R. J., Zarafonetis, C. J. D.: Histoplasmosis in man: Report of seven cases and a review of seventy-one cases. Arch. Int. Med. 75:1, 1945.

16. Merz, W. G., et al: Laboratory evaluation of serological tests for systemic candidiasis: A cooperative study. J. Clin. Microbiol. 5:596, 1977.

17. Remington, J. S., Gaines, J. D., Gilmer, M. A.: Demonstration of Candida precipitins in human sera by counterimmunoelectrophoresis. Lancet 1:413, 1972.

18. Thorley, J. D., Megna, M. J., Reinarz, J. A.: Evaluation of Candida antibodies in the diagnosis or exclusion of invasive candidiasis. Clin. Res. 25:30A, 1977 (Abstract).

19. Weiner, M. H., Yount, W. J.: Mannan antigenemia in the diagnosis of invasive Candida infections. J. Clin. Invest. 58:1045, 1976.

20. Harding, S. A., Sandford, G. R., Merz, W. G.: Three serologic tests for candidiasis. J. Clin. Path. 65:1001, 1976.

29: WHOOPING COUGH
by H. Thadepalli


Whooping cough is an acute communicable disease of the respiratory tract that affects children, characterized by paroxysms of cough ending in the typical "whoop", an inspiratory effort. Adults are not immune to this infection; in fact, nurses and pediatricians can develop this disease with or without the whoop.[1] It is caused by Bordetella pertussis, a capsulated, non-motile, non-spore-forming coccobacillary organism of size 0.5 to 1 $\mu$ in length. It is a droplet infection, pandemic in distribution. It is not a reportable disease in the United States.

## CLINICAL FEATURES

The incubation period is one to ten days. The disease marches through three phases:

1) Early or pre-paroxysmal phase may be no different than any other upper respiratory tract infection, associated with nasal and lachrymal discharge; cough is present but may not be typical.

2) Paroxysmal phase is characterized by intermittent, progressively worsening bouts of violent paroxysms of unproductive cough, ending with the loud squeaking, prolonged inspiration, a "whoop", caused by laryngeal spasm. An unfortunate victim may suffer 40 to 50 such bouts of this spasmodic attack of cough. The patient appears normal between the attacks. Fever does not occur unless secondarily infected. Physical examination of the chest may be normal or at worst may reveal a few crackles or moist rales. Epistaxis, subconjunctival petechiae can occur due to breakage of small blood vessels secondary to increased pressure due to paroxysmal cough. A small ulcer may be noted on the frenum of the tongue in children who have a lower set of incisors.

3) Convalescent phase follows within two to three weeks, with progressive, definite and rapid recovery to normalcy.

## DIAGNOSIS

There are seven types of B. pertussis, of which types I and III are prevalent in the U.S. B. pertussis passes through phases I to IV, of which phase I strains are the most virulent.

1) Clinical syndrome of paroxysmal cough, as described without fever in a child, should suggest the diagnosis. Eighty to 90% of the patients are less than ten years old. Neonates are often susceptible, apparently because of the lack of antibodies in the mother.

2) Leukocytosis: The WBC count usually increases to 15,000 to 30,000 with absolute (50% to 70%) lymphocytosis. The total WBC count may at times increase to 100,000 to 300,000/cu. mm. and be mistaken for leukemia. Premature cells are rare in pertussis. As the clinical disease progresses and the chances for cultural yield decrease, the leukocyte count increases.

3) Erythrocyte sedimentation rate (ESR): The ESR in pertussis is either normal or decreased, rarely elevated when complicated by secondary infection.

4) Chest roentgenogram: In pertussis, this is often normal. Occasionally, it may show peri-hilar infiltrates obscuring the borders of the cardiac silhouette, appearing like a "shaggy heart". Peri-bronchial infiltration and areas of patchy atelectasis may also be seen. The diaphragm may appear flattened. Many areas of the lung may show areas of fleeting collapse; rarely there is evidence for middle lobe or upper lobe collapse. It mostly involves the lower lobes.

5) Cultures: Cough plate method, post-nasal or nasopharyngeal culture and pernasal methods are some of the methods employed for culture of B. pertussis. Pernasal methods are the mostly widely recommended techniques, which involve passing a wisp of cotton wool attached around the end of a length of a fine nichrome wire to the pharynx. It is positive in nearly 60% to 80% of the cases. Nearly 90% are positive during the pre-paroxysmal phase, 60% to 70% during the paroxysmal phase and 50% during convalescence.

B. pertussis grows well on Bordet-Gengou medium (contains glycerin and potato and blood agar and penicillin) when incubated at 35°C. within 48 to 72 hours, forming the typical pearly white or silvery white colonies, resembling broken drops of mercury.

6) Fluorescent antibody (FA) test: This is done with conjugated pertussis antiserum. FA method can be used for the rapid detection of B. pertussis in the sputum (60% to 80%).[2]

7) Complement-fixation test (CFT): The CFT titers become positive after three weeks, therefore, they have no diagnostic usefulness for immediate patient care.

8) Agglutinins: A slide test with type I organisms can be done. The antigen employed is an extract of B. pertussis adsorbed onto tanned sheep erythrocytes. A negative test indicates absence of previous vaccination or infection.

Of all the tests mentioned, the pernasal swab culture is the most reliable one and if positive, diagnostic.

## DIFFERENTIAL

A previous history of immunization does not rule out the diagnosis. Other etiologic agents that mimic whooping cough, like B. parapertussis, B. bronchiseptica and adenoviruses should be excluded. It is important to note that adenoviruses can cause whooping-cough-like syndrome as reported, [3] but whooping cough is not a viral disease; it is caused by B. pertussis. The clinical syndrome produced by B. parapertussis is similar. The differentiation is made by culture. Absence of fever, normal ESR and relative lymphocytosis should distinguish pertussis and parapertussis from adenovirus infection and allergic bronchitis.

## TREATMENT

"Whooping cough remains one of the most severe and distressing diseases of the childhood. We have no drugs or therapeutic measures that have any specific effect on its course, but this is no reason to exhibit drugs that are useless."

-A. B. Christie [4]

None of the antibiotics have any significant effect on the course of the illness.

Immunoprophylaxis is the key for the prevention of this otherwise distressing disease of children. It causes more deaths during the first year of life than infectious hepatitis, scarlet fever, poliomyelitis, chickenpox and mumps combined. [5] In older children, it carries excellent prognosis; the overall mortality is around 0.8% to < 1%. Vaccination offers greater than 95% immunity. [6]

## REFERENCES

1. Linneman, C. C. , Nasenberg, J. : Pertussis in the adult. Ann. Rev. Med. 28:179, 1977.

2. Donaldson, P. , Whitaker, J. A. : The diagnosis of pertussis by fluorescent antibody scanning of nasopharyngeal smears. Am. J. Dis. Child. 99:423, 1960.

3. Connor, J. D. : Evidence for an etiologic role of adenoviral infection in pertussis syndrome. New Eng. J. Med. 283:390, 1970.

4. Christie, A. B. : Whooping Cough. Infectious Diseases, Epidemiology and Clinical Practice. E&S Livingstone, Ltd. , Edinburgh, 1969.

5. Brooksales, F. , Nelson, J. D. : Pertussis: A reappraisal and report of 190 confirmed cases. Am. J. Dis. Child. 114:389, 1967.

6. Preston, N. W. : Protection by pertussis vaccine. Lancet 1:1065, 1976.

SECTION C: INFECTIONS OF THE NERVOUS SYSTEM

30: MENINGITIS
by Gary Overturf

INTRODUCTION

The essential elements of accurate etiologic diagnosis of meningitis require careful attention to clinical history and cerebrospinal fluid (CSF) indices. Although many specialized
laboratory techniques have been introduced, they contribute
little to the standard methods of diagnosis. The speed and
accuracy of diagnosis demand that the physician be familiar
with the fundamentals of differential diagnosis and personally
supervise the examination of the CSF. Sound clinical knowledge, coupled with close cooperation with laboratory professionals, is mandatory.

BACTERIAL MENINGITIS

Some assistance in the etiologic diagnosis of meningitis can be
gained by a recognition of the epidemiologic and age patterns
characteristic of the causative bacterial microorganisms (Table
18). Approximately 70% of all episodes of bacterial meningitis
occur in children less than ten years of age. Further, the risk
of bacterial meningitis is greatest in newborn infants (i.e., $\leq 2$
months of life) with an attack rate of one to two infections per
1,000 newborns; this rate is approximately one-third to one-
half that of bacterial sepsis at this age. In many centers, meningitis due to group B Streptococci predominates in the neonates,
although E. coli, other enteric bacteria and Listeria occur frequently in this age group. [1]

The peak age incidence of the major bacterial pathogens is
strikingly repetitive and largely confined to the pediatric age
groups. Mathies reported the etiologic incidence of meningitis
by age and noted that Haemophilus and meningococcal infections
are largely confined to young children, with peak incidence at
about one year old; in contrast, pneumococcal infections demonstrated two peaks, one in children less than one year old
and subsequently in individuals greater than 40 years old. [2]
Pneumococcal infections also occur sporadically in association

TABLE 18: APPROXIMATE RANK ORDER OF BACTERIAL ETIOLOGY OF MENINGITIS

|  | NEONATES | CHILDREN | ADULTS |
|---|---|---|---|
| Gram-positive | Group B Streptococci<br>Streptococci,(other)<br>Staphylococci<br>Listeria<br><u>S. pneumoniae</u> | <u>S. pneumoniae</u><br>Streptococci,(other) | <u>S. pneumoniae</u><br>Streptococci,(other)<br>Staphylococci<br>Listeria* |
| Gram-negative | <u>E. coli</u><br><u>K</u>lebsiella<br>Proteus<br>Pseudomonas<br>Other | <u>H. influenzae</u>, typable<br><u>H. parainfluenzae</u><br><u>G</u>ram-negative* | <u>H. influenzae</u><br><u>E. coli</u>*<br><u>K</u>lebsiella*<br>Pseudomonas*<br>Other* |

*Rare; occurs in compromised host or post-surgically

with predisposing factors, such as head trauma with co-existent fracture, sickle cell disease, surgical asplenia, or congenital or acquired immunologic or phagocytic defects. Infections due to gram-negative enteric bacteria may occur in adult patients, particularly those with compromised host defenses. Infections due to E. coli and group B strepto-cocci are more frequent among adult diabetic patients; similar-ly, Listeria infections are more frequent in patients with can-cer or other immune compromised states. Meningitis due to S. epidermidis, S. aureus and gram-negative organisms are the common infections following placement of ventricular shunts; other neurosurgical procedures may also be complicated by gram-negative or staphylococcal infections. Many fungal CNS infections are also associated with iatrogenic factors or com-promise of host responses. Tuberculosis remains a significant problem throughout much of Southern Asia and South America; a clinical history of prolonged travel or residence in these areas should raise suspicion of this disease, or residence with an-other person with symptoms suggestive of active pulmonary tuberculosis.

Bacterial meningitis in the neonate presents with subtle, often non-specific, clinical signs. [1] Hypo- or hyperthermia occurs in only 30% to 40% of patients. A change in the feeding pattern, seizures or respiratory distress are the next most frequent signs. Definable meningeal signs are almost absent at this age. The reliability of classical meningeal signs becomes more prominent with increasing age and is usually apparent in most patients by six to twelve months of age. Virtually any deviation from a normal neonatal course must provoke consideration of meningitis and lead to the performance of a diagnostic lumbar puncture.

Fever and altered mental status are the most consistent signs of bacterial meningitis in older patients; headache, nausea, vomiting and photophobia are also common symptoms and may reflect increased intracranial pressure (ICP) or cerebral in-flammation. Since increase in intracranial pressure is an acute phenomenon in bacterial disease, funduscopic signs and symp-toms related to ICP may be the dominant clinical presentation in chronic or subacute bacterial meningitis.

A wide range of neurological signs may be present. Approxi-mately one-third of patients will present with convulsions or coma. [3,4] Focal neurologic signs may be manifestations of cerebritis, but should cause suspicion of a focal purulent proc-ess, such as cerebral venous thrombosis, abscess, subdural effusion or empyema, depending upon the age of the patient. Fever is present in 80% of the patients and may be more than 105°F. or only mildly elevated. Ten to twenty per cent of patients may have no fever, either due to mild disease or prior antipyretic therapy.

Nuchal rigidity is a classical finding in patients with meningitis and is indicative of meningeal inflammation. Signs which are helpful include:

1) Brudzinski's sign; flexion of the neck results in knee and hip flexion,

2) Kernig's sign; pain and difficulty extending the knee is experienced when the patient is supine with the thigh perpendicular to the trunk.

Meningismus (i.e., pain with passive neck flexion, without meningeal inflammation) may be confused with nuchal rigidity due to meningitis and may be present in septicemia, lobar pneumonia, cervical adenitis, mastoiditis, paratonsillar or cervical abscesses or cervical osteomyelitis. Some investigators have commented on the frequent association of cranial bruits in purulent meningitis in childhood;[5] although this observation has not been confirmed, it may be heard in children.

In meningococcal meningitis, a characteristic rash may be observed and allows a diagnosis solely on clinical evaluation. Five types of cutaneous lesions may be observed:

1) Early in the febrile course, a fleeting maculopapular rash may be present on the trunk. If therapy is instituted early, this rash may fade rapidly and no further cutaneous manifestations may be seen.

2) The characteristic petechial rash is diagnostic (Fig. 43); early on, the petechiae are small, scattered and raised and may blanch. Early petechiae can be scraped by a scalpel until they bleed, and Gram's stain will demonstrate gram-negative diplococci in approximately one-third to two-thirds of the lesions.

3) The petechial rash progresses to pleomorphic areas of purpura (Fig. 44), which may subsequently become so large and necrotic that the areas of skin involved may require surgical repair.

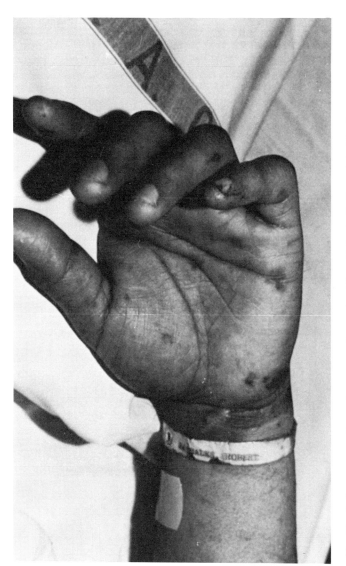

FIG. 43:  Rash in a case of meningococcal meningitis.  It is indistinguishable from vasculitis due to Gonococcus.

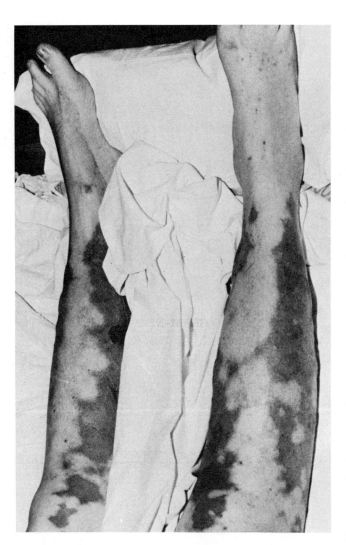

FIG. 44: Disseminated intravascular coagulation and areas of patchy ecchymosis seen in a case of meningococcemia.

4) Occasional patients have progression of purpuric lesions to bullae; and

5) A few patients may present with classical erythema nodosum.

Recognition of the first three lesions is vitally important, since they may lead to the diagnosis and early institution of appropriate therapy.

## PNEUMOCOCCAL AND HAEMOPHILUS MENINGITIS

Individual clinical characteristics for bacterial etiologies of meningitis do not exist. Pneumococcal and Haemophilus meningitis appear clinically equivalent in patients of the same age. In general, pneumococcal infection is usually more severe (i.e. , greater frequency of seizures and coma), and will frequently be associated with pneumonia, whereas Haemophilus infections are more frequently preceded by otitis media. Either of these infections may be preceded or coexistent with any upper or lower respiratory infection, i.e., pneumonia, otitis, sinusitis. Pneumococcal infections may coexist with endocarditis. Haemophilus infections are sometimes (5% to 10%) associated with cellulitis or septic arthritis in young children; facial or upper extremity cellulitis is more common, whereas septic arthritis may be in any joint, usually the knee, hip or ankle.

## MENINGITIS DUE TO GRAM-NEGATIVE BACILLI

The clues to infection due to gram-negative rods lie largely in the clinical context one finds the patients. These infections should be suspected in the following situations, where meningitis has been diagnosed:

1) The neonate, particularly in those infants less than seven days old

2) The adult with gram-negative sepsis, particularly in those with chronic or acute urinary tract infections or gram-negative pneumonias

3) Patients on immunosuppressive therapy, and

4) Patients within 48 to 72 hours of trauma with or without surgery of the central nervous system, or those who are convalescing from elective neurosurgical procedures

Gram-negative meningitis may be associated with endocarditis from these organisms. Clinical features are indistinguishable from other CNS infections and, therefore, the diagnosis must be established by appropriate cultures. Due to the wide variability of antibiotic susceptibility of these organisms, successful therapy will rest upon recovery and susceptibility testing of these organisms. Salmonella infections of the CNS are rare, except in cases of advanced typhoid fever and certain other virulent strains, such as S. cholera suis; a preceding or concomitant gastroenteritis might provide a clinical clue in some cases.

## STAPHYLOCOCCUS AUREUS AND LISTERIA

Staphylococcus (S. ) aureus is a rare CNS pathogen. Clinically, it may present during the postoperative period following neurosurgical procedures, or it may represent a complication of a parameningeal infection, such as a disc space infection, renal abscess, osteomyelitis or sinusitis. In the case of the latter predisposing infections, clinical signs may point to a localized abscess.

Listeria infections may be quite insidious or mimic pneumococcal infections. Although they are more frequent in the newborn and in adults with immunocompromised status, they also occur sporadically in normal persons. A frequent human reservoir for this disease is from asymptomatic colonization of the cervicovaginal canal. CSF pleocytosis tends to be less in respect to total cell count than other cases of purulent meningitis. Although monocytic CSF responses are typical of infection due to this organism in other animal species, this is only infrequently the case in man.

The characteristic CSF changes in bacterial meningitis, compared to those of other etiologies, are shown in Table 19. More discussion of the differential value of spinal fluid findings will be dealt with later. In general, patients with bacterial meningitis present with > 1,000 WBC/cu. mm., protein concentration of > 100 mg/dl and low glucose concentrations. The diagnosis of bacterial meningitis requires recovery of the etiologic agent; cultures and Gram's stains should be done without fail; and will reveal the organism in 80% to 90% of the patients.

## FUNGAL INFECTIONS

Fungal infections should be suspected by a chronic clinical presentation coupled with characteristic CSF changes. The

TABLE 19: CLASSICAL CHARACTERISTICS OF SPINAL FLUID BY ETIOLOGY

| TYPE OF MENINGITIS | CELLS/cu. mm. | PER CENT POLYMORPHS | GLUCOSE | PROTEIN |
|---|---|---|---|---|
| Bacterial | 500 to >1,000 | >80% | < 20 mg/dl | Increased |
| Fungal or tuberculous | 25 to 500 | <20%* | Normal to <10 mg/dl | Much increased |
| Viral infections | 25 to 500 | <10%* | Normal | Mildly increased |

*Early in the course, number of PMNs may be predominating

relatively slow onset of mental dysfunction or meningeal signs, and the more frequent symptoms of increased intracranial pressure, typify patients with chronic meningitis, such as those due to fungi (cryptococcal and coccidioidomycosis), cysticercosis or tuberculosis. The onset is frequently insidious and becomes apparent over several weeks, rather than a few hours or days. Coma is less frequent as a presenting sign, but cranial nerve signs are commonly present due to increased intracranial pressure; III, VI and VII are frequently involved. [6,7,8] Apathy and neck stiffness are prominent signs, but fever is much less regularly present. Associated systemic electrolyte disturbances may be prominent among patients with chronic meningitis. The syndrome of inappropriate ADH secretion associated with hyponatremia may provide a clue to these etiologies.

There is a wide variation in CSF indices; for example, Butler and colleagues found that the percentage of lymphocytes varied from 8% to 100% and the number of total leukocytes from 0 to 808/cu. mm. in cryptococcal meningitis. [6] In addition, glucose concentrations were $\geqslant 40$ mg/dl in nearly half of the patients, and protein concentrations were normal in 15% of the patients. Other chronic infections may also have these variations in CSF findings. Variations are largely a function of time that the disease has been present, and the majority of patients with fungal meningitis will, at some time during the course of their disease, manifest elevated CSF pressures, moderate CSF leukocytosis, a low CSF glucose and high CSF protein. Infections due to coccidioidomycosis do not differ significantly from cryptococcal infections. Patients with coccidioidomycosis are found within a restricted endemic area (i.e., southwestern U.S. and northern Mexico), and there is a higher incidence of disseminated infections among Blacks, Philippinos and Orientals. Histoplasmosis and sporotrichosis only rarely cause CNS infections; they need only infrequently be considered in the differential diagnosis of chronic meningitis. Blastomycosis and Candida may involve the CNS in disseminated cases and must be differentiated from other causes of fungal meningitis.

The diagnosis of suspected fungal meningitis relies on demonstration of a specific organism, its antigen or specific antibody, in the CSF. India ink smears may demonstrate the large encapsulated cells of Cryptococcus neoformans; Gram's stains also characteristically reveal the large gram-negative staining capsule. Large amounts of spinal fluid in excess of 25 ml. may be required for fungal cultures, and some suggest obtaining CSF by cisternal puncture, thereby increasing chances of recovering the organism. Although there are alternate methods to demonstrate the presence of Cryptococci, recovery of the organism is desirable to perform in vitro susceptibility studies.

CSF and serum can be directly analyzed for both cryptococcal antigen and antibody; although firm diagnostic criteria are not available, tentative guidelines have been established and are reviewed elsewhere.[9] Tests for cryptococcal antigen are more sensitive and specific; regardless of what technique is used, its presence in CSF is synonymous with CNS infection. Serological and CSF tests for complement-fixation antibody against coccidioidomycosis can be roughly correlated with the chance of disseminated disease, i.e., a titer of $\geqslant$ 1:32 is frequently associated with dissemination; therefore, if other signs, symptoms and CSF laboratory data are compatible with meningitis due to coccidioidomycosis, a serum titer of this magnitude may reflect active CNS disease. Similar to cryptococcal disease, a positive titer in the CSF is essentially proof of meningitis due to this organism. Serologic tests are also available for blastomycosis, histoplasmosis and Candida, and these tests may be performed by the Center for Disease Control, Atlanta, Georgia. Skin tests are unreliable in the diagnosis of acute fungal infections; so they should be avoided to prevent cross reactions with serological tests.

Fungal infections may present with a picture compatible with cerebral abscess. Intracranial pressure will often be elevated and focal neurologic signs may be present; CSF pleocytosis, and changes other than high CSF protein may be absent. Mucormycosis and other rhinocerebral phycomycoses frequently involve the paranasal sinuses and produce orbital cellulitis, with or without associated proptosis and ophthalmoplegia.[10] Extension of the process may be associated with classic signs of cavernous venous thrombosis; i.e., oculomotor palsies, unilateral papilledema, chemosis and eye pain. Smears, scrapings or, preferably, direct biopsy will demonstrate the characteristic broad non-septate hyphae.

Nocardia is a bacterium, not a fungus but clinically it resembles fungal infections. Nocardia infections may follow penetrating trauma to the skull, or occur as a complication of a primary pulmonary process.[11] Nocardia can be identified in aspirates by the appearance of its narrow, gram-positive, fragmenting filaments; some may be bacillary or coccal forms and some may be acid-fast. Actinomycosis, which may have a similar pathogenesis, differs morphologically from Nocardia in that it is an obligate anaerobic bacteria and never acid-fast, although it may have gram-positive filamentous forms. Both Nocardia and Actinomyces are frequently associated with concomitant anaerobic infections. Actinomycosis and aspergillosis are infrequent invaders of the central nervous system.[12, 13]

Disseminated Candida infections with involvement of the central nervous system may occur, particularly in compromised hosts.

Candida infections of the CNS are rare. They can be diagnosed by recovering the non-encapsulated, budding yeasts or hyphal elements from CSF. Endophthalmitis with characteristic white, glistening, raised, round deposits may also provide a clue to diagnosis.[14]

## TUBERCULOSIS

In general, the clinical presentation of an insidious onset of symptoms, with progression to local and then diffuse neurological involvement, is characteristic of tuberculous meningitis.[15,16] The time from onset of symptoms until death may be as short as one to two weeks in adults and six to eight weeks in children. Early symptoms are non-specific; apathy, lethargy or anorexia may be prominent during the first stage. Subsequently, distinct neurologic signs develop (second stage), frequently, ophthalmoplegia or facial paralysis may develop. Terminally (third stage), frank neurologic involvement becomes apparent and convulsions, vomiting or coma may be indications of rapidly increasing intracranial pressure (ICP) due to hydrocephalus.

Results of intradermal skin tests (intermediate strength) cannot be relied upon solely to indicate the presence or absence of tuberculous meningitis. Similarly, approximately 20% of patients will have no evidence of any other focus of tuberculosis, and approximately this number will have a normal chest x-ray. A presumptive diagnosis must be made with a combination of suggestive history, suspected tuberculosis exposure characteristic of CSF findings and any supporting ancillary data, such as a positive tuberculin reaction or radiographic evidence of pulmonary tuberculosis. A CSF WBC of $> 1,000$/cu. mm. is unusual, but low CSF cell counts of less than 100/cu. mm. are not uncommon. Although the pleocytosis is predominantly monocytic, a small percentage of polymorphonuclear leukocytes (2% to 30%) is the rule. Early in the course, intracranial pressure and CSF sugar and protein may be normal; however, these findings will change in association with signs suggestive of ICP, i.e., CSF sugar will fall to $\leq 5$ mg/dl and protein concentrations may rise sharply to levels $> 1.5$ mg/dl with marked hydrocephalus. Smears for acid-fast bacilli (AFB) are rarely helpful, being positive for acid-fast bacilli in < 20% of patients. Cultures may yield the organisms in the majority of patients in three to six weeks, but a diagnosis must be made to initiate appropriate therapy prior to substantiation by culture.

## VIRAL INFECTIONS

Viral meningitis is usually much milder. Increased intracranial pressure is never present unless there is an associated encephalitis. Similarly, convulsions signal cerebral involvement. Nuchal rigidity, photophobia and headache are frequent. Fever is generally less severe; most patients have fever less than 102°F. , however, children with aseptic meningitis or adult pediatric patients with encephalitis may have temperatures exceeding 105°F. Occasional episodes due to certain enteroviruses may have mild to severe neurologic involvement, particularly in young children. [17] This disease is self-limiting without specific therapy, whereas rapid deterioration of the patient's clinical status is characteristic of bacterial infections. If CSF examination is non-diagnostic, careful clinical observation coupled with repeated lumbar puncture at eight to twelve hours may better define a viral versus bacterial etiology.

Viral encephalitis may be confused with viral, fungal or tuberculous meningitis. CSF pleocytosis can range from 0 to rarely >500 cells. Cells are generally mononuclear. However, in any viral process, the lumbar puncture may yield a predominantly polymorphonuclear response. Feagin and Shackleford showed the value of repeat lumbar punctures; [18] these investigators documented a significant reduction of polymorphonuclear leukocytes in CSF obtained at six to eight hours in 87% of patients subjected to repeat lumbar punctures. CSF protein concentrations are usually mildly to moderately elevated in patients with encephalitis, but CSF glucose is virtually always normal. The diagnosis of encephalitis is made solely on a clinical basis; CSF may be normal and the only abnormalities may be mild to severe mental alterations (including coma) and fever. Increased ICP may also be present. Although EEGs may be helpful, they cannot be depended upon to exclude non-infectious etiologies of encephalopathy, such as those due to metabolic disorders or toxins; in addition, EEGs may be normal with acute viral encephalitis. Since specific tests for encephalitis are not available, other treatable diseases should be excluded before one is content to make this diagnosis.

Encephalitis due to Herpes virus is particularly difficult to diagnose. In addition to pleocytosis and elevated protein characteristic of other fungal infections, herpetic infections may produce hemorrhagic necrosis with resulting xanthochromia or the presence of red blood cells. [19] A mass effect with associated hemiplegia in the temporoparietal region may also be characteristic of herpetic infections. Brain biopsy with demonstration of characteristic intranuclear inclusion bodies is essential to substantiate the diagnosis.

## LOCALIZED PYOGENIC INFECTIONS

Cerebral abscess (Chapter 31) may be confused with meningitis. These infections may complicate congenital heart disease, endocarditis or paracranial infections, such as otitis media or sinusitis. [20,21] Eighty-five per cent of brain abscesses are due to anaerobic organisms and may be associated with chronic foci of anaerobic infections; in addition, these infections may follow surgical procedures. Patients are frequently young, usually in the first four decades of life. In brain abscess, results of lumbar puncture are inconsistent, and the associated potential hazard of uncal herniation prohibits its use when this diagnosis is suspected. [21] In the event that lumbar puncture is performed, elevated pressures and protein concentrations are the most consistent abnormalities of CSF, but WBC may be absent, low or consistent with bacterial meningitis and either lymphocytes or granulocytes may predominate.

Radionuclide brain scanning, computerized tomography or angiography should be performed in those patients with acute onset of fever associated with focal neurological signs or convulsions, to exclude the possibility of a mass lession. Computerized axial tomography (CAT) provides the most definitive data on anatomy and location of most cerebral abscesses. However, subdural or epidural pyogenic abscesses may be missed by CAT and angiography should be utilized when these specific anatomic lesions are suspected. Routine radiography should be relied upon to demonstrate associated mastoid or sinus infections.

## PARAMENINGEAL INFECTIONS

Parameningeal foci of infections may produce changes in CSF consistent with inflammatory disease. Sinusitis, otitis media with or without mastoiditis, skull and spinal osteomyelitis, posterior pharyngeal abscess with or without esophageal perforation, or rarely, retroperitoneal abscesses, may produce changes in the CSF similar to those of cerebral abscess. Central nervous system signs and symptoms are generally not present. Increased intracranial pressure is not frequently present in these syndromes. Focal signs or symptoms and non-diagnostic CSF values in association with a predisposing condition may lead to a suspicion of these infections. Intravenous drug abuse may lead to staphylococcal or gram-negative infections of the intervertebral disc space; chronic sinusitis or otitis media may also be predisposing infections. If the examining spinal needle is in close approximation to the area of inflammation or if a spinal block has occurred in the subarachnoid space proximal to the needle, then highly elevated CSF protein concentrations can be expected. If the parameningeal process has spread to form an abscess, i.e., epidural abscess, then the needle may sample material directly from within the abscess cavity. In the latter case, the CSF sample may be thick and viscid, and impossible to withdraw. High numbers of polymorphonuclear leukocytes and high protein concentrations are found in such samples.

## DIFFERENTIAL DIAGNOSIS

Chemical meningitis may occur following the injection of a toxic substance or drug, or following a neurosurgical or diagnostic study. Fever, headache and nuchal rigidity are indistinguishable from purulent meningitis;[22] CSF glucose may be low, protein concentrations elevated and WBC counts increased with a predominance of polymorphs. Pantopaque myelography, I-131 serum albumin, spinal anesthesia, chemotherapeutic and certain antimicrobial agents (amphotericin) have been incriminated. The patient is conscious and complains bitterly of headache. Diagnosis is suspected by the history of recent intrathecal injection of a meningeal irritant (within 48 hours) and negative spinal fluid cultures.

Although cysticercosis (see page 241) is a rare disease in the United States, it is common in many parts of the world.[23] Patients may present with convulsions of recent onset, headache, symptoms suggestive of hydrocephalus, or, rarely, a mass lesion. CSF findings are similar to those of chemical meningitis. Nuchal rigidity and fever may accompany periodic episodes of ruptured cerebral cysts. However, low levels of CSF glucose and CSF pleocytosis may be seen in patients with no acute symptoms. An indirect hemagglutination test is available through consultation with the Center for Disease Control, Atlanta, Georgia. Computerized tomography may reveal multiple areas of calcification and cystic structures. Other parasitic infections of the CNS are sufficiently rare to be excluded from general discussion, but include: meningitis due to Naegleria gruberi, amoebic abscess due to Entamoeba histolytica, cerebral malaria, trichinosis encephalitis, Echinococcus cysts, and trypanosomiasis.

Endocarditis patients frequently have involvement of the central nervous system (see page 297); 20% of patients present with CNS signs and symptoms. [24] Types of CNS involvement range from subarachnoid hemorrhage to cerebral infarction to mycotic aneurysm or frank bacterial meningitis. Therefore, symptoms may be focal or diffuse, and CSF findings vary widely. Acute neurological symptoms during the course of endocarditis should prompt a rapid evaluation with computerized axial tomography or angiography to exclude a surgically accessible aneurysm or abscess (see page 272).

CNS neoplasia (primary or metastatic) and cerebral hemorrhage may mimic CNS infections. Cerebral carcinomatosis in adult patients, and acute lymphoblastic leukemia in children may produce elevated CSF protein and monocytic pleocytosis; glucose concentrations are occasionally depressed. Subarachnoid hemorrhage may produce inflammatory response with white blood cells. CSF protein may be elevated, and in severe CSF hemorrhage, glucose may be depressed. Focal hemorrhage, such as subdural hematoma, may present with CSF changes ranging from strikingly elevated protein concentration to xanthochromia to a purulent process if the hematoma becomes infected, i.e., subdural empyema.

## ROUTINE LABORATORY

Most routine laboratory data are not helpful in the differential diagnosis of central nervous system infection. Although bacterial infections tend to have an associated peripheral leukocytosis ($\geqslant$20,000/cu. mm.) with extreme shift to the left, this may also be observed in early severe viral infections; overwhelming bacterial meningitis may be associated with a leukopenia ($\leqslant$5,000/cu. mm.). Characteristic changes of disseminated intravascular coagulation may be seen during any bacterial meningitis. Thrombocytopenia is also common with severe bacterial infections; this may also accompany severe viral infections. Patients with tuberculosis may have a monocytosis with 1,000 to 2,000 absolute monocyte counts; disseminated coccidioidomycosis may have a slight eosinophilia. Normocytic normochromic anemia may be a reflection of chronic infection.

Erythrocyte sedimentation is rarely elevated during acute viral infections of the CNS, but it is often strikingly elevated during bacterial infections.

Disturbances of electrolytes may be associated with acute or chronic meningitis. Vomiting may produce hyponatremia and hypokalemia. Diarrhea may be associated with acute infections of childhood and may prove to be sufficiently severe to result in dehydration. Hyponatremia, as mentioned previously, may reflect inappropriate secretion of ADH, particularly in chronic meningitis associated with increased intracranial pressure due to hydrocephalus.

Standard radiography is useful in diagnosis of associated or predisposing causes of bacterial meningitis, such as sinusitis, mastoiditis or osteomyelitis. Radionuclide brain scanning, computerized axial tomography or angiography may also be helpful in the diagnosis of suppurative complications.

## CEREBROSPINAL FLUID

The considerable overlap of clinical findings and the necessity for making a specific etiologic diagnosis makes examination of the spinal fluid mandatory. Little clinical provocation is required to justify the performance of a lumbar puncture (LP); suspicion alone of a central nervous system infection is adequate reason. The only absolute contraindication to LP is infection overlying the lumbar site; relative contraindications include the presence of increased intracranial pressure with a suspected mass lesion; spinal cord tumor; or a bleeding diathesis. Whenever time permits, and facilities are available, these relative contraindications should be excluded prior to performing LP. However, since the diagnosis of purulent meningitis is a medical emergency, undue delay should not jeopardize the institution of appropriate antimicrobial therapy.

PERFORMANCE OF THE LUMBAR PUNCTURE: Positioning the patient correctly is the single most important step in assuring a successful lumbar puncture. The patient is placed on his side, with hips and shoulders resting at the edge of a firm surface. The spine must be parallel with the edge of the surface, and the spine should be flexed as much as possible to open the space between the spinous processes; knees and hips should be fully flexed. Adequate restraint by an assistant is necessary to assist the patient in maintaining this posture. Although restraint systems are available for pediatric patients, they are usually not necessary and may unnecessarily impede view of the patient. After an antiseptic scrub and appropriate sterile draping of the LP site, the left hand is placed on the iliac crest and the thumb is dropped perpendicular to the bed; this will define either the fourth or fifth lumbar space. One should usually use this space for insertion of the needle or the one immediately above or below this line. The tap can be done from L5-S1 to L2-3. Higher interspaces are too close to the spinal cord, which ends at L1 and L2 (Fig. 45).

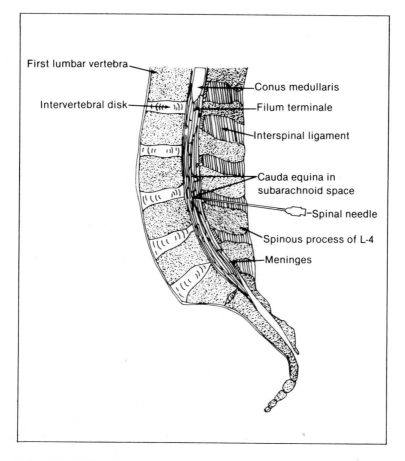

First lumbar vertebra

Intervertebral disk

Conus medullaris

Filum terminale

Interspinal ligament

Cauda equina in subarachnoid space

Spinal needle

Spinous process of L-4

Meninges

FIG. 45: Midsagittal section of spinal column with spinal needle between spinous processes of L-3 and L-4. Note the ascending direction of the needle. The needle has pierced the ligaments and the meninges to the sub-arachnoid space.

Local anesthesia may be used with local skin infiltration and then deeper infiltration; this is usually unnecessary in children and often only prolongs the procedure. In children less than three years old, a 22-gauge styleted needle, $1\frac{1}{2}$ inches, is usually adequate whereas in adults, a 20-gauge, 3-inch styleted needle is usually required. Place the needle through the skin, parallel to the surface. Once the needle has pierced the skin and subcutaneous tissue, it should be directed cephalad toward the umbilicus. It may then be advanced slowly until the dura is penetrated ("pop") entering the subarachnoid space. If bone is encountered, this may be due to a deviation from midline, or it may be directed cephalad and have encountered the spinous process. Therefore, establishing the midline is essential to the procedure. It may be helpful to maintain palpation with the index and middle fingers of the upper and lower spinous processes of the interspace with the left hand, while inserting the needle.

If bloody fluid is obtained, do not assume a bloody tap; wait for clearing and perform all studies normally done on spinal fluid. In very ill patients, particularly children, prolonged positioning in a tuck position may compromise respiration and lead to post-tap problems of cyanosis, apnea and respiratory arrests. These problems are more frequent than uncal herniation, and the patient must be stabilized before transport. Complaints of headache and backache may be frequent, usually beginning six to twenty-four hours after the procedure; reassurance and bed rest are all that is usually necessary. Infection following LP is extremely rare, but when it occurs, it is devastating; organisms frequently involved are normally saprophytes, such as Pseudomonas.

The classical characteristics of cerebrospinal fluid according to etiology are shown in Table 19. Overlap between each syndrome may be great, and no single spinal fluid value can confirm the diagnosis. For instance, leukocytes in excess of 1,000/cu. mm., polymorphonuclear leukocyte responses of greater than 75%, glucose concentration $\leqslant$ 40 mg. % and protein concentrations $\geqslant$ 150 mg. % strongly indicate bacterial meningitis. However, in a recent prospective survey for one year, of all bacterial meningitis in Los Angeles county (ages from birth to old age), 19% of patients had CSF glucose $\geqslant$ 60 mg/dl, 43% had CSF protein $\leqslant$ 150 mg/dl and 35% had CSF white blood counts (WBC) of $\leqslant$ 1,000 cells/cu. mm. [25] In addition, a variety of CNS degenerative processes, CNS hemorrhage, neoplasms and parameningeal infections or inflammatory conditions may produce changes in CSF identical to those observed in patients with a variety of infections.

CSF PRESSURE: Often overlooked are the measurements of
opening and closing pressures. Normal opening pressure in
the relaxed adult patient is rarely greater than 250 mm. water.
Patients with viral meningitis, as noted previously, do not have
ICP, while approximately one-half to two-thirds of patients
with bacterial meningitis will have ICP. The measurement of
pressure in children is rarely possible. Patients with chronic
meningitis may have markedly increased pressure or associated
CSF block as indicated by high protein concentrations, i.e.,
$\geqslant 1.0$ mg/dl.

CSF APPEARANCE: The inspection of spinal fluid to exclude
bacterial infection is the chief priority. Spinal fluid should be
examined for clarity and color. Approximately 500 leukocytes/
cu. mm. are required to make the fluid appear slightly turbid,
i.e., "ground glass appearance", or approximately 1,000 to
2,000 red blood cells/cu. mm. in the absence of leukocytes. If
meningitis is early in the course, bacteria alone may be present and turbidity will not be appreciated until concentrations
of approximately $10^7$ bacteria/ml. are attained. Also, changes
in protein and glucose concentration will generally not be observed in the presence of bacteria alone. Therefore, a careful Gram's stain and culture of centrifuged spinal fluid (2000 rpm
x 15 minutes) must be done, even in the absence of white cells
or abnormal protein or glucose concentration. Neonates frequently do not have diagnostic changes in spinal fluid in the
presence of bacterial infections; Gram's stains and culture are
the most reliable parameters of bacterial infection in this age
group. [1]

CSF RED BLOOD CELLS (RBC): The differential diagnosis of
a cerebral hemorrhage from meningitis can be aided by noting
the color of CSF. Degenerated RBCs will stain CSF red, and
centrifuged CSF should be compared to a water blank against
a white background to determine if xanthochromia is present.
The ratio of peripheral blood WBCs to RBCs should be determined. If bleeding occurs during the LP and fails to
clear during the procedure, and the CSF WBC:RBC ratio is
less than the peripheral blood ratio, a traumatic tap is unlikely. CSF supernatant of patients with cerebral hemorrhage is frequently xanthochromic, whereas a traumatic tap
will have a clear supernatant. Protein concentrations in
excess of 200 mg/dl may also cause a xanthochromia, which
is characteristically more yellow in color than that due to
hemorrhage.

CSF CELL COUNT: The white cell count may vary widely at the time of diagnosis, ranging from zero to greater than 50,000 /cu. mm. At least two-thirds will have more than 1,000 white cells/cu. mm. with polymorphonuclear leukocytes predominating. A CSF differential of less than 70% PMNs on the initial LP makes the diagnosis of bacterial meningitis doubtful, even if there has been some antibiotic therapy prior to admission. It is important to recognize that in early or in overwhelming infection, there may be as few as three to four white cells/cu. mm. However, in these cases, CSF chemistries may be diagnostic, and the Gram's stain is frequently positive.

CSF SUGAR AND PROTEIN (Table 20): Chemistries should always be obtained. A low CSF glucose concentration is characteristic of acute bacterial meningitis. The convention is that a CSF glucose concentration higher than 60% of the simultaneous blood sugar concentration is normal, while one less than 40% is reduced. The CSF protein concentration is nearly always elevated (i.e., greater than 50 mg/dl). The elevation may be dramatic and, generally, higher levels parallel the severity of disease. Moreover, high levels, particularly high levels that persist while other variables are improving during therapy, may indicate the presence of suppurative complications. CSF glucose may be artificially low, if red and white cells which continue to utilize the glucose are not separated from the CSF. Protein may be elevated if large numbers of red cells lyse in the CSF. In general, an elevation of 1 mg/dl will occur for every 1,000 cells/cu. mm. in an unspun specimen. Even if all cells are removed from the CSF, the glucose in an old specimen is unreliable. Usually a 3 to 4 mg/dl per hour decrease in CSF glucose will occur at room temperature (refrigeration may retard this degradation). CSF chlorides, although routinely done by most laboratories, have limited usefulness; they tend to be low in chronic (tuberculous and fungal) and bacterial meningitis.

CSF CULTURES: Although a presumptive etiologic diagnosis can be made by examination of the spinal fluid leukocyte determination and chemical values, a specific diagnosis requires recovery of the organism or identification of the organism on smear, or by indirect immunologic methods. When a specific diagnosis is required for a viral process, consultation with a trained virologist is necessary; these services are usually available through regional health laboratories. In general, a viral etiology is usually assumed after the exclusion of other definable agents, such as bacteria or fungi. Culture and Gram's stains of all CSF sediments are mandatory. Either or both will

## TABLE 20: EXAMPLES OF DIFFERENTIAL CHARACTERISTICS OF CSF PROTEIN AND GLUCOSE

| CSF PROTEIN (Normal, < 50 mg/dl) | CSF GLUCOSE (Normal, > 50% serum glucose) |
|---|---|
| 1. Increased (55 to 1,000 mg/dl) <br> All types meningitis <br> Viral encephalitis <br> Syphilis, degenerative disease <br> Neoplasia (primary, metastatic) <br> Abscess (intracerebral, osteomyelitis) <br> Hemorrhage, subdural hematoma <br> Polyneuropathies (diphtheria) <br> Myxedema, diabetes mellitus <br> Hyperparathyroidism | 1. Marked Increase <br> Hyperglycemic coma |
| 2. Marked Increase (>1,000 mg/dl) <br> Some fungal, TB meningitis <br> Spinal-subarachnoid block <br> Guillain-Barre syndrome | 2. 20 to 50 mg/dl <br> Early TB or fungal <br> Bacterial (early) <br> Meningeal carcinomatosis <br> Severe hemorrhage <br> Systemic hypoglycemia |
| 3. Increased Gamma Globulins <br> SSPE (specific antibodies) <br> Multiple sclerosis <br> Tuberculosis <br> Tabes dorsalis <br> Multiple myeloma | 3. <20 mg/dl <br> Late TB or fungal <br> Bacterial (advanced) <br> Ruptured abscess <br> Diabetic ketoacidosis <br> Cysticercosis |

define the etiology in 85% of patients with bacterial meningitis. There must be $10^5$ to $10^6$ organisms per ml. of unspun CSF for the Gram's stain to be positive. Visualization of organisms on Gram's stain can be facilitated by centrifugation, usually for 20 to 30 minutes (2,000 to 3,000 rpm) in the standard hematologic centrifuge. Supernatant is removed and again may be used for chemical studies. The sediment is resuspended in a drop of CSF; this suspension is then placed on a microscopic slide and allowed to air dry. This drying process may be hastened with the heat of a 60-watt incandescent bulb. Occasionally, if the suspension is thin, it is desirable to layer several drops of suspension over the previous one on the slide, thereby further concentrating the specimen. Techniques of Gram's staining are varied, and a rapid method[24] can be employed with good results.

BLOOD CULTURES: Two to three blood cultures should be obtained because of the high incidence of associated septicemia; in our experience, as high as 65% to 70% are positive in Haemophilus influenzae type B and we have had 71% positive in Streptococcus pneumoniae, 53% positive in Neisseria meningitidis and 45% positive in Haemophilus influenzae in a recent survey. Occasionally, the blood culture is positive, and CSF cultures fail to yield an organism. Cultures from sites other than CSF or blood are not reliable indicators of meningitis.

Cultures for bacteria should routinely be placed on sheep blood agar and chocolate blood agar with Fildes enrichment or 1% supplement B. Staphylococcal streaking of chocolate blood agar may not be adequate to isolate small numbers of Haemophilus influenzae.

The quellung reaction may be done with type-specific rabbit antisera against Haemophilus (types A, B, C, D, E, F) or pneumococcal organisms (omnisera or types 1 to 83); most laboratories specifically utilize type B Haemophilus antisera only, and some may use pneumococcal omnisera. A heavy suspension of organisms from CSF or culture (preferably young, log phase cultures) can be mixed with approximately equal amounts of antisera with or without additional contrast dye, such as methylene blue. Cross reactions do occur, but they are sufficiently rare to be of little concern in CNS infections. When the precipitate formed by the union of a capsular polysaccharide with its homologous capsular antibody is viewed microscopically, it has a different refractile property, giving the appearance of "capsular swelling". More specific techniques for the quellung reaction are detailed elsewhere. [41]

A rapid test for detection of beta-lactamase by Haemophilus
influenzae is available. [26] A reagent of phenol red (2 ml. of
solution of 0.5%) is added to 16.6 ml. sterile distilled water;
this solution is then added to a vial containing 20 million units
of potassium penicillin G and pH of the solution is adjusted to
pH 8.5 with sodium hydroxide. The test is performed against
a known positive and negative control Haemophilus strain and
the test strain. One to three colonies of an organism is added
to 1 to 2 cm. of solution in a capillary tube and incubated in a
vertical position. A positive result is a color change, consisting of a bright yellow color, in five to fifteen minutes. The
test is dependent on the ability of beta-lactamase to decompose
penicillin G to penicilloic acid and cause a pH depression.

PARTIAL TREATMENT AND REPEAT LP: Partial treatment
of bacterial meningitis rarely causes difficulty with diagnosis.
Numerous investigators have shown that there is little alteration of the expected CSF changes in glucose, protein and leukocytes in partially treated bacterial meningitis. [27,28,29] Although there is a trend for higher CSF glucose concentrations
and lower CSF protein concentrations following partially effective therapy, there is little effect on other parameters. Prior
treatment may slightly affect the rate of positive cultures in
meningococcal or pneumococcal meningitis, but antibiotic therapy has little effect on the recovery of H. influenzae. Similarly, the percentage of polymorphonuclear (PMN) leukocytes is
rarely less than 50% of the total CSF WBC with partially effective therapy. Indeed, in patients undergoing appropriate
therapy, a reduction of polymorphonuclear leukocytes to less
than 50% of the total CSF white blood cell counts required five
to ten days of therapy.

Depending upon the clinical status of the patient, therapy should
be delayed and a repeat lumbar puncture should be performed.
Accuracy of diagnosis may avoid unnecessary treatment of some
patients with viral meningitis, and will help diagnose the etiology of bacterial meningitis. In adult patients, intervals of six
to twelve hours prior to repeat LP may be helpful; in children,
this period of observation may need to be less. In established
cases of bacterial meningitis, LPs after twenty-four to forty-
eight hours of therapy should always be done; with appropriate
therapy, Gram's stain and cultures should be negative and the
glucose will have begun to return to normal. The CSF cells may
be variable, either up in total count (one-half to two-thirds of
patients), or down, and the number of cells will continue to be
predominantly polymorphonuclear at this time. It is also wise
to perform another LP near the end of therapy, i.e., ten to

fourteen days, to have a baseline set of LP values to compare with if problems arise during the patient's convalescence requiring another LP.

## SPECIAL STUDIES

Because the traditional symptoms, signs and laboratory data for CNS infections are not specific, interest has been generated in a variety of laboratory tests to distinguish bacterial disease processes from those due to other agents (Table 21). Currently, only a few of these tests are sufficiently promising to be of special note.

---

### TABLE 21: ADJUNCTIVE LABORATORY TESTS FOR THE DIAGNOSIS OF BACTERIAL MENINGITIS

---

Biochemical Substances
Amylase
Isocitric dehydrogenase
Glutamic acid, glutamine, gamma-amino butyric acid
Glutamic oxalacetic acid transaminase
Lactic dehydrogenase
Volatile acids (lactic acid)

Endotoxin (limulus) Assays

Nitroblue Tetrazolium

Immunologic Markers
Immunoglobins, complement
Counter-current immunoelectrophoresis
Fluorescent antibodies

---

The nitroblue tetrazolium (NBT) reduction test has been reviewed by Park.[30] Although Fikrig, et al.[31] felt the test adequately distinguished bacterial meningitis from that due to viral or tuberculous meningitis, there was occasional overlap between the various entities. These investigators also pointed out the failure of NBT to diagnose bacterial infections in sickle cell disease, and recommended that it not be relied upon in these patients.

Endotoxin assays have been proven to be cheap, practical and reliable for the diagnosis of meningitis due to gram-negative organisms (including H. influenzae and N. meningitidis) in older infants, children and adults. False-positive results in gram-positive meningitis or viral meningitis did not occur in 146 suspected cases investigated.[32] However, this test is obviously limited by the inability to detect meningitis due to gram-positive organisms. Also, McCracken has noted a rate of 31% false-negative results in culture proven gram-negative meningitis in neonates.[33]

Counterimmunoelectrophoresis (CIE) has been examined by a number of investigators. Shackleford and colleagues showed that CIE was most accurate in diagnosis of H. influenzae meningitis; poorest correlation was observed in pneumococcal meningitis. However, only 38 of 59 culture proven cases of bacterial meningitis had positive CIE results.[34] Others[35] have shown better correlation and have quantitated the level of antigen present. In general, CIE is approximately as reliable as optimally performed standard bacteriology, and may add little to conventional laboratory tests.

Concentrations of CSF of various enzymes, such as LDH,[36,37] SGOT,[38] isocitric dehydrogenase[39] and amylase have been examined. All rise in infections due to bacterial agents; only LDH and SGOT have been studied in definitive detail. However, CSF rises in these enzymes have been ascribed to increased blood-brain barrier permeability. Therefore, considerable overlap between bacterial and viral etiologies may occur. Thus, the tests are somewhat dubious for individual patients where the diagnosis is in doubt.

Volatile acids, particularly lactic acid, have been examined in CSF utilizing liquid-gas chromatography.[40] Lactic acid has been shown to be more specific for bacterial meningitis. Rises do not correlate with other elements of inflammation, such as total number of WBC or protein concentration.

Immunoglobulins have been inconsistently correlated with bacterial meningitis. Also, CSF pH is not reliable. Although CSF pH tends to decline more in bacterial disease, it is a nonspecific sign of inflammation and, therefore, is unreliable in individual patients.

### INITIATION OF ANTIBIOTICS (Table 22)

Our current recommendations for initiation of antibiotic therapy are as follows:

TABLE 22: PARENTERAL ANTIBIOTIC DOSAGE
SCHEDULES*

| DRUG | DOSAGE | INTERVAL |
|---|---|---|
| Ampicillin | 200 mg/kg/day | Every 4 hours |
| Penicillin G | 200,000 units/kg/day | Every 4 hours |
| Chloramphenicol | 100 mg/kg/day (maximum 4 grams) | Every 6 hours |
| Methicillin | 200 mg/kg/day (maximum 14 to 16 grams) | Every 4 hours |
| Gentamicin | 5 to 7 mg/kg/day | Every 8 hours |

*Excludes neonates

1) In all patients with culture or Gram's stain proven pneumococcal or meningococcal meningitis, treatment may be initiated with ampicillin (200 mg/kg/day) or aqueous penicillin G (200,000 units/kg/day).

2) In all patients with culture or Gram's stain confirmed meningitis due to H. influenzae, type B treatment may be initiated with chloramphenicol, 100 mg/kg/day until sensitivity testing and/or beta-lactamase assay demonstrates susceptibility to ampicillin; thereafter, ampicillin may be used
as noted previously.

3) In all patients with suspected but unconfirmed purulent
meningitis, i.e., initial Gram's stain negative, due to the
major three pathogens, treatment should be initiated with
ampicillin, 200 mg/kg/day. All penicillin-allergic patients
should receive chloramphenicol (100 mg/kg/day) to a maximum daily dose of 4.0 grams, unless disease is suspected
to be due to a non-susceptible organism.

DOSAGE: We employ an initial loading dose of 50 to 75 mg/kg
of ampicillin, 50,000 to 75,000 units/kg of penicillin G or 25
to 35 mg/kg of chloramphenicol by intravenous push. Thereafter, maintenance dosage and dosing intervals are as summarized in Table 22. There is some disagreement among au-
thorities as to total dosage of ampicillin. Those who advocate
a high dosage schedule (400 mg/kg/day) do so under the assumption that with improvement, decreased meningeal inflammation

will result in lowering of CSF concentrations, possibly below therapeutic levels. Although true, this may be a more theoretic than real concern. A clinical study conducted at the Los Angeles County University of Southern California Medical Center compared 150 mg/kg/day versus 400 mg/kg/day dosage schedules of ampicillin (Overturf, et al., unpublished data). A total of 89 patients with meningitis due to H. influenzae, type B were studied; 37 received the lower and 45 the higher dosage; 7 were excluded. Sex, age, severity of disease and prior treatment with antibiotics were equivalent for both groups. Mortality, residua, length of hospital stay, cultures positive after 24 hours of therapy and complications were not significantly different for either group. Fever was present on the average one day longer in the low dose group, while eosinophilia and rash were increased in the high dose group. This suggests that 150 mg/kg/day schedule is sufficient for infections due to susceptible strains and that higher dosage is unnecessary.

ROUTE: Intravenous (IV) administration of antibiotics is preferred. However, if for some reason an IV line is not functional, rather than delay an individual dose, it may be given intramuscularly. Wilson and Haltalin[42] compared the two routes after initially treating patients with five days of IV therapy. No significant clinical or pharmacologic (i.e., CSF levels) differences were noted. We recommend the use of scalp vein needles for IV infusion, and these should be changed every 48 hours. Cutdowns and indwelling polyethylene catheters should be avoided if at all possible.

## SUMMARY

In summary, the diagnosis of meningitis must rely on a thorough evaluation of the clinical history and physical examination in addition to examination of the spinal fluid. Special attention should be given to the presence or absence of meningeal signs, focal neurologic signs and the presence or absence of signs and symptoms related to increased intracranial pressure. These factors, in association with the characteristics of spinal fluid, should lead to an etiologic or anatomic diagnosis in the vast majority of infections. The physician's first obligation is to exclude the potentially treatable conditions and, therefore, speed of diagnosis is critical. The performance of a lumbar puncture is mandatory to establish an etiologic diagnosis of most central nervous system infections; the overlap between various clinical syndromes requires its performance without delay. Only the presence of signs of acute increased intracranial pressure and focal neurologic signs should deter one from performing the LP. In this latter case, appropriate anatomic studies should be performed to exclude a mass lesion.

## REFERENCES

1. McCracken, G. H.: Neonatal septicemia and meningitis. Hosp. Prac. 11:89, 1976.

2. Mathies, A. W.: Penicillins in the treatment of bacterial meningitis. J. Roy. Coll. Phys. Lond. 6:139, 1972.

3. Smith, A.: Diagnosis of bacterial meningitis. Pediatrics 52:589, 1972.

4. Seligman, S. J.: The rapid differential diagnosis of meningitis. Med. Clin. N. A. 57:1417, 1973.

5. Macc, J. W., Peters, E. R., Mathies, A. W.: Cranial bruits in purulent meningitis in childhood. New Eng. J. Med. 278:1420, 1968.

6. Butler, W. T., et al: Diagnostic and prognostic value of clinical and laboratory findings in cryptococcal meningitis. New Eng. J. Med. 270:59, 1964.

7. Winn, W. A.: Coccidioidal Meningitis: A Follow-up Report, Coccidioidomycosis. Proceedings of the Second Coccidioidomycosis Symposium, (Ed.) L. Aje-lo. University of Arizona Press, Tucson, p. 55, 1967.

8. Idriss, Z. H., Sinno, A., Kronfol, N. M.: Tuberculous meningitis in childhood. Am. J. Dis. Child. 130:364, 1976.

9. Bucchner, H. A., et al: The current status of serologic, immunologic and skin tests in the diagnosis of pulmonary mycoses: Report of the committee of fungus disease and subcommittee on criteria for clinical diagnosis. Chest 63:259, 1973.

10. Meyer, R. D., Rosen, P., Armstrong, D.: Phycomycosis complicating leukemia and lymphoma. Ann. Int. Med. 77: 871, 1972.

11. King, R. B., et al: Nocardia asteroides meningitis. J. Neurosurg. 24:749, 1966.

12. Eastridge, C. E. , et al: Actinomycosis: 24-year experience. So. Med. J. 65:839, 1972.

13. Prystowsky, S. D. , et al: Invasive aspergillosis. New Eng. J. Med. 293:655, 1976.

14. Weinstein, A. J. , Johnson, E. H. , Moellering, R. C. : Candida endophthalmitis. Arch. Int. Med. 132:749, 1973.

15. Lincoln, E. M. : Tuberculosis in Children. McGraw-Hill, Inc. , New York, 1963.

16. Chapman, P. T. , revised by Eickhoff, T. C. : Tuberculosis in Communicable and Infectious Diseases, 8th Edition, (Ed. ) P. F. Wehrle. C. V. Mosby Co. , St. Louis, 1976.

17. Sells, C. J. , Carpenter, R. L. , Ray, C. G. : Sequelae of central nervous system enterovirus infection. New Eng. J. Med. 293:1, 1975.

18. Feagin, R. D. , Shackleford, P. G. : Value of repeat lumbar punctures in the differential diagnosis of meningitis. New Eng. J. Med. 289:571, 1973.

19. Sarubbi, F. A. , Sparling, F. , Glezen, W. P. : Herpes hominis encephalitis. Arch. Neurol. 29:268, 1973.

20. Carey, M. F. , Chou, S. M. , French, L. A. : Experience with brain abscesses. J. Neurosurg. 36:1, 1972.

21. Samson, D. S. , Clark, K. : A current review of brain abscess. Am. J. Med. 54:201, 1973.

22. Austin, D. , Sokolowski, J. N. : Postlumbar puncture chemical meningitis. N. Y. State J. Med. 68:2444, 1968.

23. Dixon, H. B. F. , Lipscomb, O. B. E. : Cysticercosis: An analysis and follow-up of 450 cases. Med. Research Council Report Series, No. 229, 1961.

24. Ziment, I. : Nervous system complications; bacterial endocarditis. Am. J. Med. 47:593, 1969.

25. Baraff, L. B. , Wehrle, P. F. : Los Angeles County Meningitis Surveillance Program, 1975-1976 (unpublished data).

26. Thornsberry, C. , Kirven, L. A. : Ampicillin resistance in Haemophilus influenzae as determined by a rapid test for beta-lactamase production. Antimicrob. Agents Chemother. 6:653, 1974.

27. Dalton, H. P. , Allison, M. J. : Modifications of laboratory results by partial treatment of bacterial meningitis. Am. J. Clin. Path. 49:410, 1968.

28. Harfer, D. H. : Preliminary antibiotic therapy in bacterial meningitis. Arch. Neurol. 9:343, 1963.

29. Winkelstein, J. A. : The influence of partial treatment with penicillin on the diagnosis of bacterial meningitis. J. Pediatrics 77:619, 1970.

30. Park, B. H. : The use and limitations of the nitroblue tetrazolium test as a diagnostic aid. J. Pediatrics 78: 376, 1971.

31. Fikrig, S. M. , et al: Nitroblue tetrazolium dye test and differential diagnosis of meningitis. J. Pediatrics 82:855, 1973.

32. Berman, N. S. , Siegel, S. E. , Nachum, R. , et al: Cerebrospinal fluid endotoxin concentrations in gram-negative bacterial meningitis. J. Pediatrics 88:553, 1976.

33. McCracken, G. H. , Sarff, L. D. : Endotoxin in CSF: Detection in neonates with bacterial meningitis. J. A. M. A. 235:617, 1976.

34. Shackleford, P. G. , Campbell, J. , Feigin, R. D. : Counter current immunoelectrophoresis in the evaluation of childhood infections. J. Pediatrics 85:478, 1974.

35. Coonrod, J. D. , Ryfel, N. W. : Determination of etiology of bacterial meningitis by counter immunoelectrophoresis. Lancet 1(2):1154, 1972.

36. Feldman, W. E. : CSF lactic acid dehydrogenase activity. Am. J. Dis. Child. 129:77, 1975.

37. Neches, W. , Platt, M. : CSF LDH in 287 children, including 53 cases of meningitis: Bacterial and non-bacterial etiology. Pediatrics 41:1097, 1968.

38. Lending, M. , Slobody, L. B. , Mestern, J. : CSF glutamic oxalacetic transaminase and lactic dehydrogenase activities in children with neurologic disorders. J. Pediatrics 65:415, 1964.

39. Van Rymenant, M. , Robert, J. , Otten, J. : Isocitric dehydrogenase in the CSF: Clinical usefulness of its determination. Neurology 16:351, 1966.

40. Controni, J. G. , et al: Rapid diagnosis of meningitis by gas-liquid chromatographic analysis of CSF lactic acid. Presented at the 75th Annual Meeting Am. Soc. Microbiol. , April, 1975.

41. Austrian, R. : S. pneumoniae, Chapter 8 in Manual of Clinical Microbiology, 2nd Edition, (Eds. ) Cennetu, E.H., Spaulding, E. H. , Thuart, J. P. Am. Soc. Microbiol. , Washington, D. C. , 1974.

42. Wilson, A. D. , Haltalin, K. C. : Ampicillin in H. influenzae meningitis. Am. J. Dis. Child. 129:208, 1975.

## 31: BRAIN ABSCESS
### by Gary Overturf

Pyogenic infections of the central nervous system may manifest as:

1) Bacterial meningitis (Chapter 30)
2) Cerebral abscess
3) Subdural empyema
4) Epidural (cerebral or spinal) abscess
5) Septic thrombophlebitis of the cortical veins or major cerebral venous sinuses

The brain abscess occurs during the first ten years of life and between the twentieth and forty-fifth years, more frequently among men. [1]

The brain abscess usually presents as an intracranial space-occupying lesion with or without fever. The symptoms include nausea, vomiting, headache and occasionally nuchal rigidity. It is often preceded by sinusitis, middle ear infection or heart disease (20%). [1] The diagnosis can be missed initially in 77% of the patients and mistaken for other diseases;[2,3] therefore, the clinical symptomatology alpha is rarely diagnostic.

The symptomatology of the frontal lobe abscess is indistinguishable from a frontal lobe tumor, such as headache, drowsiness, inattention, impaired higher intellectual functions and the increased grasp and suck reflexes. Similarly, a temporal lobe abscess may present with nominal aphasia, homonymous quadrantic hemianopsia, or weakness of the contralateral side of the face and the hand. Brain abscess, when ruptured, may present as acute meningitis.

### INVESTIGATIONS

Blood cultures are rarely rewarding in the diagnosis of brain abscess. The exception is endocarditis with septic emboli.

Roentgenograms of the skull, chest, sinuses and mastoid should be routinely obtained in all cases of suspected brain abscess. The chest may, on occasion, show evidence of lung abscess. The skull should be examined for evidence of fracture, shift of the pineal body, opacification of the sinuses, osteomyelitis and, rarely, gas formation. The skull x-rays are of diagnostic benefit in only 40% of the patients. [4]

The brain scan done with technetium, Tc-99m pertechnetate, if interpreted within the clinical context, is highly accurate. [5] Normal scan indicates an intact blood-brain barrier. When the disease causes a breach in this barrier, technetium accumulates in the pathologic brain tissue. The diagnostic accuracy of brain scan alone in the detection of brain abscess is close to 80%.

Angiography, especially of the carotid artery, may demonstrate the site of lesion in nearly 90% to 96% of the cases. Almost all cases of brain abscess can be diagnosed by combining angiography and brain scan. [6,7]

Ventriculograms are useful in establishing the diagnosis, but are uncomfortable to the patient and rarely required.

The electroencephalogram may show high voltage, slow waves, with occasional spike discharges over the surrounding area of the abscess. Its accuracy is close to that of the brain scan, nearly 80%. [2]

Computerized axial tomography (CAT) is also extremely helpful in the localization and the determination of the size of the brain abscess (see page 814). CAT scans can be more helpful than the carotid angiograms. They are of immense value in the localization of intracerebral lesions. The overall limitations of CAT scan in the diagnosis of brain abscess is unclear. I have seen cases of extradural and subdural empyemas missed by CAT scan.

Lumbar puncture: When brain abscess is clinically suspected, lumbar puncture should be postponed in favor of other diagnostic procedures. Lumbar puncture may precipitate catastrophic events. Fortunately, brain abscess is not as common as meningitis, and the latter should be diagnosed without delay. When meningitis is a diagnostic consideration, lumbar puncture should be done promptly without hesitation.

Papilledema is a delayed feature of brain abscess and, therefore, should neither be used for the diagnosis of brain abscess nor to differentiate it from meningitis. When papilledema is present, lumbar puncture should be deferred to a neurosurgeon.

The cerebrospinal fluid cell count might range from 25 to 400 cells/cu. mm. with 80% polymorphs. [1,2,3] When the abscess ruptures into the ventricle (Figs. 46, 47), it may appear purulent and the cell count may abruptly rise to 1,000 to 25,000 cells/cu. mm. The spinal fluid sugar may be normal in brain abscess, whereas it is decreased in meningitis, but the protein content

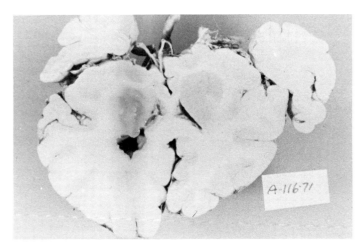

FIG. 46: Coronal section of the brain showing an area of abscess formation in the right cerebral hemisphere, in the region of the basal ganglia, with rupture into the third ventricle.

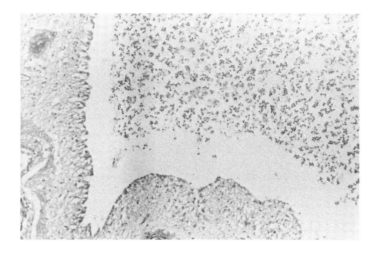

FIG. 47: Section of the same brain showing the ependymal lining of the third ventricle, which contains purulent exudate.

is very high in cases of brain abscess. The chlorides are of no diagnostic value. Gram's stains may fail to reveal the organisms in nearly 75%; nevertheless, they should be performed in all cases of purulent meningitis. In general, patients with positive smears and cultures of the spinal fluid carry worse prognoses than those who have no demonstrable organisms.

## MICROBIOLOGY

The etiologic agent should be suspected on the basis of the predisposing cause. The aerobes, especially Staphylococcus aureus, cause brain abscess secondary to a neurosurgical procedure.[8] No detectable primary focus may be present in nearly 70% of the cases of brain abscess caused by anaerobic bacteria. Spinal fluid specimens in cases of suspected brain abscess should be routinely processed for anaerobic bacteria, as well.

Streptococcus viridans, microaerophilic and anaerobic streptococci (Peptostreptococcus, Peptococcus) are the most frequent isolates. [6,7,8] They are susceptible to penicillin. Bacteroides fragilis, a penicillin-resistant organism, is an infrequent isolate of almost all intracranial infections, including brain abscess.

Actinomyces israelii, Fusobacterium and Clostridium are rare causes. [7] Enterobacteriaceae group of organisms is isolated much less frequently.

## LOCATION OF THE ABSCESS

Frontal and temporal lobes are more frequently involved than the parietal. Occipital lobe involvement is the least common. In children, cerebellar involvement is common. [9]

## DIFFERENTIAL DIAGNOSIS

The brain abscess should be differentiated from other intracranial lesions, including epidural abscess and subdural empyema. These differentiations are often of academic importance because they all require surgery. Without surgical drainage, the brain abscess, subdural and epidural abscesses are invariably fatal. In spite of surgical drainage, the mortality is around 20% to 50%.

## PROGNOSIS

The greatest danger of brain abscess is the mass effect first, and the infection second. In spite of the administration of anti-biotics known to be effective against the organisms isolated from the site of infection in cases of brain abscess, in several instances, the bacteria may still be persistent in an undrained abscess.

## MORTALITY FACTORS [10]

Following are poor prognostic indicators:

1. Coma on admission
2. Multiple brain abscesses
3. Rupture of the abscess into the ventricle
4. Inaccurate or missed diagnosis

It is also poor among those with:

5. Positive spinal fluid cultures
6. Brain abscess secondary to remote primary focus of infection
7. Absence of focal signs
8. Seizures
9. Symptoms of meningitis early in the illness

The prognosis is more favorable among those who are not in coma on admission, and who had prior cranial injury or surgery with contiguous infection.

## ANTIBIOTICS

Penicillin in large doses (20 million units) is effective against most bacteria isolated from brain abscess. When in doubt, because of the possibility of the associated Bacteroides fragilis, generally resistant to penicillin, chloramphenicol should be used. Chloramphenicol is recommended to be administered alone and not to be combined with penicillin; the combined effect of these antibiotics may be inferior to that of either one of them used alone.

## SUBDURAL EMPYEMA

Sinusitis, mastoiditis, chronic suppurative otitis media and septic endocarditis (paradoxical emboli with congenital heart disease) are some of the common predisposing causes for subdural empyema. [10,11] Most of them are due to anaerobic bacteria, anaerobic streptococci being the most frequent. Subdural empyema accounts for one-fifth of all cases of intracranial suppuration. The clinical features and physical signs are indistinguishable from brain abscess. In children, the subdural effusion may be complicated by empyema of the chest.

Lumbar puncture is hazardous. A straight x-ray of the skull and sinuses should be done in all cases. Arteriography is one of the most reliable methods for diagnosing subdural empyema. Subdural empyemas should be diagnosed promptly and surgically drained, or else the outcome is fatal. The most common cause of death in subdural empyema is failure to recognize the disease process during the first week of illness.

An x-ray of the skull might show opacification of the frontal sinuses, osteomyelitis of the skull bones and sometimes an intracranial epidural gas at the site of infection.

## CRANIAL EPIDURAL ABSCESS

Epidural abscess may result from mastoiditis or sinusitis or cranial surgery. [12] The clinical signs of epidural abscess may be more subtle than a brain abscess. On occasion, a patient may have no more than a headache or pain at the site of infection with fever. The cerebrospinal fluid, as in the case of brain abscess, may be sterile or contain 25 to 400 cells, predominantly lymphocytes with normal sugar and increased proteins.

Case History of Subdural Abscess: A 19-year-old male was admitted with two weeks' history of fever and chills associated with headaches. He was stuporous on admission. It was later found that two months prior to admission, he had an attack of pneumonia and a week prior to admission, he had dental extraction.

He appeared acutely ill with fever of 105.6°F., pulse 84, blood pressure 112/70, respiration 24. His ear, nose and throat examination was unremarkable, except that he had stiffness of the neck. He was awake but not alert. Lumbar puncture was performed for diagnosis.

The peripheral WBC count was 22,400/cu. mm.; otherwise, the remaining laboratory tests were unremarkable. He was started on dexamethasone, mannitol and chloramphenicol. The spinal fluid showed a white cell count of 317/cu. mm. with 40% polymorphs and 60% lymphocytes and 2,000 red blood cells. Angiography was unremarkable. The brain scan was abnormal. One hour later, he developed fixed, dilated pupils with papilledema and decerebrate rigidity accompanied by bilateral plantar extensor responses. At this time, burr holes were performed on both sides of the skull, and he was discovered to have epidural and subdural empyema. He had a stormy postoperative course and died one week later. At autopsy, purulent material was found in the subdural and epidural areas, which was greenish in color, in addition to evidence of increased intracranial tension, such as uncus herniation.

COMMENT: The preceding case history suggests the typical outcome of subdural empyema or brain abscess when the diagnosis is delayed.

The pus cultures obtained at surgery grew Bacteroides fragilis and Peptococcus magnus, both susceptible to chloramphenicol at less than 5 mcg./ml. dilution.

## SPINAL EPIDURAL ABSCESS

Spinal epidural abscess may be found in association with vertebral osteomyelitis. Spinal epidural infections are infrequent.

Staphylococcus aureus is the most common etiologic agent, followed by Streptococcus, Pneumococcus, Salmonella and other gram-negative organisms. Among addicts, Pseudomonas and Serratia organisms are frequently implicated. In most parts of the world, Mycobacterium (M.) tuberculosis is the most common cause of spinal epidural abscess. Bacterial infections other than M. tuberculosis are more common in North America.

A careful physical examination should be performed on all those patients who complain of fever and chills; chronic low back pain with tenderness. Physical examination may show limitation of movement. Skin infections are occasionally the primary focus of infection. On occasion, the primary focus may be either a pneumonia or urinary tract infection.

When the disease is in progress, it may cause backache, followed by root pains and weakness of the limbs, later followed by paralysis. Fever, backache and local tenderness are common with spinal epidural abscess.

The spinal fluid may reveal pus cells and increased protein, normal or low sugar, with or without bacteria on Gram's stain. The white cell count may range from 0 to 800 cells/cu. mm., predominantly polymorphonuclear. The protein is markedly increased, usually greater than 400 mg. %, but the glucose is usually within normal limits. Roentgenographic examination of the spine may be consistent with osteomyelitis.

Myelograms may show a block or may be abnormal, with compression or obstruction to the flow of the contrast material.

The scans with Tc-99m and Ga-67 may show increased uptake in these areas. [9]

Signs of cord compression require myelography; evidence of block, when found, should be promptly followed by laminectomy, and abscess drainage to prevent paralysis. Semisynthetic penicillins or cephalosporins are the drugs of choice.

## THROMBOSIS OF THE CEREBRAL VENOUS SINUSES

It is a rare complication which can occur within three to ten days after the onset of meningitis. Clinically, it is indistinguishable from bacterial cerebral abscess, except that it responds to antibiotic therapy alone; no surgery is required.

## REFERENCES

1. Balakrishnan, D. , Natarajan, M.: Intracranial abscesses. J. Indian Med. Assoc. 57:87, 1971.

2. Brewer, N.S. , MacCarthy, C.S. , Wellman, W.E.: Brain abscess: A review of recent experience. Ann. Int. Med. 82:571, 1975.

3. Samson, D.S. , Clark, K.: A current review of brain abscess. Amer. J. Med. 54:201, 1973.

4. Handel, S.F. , Klein, W.C. , Kim, Y.W.: Intracranial epidural abscess. Radiology III:117, 1974.

5. Crocker, E.F. , et al: Technetium brain scanning in the diagnosis and management of cerebral abscess. Amer. J. Med. 56:192, 1974.

6. Heineman, H.S. , Braude, A.I.: Anaerobic infections of the brain. Amer. J. Med. 35:682, 1963.

7. Swartz, M.N. , Karchmer, A.W.: Infections of the Central Nervous System. Anaerobic Bacteria: Role in Disease, (Eds. ). A. Balows, et al. Charles C Thomas, Springfield, p. 309, 1974.

8.   Fleurette, J. , Riou, R. :  Etude bacteriologique de 44
     cas d'absces du cerveau observes de 1970 a 1973. Lyon
     Medical 233:1141, 1975.

9.   Editorial: Subdural suppuration. Lancet 2:1299, 1972.

10.  Karandanis, D. , Shulman, J. A. :  Factors associated with
     mortality in brain abscess. Arch. Int. Med. 135:1145,
     1975.

11.  Yoshikawa, T. T. , Chow, A. W. , Guze, L. B. : Role of
     anaerobic bacteria in subdural empyema. Am. J. Med.
     58:99, 1975.

12.  Baker, A. S. , et al: Spinal epidural abscess. New Eng. J.
     Med. 293:463, 1975.

## 32: TICK PARALYSIS
### by H. Thadepalli

Tick paralysis is not an infectious disease; it is a toxin-produced paralysis, caused by a tick, that can also transmit Rickettsia and leptospirosis. The paralysis caused by the tick mimics Guillain-Barre syndrome.

### THE TICK

The female pregnant wood tick, Dermacentor (D.) andersoni, in the West, and D. variabilis, the dog tick, in the eastern portion of the United States, causes this disease. It liberates a neurotoxin which can block the production of acetylcholine [1] from the neuromuscular junctions.

### CLINICAL FEATURES

Dramatic and rapidly progressive ascending paralysis, beginning with the feet up, is the rule. When not diagnosed promptly, it progresses to bulbar palsy and death. The sensory system is intact and the mental status is undisturbed. Tick paralysis is prevalent in children because of their tendency to pet animals. It tends to be more severe in women, because the tick may remain undetected longer in the scalp hair of girls than in that of boys. The victim is afebrile to the end.

### DIAGNOSIS

A history of being near animals or being in certain known tick zones in the country, and awareness of the entity, are the clues to the diagnosis. At present, there are no laboratory tests to detect this disease. The spinal fluid is unremarkable. When the diagnosis is clinically suspected, one must carefully look for the engorged tick in the scalp, ears, behind the ears, under the breasts, groin or perineum. [2]

THERAPY: This consists of removal of the tick with its mouth parts intact.

PROGNOSIS: Death can occur in 12% to 14% of the cases. [3]

### REFERENCES

1. Murnaghan, M. F.: Site and mechanism of the tick paralysis. Science 131:418, 1960.

2. Abbott, K. H.: Tick paralysis. Review I & II: Proc. Mayo Clin. 18:39-45, 59-64, 1943.

3. Rose, I.: A review of tick paralysis. Can. Med. Assoc. 70:175, 1954.

## 33: BOTULISM
by H. Thadepalli

### THE ORGANISM

Botulism is a paralytic disease of the vertebrates. It is a disease of intoxication, not infection. Botulism is caused by the gram-positive anaerobic bacilli, Clostridium (C.) botulinum, which has a subterminal spore. Its spore is heat-resistant, and, by itself, is incapable of causing the disease. Its toxin is heat-sensitive and is the most lethal known toxin. A mere taste of food with this toxin would be fatal. C. botulinum is a normal flora of the intestinal tract of some animals and birds. It produces eight varieties of toxin, simply called A, B, $C_1$, $C_2$, D, E, F, and G, but most human intoxications are caused by A, B or E. They are designated as C. botulinum types A to G. The bacteriophages can change type C to D or change it to an altogether different species, Clostridium novyi type A. The disease is acquired by eating canned or improperly stored food. Three-fourths of the outbreaks in the United States are caused by mushrooms and other vegetables. The sausages (botutinus), after which the disease is named, are responsible for less than 15% of the outbreaks. The "izushi" food in Japan (soaked, salted and fermented fish) caused 57 outbreaks in 17 years. Eggs of the salmon fish were the source of several epidemics among the Eskimos.[1]

### CLINICAL FEATURES

Botulism may present as:

        A. Food poisoning
        B. Wound botulism
        C. Infant botulism

A. FOOD POISONING: The outbreak may attack a group of people in a party or a household or occasionally an individual, generally 18 to 36 hours (even up to 8 days) after the ingestion of a botulogenic food.

The clinical picture is characterized by four positive and four negative signs. They are the presence of the following:

1) Visual disturbances (mydriasis, external ophthalmoplegia) such as blurring of vision, diplopia
2) Speech disturbances (dysphonia, dysarthria)

3) Dysphagia
4) Bilateral, symmetrical descending motor paralysis

It is further characterized by the absence of the following:

1) Diarrhea: Although it is a form of food poisoning, diarrhea seldom occurs in botulism. Constipation is the rule.
2) Sensory disturbances are absent.
3) Mentation is clear to the point of death. It is one of the most pathetic deaths known.
4) Fever is rare, unless the patient develops secondary infection due to aspiration pneumonia. Death can occur within a few hours to ten days in 40% to 50% of the cases. [1]

B. WOUND BOTULISM: Open wounds can be contaminated with C. botulinum from the soil. In most instances, it is of no consequence.[2] On occasion, C. botulinum types A and B notably can produce toxins and produce the syndrome of botulism. The contagion can be introduced through improperly sterilized catgut.

C. INFANT BOTULISM:[3] Infant botulism is a form of "floppy" baby syndrome, characterized by acute and progressive weakness which occurs in infants and young children. Soon the infant is unable to suck or swallow, loses head control and cries very feebly. Close examination may reveal ptosis, sluggish reaction to pupils, decreased extra-ocular and facial movements and depressed gag reflex. Nearly a third of them develop respiratory arrest.

## DIAGNOSIS

The syndrome of acute onset of diplopia, dysphagia, and dysphonia without fever or mental disturbances, and history of a potentially botulogenic food, should lead one to consider the possibility of botulism. The following investigations may reveal diagnostic clues:

1) Blood for levels of botulism toxin. Withdraw 20 ml. of blood for this purpose before administering the antitoxin. This is useful in all three types of botulism described.

2) Feces can be examined for the botulism toxin. It is rewarding in cases of infant botulism and food poisoning, but not in wound botulism. The botulism toxin can be recovered from the feces for several weeks after the patient has become totally asymptomatic.

3) Fecal culture for Clostridium botulinum

4) Fluorescent antibody is an extremely useful and a relative- ly quick way to detect C. botulinum in the stool. It can also be used for the detection of these organisms in the wound.

5) Wound cultures: All dirty wounds in the presence of a clin- ical picture suspicious of botulism should be cultured.

6) Gastric aspirates and the suspected food should also be cul- tured and processed for the detection of botulinum toxin by mouse neutralization test. Honey was suspected to be the source of botulism toxin for infant botulism.

The final detection of the toxin, and the identification of the organism, may require intraperitoneal inoculation in ani- mals for the demonstration of toxicity of the organism. If not, it can be mistaken for 70 other named and a couple of hundred innominate, Clostridia. Gas-liquid chromatography and biochemical reactions in the pre-reduced media are also useful. C. botulinum can also be detected by rapid gas chromatographic technique in contaminated food.[4]

7) Electromyography (EMG) is extremely useful to differen- tiate it from Guillain-Barre syndrome. In botulism, the amplitude of the muscle action potential is usually dimin- ished in response to a single supramaximal stimulus. But, when paired or repetitive supramaximal stimuli at rates of 25 to 50/second are applied, facilitation of the action potential occurs.[5]

## DIFFERENTIAL

Botulism should be differentiated from the following:

1) Myasthenia gravis: By its response to tensilon test
2) Antibiotic toxicity: Aminoglycoside antibiotics may rarely cause a sudden onset of such paralysis.
3) Diphtheria
4) Tick paralysis (see page 268)
5) Guillain-Barre syndrome
6) Hypermagnesemia
7) Hypocalcemia
8) Cobra bite: Ptosis is a late feature of cobra poisoning.
9) Paralytic shellfish poisoning
10) Belladonna or atropine intoxication: The mouth is dry and fever is usually present.

11) Mushroom (muscarine) poisoning
12) Carbon monoxide poisoning
13) Lambert-Eaton syndrome

## TREATMENT

Complete recovery can occur in botulism without therapy over a period of weeks. Antitoxin therapy often prevents the further progression of the disease, but dramatic improvement is not expected.

1) The antitoxin: If the type of the organism is known, one may use monovalent serum (50,000 units). If not, trivalent (against types A, B and E), 100,000 units, should be used.

2) Guanidine: This, which enhances the release of acetylcholine at the nerve terminal, was also found to be effective in the treatment of botulism. [7]

## REFERENCES

1. Dolman, C. E.: Human botulism in Canada. C. M. A. Journal 110:191, 1974.

2. Hall, I. C.: The occurrence of Bacillus botulinus type A and B in accidental wounds. J. Bacteriol. 50:213, 1945.

3. Arrow, S.S., et al: Infant botulism. J.A.M.A. 237:1946, 1977.

4. Mayhew, J.W., Gorbach, S.L.: Rapid gas chromatographic technique for presumptive detection of Clostridium botulinum in contaminated food. Appl. Microbiol. 29:297, 1975.

5. Merson, M. H., et al: Current trends in botulism in the United States. J.A.M.A. 229:1305, 1974.

6. Cherington, M.: Botulism. Ten years experience. Arch. Neurol. 30:432, 1974.

34: TETANUS
by H. Thadepalli


THE ORGANISM

Tetanus is caused by Clostridium (C.) tetani, a motile anaerobic, gram-positive tennis racket shaped organism with a size of
0.5 x 2.5μ, with a terminal spore. It produces one of the most
deadly toxins (next only to C. botulinum), called tetanospasmin, an exo-neurotoxin which can inhibit the production of
acetylcholine at neuromuscular and neuroneuronal junctions,
producing the tetanic spasms of voluntary striated muscles. C.
tetani is a normal flora of the stools of many living creatures,
including man. Like most Clostridia, it is a soil organism,
which can be found as a wound contaminant in 1% of open wounds
without producing tetanus.


THE DISEASE

Nearly half a million people die every year worldwide because
of this disease. It is the commonest disease of the neuromuscular system in the tropics. About 100 cases of tetanus are reported per year in the United States.

Predisposing causes include trauma, surgery, tooth extraction,
otitis media, circumcision, deliveries conducted at home with
cutting of the umbilical cord with contaminated instruments,
dirty splinters, gunshot or knife wounds, septic abortion and
heroin or other drug addiction.[1]

The tetanospasmin is generated during the germination of the
spores of C. tetani, which spreads centripetally through the
bloodstream, lymphatics and neurons, and finally fixes to the
neuromuscular and neuroneuronal junction.


MORTALITY

It is a highly fatal disease, with 20% to 90% mortality in the
neonates, and 16% to 60% in the adult over 45 years of age.

The incubation period can be as short as three to ten days, but
is generally ten to fourteen days. The shorter the incubation
period, the graver the prognosis. The nearer the site of the
wound to the face, the faster the onset of the lockjaw, which is
the characteristic sign of tetanus.

## CLINICAL FEATURES

Muscle spasms elicited by even the slightest stimulation, slight noise or change in brightness of the room, or the slightest bodily movement, can provoke a spasmodic fit. Tetanus can begin at any part of the body and spread centripetally and produce lockjaw, or it may begin with a lockjaw. The lockjaw, as it is meant, is literally the inability to open the mouth because of spasms of the masseter muscles. The mentation is clear to the end.

NEONATAL TETANUS: This can manifest within a week to ten days after birth, sometimes with fever ($101^O$ to $104^O$F. ). The infant is unable to suck because of the spasms and the contractions of the facial muscles, which give a characteristic caricature of an unhappy face, called risus sardonicus. Neonatal tetanus is often due to umbilical cord contamination. In Araku Valley, Andhra, India, where I worked as a physician for one of the hill tribes called Khonds (hill-loving people), they had a habit of cutting the cord with a sickle if it were a girl (that she would reap good harvests in the field), and with an arrow (that he would be a good hunter) if it were a boy. Neonatal tetanus was a common disease among them.

LOCAL TETANUS: When tetanus starts at the site of injury, it causes reflex spasms of the muscles in the vicinity, but may not cause lockjaw. However, a reflex trismus can occur when the jaw is suddenly depressed.

CEPHALIC TETANUS: This is a disease with grave prognosis. The site of infection is the middle ear or a wound in the head and neck region. Cephalotetanus begins with lockjaw, and various cranial nerves, III, IV, VI, VII and XII, may be involved. Seventh nerve involvement is the most frequent. The remaining nerves are not that commonly involved. Cephalotetanus is a rare disease. Vakil encountered 23 cases of cephalotetanus among 1025 cases of tetanus.

CHRONIC TETANUS: An attack of tetanus does not confirm immunity from future attacks. Fortunately, it is not common, but it can recur and produce a second and even a third episode. [3]

## INVOLVEMENT OF THE SYMPATHETIC SYSTEM

When the lateral horn cells of the spinal cord are involved by tetanospasmin, excitation of the sympathetic nervous system occurs. It is characterized by hyperhydrosis, tachycardia,

cardiac arrhythmias, periodic, but brief, episodes of hyper-
or hypotension, fever, and increased output of urinary cate-
cholamines. [4, 5]

Some of the previously mentioned symptoms can be due to recurrent minute pulmonary emboli.

## DIAGNOSIS

Tetanus is often a clinical diagnosis; the organism is difficult
to isolate.

A.  CULTURES: Nearly a third of the wound cultures in tetanus are said to be positive. The specimen can be smeared
on a slide, gram-stained and examined for Clostridia with
a terminal spore (Fig. 48). Often, it is found in the company of other Clostridia of other subspecies and other aerobic and anaerobic organisms. Isolation of C. tetani in pure
culture is often a formidable task.

At one time, I collected all four gangrenous toes, resected
in a patient suffering from tetanus and cultured for aerobic
and anaerobic bacteria. The patient was a 35-year-old American Indian who was a garbage collector, in Chicago. After
a drinking spree between Christmas and the New Year of
1972, he felt warm enough to walk in the snow, without shoes,
on a cold and windy day. He picked up a garbage can and
accidentally dropped it on his feet. He found that his toes
had changed color the next day, but since he felt no pain,
he did not seek medical help until the holiday season was
over. He was admitted during the first week of January for
gangrene of his toes. The nurse found that the patient was
unable to eat his breakfast because of the inability to open
his mouth. Tetanus was suspected and the gangrenous toes
were amputated.

Gram's stain of the specimens from the gangrenous toes
(see Fig. 48) showed a variety of bacteria and a Clostridium
with a terminal spore. On culture, it yielded Proteus mirabilis, Escherichia coli, Enterococcus, Enterobacter hafniae,
and Pseudomonas aeruginosa, in addition to C. perfringens,
C. bifermentans, C. novyi, C. sporogenes and C. subter-
minale. We failed to isolate C. tetani, in spite of rigorous
and meticulous culturing with sophisticated anaerobic techniques and other recommended techniques for culturing this
organism. This illustrates the practical difficulties in isolating C. tetani.

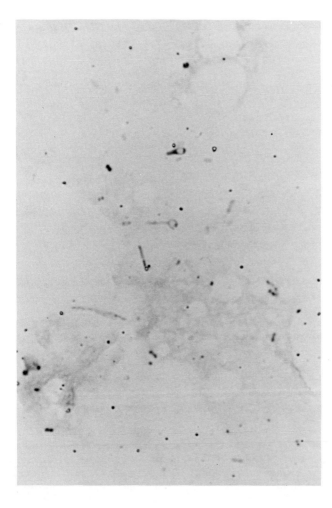

FIG. 48: Gram's stain from a case of tetanus showing Clostridium (C) tetani, seen as thin, tennis racket shaped, sporebearing bacillis to the left, of which there is another Clostridium species (not tetani). Five other species of Clostridia were also isolated from this specimen. See text for case report.

This case also illustrates certain difficulties encountered in the clinical management of tetanus. The toes were amputated under general anesthesia because of an unsuccessful attempt to do local nerve block. When he recovered from anesthesia, the endotracheal tube was removed. It, in turn, excited a severe laryngospasm, creating asphyxia and cardiac arrest, for which reason an immediate tracheostomy was done. The patient never recovered from the brain damage during this episode and remained dependent on the respirator for nearly a month. During this period, he developed disseminated intravascular coagulation secondary to antibiotics administered to suppress secondary bacterial infections. He finally died of accidental disconnection from the respirator.

B. MOUSE INOCULATION: The tissue should be coarsely ground in normal saline and the specimen centrifuged. The fluid should be injected into four mice, two of which are immunized with tetanus antitoxin several hours prior to intraperitoneal inoculation of the test material, and two are used as unprotected controls. If the unprotected animals die within three days, and those immunized do not, the diagnosis of tetanus is almost certain. It should, of course, be confirmed by culture. Occasionally, contamination from other toxigenic Clostridia, such as C. perfringens, may kill all four animals when the diagnosis is uncertain.

C. FLUORESCENT ANTIBODY TEST: This test can be used for the detection of C. tetani in tissue specimens.

D. ANTITOXIN ASSAY: In the serum, this can be done by hemagglutination inhibition test or mouse neutralization test. Demonstration of 0.01 I. U. of antitoxin/ml. is considered protective.

E. DEMONSTRATION OF NEUROTOXIN: This is required to confirm the diagnosis, even if C. tetani is isolated from a wound. All strains of C. tetani are not toxigenic.

F. OTHER LABORATORY TESTS: The leukocyte count may be normal or increased; platelets and fibrinolysin content may also be decreased. Prothrombin and thrombin generation time; enzymes, like SGOT, SGPT and CPK; aldolase and alkaline phosphatase may be increased. The iron content is decreased with increase in iron-binding capacity. The serum calcium, magnesium, inorganic phosphorous and leucine aminopeptidase may be normal. Metabolic

acidosis is frequent. The cerebrospinal fluid is normal.
Electroencephalogram and electromyelography are useless
for diagnosis. Electrocardiogram may reveal nodal or sinus tachycardia, nodal bradycardia, AV node delay with
first degree blocks, U wave, extrasystoles and decreased
voltage patterns and changes in axis.

## DIFFERENTIAL

Fever is not an early feature of tetanus, which distinguishes
it from other febrile illnesses, such as quinsy (peritonsillar
abscess). It should be distinguished from dislocated mandible,
rabies (see page 674), and dental abscess. Tetany (hypocalcemia) has the characteristic carpopedal spasm (Trousseau's
sign). Allergic disorders, due to phenothiazines can cause an
extra-pyramidal disease with trismus; it can be diagnosed by
the red-purple reaction of the urine with 10% ferric chloride;
it improves on intravenous benadryl which distinguishes it
from tetanus.

## THERAPY

There is no treatment for tetanus. If the patient survives the
first 21 days, recovery can be expected. Masterful management during this time is the most important. C. tetani is susceptible to penicillin, but penicillin will not cure the disease.
Antibiotics, perhaps, kill the tetanus bacillus by eradicating
the other associated organisms from the sites of infection that
promote a congenial environment for the growth of C. tetani.
Antitoxin will destroy the circulating toxin, if any, but has no
effect on fixed toxin. I believe that 2,000 units of antitoxin is
just as good as 120,000 I. U. In my opinion, tetanus should
be regarded as dangerous even if it is just a single muscle
twitch to begin with. A benign twitch can soon become
universal and march down to the grave.

For cases of clinical tetanus, we give 500 units of tetanus immune globulin on one arm and 50,000 units of toxoid on the
other. They should not be given in the same arm or mixed in
the syringe, for when toxoid is mixed with immune globulin,
they can be neutralized.

REFERENCES

1. Weinstein, L.: Tetanus. New Eng. J. Med. 289:1293, 1973.

2. Vakil, B.J., et al: Cephalic tetanus. Neurology 23:1091, 1973.

3. Vakil, B.J., Mehta, A.J., Tulpule, T.H.: Recurrent tetanus. Postgrad. Med. J. 40:601, 1964.

4. Corbett, J.L., Spalding, J.M.K., Harris, P.J.: Hypotension in tetanus. Brit. Med. J. 2:423, 1973.

5. Kerr, J.H., et al: Involvement of the sympathetic nervous system in tetanus. Lancet 2:236, 1968.

# SECTION D: HEART

## 35: PERICARDITIS AND PERICARDIAL EFFUSION
by H. Thadepalli

## PHYSICAL EXAMINATION

PAIN: Acute crunching, or nagging periodic, or constant peri-cardial pain, with or without radiation to the back or the shoul-ders, that is aggravated by lying on the back but relieved by the prone position, is very characteristic of pericarditis. The patient might assume the "Namaz pose" or knee-elbow position, as though praying in a mosque, to obtain relief of the chest pain. Generalized anasarca is rare, but, when present, can be mis-taken for nephrotic syndrome, cirrhosis of the liver or poly-serositis.

FEVER: Fluctuating fever up to $103^{\circ}$ to $104^{\circ}$F. with or without chills, associated with leukocytosis and increased sedimenta-tion rate, is usually present.

The cervical veins appear distended and the anterior intercos-tal spaces may appear full.

On palpation, the pericardial rub may be palpable in the pre-cardial area.

On percussion, there may be dullness over the right border of the heart for three to four centimeters beyond the right sternal border in the fourth and fifth intercostal spaces. The heart sounds are often distant, normal or loud, or often muffled. Cardi-ac murmurs may or may not be heard. A to-and-fro, or a sin-gular "systolic scratch" heard in the pericardium, may suggest pericarditis. A pericardial rub may be heard even in mas-sive pericardial effusions.

Dullness to percussion over the right infra and mid-scapular zones of the chest, due to consolidation of the right middle or lower lobes of the lung (Ewart's sign), may be present. It is attributed to the obstruction of lymphatics in the adjacent lung. Ar-thritis or meningitis may be present in Haemophilus influenza or meningococcal infection and occasionally viral infections like Rubella and Herpes. In most instances (greater than 60%), the etiology of pericarditis and effusion may remain undetermined. Such cases are referred to as "acute idiopathic pericarditis".

BLOOD CULTURES: These should be obtained in all suspected cases of pericarditis. The blood culture isolate is often, but not necessarily, the etiologic agent of pericarditis.

VIRUS CULTURES: Viruses may be cultured from the stool or from the pericardial fluid. A four-fold rise in viral antibody titers in the serum, and/or pericardial fluid or culture of the virus from the stool, or from the pericardial fluid, strongly favors the viral etiology.

CHEST ROENTGENOGRAM: It may show increased size in the cardiac silhouette, associated with bulging of the left border of the heart, resembling an aneurysm of the left ventricle. When the cardiac silhouette is much larger than the actual size of the heart, as determined clinically by location of the apical impulse, pericardial effusion should be considered as the most likely diagnosis.

ECHOCARDIOGRAPHY: This is a non-invasive diagnostic procedure, very useful in the diagnosis of pericardial effusion. Demonstration of echo-free space behind, below or in front of the heart is suggestive of pericardial effusion.

CARDIAC CATHETERIZATION: When the catheter is lying in the right atrium, it may demonstrate the space between the catheter and the lung and indicate the presence of fluid in the pericardial sac. During catheterization, one might inject a radiopaque material into the right atrium and demonstrate the increased gap between the right atrium and the lung.

CARBON DIOXIDE ANGIOGRAPHY: Insufflation of carbon dioxide into the right atrium may demonstrate the pericardial sac space between the right side of the heart and the lung.

PERICARDIOCENTESIS: Aspiration of 30 ml. or more of fluid by pericardiocentesis is the sine qua non of pericardial effusion. The clinical, radiologic, echocardiographic and scintigraphic techniques are not foolproof diagnostic methods. Aspiration of the pericardial fluid should be performed, taking all aseptic precautions. A 16-gauge needle attached to the EKG machine may be used for this purpose. Pericardiocentesis may be done through the infra-xiphisternal route, with the needle directed upwards or through the fourth or fifth intercostal space to the right of the sternum, or from the back of the chest. I prefer the infra-xiphisternal route. Arrhythmia may occur during peri- cardiocentesis. One should be prepared to manage arrhyth- mias. The normal pericardium may contain up to 25 to 30 ml. of fluid. In acute pericarditis with effusion, nearly 250 to 300 ml. may be found. In chronic pericardial effusions secondary to tuberculosis or malignancy, however, a full liter of fluid may accumulate in the pericardial sac. Pyogenic pericardial effu- sions generally contain up to 300 to 500 ml. of pus.

Characteristics of the pericardial fluid: The aspirate is usu- ally serosanguineous in tuberculous pericardial effusion. It is turbid or frankly purulent in pyogenic pericarditis. It may be hemorrhagic in tuberculous pericardial effusion, due to rup- ture of granulation tissue and postmyocardial infarction syn- drome. It is cloudy yellow in myxedema.

Gram's stains of aspirated pericardial fluid should be examined in all instances. Acid-fast stains should also be done routine- ly, but they are rarely rewarding. The acid-fast stains may be done on the centrifugate. Alternatively, the pericardial fluid may be left standing for several hours. A "web" forms on the top of the fluid on standing. This web may be removed with the tip of a needle and transferred to the surface of a clean glass slide, heat-fixed and stained for acid-fast bacilli. An aliquot of all the specimens should also be sent for cultures.

The sugar content of pericardial fluid is low in bacterial peri- carditis but normal in others. The characteristics of fluid in exudative pericarditis are similar to those of exudative pleural fluid. In pericarditis, the cell counts may be increased up to 400 to 500 cells; occasionally up to several thousands of cells per ml. of sample. The protein content of the fluid is at least about 4 gm./100 ml. In infection, the LDH may be elevated. The leukocytic response is predominantly polymorphonuclear in acute bacterial pericarditis. It may be mononuclear in chronic pericarditis and tuberculous pericarditis.

COUNTER-CURRENT IMMUNOELECTROPHORESIS (CIE): This is extremely useful in the diagnosis of partially treated bacterial pericarditis. CIE may also be used for the rapid de- tection of bacteria in pericardial effusion.

PERICARDIAL BIOPSY: This is very useful in the diagnosis of tuberculous pericarditis and pericarditis secondary to ma- lignancy. Pericardial biopsy may be obtained by either a closed or open needle biopsy.

## TUBERCULOUS PERICARDITIS

Tuberculosis should be considered in the diagnosis of pericardial effusions, although only 10% of the cases are caused by tuberculosis. In 60% of the cases, the cause of effusion is unknown. The primary focus of tuberculosis is often clinically obscure. A chest roentgenogram may show old lesions, rarely pneumonia or cavitation. At autopsy, the mediastinal lymph nodes are almost always found to be involved in tuberculous pericarditis. Fever, tachycardia, cardiomegaly, hepatomegaly, positive Ewart's sign, and increased venous pressure that is greater than 100 mm. of water are some of the signs of tuberculous pericardial effusion. It is more common among men at the ages of 20 to 40. Symptoms of weight loss, cough, dyspnea, chest pain and fever are frequently present. Most patients will have a positive skin test ( >10 mm. induration) when tested with intermediate strength PPD. M. tuberculosis may be cultured from the gastric aspirates and, in one-half of the patients, from the pericardial fluid itself.[1,2]

The bacterial causes of pericarditis in children are M. tuberculosis, Haemophilus influenzae, meningococcus and pneumococcus. Some may present with simultaneous meningitis and pericarditis, or as pericardial effusion without meningitis. [3]

In compromised patients, such as those with lupus erythematosus and uremia, Staphylococcus aureus pericarditis is more common.

In certain cases of septicemia due to Staphylococcus aureus or gram-negative bacilli, a delayed febrile pleuro-pericarditis-like syndrome resembling the post-cardiotomy syndrome may develop, [4] presumably due to an allergic reaction to the circulatory bacterial proteins. Such patients frequently respond to antibiotic therapy directed against the primary infection.

Pericardial tamponade is the most dreaded complication of pericardial effusion. The accompanying clinical distress is not always proportional to the quantity of accumulated pericardial fluid. Whereas rapid accumulation of 250 ml. of fluid in the pericardium can cause an immediate deterioration, often a slow accumulation of even up to 1,000 ml. over a period of one month may remain silent. While I was in India, one of my patients walked into the hospital without any complaints other than mild pericardial discomfort. On physical examination, he had pericardial fullness with "silent heart". Because of the shortage of radiographic film, fluoroscopy was done, which revealed a massive, but immobile, cardiac silhouette

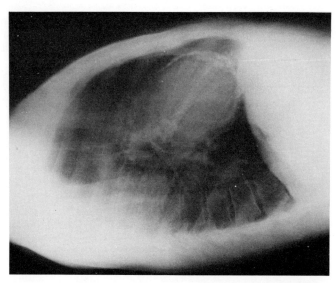

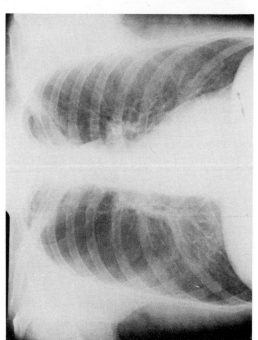

FIG. 49: Calcific pericarditis due to tuberculosis. Note the calcified rim of pericardium in the lateral view.

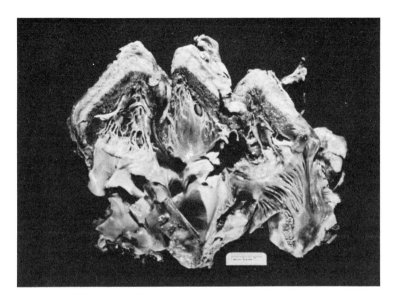

FIG. 50: Tuberculous pericarditis. The pericardium is markedly thickened, fibrotic and has a granular whitish-
gray appearance.

with clear lung fields. Pericardiocentesis revealed 1,100 ml.
of straw-colored fluid withdrawn from the pericardial sac,
which, on culture, grew M. tuberculosis.

Constrictive pericarditis is a delayed complication of tuberculous, uremic or hemorrhagic pericarditis. Tuberculosis is
perhaps the leading cause of pericardial constriction. On occasion, constrictive pericarditis might become adhesive to the
myocardium or thickened; sometimes even calcified (Figs. 49,
50). This calcification can be readily appreciated on a plain
roentgenogram of the chest. The pericardial constriction may
eventually shrink and profoundly disable the heart, muffle its
tone and incapacitate the myocardium to such an extent that it
can no longer compensate either by hypertrophy or dilatation.
The overall mortality in tuberculous and other pericarditis with
or without constriction is still close to 40% to 50%.

Amoebic pericarditis occurs as a complication secondary to
rupture of the liver abscess, more commonly from the left
lobe of the liver. It may be preceded by a pre-suppurative
phase, wherein the fluid is serosanguineous. Suppurative

pericarditis may follow shortly thereafter. The pus in the amoebic pericarditis is odorless and has the characteristic anchovy-sauce color. In amoebic pericarditis, both pericardium and the liver should be drained. Contrast material, like air or radiopaque material, may be injected to delineate the liver abscess. Amoebic pericardial effusion, if not promptly drained, is invariably fatal. Rheumatoid, malignant and uremic pericardial effusions, unless secondarily infected, are sterile.

## REFERENCES

1.  Rooney, J. J. , Crocco, J. A. , Lyons, H. A. : Tuberculous pericarditis. Ann. Int. Med. 72:73, 1976.

2.  Matsuo, T. , Yao, T. , Ishihama, Y. , Miyasaki, K. : So-called primary tuberculous pericarditis. Jap. Circ. Journal 37:1371, 1973.

3.  Van Reken, D. , et al: Infectious pericarditis in children. J. Pediat. 85:165, 1974.

4.  Miler, G. C. , Witham, C. : Delayed febrile pleuro-pericarditis after sepsis. Ann. Int. Med. 79:194, 1973.

## 36: INFECTIVE ENDOCARDITIS
### by H. Thadepalli

The clinical spectrum of bacterial endocarditis is kaleidoscopic. Any description of this disease can be outdated within the same decade. The most common cause of endocarditis in the United States today is intravenous drug abuse and the classic "subacute bacterial endocarditis" occurs far less frequently. "Acute endocarditis" in addicts is an entity to be considered by itself.[1,2] Early antibiotic therapy of addict endocarditis carries excellent prognosis, but when delayed, the mortality rate is high.[3,4] In endocarditis, early diagnosis is therefore of paramount importance.

### ACUTE BACTERIAL ENDOCARDITIS IN ADDICTS

Fever, cardiac murmur, pneumonia, anemia, and positive blood cultures are some of the features of infective endocarditis.[1] The fever may or may not be associated with chills and rigors. Nearly one-half of them are afebrile on admission. Cardiac murmurs are heard in nearly a third of these patients on admission, although they become audible generally within five days in the remaining. Precious time is lost, and often the diagnosis is delayed for want of cardiac murmur. The murmurs, when heard, are of changing character; heard one day but not on the other, or heard by one person and not by the other. One should, therefore, presumptively treat all drug addicts admitted for fever with lung infiltrates (after obtaining blood cultures) for endocarditis. Later, if blood cultures become positive and cardiac murmur appears, the treatment should be continued for the traditional four to six weeks. If blood cultures remain negative, the antibiotics are discontinued after five days. Splenomegaly is an inconstant feature[1] (less than 10%). When treatment is delayed, it becomes palpable within two weeks of hospitalization. Anemia, mostly normocytic, is a constant feature. Hypochromic microcytic anemia due to iron deficiency is more common with subacute bacterial endocarditis.

Many patients with endocarditis have metastatic skin lesions on admission. These lesions should be aspirated and Gram's stained. Often, valuable clues can be obtained from these lesions.

SKIN LESIONS: Petechiae, Osler's nodes, Janeway's lesions and subcutaneous abscesses are common skin manifestations of endocarditis. The Osler's nodes are erythematous, painful and tender lesions on the palmer and plantar surfaces, and tips of the fingers and toes, with intact skin surface and palpable nodules underneath the lesions (Figs. 51, 52). Janeway's lesions are similar to Osler's nodes, except that they are painless (Fig. 53). Such lesions, if found elsewhere on the body, are simply called subcutaneous lesions. These lesions should be routinely aspirated and Gram's stained for bacteria. The general belief that Osler's nodes and Janeway's lesions are sterile is incorrect.

A skin lesion is considered positive (+) when the Gram's stained slide prepared from the needle aspirate of the lesions shows polymorphonuclear leukocytes in addition to bacteria. When neither bacteria nor polymorphs are seen within the first five to ten consecutive high power fields, it is regarded as negative. Contrary to general belief, Osler's nodes, Janeway's lesions and other skin lesions in staphylococcal endocarditis of addicts are often positive. Bacteria can also be found in cases of gram-negative and fungal infections of the heart. My experience with 26 such patients is summarized in Table 23. [5] The following are two such examples:

Case History 1:  A 43-year-old heroin addict was seen for shortness of breath and edema of both legs. On admission, he was afebrile, the blood pressure was 150/70 mm. of Hg. , and pulse was 108/minute. The jugular veins were distended with increased central venous pressure. He had a loud third sound and a grade III/IV non-radiating systolic murmur on the left sternal border. The liver and spleen were palpable two to three finger breadths below the costal margins. On closer examination, a 3 x 8 mm. size pustule with surrounding erythematous reaction was found on the right infraclavicular area. It was aspirated and Gram's stained, which showed several polymorphs and gram-positive bacilli. Several blood cultures yielded gram-positive bacilli, later identified as Lactobacillus species.

Case History 2:  A 35-year-old man was admitted with chest pain and hemoptysis. He had lobar pneumonia and arthritis. He had Osler's nodes, arteritis and subcutaneous abscesses (Fig. 54). Needle aspiration of the joint fluids and subcutaneous abscesses all showed several polymorphs and gram-positive cocci. Two days later he developed empyema, which also showed gram-positive cocci. Blood cultures later grew Staphylococcus aureus.

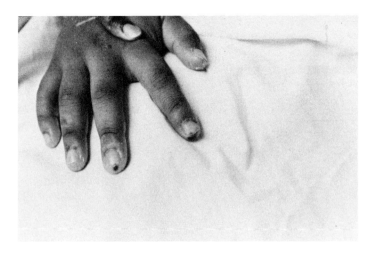

FIG. 51: Osler's nodes in a child with subacute bacterial endocarditis secondary to congenital heart disease. These lesions were not cultured.

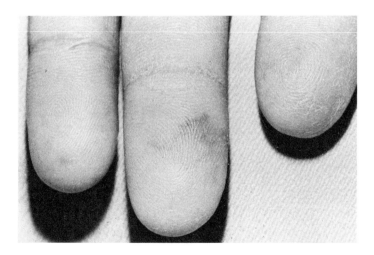

FIG. 52: Osler's nodes on the tips of the fingers in a case of acute bacterial endocarditis due to Staphylococcus aureus in a drug addict. Gram-positive cocci were demonstrated in the needle aspirates of these lesions.

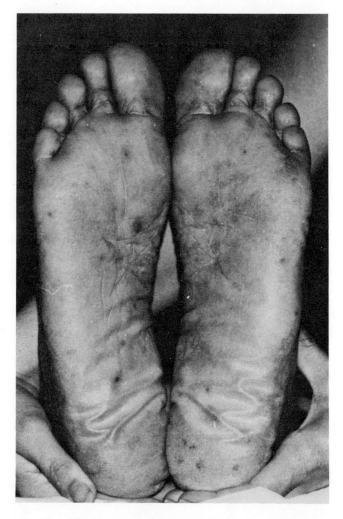

FIG. 53: Janeway's lesions on the soles of the feet in a
case of acute bacterial endocarditis in a drug
addict. Needle aspirates from these lesions
showed gram-positive cocci, and blood cultures were positive for Staphylococcus aureus.

TABLE 23: EXTRAVASCULAR CULTURE SITES IN 17 CASES OF ADDICT ENDOCARDITIS

| Serial Number | Causative Organism | Affected Valves | Osler & Janeway Lesions | Subcutaneous Abscess | Pleural Fluid | Joint Fluid | Trans-tracheal Aspiration | Spinal Fluid | Peri-cardial Fluid | Muscle Abscess | Endome-trium |
|---|---|---|---|---|---|---|---|---|---|---|---|
| 1 | Staphylococcus aureus (S.A.) | Mitral (M) | | | | | | + | + | | |
| 2 | S.A. | Tricuspid (T) | + | + | + | | | | | | |
| 3 | S.A. | M and T | + | + | | + | | + | | | |
| 4 | S.A. | T | + | + | + | | | | + | | |
| 5 | S.A. | M and T | + | + | | | | | | | |
| 6 | S.A. | M | + | + | + | | | | | | |
| 7 | S.A. | Aortic (A) and M | + | + | + | | + | + | | | |
| 8 | S.A. | Pulmonary (P) | + | + | + | | | | | | |
| 9 | S.A. | T | + | | | | | | | + | |
| 10 | S.A. | M and T | + | | | + | | | | | |
| 11 | S.A. | A | + | | + | + | | | | | |
| 12 | S.A. and alpha Streptococcus (A.S.) | T | | | + | | + | | | | |
| 13 | A.S. | A | + | | | | | | | | + |
| 14 | Serratia | Tricuspid | | | | | | | | | |
| 15 | Pseudomonas | A and M | | | + | | + | | | | |
| 16 | Lactobacillus and Entero-coccus | A | | + (Gram-positive rods only - no cocci seen) | | | | | | | |
| 17 | Enterobacter | M | | + | | | | | | + | |

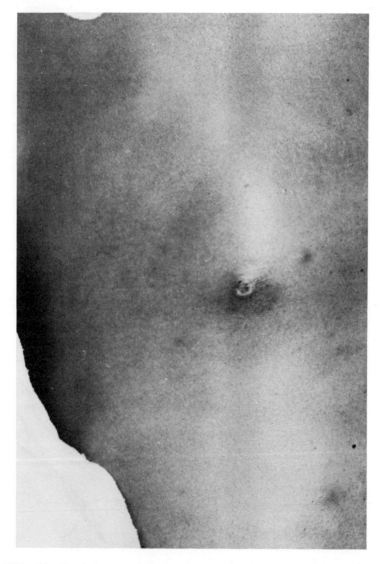

FIG. 54: Pustular lesion on the chest wall in a patient suspected to have endocarditis. Gram stain of the needle
aspirate from this lesion showed gram-positive cocci;
later on, Staphylococcus aureus was cultured from
this lesion, as well as from blood cultures.

More than one site may yield bacteria in cases of endo-carditis and, therefore, every available site should be ex-amined for potential clues.

Joint fluid aspirates may be an important source of diagnosis in patients presenting with arthritis. Clubbing of fingers oc-curs frequently with subacute and chronic bacterial endocar-ditis, but they are infrequent with acute endocarditis. Splinter hemorrhages under the nail-bed, as if a sliver had been run in, may occur with endocarditis. They are not characteristic of endocarditis. Splinter hemorrhages, may also occur in the conjunctiva (Fig. 55) or the retina (Roth's spots). It is unknown if these lesions are due to vasculitis or due to septic emboli. Hemorrhagic lesions of the skin of the fingers and toes com-monly occur due to septic emboli, which are due to acute staph-ylococcal endocarditis in heroin addicts (Fig. 56).

VALVULAR INVOLVEMENT: Tricuspid murmurs are the most frequent with endocarditis in addicts. The mitral valve is in-volved just as frequently as the tricuspid. Aortic and pulmo-nary valves are less frequently involved.

RENAL ABNORMALITIES: Nearly a third of the chronic her-oin addicts have abnormal kidney function tests and proteinuria. Endocarditis, by itself, may depress the renal function. The semisynthetic penicillins frequently used in the treatment of staphylococcal endocarditis are also potentially nephropatho-genic. The kidneys of a heroin addict with staphylococcal en-docarditis, treated with semisynthetic penicillins, are, there-fore, under triple jeopardy. Membrano-proliferative glomer-ulonephritis and binding of IgM beta 1-C are typical of heroin nephropathy. [2] A heroin addict having endocarditis, with edema and proteinuria, is likely to have this syndrome.

PLEUROPULMONARY: Pleuropulmonary involvement is fre-quent with endocarditis. A heroin addict with pneumonia and/or pleural effusion should be considered to have endocarditis and treated as such for at least five to seven days until it is proven otherwise.

Transtracheal aspiration (TTA) was found to be a useful diag-nostic procedure in such patients. The transtracheally aspirated specimen, on Gram's stain, may show the causative agent in pa-tients with pneumonia, associated with staphylococcal endo-carditis [5] (see Table 23). In my experience, the TTA was posi-tive in both staphylococcal and also gram-negative endocardi-tis, but it was negative in cases of pneumonia associated with enterococcal endocarditis. In cases of empyema, the pleural fluid may yield the organisms.

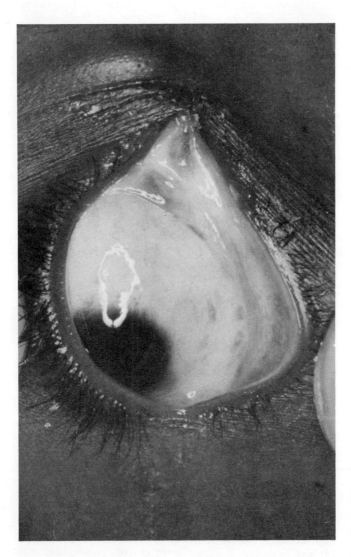

FIG. 55: Subconjunctival hemorrhagic spots in a case of endocarditis. This patient died of Staphylococcus aureus endocarditis and meningitis.

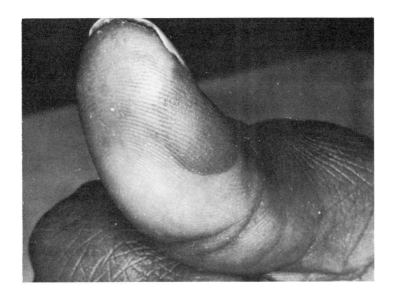

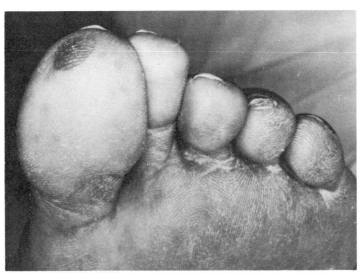

FIG. 56: Hemorrhagic lesions on fingers and toes found in a case of acute <u>Staphylococcus aureus</u> endocarditis. Gram-positive cocci were seen from the needle aspirates of the lesions.

PULMONARY EDEMA DUE TO HEART FAILURE: Aortic valvulitis may cause acute pulmonary edema; therefore, when aortic
valvulitis is suspected, a cardiac surgeon should be consulted.
When the aortic incompetence is severe, the murmurs are
masked by the surrounding noisy rales due to pulmonary edema.
Acute pulmonary edema may, at times, be mistaken for bronchial asthma or hypersensitivity to intravenous drugs.

CLUBBING OF FINGERS:  This is frequent with endocarditis
secondary to congenital heart disease.  Clubbing of fingers may
also be acquired in endocarditis secondary to drug abuse. It is
thought to be due to increased capillary blood flow in the digital
terminals. [6] Clubbing of fingers may also be due to changing
supply of nutrition to the fingers.  Acquired clubbing in endocarditis is reversible.

SPLENIC ABSCESS:  Endocarditis is the most common cause
of splenic abscess.  It is often solitary, large, and diagnostically challenging.  Its recognition and prompt splenectomy averts
the otherwise formidable mortality.  Pain in the left upper abdominal quadrant radiating to the shoulder, weight loss, persistent leukocytosis with fever, and night sweats should suggest splenic abscess, even if there is no palpable mass in the
left upper quadrant. Elevation of the left dome of the diaphragm,
as seen on the plain roentgenogram of the abdomen and a ra-
dionuclide-defective uptake in the liver-spleen scan, confirms
this diagnosis.

OSTEOMYELITIS: Osteomyelitis of the lumbar spine is a known
complication of drug abuse.  When an addict complains of lower
back pain, even if diagnosis is endocarditis, consider the possible association of osteomyelitis.  Appropriate investigations
should be done to exclude this possibility.

FUNDUS EXAMINATION:  This is mandatory in all cases of
suspected endocarditis.  Examine the conjunctiva for hemorrhages.  The fundus might show:

a)  retinal hemorrhages
b)  degeneration of the nerve fiber layer (Roth's spots)
c)  obstruction of the retinal artery, or
d)  optic neuritis

These lesions may be seen in both acute and subacute endocarditis.  Amaurosis fugax, a term used for intermittent blindness, may occur due to multiple minute retinal artery emboli.
The emboli in transit may or may not be readily obvious on a
single funduscopic examination.

NERVOUS SYSTEM: Endocarditis may present as peripheral neuritis, stroke, transient paresis, or paraplegia. The spinal fluid analysis may be normal. Only a third of my patients with these complications had positive spinal fluid cultures. The following two case histories illuminate the Guillain-Barre type of syndrome, an unusual complication occurring in endocarditis.

Case History 1: A 16-year-old was admitted with the following history. On the night prior to admission, he self-administered a "fix" of heroin and fell asleep in his apartment. On awakening, he thought that his room was dark, but soon realized that he was totally blind because he was "running into things". On admission, he was found to have bilateral retinal artery thrombosis and a left parasternal pansystolic murmur (grade IV/VI) and fever. The next day, he developed a sudden onset of lower motor neuron type of weakness in both upper limbs. A week later, it extended to both lower limbs. All of his blood cultures were negative. The spinal fluid was unremarkable. He was on antibiotic therapy for four weeks. One month later, he developed respiratory arrest, for which he was intubated, but two days later, he developed cardiac arrest and died. At autopsy, he was found to have vegetations in the mitral valve (Fig. 57), which grew out Enterobacter on culture.

Case History 2: A 40-year-old multipara was transferred from another hospital for the treatment of endocarditis. Multiple blood cultures were positive for Staphylococcus aureus, and she also had a heart murmur. She was treated with a semi-synthetic penicillin. Four weeks later, she developed progressive paresthesias, ending in quadriplegia of lower motor neuron type. The spinal fluid was sterile, but protein levels were markedly elevated. She improved over a period of one year, followed by an almost complete recovery in eighteen months.

MAJOR BLOOD VESSEL BLOCKAGE: It is a characteristic feature of fungal endocarditis; notably Candida and Aspergillus organisms. Massive emboli might block the bifurcation of the aorta (Leriche's syndrome), the retinal, brachial or femoral arteries.

### SUBACUTE BACTERIAL ENDOCARDITIS
(The Classic Form of Endocarditis)

The clinical syndromes of subacute bacterial endocarditis (SBE) and endocarditis in addicts are similar, except that the subacute form is indolent in onset and in its clinical course.

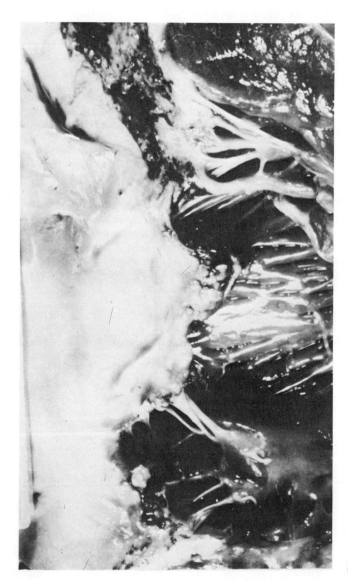

FIG. 57: Subacute bacterial endocarditis. Mitral valve showing some fibrous shortening of the chordae tendineae and small friable vegetation attached to the valve at the line of closure.

Splenomegaly, anemia and fever are common clinical manifestations of the subacute bacterial endocarditis and the predisposing factors are congenital and rheumatic heart diseases. The
bicuspid or quadricuspid aortic valves, ventricular septic defect,
tetralogy of Fallot and patent ductus arteriosus are vulnerable
to infection. Atrial septic defect of primary or secondary types
is not. Endocarditis in the elderly patient is of subacute onset,
usually secondary to arteriosclerotic or rheumatic endocardial
disease. Alpha-hemolytic Streptococcus (Streptococcus viridans) is the common cause of SBE.

PERIPHERAL MANIFESTATIONS: The spleen is palpable in
50% to 75% of cases of SBE. Heart murmurs are almost always heard on admission to the hospital in SBE. Microscopic
hematuria is also a constant feature. Peripheral embolic phenomena, like splinter hemorrhages, Roth's spots, clubbing of
fingers and toes, splenomegaly, and cerebral vascular lesions
are some of its delayed sequelae. In SBE, purulent arthritis
and pulmonary emboli manifesting as pneumonia are infrequent.

### DIAGNOSTIC METHODS

BLOOD CULTURES IN ENDOCARDITIS: Bacteremia in endocarditis is continuous; therefore, timing of the sample is not
critical. Blood cultures should not be drawn following manipulation of contaminated tissues, abscess drainage, dental extraction, bronchoscopy, proctoscopy, sigmoidoscopy, needle
biopsy of the liver, genitourinary tract manipulation and other
such procedures known to cause bacteremia.

Three sets of blood cultures drawn in one to two hourly intervals are sufficient. Nearly 80% of the positive blood cultures can be identified by the first set, 89% by the first two
sets, and 99% by the first three sets.[7] Very little additional
benefit is, therefore, expected by drawing any more than
three blood cultures.

The satisfactory critical volume for each blood sample is 10
ml. of blood injected into 100 ml. of broth. Some investigators recommend as small a volume as 2 ml. for fear of
antimicrobial substances in the larger volume of blood which
may interfere with bacterial growth. The blood culture bottles
are now supplemented with sodium polyanethole sulfonate, called
SPS or liquoid, to neutralize this bactericidial effect of human

serum; therefore, 10 ml. of blood can be added to 100 ml. of broth. Generally, two bottles are used for each set of blood cultures, in which case, 20 ml. of blood should be drawn and divided into two separate bottles. [7] In the laboratory, one bottle should be vented and the other left unvented on a routine basis to ensure recovery of aerobic and facultative anaerobic organisms. Venting of the culture bottles is critical for the early isolation of Pseudomonas and Candida organisms. If the amount of blood collected is less than 10 ml. , it should be inoculated into one bottle (for aerobes and facultatives) only.

Scrupulous antiseptic precautions should be taken to cleanse the skin before the cultures are obtained; first, with 70% alcohol, and second, with 1% to 2% idophor solution. Together, they decrease, by 90%, the skin microflora but do not sterilize the skin. The intended site of venipuncture should not be touched after cleansing. After the collection of blood, change the needle before the blood is injected into the culture bottle.

POUR PLATE TECHNIQUES: This technique involves mixing the patient's blood with moulten agar and pouring of the plates at the bedside. They are useful to differentiate between positive cultures due to skin contamination from the actual bacteremic patients. Generally, the yield is much lower with pour plates than with regular liquid culture media.

The routinely used blood culture media are tryptic digest of casein soy broth (TSB) and thioglycolate, or thiol bottled under vacuum with $CO_2$. I found no advantage whatsoever in the pre-reduced medium (PRAS) over the conventional thiol medium for isolation of anaerobes in the blood cultures.

HYPERTONIC LIQUID MEDIA: These may be employed when routine blood cultures are negative and when endocarditis is still suspected. Hypertonic liquid media, with 10% to 15% sucrose, are used to detect the L-forms or cell wall deficient organisms that may be found in association with partially treated cases of bacterial endocarditis.

PENICILLINASE: Routine addition of penicillinase to blood cultures is not recommended because it may increase the risk of contamination of the blood cultures. A small fraction of all febrile patients, regardless of the cause of fever, may have positive blood cultures; therefore, caution should be exercised in the interpretation of culture results.

BUFFY-COAT EXAMINATIONS: [8] A smear of leukocytes from
the buffy-coat layer of the peripheral blood is used for early
diagnosis of endocarditis. While collecting blood for culture,
an aliquot of EDTA, 5 ml., is added, and left in a Wintrobe
hematocrit tube; centrifuge and transfer a few drops of the supernatant buffy-coat layer of leukocytes with a capillary tube
onto a clean glass slide to make an even smear. Air dry two
such smears - one for Gram's stain and the other for Wright's
stain. The Gram's stained smears may show bacteria in cases
of endocarditis and septicemia.

The overall yield by these smears is very low. In one study,
it was positive in only five of eleven patients with bacteremia. [8]
The presence of intraleukocytic bacteria may suggest poor
prognosis. A high percentage of the EDTA coated blood collection tubes were found to be contaminated during the process
of manufacturing.

LEUKOCYTE MONOLAYER EXAMINATION: This is a simple
and rapid technique. Draw a sample of venous blood and place
a drop on a clean glass cover slip, incubate for 25 minutes, at
37°C., in a moist Petri dish. Remove the clot gently with normal saline. Immerse the cover slip with the attached leukocytes
in 2% glutaraldehyde fixative; wash in distilled water and de-
hydrate sequentially in 30%, 70% and absolute ethanol for one
minute in each. The cells are later stained for 30 minutes with
2% Giemsa stain, washed, air-dried and mounted for viewing.
A 30-minute scan is satisfactory. This test is useful in nearly
60% of the patients.

TEICHOIC ACID ANTIBODIES: Teichoic acids are major cell
wall components of staphylococci. Teichoic acid precipitin may
be found in all adult sera. The concentration of the precipitin
in uninfected patients is too low to detect by gel diffusion plates,
but in patients with staphylococcal infection, they are in high
enough quantities. Fourteen of fifteen patients with S. aureus
endocarditis, in one study, had detectable teichoic acid pre-
ciptin. [10] A positive test, therefore, clearly distinguishes between staphylococcal endocarditis and endocarditis due to other
organisms, but it will not differentiate staphylococcal endocarditis from bacteremia. The precipitin lines form within four to
seven hours after the antigens, and sera are added to the gel
diffusion plates. This test is relatively more rapid than blood
cultures. Successful therapy reverses the titers to undetectable
levels.

COMPLEMENT CONTAINING CIRCULATING IMMUNE COM-
PLEXES (CIC): The CIC can be measured by Ragi-cell line
assay. Levels above 12 mcg/ml. serum are considered abnormal. CIC appears in most cases of endocarditis with extravascular manifestations. [11] The longer the duration of the
disease, the higher are the levels. The CIC disappears after
surgery or successful therapy.

Unacceptably high levels of positive tests occur among narcotic addicts even without infection, and addicts with infection
but not endocarditis. The value of CIC in the "culture-negative"
infective endocarditis is not known. This test, when verified
by further trials, may have a place in the diagnosis of right-
sided endocarditis in narcotic addicts (pending blood culture
results) and among those with endocarditis without cardiac
murmurs and no detectable embolic phenomena. Whereas high
levels of CIC (100 mcg/ml. or more) suggest the diagnosis of
infective endocarditis, they don't exclude connective tissue disease and lupus erythematosus.

ECHOCARDIOGRAPHY (see Fig. 134, page 771 ): Echocardiography is of limited value in the diagnosis of endocarditis.
Twenty out of twenty-two patients, with vegetations of size recognized by echocardiography, either underwent cardiac surgery or died. The diagnosis was delayed by an unacceptably
long time interval of twenty-two days after admission.[12] When
the patients had no vegetations of size which could be recognized by echocardiography, none required cardiac surgery and
there were no deaths. By the time endocarditis is diagnosed
by echocardiography, the disease process appears to be far
advanced and therefore, it appears to be of little diagnostic
value in endocarditis.

GALLIUM SCANS: In our study, 12 patients with suspected
endocarditis, with pneumonia, had Ga-67 scans. Increased
accumulation of gallium in the lung was noted in nine patients,
and three showed no uptake.[21] All three patients with gallium-
negative lung scans had sterile transtracheal aspirates; in contrast, five patients with increased uptake of gallium in the lung
had Staphylococcus aureus isolated from TTA or thoracentesis
specimens (see Figs. 150, 151, pages 803, 804). Gallium
scans are non-specific and, therefore, of limited diagnostic
value. Positive gallium scans may be found in other disorders.
An abnormal gallium scan, when associated with an abnormal
roentgenogram of the chest, suggests an active inflammatory
process. The value of gallium scans in bacterial pneumonia is
discussed elsewhere.

## GROUP D STREPTOCOCCAL ENDOCARDITIS

Group D streptococcal endocarditis is the second most frequent cause of endocarditis in addicts. It is important to recognize this entity, because some of the group D strains of streptococci are extremely susceptible to penicillin. Among group D streptococci, only enterococcus needs to be treated with an additional antibiotic, streptomycin.

Enterococcus is not as invasive as S. aureus, and, therefore, infrequently causes peripheral manifestations like microscopic hematuria, pneumonia due to septic emboli, and subcutaneous lesions, like Janeway's lesions or Osler's nodes. These skin stigmata, if present, rarely show organisms in cases of enterococcal endocarditis. In a small number of cases I studied, the aspirates were also sterile. The clinical syndrome of enterococcal endocarditis, however, is indistinguishable from S. aureus endocarditis.

To choose proper therapy, it is important to distinguish enterococcus (Streptococcus fecalis) from other group D streptococci.[13,14] Streptococcus bovis, also a group D organism, is highly susceptible to penicillin. Additional aminoglycoside is seldom required for the treatment of S. bovis endocarditis. Table 24 shows the differentiating biochemical characteristics of Streptococcus bovis and enterococcus.

## GRAM-NEGATIVE ENDOCARDITIS

Gram-negative endocarditis can occur on either side or both sides of the heart. Genitourinary infections frequently predispose to gram-negative endocarditis. The clinical history and physical signs of gram-negative endocarditis are similar to those of S. aureus endocarditis.

Certain types of gram-negative endocarditis appear to be regional in distribution, such as Pseudomonas endocarditis in Detroit,[15] and Serratia endocarditis in San Francisco.[16]

Left heart involvement in gram-negative endocarditis frequently requires surgical replacement of the infected valve, and more so if the aortic valve is affected. Tricuspid valve infection can be cured with medical treatment alone. Surgical treatment is rarely required.

## TABLE 24: BIOCHEMICAL CHARACTERISTICS OF STREPTOCOCCUS BOVIS AND ENTEROCOCCI

| Reaction | Streptococcus bovis | Enterococci |
|---|---|---|
| Group D Reaction | + | + |
| Bile esculin hydrolysis | + | + |
| S. fecalis broth | + or O | + |
| 6.5% NaCl broth | O | + |
| Eosin Methylene Blue Agar | O | + |
| MIC of Penicillin G in mcg/ml. | < 0.5 | > 2 |
| Starch hydrolysis | + | O |
| Arginine hydrolysis | O | + |
| Resist tellurite | O | + |
| Clot in litmus milk | + | + |
| Acid from melibiose | + | O |
| Acid from melezitose | O | + |
| MIC of Cephalothin (mcg/ml.) | Susceptible | Resistant |
| MIC of Clindamycin (mcg/ml.) | Susceptible | Resistant |

O = No growth
+ = Growth

## FUNGAL ENDOCARDITIS

Fungal endocarditis may occur among drug addicts following cardiovascular surgery, [17] prolonged periods of intravenous hyperalimentation, long-term broad spectrum antibiotic treatment, or among compromised hosts, such as renal transplant and immunosuppressed patients. Among addicts, Candida parapsilosis infections are common. Despite cardiac surgery and effective antifungal therapy, the prognosis of fungal endocarditis is generally poor. Prompt diagnosis and treatment is, therefore, important. Serum Candida antibody titers may be useful when the blood cultures are negative.

## PROSTHETIC VALVE ENDOCARDITIS

Even with stringent pre-operative techniques, the incidence of prosthetic valve endocarditis is around 2%. It is caused by

such usually benign organisms as Staphylococcus (S. ) epidermidis, Diphtheroides, Candida or Lactobacillus, or the usually
pathogenic strains of Streptococcus and gram-negative bacilli.[18]

Most postoperative infections are caused by S. epidermidis,
S. aureus, gram-negative bacilli or Candida organisms. Delayed (more than four weeks after surgery) post-operative infections are frequently due to Streptococcus. Isolation of any
organism from the blood cultures of a patient with a prosthetic
valve implant should be taken seriously, and the blood cultures
should be repeated for confirmation and therapy promptly instituted.

Diphtheroides (Corynebacterium) is a gram-positive, non-motile
catalase-positive, pleomorphic rod. It is a normal flora of the
surface skin and feces. On Gram's stain, they resemble Listeria,
streptococci and clostridia. Diphtheroides are resistant to most
of the traditionally used antibiotics, like penicillin and cephalosporins.[19] Removal of the infected prosthetic valve may be
required to accomplish cure.

It is often difficult to distinguish the prosthetic valve infection
from the post-operative extra-cardiac infection. Delayed onset
of gram-positive cocci bacteremia beyond the twenty-fifth post-
operative day, often due to organisms susceptible to the antibiotics prophylactically administered to the patient, is likely
to be due to prosthetic valve infection. However, each patient
should be carefully examined for possible extra-cardiac source
of bacteremia. It is conceivable that one might develop endocarditis following an extra-cardiac infection or vice versa. It
is my practice to treat all patients with suspected intra- or extra-cardiac infection for not less than a four to six-week period,
starting on the very first day of the post-operative febrile illness. At the end of therapy, the blood cultures are repeated for
evaluation.

## INFECTIVE ENDOCARDITIS CAUSED
## BY ANAEROBIC BACTERIA

Propionibacterium (P. ) acnes, Bacteroides (B. ) fragilis and
Clostridium were reported to cause endocarditis.[20] Cardiac
surgery was the most common predisposing cause for P. acnes
endocarditis. B. fragilis endocarditis apparently developed following gastrointestinal or female genital tract surgery. The
blood culture isolates of anaerobic bacteria are generally less
fastidious; they can be isolated by drawing blood cultures into
routine thioglycolate and thiol media.

Infective endocarditis due to anaerobic bacteria is a rare disease. The Center for Disease Control, which receives unusual bacterial isolates from many parts of the United States, accumulated 48 such cases over a seven-year period.

During the past seven years, I have examined most of our patients with positive blood cultures, including those with anaerobic organisms, and found that 8% (620 patients) of all positive blood cultures were due to anaerobes. During this period, we have also prospectively evaluated and treated nearly 120 patients with proven bacterial endocarditis, due to aerobic bacteria. I have not yet seen a proven case of endocarditis due to anaerobic bacteria. In all instances of suspected endocarditis due to anaerobes, the anaerobic septicemia was secondary to infection elsewhere. An aerobic septicemia was almost always of extra-cardiac origin. Endocarditis due to anaerobic bacteria, at least in my experience, is another unicorn of medicine believed to exist but hard to find.

## REFERENCES

1. Kaye, D. (Ed. ): Infective Endocarditis. University Park Press, Baltimore, 1976.

2. Learner, P. I. , Weinstein, L. : Infective endocarditis in the antibiotic era. New Eng. J. Med. 274:199-206, 259-266, 323-331, 388-393, 1966.

3. Cherubin, C. E. , et al: Infective endocarditis in narcotic addicts. Ann. Int. Med. 69:1091, 1968.

4. Menda, K. B. , Gorbach, S. L. : Favorable experience with bacterial endocarditis in heroin addicts. Ann. Int. Med. 78: 25, 1973.

5. Thadepalli, H. , et al: Diagnostic clues in metastatic lesions of endocarditis in addicts. West J. Med. 128:1-5, 1978.

6. Racoceanu, S. N. , et al: Digital capillary blood flow in clubbing - 85 Kr studies in hereditary and acquired cases. Ann. Int. Med. 75:993, 1971.

7. Washington, J. A. , II: Blood cultures: Principles and techniques. Mayo Clin. Proc. 50:91, 1975.

8.  Brooks, G. F. , Pribble, A. H. , Beatty, H. N.: Early diagnosis of buffy-coat examination. Arch. Int. Med. 132: 673, 1973.

9.  Powers, D. L. , Mandell, G. L.: Intraleukocytic bacteria in endocarditis patients. J. A. M. A. 227:312, 1974.

10. Crowder, J. G. , White, A.: Teichoic acid antibodies in staphylococcal and non-staphylococcal endocarditis. Ann. Int. Med. 77:87, 1972.

11. Bayer, A. , et al: Circulating immune complexes in infective endocarditis. New Eng. J. Med. 295:1500, 1976.

12. Wann, L. S. , et al: Echocardiography in bacterial endocarditis. New Eng. J. Med. 295:135, 1976.

13. Hoppes, W. L. , Lerner, P. I.: Non-enterococcal group D streptococcal endocarditis caused by Streptococcus bovis. Ann. Int. Med. 81:588, 1974.

14. Moellering, R. C. , Jr. , et al: Endocarditis due to group D Streptococci. Amer. J. Med. 57:239, 1974.

15. Reyes, M. P. , et al: Pseudomonas endocarditis in the Detroit Medical Center. Medicine 52:173, 1973.

16. Mills, J. , Drew, D.: Serratia marcescens endocarditis: A regional illness associated with intravenous drug abuse. Ann. Int. Med. 84:29, 1976.

17. Rubinstein, E. , et al: Fungal endocarditis: Analysis of 24 cases and review of the literature. Medicine 54:331, 1975.

18. Sande, M. A. , et al: Sustained bacteremia in patients with prosthetic cardiac valves. New Eng. J. Med. 286:1067, 1972.

19. Davis, A. , et al: Diphtheroid endocarditis after cardiopulmonary bypass surgery for the repair of cardiac valvular defects. Antimicrob. Agents and Chemother. 3:643, 1963.

20. Felner, J. M.: Infective Endocarditis Caused by Anaer-
    obic Bacteria. Anaerobic Bacteria: Role in Disease,
    (Eds. ) Balows, A. , DeHaan, R. M. , Guze, L. B. Charles
    C Thomas, Springfield, Ch. XXVI, pp. 345-352, 1974.

21. Thadepalli, H. , Mishkin, F. S.: Gallium-67 scans in en-
    docarditis, differentiation of septic from aseptic pulmonary
    emboli. Applied Radiology, 7:226-231, 1978.

## SECTION E: GENITOURINARY INFECTIONS

## 37: URINARY TRACT INFECTIONS
by II. Thadcpalli

It is estimated that approximately 1% of schoolgirls, 4% of young women and 7% of women above 50 have bacteriuria. Bacteriuria in men occurs one-tenth as frequently as in women. A single positive "clean catch" (midstream urine) culture with colony count of 100,000/cu. ml. or more is considered to represent urinary tract infection (UTI), even in asymptomatic patients.

There are various causes for UTI, of which the most frequent are ascending or descending infections secondary to:

1) Obstruction: Diseases of the prostate, calculus, stricture, tumors, congenital defects or stenosis of the urethra.

2) Non-obstructive causes: Diabetes mellitus, analgesic abuse, sexual intercourse (honeymoon cystitis), bacteriuria in pregnancy and oral contraceptives. Mere constipation in children can cause UTI.

### MICROBIOLOGY OF UTI

Escherichia (E.) coli leads the list, followed by other species of Enterobacteriaceae. Emphysematous cystitis in diabetics is caused by E. coli (Fig. 58). Gram-positive cocci, like Staphylococcus epidermidis (coagulase-negative Staphylococcus) and Micrococcus subgroup 3, are perhaps more prevalent than recognized.[1] Micrococcus group 3 is not a part of the normal flora of the stool, cervix, or male urethra; yet, it was reported as the second most common pathogen in UTI. Anaerobes and viruses rarely cause UTI. Anaerobic bacteria cannot tolerate the oxygen in urine, but can invade the bladder and cause cystitis. Adenovirus types 11 and 21 and rarely Papova virus, can cause hemorrhagic cystitis. The role of anaerobic bacteria in prostatic abscess is described elsewhere. It is beyond the scope of this book to describe in detail the clinical and radiologic features of UTI. The main focus is on the laboratory diagnosis when UTI is suspected.

309

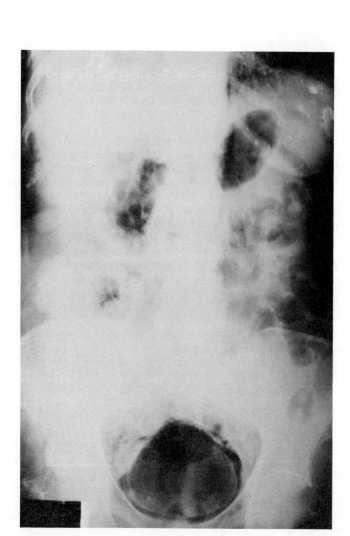

FIG. 58: Emphysematous cystitis. Note the air bubbles in the bladder wall, secondary to urinary tract infection due to Escherichia coli in an elderly woman with diabetes mellitus.

It is necessary to emphasize that all children and males with the very first attack of UTI should have a thorough radiologic examination of the urinary tract. In addition, all children with UTI should have a micturating cystourethrogram. Further, all women with UTI must have a pelvic examination. Nearly 20% of the asymptomatic women and 50% of neonates and children with UTI will have vesicoureteric reflex.

DIAGNOSTIC TECHNIQUES

A. MIDSTREAM URINE: It is important to obtain a clean voided specimen - known as "clean catch" in the U.S. and as midstream urine (MSU) in other parts of the world -for urinalysis. The physician should explain to the patient every step involved in the collection of MSU. The patient should have no vaginal discharge and should not be menstruating at the time of the specimen collection. She should separate the labia and clean from front to back with a soft rubber sponge (not cotton wool) soaked with distilled water (no antiseptic should be used.) The process is repeated and a little urine is voided in the toilet and the midstream specimen collected into a sterile container before emptying the bladder. Men should retract the prepuce (if uncircumcised), clean the glans and void a little urine in the toilet before collecting the specimen.

A preliminary examination of the midstream urine specimen should be carried out in the office. Demonstration of numerous squamous cells denotes vaginal contamination; such a specimen is useless for culture. Numerous white cells and bacteria, seen in an unspun specimen, denote UTI. A drop of unspun urine can be gently heat-fixed (avoid boiling), gram-stained and examined for bacteria. An experienced clinician may be able to determine from this preliminary examination whether or not the patient has a urinary tract infection, and whether it is caused by a gram-negative rod or gram-positive cocci, and initiate appropriate therapy. Proper cultures are mandatory to confirm this initial clinical suspicion.

B. SEGMENTAL LOCALIZATION OF CULTURE IN MALES: The purpose of this procedure is to differentiate between urethritis, cystitis and prostatitis. The procedure briefly involves collection of 10 cc. of the first voided urine in the first container, and then to almost, but not completely,

empty the bladder and to catch another specimen of urine
in the second container for culture. Then the patient stops
voiding and bends forward and milks out the urine from
the urethra, and holds a third container for collection of
prostatic secretions. The physician then massages the
prostate. In the fourth container, the patient voids 10 ml.
of urine. Qualitative and quantitative cultures are done
on all four specimens. If the third and the fourth containers contain greater numbers of bacteria than the first
and the second, prostatitis is likely.

C. SELECTIVE URETERIC CATHETERIZATION: This is
   done to identify the source and the site of infection. Among
   women with UTI, nearly one-half of them have an infected
   kidney; one-fourth may have one kidney, and others may
   have both kidneys involved.

METASTATIC LESIONS FROM URINARY TRACT INFECTIONS:
Genitourinary manipulations at the site of an obvious septic
focus can cause metastatic septic lesions in other parts of the
body. The heart and the bone are the most common sites,
leading to endocarditis or osteomyelitis. Such lesions are
far more frequent among elderly men than young women.
Interestingly, although a majority of urinary tract infections
are caused by Escherichia coli, most cases of metastatic
lesions are caused by gram-positive cocci, namely, Streptococci and Staphylococci; metastatic lesions due to E. coli
are less frequent.[2]

SUPRAPUBIC TAP: As mentioned, catheterization carries
an inherent risk of sepsis, both local and metastatic. Suprapubic aspiration of the bladder is therefore preferable.

With the patient in the recumbent position, clean the area of
skin between pubis and the umbilicus with a local antiseptic.
Anesthetize an inch of skin with 1% xylocaine 2.5 inches
above the symphysis pubis. Pass an 18 or 21-gauge needle
through the anesthetized area with an angle of 80° towards
the bladder, with slight suction applied to the plunger of the
syringe. Aspirate the urine as needed for urinalysis and
cultures. Withdraw the syringe and change the needle before

transferring the specimen to the tubes for culture. Suprapubic tap[3] is a rapid, economical, efficient and precise
procedure with no risk of contamination, and it obviates the
need to do multiple midstream urines. It precludes the
need for quantitative cultures, because the urine in the bladder is normally sterile. Any bacteria seen on Gram's stain
of the suprapubic aspirate of urine needs prompt therapy.
The discomfort experienced by the patient is generally less
than a venipuncture. The only disadvantage of this procedure is that the patient has to wait until the bladder is
filled. Even direct microscopy of suprapubic tap (SPT)
urine can provide accurate clues to the diagnosis of urinary
tract infection in nearly three-fourths of the patients, which
is equivalent to the reliability of culture of the MSU specimen. Together, the dip slide technique, which is described
on page 317, and the SPT urine, can further increase the
diagnostic accuracy of urinary tract infection to almost
90%.

TRANSVAGINAL ASPIRATION OF THE BLADDER: Bacteriuria can be screened by this procedure. It involves direct aspiration of urine from the bladder through the anterior wall of
the vagina. There appears to be little advantage to this procedure over the suprapubic aspiration, unless the patient requires a concomitant cervical culture, or Pap smear, or such
procedure that the patient has to be in the lithotomy position.
Transvaginal aspiration provides a more accurate and reliable
specimen of urine for culture than MSU. This technique is not
yet popular. For the details of the procedure, the reader is
referred to the original publication. [4]

FOLEY CATHETER TIP CULTURE: Culture of the Foley catheter tip is mentioned here only to condemn this procedure. It
should not be cultured because it has no diagnostic value. [5]

LEUKOCYTE COUNT OF THE URINE: An unspun specimen
of the urine may be examined for leukocytes in the same
manner as one does the peripheral leukocyte count. It is
generally regarded that a white cell count greater than 10/
cu. mm. in a fresh unspun urine is diagnostic of UTI, provided gross contamination is excluded. The truth is that
only 50% of asymptomatic UTI patients have white cells. The
test is less reliable if done by the notoriously inaccurate
microscopic, quantitative counts by inexperienced personnel.

BACTERIAL CELL COUNTS: Bacterial cell counts of 100,000/ ml. or more in MSU are regarded as diagnostic of UTI.[3] Lower counts can occur due to contamination. Provided the MSU is collected properly, this assumption is correct in 80% and false-positives occur in 20% due to heavy contamination. The criterium of 100,000/ml. viable cells does not apply to neonates, infants, children, the elderly, bedridden or paraplegic patients, menstruating women, or those with vaginal discharge, post-surgical or post-partum patients, patients with increased frequency of micturition or UTI due to gram-positive organisms. It is a mistake to exclude gram-positive bacteria as contaminants when present in lower counts. One should be aware of UTI due to Staph. epidermidis and Micrococcus; they do not grow well on the conventional media used for growing Enterobacteriaceae. Counts lower than 100,000/ml. do not altogether exclude the diagnosis of UTI. Spuriously low and falsely high concentration of bacteria may be found in the urine, depending on various other factors of hydration and frequency of micturition and other factors that affect uro-concentration.

RECURRENT UTI DUE TO PROTEUS MIRABILIS: P. mirabilis, by virtue of its urea-splitting property, can alkalinize the urine (pH > 7.5), and increase the chances for formation of struvite stones. Nearly two-thirds of these stones are associated with P. mirabilis infection. Recurrent urinary tract infections, therefore, require intravenous pyelography to exclude these stones. Bacteriuria of any kind in the presence of renal stones should not be disregarded as contamination, even if bacteria are present in very low counts.

CHEMICAL TESTS: Several chemical tests have been devised as rapid diagnostic tools for bacteriuria. They give almost immediate results, but are not as reliable as conventional bacteriologic methods.

Microstix[6,7,8,9] (Griess test): The microstix is a plastic strip of size 8 x 1 cm. with three pads, one pad containing a chemical reagent called tetrazolium which detects traces of nitrate in urine, and two pads containing dehydrated agar, one of which has an inhibitory compound to suppress the growth of gram-positive bacteria, and the other without this inhibitory substance. The test is based on the fact that bacteria in urine reduce the dietary nitrates to nitrites. When nitrites are present in the urine, the colorless tetrazolium, within seconds, turns to bright pink color. The density of bacteria are indicated by the intensity of color reaction as compared with a reference chart provided by the manufacturer. Most bacteria that cause UTI, with the exception of Enterococcus, are capable of reducing nitrate.

Best results are obtained with the first voided specimen of morning urine. If urine was retained in the bladder for only a short time, false-negative results can occur. Therefore, this test should not be used to detect UTI in patients with indwelling catheters.

The test should be read within a minute. Results beyond this period are not valid. After the test is read, one should place this strip in a plastic envelop, express all air from the envelope and incubate it overnight at 37°C.

The pads that contain the culture media also include colorless tetrazolium which, when reduced by bacterial multiplication, is converted into red spots. The density of the spots indicates the number of bacteria in the urine. The final reading is based on its comparison with a graded chart provided for $10^1$ to $10^5$ bacteria/ml.

The advantage of this test is that it is rapid and it can be used by an educated patient at home or on vacation. The actual test involves dipping the stick in urine for five seconds and reading it within a minute and incubating at 37°C. for 12 to 24 hours.

Microstix is not reliable for the diagnosis of UTI due to gram-positive bacteria. False-positive tests can result if the patient is on antibiotics. Nitrite test may remain positive for some time after the elimination of bacteria from the urine. False-negative results can occur in UTI caused by Candida and Enterococcus.

Microstix nitrite color detection and the bacterial growth on the media pads are reliable (90%) when bacterial cell counts are 100,000/ml. or greater. At counts of $10^3$ or less, they are unreliable.

Microstix should not be refrigerated. It should not be stored at temperatures higher than 86°F. (30°C. ) and should not be exposed to sunlight or moisture (Microstix is manufactured by Ames Co. , Elkhart, Indiana, and also sold as Bac-U-Dip by Warner Chilcott Labs, Morris Plains, New Jersey).

Low urinary glucose indicator (Uroglox, KABI Labs, Stockholm, Sweden): It is used as a preliminary screening test for bacteriuria. This is a strip of paper coated with a glucose-specific enzyme system with a color reagent. [10,11] When sufficient glucose (greater than 1 to 1.5 mg/100 ml. ) is present, the strip turns to blue-green color. Absence of color change indicates significant bacteriuria. Bacteria in the urine decrease the normal glucose concentration, as in the CSF in cases of meningitis.

For this test, the patient empties the bladder before retiring to bed and fasts until this test is done in the morning (should not empty bladder for at least six hours after the test is commenced and the urine should be fresh to do the test). False-positives are high with this test.

Catalase screening test: Catalase is present in many bacteria (except pneumococci and anaerobes). Catalase converts hydrogen peroxide to water and oxygen. The number of oxygen bubbles produced is proportional to the density of bacteria in the urine. This test is not widely in use. Some report 92% reliability with this test. [12]

Luciferase assay: Adenosine triphosphate in the bacterial cells can be assayed with the firefly luciferin/luciferase system. It is sensitive enough to detect over 10 bacteria/ml. and it can be done rapidly. A sample of urine is incubated with triton x-100 and ATP hydrolyzing enzyme, a pyrase, which inhibits the ATP of human cells, not bacteria. It is extracted with boiling buffer and assayed by the luciferase method. [13]

Limulus assay: Limulus assay can be used for the detection of UTI due to gram-negative bacilli, but it is of no value in UTI caused by gram-positive organisms. Limulus test detected 98. 8% of UTI due to gram-negative bacilli. Gram stain alone may diagnose nearly 70% of the cases. [14]

OFFICE CULTURE TESTS:

Agar plate method: A drop of urine can be placed on the surface of a blood agar plate or selective media (eosine, methylene

blue agar on MacConkey medium), and spread with the aid of
the tip of a curved-tip eyedropper and incubated at 37°C. for
24 hours. The growth is read on the next day.

Dip slides:  The dip slides contain different bacteriologic media
on each side. Both gram-positive and gram-negative bacteria
can grow on one side, and only gram-negative bacteria on the
other. The dip slides are sold as Uricult, Orion Labs, Hel-
sinki, Finland; and Oxoid (Flow Labs, Rockville, Maryland)
and Clinicult (Smith Kline Corp. , Philadelphia). They can be
used at home or on vacation and mailed to the physician's office. This method gave no false-positive or false-negative results in one study. [15]

The dip stick or dip slide method is as reliable as the standard quantitative culture technique, suitable for office practice. It is not suitable for identification of the bacteria.

Testuria (Ayerst, New York, New York) "Mini-culture" method:  It consists of a small agar plate with a strip of filter paper
on which urine is delivered. If there are 25 colonies per plate,
it is equivalent to more than 100,000 bacteria/ml. False-positives and false-negatives can occur in about 5% of the tests. It
is not a selective medium and, therefore, does not distinguish
between the pathogenic and the non-pathogenic bacterial strains. [16]
If the bacterial cell count is less than 50,000/cu. mm. , the test
yields unacceptably high false-positives (35%). [17]

Speci-Test, an agar-cup quantitative culture method:  Speci-
Test (Ross Labs, Columbus, Ohio) for the detection of bacteriuria, consists of a 0.75" x 2" plastic cup with a nutrient
agar in a 1.5" shallow well. After the inoculation of urine, it
is incubated at 37°C. The density of the colonies on the upper
surface is then compared with photographic standards to esti-
mate the colony count. The overall specificity of the test is
around 93%, [6] but preliminary identification of the organism is
not possible with the use of this medium alone.

NON-INVASIVE TESTS TO DIFFERENTIATE BETWEEN PY-
ELONEPHRITIS AND CYSTITIS:

1) Antibody coated bacteria:  It is an immunofluorescence test
   for the detection of antibody-coated bacteria in urinary sediments to predict the site of infection. In cases of pyelonephritis, the bacteria are coated with antibodies but not in
   cases of cystitis.

Method: Centifuge 9.5 ml. of urine at 1500 g., and wash the sediment twice with phosphate buffer and treat with 0.5 ml. of fluorescence conjugated antihuman globulin of horse origin (and incubate at 37°C. for 30 minutes); rewash and examine for fluorescence.

It is positive in cases of pyelonephritis and negative in cases of cystitis. [18] The technique is sensitive and reliable. It is a non-invasive and safe method to differentiate the upper from the lower urinary tract infections. [19] It is not useful to detect UTI caused by yeast organisms. [20]

2) Water-loading test: Administration of large quantities of water by mouth or by intravenous route increases the concentration of the number of viable cells in the urine. In cases of cystitis, water loading decreases the bacterial concentration in the urine. [21] This test is cumbersome and time-consuming.

### REFERENCES

1. Haskell, R.: Importance of coagulase-negative Staphylococci as pathogens in the urinary tract. Lancet 1:1155, 1974.

2. Siroky, M.B., et al: Metastatic infection secondary to genitourinary tract sepsis. Am. J. Med. 61:351, 1976.

3. Kass, E.H.: Asymptomatic infections of the urinary tract. Trans. Ass. Amn. Phys. 69:56, 1956.

4. Simpson, J.W., McCracken, A.W., Radwin, H.M.: Transvaginal aspiration of bladder in screening for bacteriuria. Obstet. & Gynecol. 43:215, 1974.

5. Gross, P.A., et al: Positive Foley catheter tip cultures - Fact or fancy? J.A.M.A. 228:72, 1974.

6. Craig, W.A., Kunin, C.M., DeGroot, J.: Evaluation of new urinary tract infection screening devices. Appl. Microbiol. 26:196, 1973.

7. Kunin, C.M., DeGroot, J.E.: Self-screening for significant bacteriuria. J.A.M.A. 231:1349, 1975.

8. Moffat, C. M. , Brit, M. R. , Burke, J. P. : Evaluation of miniature test for bacteriuria using dehydrated media and nitrite pads. Appl. Microbiol. 28:95, 1974.

9. Litvak, A. S. , Eadie, E. B. , McRoberts, J. W. : A clinical evaluation of a screening device (Microstix) for urinary tract infections. South. Med. J. 69:1418, 1976.

10. Schertsten, B. , Fritz, H. : Subnormal levels of glucose in urine: A sign of urinary tract infection. J. A. M. A. 201: 949, 1967.

11. McDonald, J. P. : The use of an ion exchange paper strip test in gynaecological surgical practice. J. Clin. Pract. 28:61, 1974.

12. Singh, K. N. , et al: A catalase screening test for urinary tract infections. Ind. J. Med. Res. 61:1, 1973.

13. Thore, A. , Lundin, A. A. , Bergman, S. : Detection of bacteriuria by luciferase assay of adenosine triphosphate. J. Clin. Microbiol. 1:1, 1975.

14. Jorgensen, J. H. , Jones, P. M. : Comparative evaluation of the limulus assay and the direct Gram's stain for detection of significant bacteriuria. J. Clin. Path. 63:142, 1975.

15. Cohen, S. , Kass, E. H. : A simple method for quantitative urine culture. New Eng. J. Med. 277:176, 1967.

16. Medical Letter 16:13, 1974.

17. Bruppacher, R. , Domingue, G. : Experiences with a screening test for bacteriuria. Am. J. Clin. Path. 59:203, 1973.

18. Thomas, V. , Shelkov, A. , Forland, M. : Antibody coated bacteria in the urine and the site of urinary tract infection. New Eng. J. Med. 290:588, 1974.

19. Jones, S. R. , Smith, J. W. , Sanford, J. P. : Localization of urinary tract infections by detection of antibody coated bacteria in urine sediment. New Eng. J. Med. 290:591, 1974.

20. Harding, S. A. , Herz, W. G. : Evaluation of antibody coating of yeasts in urine as an indicator of the site of urinary tract infection. J. Clin. Microbiol. 2:222, 1975.

21. Papanayiotou, P. , Dontas, A. S. : Water-loading test in bacteriuria. New Eng. J. Med. 287:531, 1972.

### 38: PELVIC INFLAMMATORY DISEASE (PID)
by H. Thadepalli

## CLASSIFICATIONS

1. Post-operative - secondary to hysterectomy and cesarean section.

2. Post-abortal, post-partum and following dilatation and curettage and post-insertion of intra-uterine contraceptive device (IUCD).

3. Spontaneous (unassociated with above):
   a) Acute:
      (1) Gonococcal
      (2) Anaerobic
   b) Chronic:
      (1) Mycobacterium tuberculosis infection
      (2) Fungi and parasites

PID can be recurrent (rather than relapsing) or chronic. The internist can be confounded with spontaneous PID, because it is a common disease and the patients rarely sort themselves out before they go to the physician.

Post-surgical infections of the pelvis are frequently caused by a variety of anaerobic bacteria, normally residents in the cervix. [1,2,3]

## SYMPTOMATOLOGY

Acute pelvic inflammatory disease should be considered in the differential diagnosis of any abdominal pain in women. The pain is often bilateral and localized to both iliac fossae without radiation, associated with rebound tenderness and local guarding. PID can be unilateral. Acute PID is vastly a disease of the sexually active woman during the reproductive years. PID rarely, if ever, occurs during the second or the third trimester of pregnancy. In cases of gonococcal PID, it may begin within the first ten days of the onset of the menstrual cycle. In others, no such relationship exists between menstruation and the onset of PID. Recurrences are common with non-gonococcal PID; they are infrequent in gonococcal PID. Patients with recurrent non-gonococcal PID are less likely to become pregnant than those with gonococcal PID. [4]

## PHYSICAL SIGNS

Depending on the predisposing causes, the following signs are found in PID. At the onset, please note that the clinical diagnosis of PID can be correct in only 65% to 70% of cases (it is inaccurate in 35%).

1) Rebound tenderness in the iliac fossa is a fairly common sign.

2) Fever (101° to 103°F. ) and chills (41%). More than one-half of the patients have no fever. [5]

3) Abdominal pain is the most constant symptom found in 95% of the cases. The pain is sometimes so severe that one may lie curled up and confined to bed.

4) Right subcostal pain may occur secondary due to perihepatitis (Fitz-Hugh-Curtis syndrome); it is present in nearly a third of the cases of acute spontaneous PID due to gonococcus. [6]

5) Gonococcal PID may be associated with signs of bartholinitis or urethritis.

6) Purulent vaginal discharge may be present in 55% of the patients. [5]

7) Paralytic ileus may occur secondary to local peritonitis.

8) The size of the uterus is normal on bimanual palpation (it is enlarged in ectopic pregnancy) and manipulation of the cervix causes pain.

9) The fallopian tubes may be palpable. Normally they are not palpable.

10) Large adnexal masses suggest chronic or recurrent PID, likely to be associated with abscess formation.

### PID DUE TO INTRAUTERINE CONTRACEPTIVE DEVICES (IUCD)

The risk of PID in the IUCD wearer is at least nine-fold higher than the non-IUCD wearer. [7] Febrile PID is at least five times more likely to develop among IUCD users than the non-users. [8] PID was attributable to IUCD in 77% of IUCD users, and it was found to be a greater risk factor in the non-gonococcal PID group than in gonococcal PID.[9] Compared to non users of IUCD, PID is at least seven times greater in multigravida IUCD users and 1.7 times greater among the previously gravid IUCD users.[10] The incidence of PID does not seem to be related to the types of IUCD employed.[11] Even if IUCD does not cause PID, it seems to exacerbate the pre-existing endometritis leading to PID.[12]

The onset of pain is most frequent during menstruation. It may either begin immediately (acute PID) or after one or two weeks with a low, dull ache in the pelvis, progressively worsening over the next four to six weeks. Such a subacute onset is likely to lead to pelvic suppuration and localization of the abscess at the tubo-ovarian junction.[13] Unilateral PID may be unrelated to the use of the IUCD.[14]

## DIAGNOSIS

1) <u>Leukocyte count</u>: This may be normal or increased.

2) <u>Erythrocyte sedimentation rate</u>: This may be normal or increased.

3) <u>Hemoglobin and the hematocrit</u>: These are normal.

4) <u>Pregnancy test</u>: This should be negative. A positive test with signs of PID suggests ectopic pregnancy. Remember, PID is rare during pregnancy.

5) <u>Urinalysis</u>: This should be normal.

6) <u>Gram's stain and culture for Gonococcus</u>: The cervix, rectum, throat, urethra and vagina should be cultured for Neisseria (N.) gonorrhoeae. A non-lubricated speculum should be used to obtain cervical cultures. Sterile cotton-tipped applicator should be placed in the cervical canal and rotated and left long enough to soak, and the swab is directly streaked onto Thayer-Martin agar medium (it contains vancomycin, nystatin, and colistimethate to inhibit other flora) and transferred into a candle extinguishing jar. Care should be taken to culture the rectal mucosal smears (not feces) while obtaining rectal cultures.

The cervical and rectal cultures are often rewarding (90%) in cases of gonococcal PID. Routine urethral and vaginal cultures are not indicated. They add little to the cervico-rectal culture results. If the hymen is intact, introitus culture may be obtained.

Diagnosis should not be based upon Gram's stain results of the cervical smears. Several other bacteria may appear, like gram-negative diplococci, notably Veillonella, an anaerobe, Serratia and Acinetobacter, and occasionally Haemophilus vaginalis. The diagnosis of gonorrhea should therefore be confirmed by culture. Nearly 30% to 40% of the cases of PID will yield positive culture for N. gonorrhoeae.

7) Culdocentesis (Fig. 59): This is a reliable technique for the bacteriologic diagnosis of acute PID. [15] With the patient in the lithotomy position, cul-de-sac taps should be performed with an 18-gauge spinal needle and syringe. The needle should be replaced with a fresh needle to avoid contamination prior to discharging the contents of the syringe into the culture bottle. If there is no specimen (dry tap), irrigate the cul-de-sac with 2 to 5 ml. of sterile non-bacteriostatic saline solution. The specimen should be collected in oxygen-free carbon dioxide containers, and promptly processed for aerobic and anaerobic bacteria.

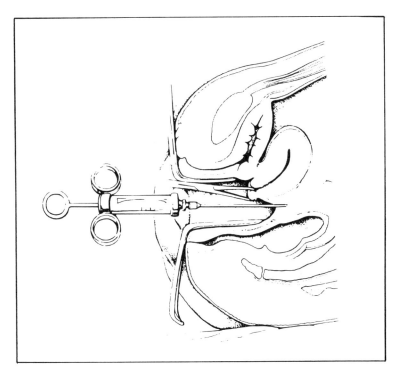

FIG. 59: Culdocentesis

The specimen should be gram-stained prior to culture. Demonstration of gram-negative diplococci in culdocentesis specimen clinches the diagnosis of acute gonococcal PID. Gram-positive cocci are more frequently seen in non-gonococcal anaerobic PID. The specimen should also be examined for leukocytes. An exudate with polymorphonuclear leukocytes is seen with cases of PID caused by bacteria; gonococcal and non-gonococcal or anaerobic bacteria. Lymphocytes and round cells without bacteria on Gram's stain may be found in cases of PID caused by viral infections, i.e., mumps, and occasionally tuberculosis. Purulent material may be obtained by culdocentesis in cases of ruptured tubo-ovarian abscess, rarely appendicitis and diverticulitis. An obviously hemorrhagic tap may suggest ectopic pregnancy, confirmed by pregnancy test.

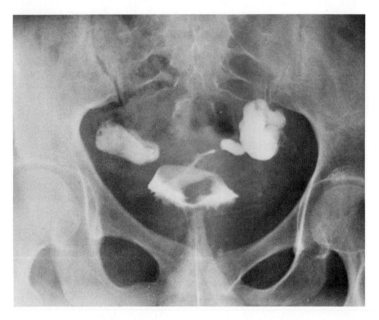

FIG. 60: Hysterosalpingogram in a patient with chronic, recurrent, pelvic inflammatory disease. Note the bilateral hydrosalpinx.

8) Laparoscopy and laparotomy:[5] Laparoscopy and laparotomy are not routinely indicated for the diagnosis of PID. They are useful adjunct procedures when the patient fails to respond to appropriate antibiotic therapy.

9) Hysterosalpingography: This is useful to determine the patency and the anatomical configuration of the tubes (Fig. 60).

## MICROBIOLOGY OF PID

It is controversial if N. gonorrhoeae causes PID. Most physicians believe that it does, and some believe that gonococcus may merely pave the way for anaerobic infection.[16] Anaerobes are the predominant flora (as verified by culdocentesis) in cases of PID; gram-positive cocci predominating.[15] Both aerobic and anaerobic bacteria can jointly or severally cause PID.[16] If the cervical cultures are negative for Gonococcus, gonococcal PID is unlikely because in most cases of gonococcal PID cervical cultures are positive for N. gonorrhoeae. Bacteroides is an infrequent cause for PID.

## REFERENCES

1. Gorbach, S. L. , et al: Anaerobic microflora of the cervix in healthy women. Am. J. Obstet. Gynecol. 117:1053, 1973.

2. Thadepalli, H. , Gorbach, S. L. , Keith, L. : Anaerobic infections of the female genital tract: Bacteriologic and therapeutic aspects. Am. J. Obstet. & Gynecol. 117:1034, 1973.

3. Swenson, R. M. , et al: Anaerobic bacteria of the female genital tract. Obstet. & Gynec. 42:538, 1973.

4. McCormack, W. H. , et al: Comparison of gonococcal and and non-gonococcal pelvic inflammatory disease. Clin. Res. 25:381A, 1977 (Abstract).

5. Jacobson, L. , Westrom, L. : Objectivized diagnosis of acute pelvic inflammatory disease: Diagnostic and prognostic value of routine laparoscopy. Am. J. Obstet. Gynecol. 105:1088, 1969.

6. Eschenbach, D. A. , Holmes, K. K. : Acute pelvic inflammatory disease. Current concepts of pathogenesis, etiology, and management. Clin. Obstet. & Gynec. 18:35, 1975.

7. Targum, S. D. , Wright, N. H. : Association of the intrauterine contraceptive device and pelvic inflammatory disease. A retrospective pilot study. Am. J. Epidemiol. 100: 262, 1974.

8. Falkner, W. L. , Ory, H. W. : Intra-uterine devices and acute pelvic inflammatory disease. J. A. M. A. 235:1851, 1976.

9. Eschenbach, D.A., Harnisch, J.P., Holmes, K.K. : Pathogenesis of acute pelvic inflammatory disease: Role of contraception and other factors. Am. J. Obstet. & Gynecol. 128:838, 1977.

10. Westrom, L. , Bengstsson, L. P. , Mandh, P. A. : The risk factors of pelvic inflammatory disease in women using intra-uterine contraceptive devices as compared to nonusers. Lancet 2:221, 1976.

11. Mead, P. B. , Beecham, J. B. , Maeck, J. V. S. : Incidence of infection associated with the intra-uterine contraceptive device in an isolated community. Am. J. Obstet. Gynec. 125:79, 1976.

12. Gray, R. H. : Pelvic inflammatory disease and intra-uterine contraceptive devices. Lancet 2:521, 1976. (Letter).

13. Taylor, E. S. , et al: The intra-uterine devices and tubo-ovarian abscess. Am. J. Obstet. Gynec. 123:338, 1975.

14. Golde, S. H. , Israel, R. , Ledge, W. J. : Unilateral tubo-ovarian abscess: A disease entity. Am. J. Obstet. Gynecol. 127:807, 1977.

15. Chow, A. W. , et al: The bacteriology of acute pelvic inflammatory disease. Am. J. Obstet. Gynecol. 122:876, 1975.

16. Eschenbach, D. A. , et al: Polymicrobial etiology of acute pelvic inflammatory disease. New Eng. J. Med. 293:166, 1975.

39: LISTERIOSIS
by H. Thadepalli

Listeriosis is caused by Listeria (L.) monocytogenes, a gram-positive coccobacillary diplobacillus of size $1.0$ to $2.0$ x $0.5$ $\mu$m, with peritrichous flagellae. It grows well in both aerobic and $CO_2$ environment. Characteristically, it grows at $4^0$ as well as at $37^0$ and $42^0C$. It exhibits tumbling movements by which it is readily differentiated from diphtheroides, which it otherwise strongly resembles. It requires no special media for culture and grows well within the first 48 hours of incubation. As its name implies, it causes monocytosis in rabbits but not in humans. It is a facultative intracellular parasite; therefore, its prevalence in patients with T-cell dysfunction.

RESERVOIR: There are at least 37 mammalian reservoirs described, both domestic and wild. It is found in fowl, fish, ticks and crustaceans; it was found in mud and sewage where it can live for almost a year.

CARRIERS: Healthy fecal carriers exist among men and cattle [1] (Table 25).

CLINICAL MANIFESTATIONS

The clinical presentations of L. monocytogenes can be divided into three major clinical categories:

   A) Abortion
   B) Meningitis of the healthy newborn, and
   C) Meningitis in the compromised host

A) ABORTION: Queen Ann of England, who conceived 17 pregnancies but had no heir to the throne, probably had Listeria. In some parts of the world nearly 2% of healthy pregnant women harbor L. monocytogenes in the cervix (see Table 25). [2] Habitual abortion is a common feature of Listeria infection. Listeriosis should be considered in the differential diagnosis of FUO during the latter half of the pregnancy and delivery. Listeria can cause abortion, premature delivery and neonatal death. Maternal mortality due to Listeria is rare. [3]

TABLE 25: RECOVERY RATE OF LISTERIA
MONOCYTOGENES IN CATTLE AND HUMAN BEINGS[1-3]

| FECES | PER CENT POSITIVE |
|---|---|
| Cattle: | |
| Asymptomatic herds without infection | 1. 7 |
| Asymptomatic herds with previous Listeria infection | 6. 7 |
| Cattle with meningitis | 14. 1 |
| Cattle with abortion due to Listeria | 24. 2 |
| Humans: | |
| Men working in slaughterhouses and canned-food factories | 4. 6 |
| Women working in slaughterhouses and canned-food factories | 5. 4 |
| Patients admitted to medical wards and Ob/Gyn wards not suspected to have listeriosis | 1. 0 |
| Patients admitted to pediatrics | 0 |
| Patients with diarrhea | 1. 0 |
| Miscellaneous: | |
| Cervical samples positive during normal pregnancy | 2. 0 |
| Listeria isolated from the placenta of random pregnancies | 0. 3 |

B) NEONATAL MENINGITIS: Nearly 80% of Listeria infections manifest as meningitis, of which 40% are either newborn or older than 40 years. A great proportion of the latter have debilitating illnesses. Listeria is responsible for 17.4% of all cases of neonatal meningitis and 5% of the perinatal deaths. Nearly one of every 300 placental samples obtained at random contained Listeria. [4] Listeria can be venereally transmitted. It has been demonstrated in the semen of the husbands of some of the habitual aborters due to Listeria. While examining for the source in cases of neonatal meningitis, one should therefore, examine both parents.

The clinical features and the cerebrospinal fluid (CSF) findings in Listeria meningitis are similar to any other pyogenic meningitis. The neonates with Listeria infection may have hepatosplenomegaly and dark red papules on the lower extremities. Neonatal meningitis should be suspected if the mother had previous abortions, and/or gram-positive bacilli are seen in the CSF of the child. It is a highly fatal disease; the mortality in neonatal meningitis due to Listeria is close to 90%.

C) COMPROMISED HOST: Listeria should be considered in the differential diagnosis of meningitis in all cases of compromised host. [5] This includes post-splenectomy (see page 523), renal transplant, multiple myeloma, carcinoma of the lung, chronic renal failure, pregnancy, newborn, old age and those on steroid therapy. In the United Kindgom and Ireland, the incidence was higher above age 45, with an overall mortality of 16%. Nearly 100 cases in the U.S.A. and 20 cases in the U. K. are reported each year. The clinical picture is that of any other pyogenic meningitis. It carries nearly 50% to 75% mortality. Listeria has a special predilection to the central nervous system. Frequently there is history of febrile pharyngitis, cervical adenopathy, cough, coryza and gastrointestinal symptoms. Occasionally, listeriosis may disseminate and cause pleural or pericardial effusions and visceral granulomas or abscesses. Listeriosis should be considered in the diagnosis of FUO in cases of compromised host.

Listeriosis may also manifest in:

1) Septicemic form

2) Oculoglandular form - conjunctivitis with cervical lymph-adenopathy

3) Cervicoglandular - enlarged cervical lymph nodes and sore throat, resembling infectious mononucleosis, but the Paul-Bunnell reaction is negative

4) Pneumonia-like - as in typhoid fever, and, rarely,

5) Cutaneous form with multiple abscesses, and

6) Urethritis in men.

In general, the above six forms of Listeriosis carry favorable results.

## INVESTIGATIONS

BLOOD CULTURES:  Blood cultures should be obtained in all cases.  All gram-positive non-spore-forming diphtheroid-like organisms isolated from the blood and CSF cultures within the first 48 hours must be routinely tested for the possibility of Listeria, or else it will be missed.  The "tumbling test" and its growth at 4°C. are confirmatory.

CEREBROSPINAL FLUID: Listeria is the most likely organism if gram-positive bacilli are seen in the CSF of the newborn. Centrifuge 2 ml. of the CSF at 1500 g. for 15 minutes and re-move all supernatant except for 0.4 ml. of the sediment. Ex-amine the latter for gram-positive intra- (or extra-) cellular coccobacilli (or diplobacilli). Listeria may sometimes stain unevenly and resemble H. influenzae. It should be confirmed by culture.

CERVICAL SWABS:  The cervical swabs may be transported in Stuart's medium, transferred to a tryptic soy broth and in-cubated at 4°C. Cervical swabs should be obtained for culture of Listeria from all mothers who had abortion, or whose new-born had developed meningitis. It should also be obtained from women who have high fetal loss.

FECES:  Fecal samples (approximately 1 gm of stool) can be collected in glycerol saline medium and incubated at 4°C. and examined and transferred to another medium once a month for three months.

TISSUE CULTURES:  Biopsies of the tissue samples should be homogenized and the homogenate transferred to the blood agar plates and incubated at 35°C. An aliquot of this should also be

kept in broth culture in a cold environment (4°C.) and transferred once a month.

ANIMAL INOCULATION: Listeria is lethal to mice on intraperitoneal injection. When in doubt, to differentiate between
diphtheroid and Listeria, mouse peritoneal inoculation is indicated. Listeria will cause peritonitis and death in mice within a day or two, diphtheroids do not.

ANTON TEST: When a culture of suspected Listeria is applied
to the conjunctiva of the rabbit, purulent conjunctivitis will result. Further, the organism can be recultured from this lesion.

INDIRECT HEMAGGLUTINATION (IHA) REACTION: Serum
samples from the patients are required for this test. However,
a certain percentage of uninfected persons may also give positive reactions. Nearly one-fourth of the pregnant women with
history of abortions and premature deliveries, and one-tenth
of the full-term mothers without any clinical problems, are
IHA positive.

FLUORESCENT ANTIBODY TEST: This can also be used for
rapid presumptive identification of Listeria in the CSF samples.

## REFERENCES

1.  Bojsen-Moller, J.: Human listeriosis - Diagnostic, epi-
    demiological and clinical studies. Acta. Pathologica et
    Microbiologica Scandinavia, No. 229: (Supplement), Section
    B, 1972.

2.  Nagy, T., Mero, E.: Screening examination for listeriosis
    in pregnancy. Acta. Microbiol. Acad. Sci. Hung. 19:385,
    1972.

3.  Morosov, B.: Listeriosis and gestation. Acta. Microbiol.
    Acad. Sci. Hung. 19:399-402, 405-410, 1972.

4.  Dean, J. P., et al: Rechercha de Lesteria monocytogenes
    dans les placentas preleues en salle de travail. La Nouvelle
    Presse Medicale 3:2561, 1974.

5.  Gantz, N. M., et al: Listeriosis in immunosuppressed pa-
    tients. Am. J. Med. 58:637, 1975.

## 40: PROSTATIC ABSCESS
by H. Thadepalli

Prostatic abscess should be considered in the differential diagnosis of a patient with suspected abdominal abscess, who on physical examination, has an enlarged and tender prostate. Routine physical examination may fail to reveal any apparent source for sepsis. Increased urinary frequency, decreased caliber of the stream, strangury with pain in the perineum, and fishy and offensive odor of the urine, associated with fever and chills and rigors, are some of the features of prostatic abscess. The urine might be cloudy with or without pyuria. The diagnosis of prostatic abscess will be missed if rectal exam is not performed. Undrained prostatic abscess is almost always fatal.

## COLONY COUNTS

Perform colony counts on the urine voided before and after prostatic massage. If the colony counts in the urine collected before massage are less than the counts in the post-massage specimen, the diagnosis of prostatitis or abscess is the most likely. [1]

Semen culture and colony counts might be just as useful as the secretions collected by prostatic massage. [2]

The value of sonography (echography) in the diagnosis of prostatic abscess has not been fully evaluated; it may have a place.

## BACTERIOLOGY

Gram-negative aerobic bacilli and anaerobic bacteria are frequently found in the prostatic abscess. [3] Escherichia coli is the most frequent isolate. Among anaerobes, Bacteroides is frequent. Anaerobic bacteria are normal flora of the urethra. [4,5]

Suprapubic needle aspiration of urine from the bladder is the most reliable culture source, and it should be obtained whenever in doubt. In one study, only 1 of 19 specimens collected by suprapubic needle aspiration of the bladder contained anaerobic bacteria. [5] Quantitative anaerobic culture of the urine is of no help in distinguishing between actual infection and contamination from normal flora. In my experience, 5 of 180 patients with intra-abdominal and pelvic abscess had prostatic abscess. None were post-surgical. All five patients had anaerobes at the infected site. Two had aerobic bacteria in addition. The most common anaerobes found were Bacteroides. All five patients improved on surgical exploration and drainage. In two cases, the source of infection was unknown; routine urine cultures were negative, but the suprapubic needle aspirates yielded Peptococcus magnus (1 x $10^3$/ml. ) in one and Bacteroides fragilis (1 x $10^5$/ml. ) in the other. See page 332 for a case history of prostatic abscess.

## REFERENCES

1. Meares, E. M. J.: Bacterial prostatitis vs. "prostatosis". A clinical and bacteriological study. J. A. M. A. 224:1372, 1975.

2. Moblcy, D. F.: Semen cultures in the diagnosis of bacterial prostatitis. J. Urology 114:83, 1974.

3. Fischbach, R. S., Finegold, S. M.: Anaerobic prostatic abscess with bacteremia. J. Clin. Path. 59:408, 1973.

4. Finegold, S. M., et al: Significance of Anaerobic and Capnophilic Bacteria Isolated from the Urinary Tract. Progress in Pyelonephritis, (Ed. ) Kass, E. A. Davis Co., Philadelphia, p. 159, 1965.

5. Kumazarwa, J., et al: Significance of anaerobic bacteria isolates from the urinary tract. Invest. Urol. 13:309, 1976.

## 41: GONORRHEA
### by A. Paul Kelly

Gonorrhea (Greek for "flow of semen or seed") is an acute or chronic infectious disease caused by the gram-negative diplococcus, Neisseria gonorrhoeae and except for vulvovaginitis and ophthalmia, it is transmitted by sexual contact. Gonorrhea is found throughout the world. In the United States alone, nearly three million cases occur each year, thus, for every case of syphilis, there are 40 to 50 cases of gonorrhea. An infection confers no immunity and reinfections are common. Although it can affect any age, it is predominant during the early twenties. The male-female ratio is three to one; this discrepancy may be explained by the higher incidence of asymptomatic infections in women. Transmission of gonorrhea by way of toilet seats, bath towels, sheets, mattresses, chairs, drinking glasses, bathing, or sitting on someone's lap does not occur. These are face-saving myths.[1]

## CLINICAL MANIFESTATIONS

Gonorrhea is essentially a disease of man. Since gonococcus is unable to penetrate the normal skin, the initial attack occurs on mucous membranes. In men, the incubation period ranges from two to eight days or it may be as short as one day, or as long as three weeks. When induced experimentally, it may last for three to four weeks.

Acute gonorrhea in men presents as a urethritis, characterized by a thick, yellowish purulent discharge from the anterior urethra, preceded by uncomfortable and painful sensations along the urethra, followed by increased frequency of burning urination. Constitutional symptoms are rare. When untreated, it extends to cause posterior urethritis and later, epididymitis and prostatitis. Epididymitis may be painful and unilateral. When untreated, a chronic carrier state may result. With therapy, acute anterior urethritis promptly subsides within 24 hours, prostatitis and epididymitis respond slowly, however. In 80% to 90% of women, acute gonorrhea is asymptomatic. Occasionally, women may present with a vaginal discharge and, like men, may also have urinary frequency and dysuria. Untreated, it ascends along the fallopian tubes or spreads to the lymph nodes. Symptoms of pelvic invasion are often mild with fever and nausea, or occasionally it can be severe, with vomiting and lower quadrant pain simulating appendicitis and other acute surgical conditions. Signs of peritonitis may be present.

## DIFFERENTIAL DIAGNOSIS

Gonorrhea in men should be differentiated from non-specific urethritis and Reiter's disease, although Reiter's disease and acute gonococcal infection may coexist. In women, Tricho- monas vaginalis, candidiasis and Haemophilus vaginalis should be differentiated from gonorrhea.

## EXTRAGENITAL GONOCOCCAL INFECTION

During the past two years, there seems to be a female pre- dominance in extragenital manifestations of gonorrhea, espe- cially among those under the age of 30.[2] Over 50% of the men with extragenital gonorrhea are homosexuals, therefore, ho- mosexual men are more apt to have asymptomatic gonococcal proctitis rather than urethritis. Asymptomatic gonorrhea may go untreated for long periods, allowing greater chances for dissemination of the disease (Table 26).

TABLE 26: EXTRAGENITAL GONOCOCCAL INFECTIONS[2]

| PRIMARY | DISSEMINATED |
|---|---|
| 1. Conjunctivitis | 1. Skin |
| 2. Proctitis | 2. Arthritis |
| 3. Oral infections | 3. Perihepatitis |
|    a) Stomatitis | 4. Peritonitis |
|    b) Pharyngitis | 5. Pericarditis and myocarditis |
| | 6. Endocarditis |
| | 7. Hepatitis |
| | 8. Meningitis |

### PRIMARY EXTRAGENITAL GONOCOCCAL INFECTIONS

These result from auto-inoculation, for instance, from the genitals to the eye. The vascular and lymphatic systems and the contiguous structures are unaffected during the spread of primary infection.

### GONOCOCCAL EYE INFECTION

Ophthalmia neonatorum is acquired at birth during the passage through the birth canal of an infected mother. It is usually bi- lateral, initially presenting with a catarrhal conjunctivitis, later leading to a characteristic grayish-yellow purulent discharge from the swollen eyelids. In adults, the gonococcal conjunctivitis

can be as a result of auto-inoculation. The incubation period is the
same as in acute gonococcal urethritis, two to eight days. It
usually begins with a unilateral red, swollen and infected conjunctiva exuding a purulent yellowish discharge. If untreated,
the other eye also becomes infected within a period of one week.
Other complications include hypopyon, corneal ulceration and
early neovascularization of the cornea; thereby, there is a loss
of visual acuity within three to seven days. [3] These complications can be prevented by prompt and appropriate therapy.

## GONOCOCCAL PROCTITIS

Proctitis in men is often secondary to homosexuality. About
one-third of the women with gonorrhea develop proctitis secondary to vaginorectal contamination or from anal intercourse.
Both men and women with proctitis may remain asymptomatic,
although a slight discomfort on defecation, bloody or mucoid
or purulent stools may result with pruritus ani and the constant
urge to defecate. It may occasionally be complicated by anal
fissures, perianal abscess, and ischiorectal abscesses.

## OROPHARYNGEAL GONORRHEA

Oropharyngeal infection may be observed two to eight days after oral-genital contact (fellatio or cunnilingus). Those with
gonococcal tonsillitis and/or pharyngitis usually present with
dry mouth and sore throat, accompanied by headache, fever
and chills. Gonococcal stomatitis may present with itching,
burning, soreness and dryness of the mouth, accompanied by
headache, fever and chills with dysphagia and even trismus.
Oropharyngeal examination may reveal stomatitis as evidenced
by a bright red oral mucosa studded with areas of yellow exudates on the tonsils. Sometimes the exudate may form yellowish-
white or grayish-yellow pseudomembranes. In some cases,
genital complaints may be altogether absent.

Pharyngeal and/or tonsillar disease may show diffuse erythema and edema of the pharynx. Both the anterior and posterior
tonsillar pillars are swollen and erythematous. Tonsils may
be enlarged and inflamed, either unilaterally or bilaterally.
Sometimes this enlargement is accompanied by a yellowish
discharge located in the crypts and/or cervical adenopathy.
Occasionally, vesicles or pustules may be located on the uvula
and the anterior pillars of the tonsil.

## DISSEMINATED GONOCOCCAL INFECTION

Dissemination of gonococcal infection may occur by direct local extension or by way of the bloodstream. The gonococcal infection may disseminate by invading the bloodstream. One type of gonococcal sepsis involves mainly the skin (vesiculopustular lesions) and joints (acute polyarthritis) without urologic symptoms. This type is essentially benign. Most of the patients contract the disease two to three weeks prior to the symptomatology. Response to appropriate therapy is prompt with all signs and symptoms abating in 24 to 48 hours. When there is invasion of vital multi-organ systems, such as the heart, meninges, pleura and liver, the prognosis is poor. Thus, in those with disseminated disease, one may find skin lesions, arthritis, perihepatitis, peritonitis, pericarditis, myocarditis, endocarditis, meningitis and hepatitis, occurring either alone or in combination.

## CUTANEOUS LESIONS IN GONORRHEA

Skin lesions are almost always associated with other types of disseminated gonococcal disease, although they may occasionally occur alone. They are the second most common manifestation of disseminated gonorrhea. Three basic types of skin lesions may occur in gonorrhea:

1) Vesiculopustular lesions on an erythematous base
2) Hemorrhagic papules, and
3) Bullae [4,5,6]

Skin lesions may be solitary, or few in number, although they appear in crops. The initial lesions are tiny red papules or vesiculopustules surrounded by an erythematous base. Most of them resolve spontaneously in four to six days. They are often localized on the palms and over the joints. Most of the lesions are asymptomatic, although sometimes the lesion itself may be tender.

Culture of the organisms from skin lesions is difficult, although Kahn[7] has demonstrated gonococcal antigens in arthritis and skin lesions by immunofluorescence method. Arthritis is the most common manifestation of gonococcal dissemination. There are two clinical forms of gonococcal arthritis, but numerous variations may occur. [8] The first type, the bacteremic form, is associated with clinical and bacteriologic manifestations of gonococcal sepsis, such as fever, chills, cutaneous lesions, polyarticular arthritis, generalized sepsis and tenosynovitis. However, on smear and cultural examination of an affected joint, no gonococci can be demonstrated; this finding has led to the descriptive term "sterile joint". The second type has minimal septic manifestations, is usually mono-articular and the gonococci are found in the synovial fluid ("septic joint"). There may be accompanying pain, swelling and joint effusion. The third form of gonococcal arthritis may be accompanied by all other forms of disseminated gonococcal disease, but is most commonly associated with genital infection, skin infection, proctitis and pharyngitis. In most patients, the symptoms of acute gonococcal infection are absent, and the disease seems to progress rapidly from acute to full manifestations within 24 to 48 hours. In women, the arthritis is more apparent during menstruation and pregnancy. During pregnancy, it is more common during the second and third trimester. In men, arthritic symptoms usually appear within one to four weeks after the onset of acute primary gonococcal infection.

## GONOCOCCAL PERIHEPATITIS

Gonococcal perihepatitis, also known as the Fitz-Hugh-Curtis syndrome, is characterized by severe anterior right upper quadrant pain, which is sharp and often referred to the right shoulder, or occasionally to both shoulders. Frequent belching and nausea are common and, although less frequent, vomitting may occur. Normally, there is a three to four week period of quiescence between the onset of perihepatitis and previous pelvic inflammatory disease.

Physical findings include a slight elevation of temperature, moderate abdominal distention and decreased peristolic sounds. Marked tenderness and rigidity are noted in the anterior and lateral right upper quadrant. A positive Murphy sign may be present. The liver is often enlarged. Only minimal tenderness and rigidity are noted in the lower abdominal quadrants. [9,10] Symptoms subside in three to six weeks in untreated patients. A chronic stage may follow.

The acute phase must be differentiated from acute cholecystitis, hepatitis, pneumonia, perforated peptic ulcer, subphrenic abscess, pleurisy, nephrolithiasis and perinephric abscess. Perihepatitis is a cause of "violin string" adhesions.

## GONOCOCCAL PERITONITIS

Gonococcal peritonitis is rare. To begin with, there may be mild abdominal discomfort, followed immediately by fever, nausea with or without vomiting, abdominal pain accentuated in the lower quadrants and profuse vaginal discharge.

Appendicitis, pelvic inflammatory disease, pyelonephritis and an acute abdomen must be ruled out.

## PERICARDITIS AND MYOCARDITIS

In most patients, the diagnosis of myocarditis and pericarditis secondary to disseminated gonococcal infection is made by electrocardiographic examination; for seldom do they have any symptoms or demonstrable cardiac findings on physical examination. They often see the physician for arthritis rather than for "heart" disease. Electrocardiographic changes are similar to that of any type of acute pericarditis, including inverted T-wave, prolonged P-R interval and elevation and coving of ST segments in any or all leads. [11] With proper antibiotic therapy, the electrocardiographic changes revert to normal.

Since the myocarditis and pericarditis are usually accompanied by fever, chills, migratory polyarthritis and electrocardiographic abnormalities, rheumatic fever must be ruled out. This is usually done by the failure of disseminated gonococcemia to respond to salicylates or bed rest.

## GONOCOCCAL ENDOCARDITIS

As with gonococcal myocarditis and pericarditis, most patients with gonococcal endocarditis usually present with severe polyarthritis. Within days to weeks after the joint pains begin, they complain of chills, chest pain, dyspnea on exertion and malaise. During this stage of the disease, they have a fever of 38° to 39°C. and pathologic murmurs. Petechiae, septic emboli, anemia, splenomegaly and glomerulonephritis may also be present. Jaundice, presumably a toxic hepatitis, is present in more than half of these patients.

A biphasic febrile pattern consisting of two distinct spikes of fever during each 24-hour period (the church steeple, double quotidian pattern, the double daily hump) is seen in gonococcemia with endocarditis. A similar type pattern may be seen in kala-azar (see page 581) and in some patients with miliary tuberculosis.

The infection is commonest on the aortic valve, although the mitral, tricuspid and pulmonary can be involved alone or in various combinations. Sometimes it is associated with myocarditis.

## HEPATITIS

Gonococcal hepatitis is secondary to gonococcal bacteremia. It is usually accompanied by fever, arthritis and skin lesions, although it may occur alone. Jaundice may or may not be present. It seldom leads to any serious sequelae, but it must be differentiated from other more serious forms of hepatitis.

## DIAGNOSTIC TESTS

TRANSPORT MEDIUM: For transport to a distant laboratory, transgrow medium is recommended for cultivation of Neisseria gonorrhoeae. This medium with 10% concentration of carbon dioxide, favors the growth of N. gonorrhoeae. This medium is not ideal and it has its own limitations.

It should be remembered that in women, cultures should be obtained from the urethra and cervix, but not from the vagina. Use of surgical lubricants on the speculum or gloves of the examiner contain bacteriostatic agents and may kill gonococci present in the specimen. Also, gonococci seem to be present in greater numbers during menstruation than in the intermenstrual period.

FLUORESCENT ANTIBODY TEST (FA): There are two types of FA test, direct and indirect. The direct FA test involves a fluorescein dye conjugated with a specific globulin (antibody) against the suspected organism. A smear containing the organism is flooded with the fluorescein-tagged globulin specific for the suspected organism. If positive, there is union between the globulin and surface antigen of the organism, thereby allowing the organism to fluoresce when illuminated with ultraviolet light.

INDIRECT FLUORESCENT ANTIBODY TEST (IFA): This test is essentially used to detect antibodies by use of the fluorescein isothiocyanate-globulin conjugate.

Both the direct and indirect tests have approximately the same reliability and sensitivity as the Thayer-Martin culture. The IFA test however, requires a well-equipped laboratory, specifically trained technicians and is therefore expensive. The direct fluorescent antibody test is superior over the Thayer-Martin cultures to detect N. gonorrhoeae damaged by antibiotics. On the other hand, the IFA test seems to yield many false-positive results. Commercially labeled antigonococcus sera for IFA diagnosis is often fraught with false-positives and false-negatives because of the non-specific fluorescence of the leukocyte cytoplasm, the strong fluorescence of the granules of eosinophil and basophil granulocytes, the weak or absent fluorescence of intracellular gonococci and the non-specific fluorescence phenomena due to the mode of preparation of commercially available gonococcus antiserum.

Hare[12] reported that the delayed fluorescent antibody test was found to be more reliable and more sensitive than conventional tests. It was positive in 90% of the cases of gonorrhea in women compared with 75% for a combination of conventional smears and cultures. The direct FA test was found to be less sensitive than the delayed antibody test.

COMPLEMENT-FIXATION TEST: The gonococcal complement-fixation test (CFT) uses a standard gonococcal antigen to test for the presence of circulating antibodies. The test has drawbacks. Other members of the Neisseria family may cross react and also give a positive reaction.

OTHER TESTS: Other tests which may be of value in the future for diagnosing gonorrhea, but at present are done only in specialized laboratories with equivocal results, are the bacterial hemagglutination by Neisseria gonorrhoeae,[13] the use of gonococcal ribosomes as skin test antigens,[14] more sophisticated and updated methods of the previously described tests and the microflocculation technique. By scanning electron microscope, virulent and avirulent gonococcal colonies may be separated by their morphology.[15]

## REFERENCES

1. Fiumara, N. J.: Clinical Dermatology. Harper & Row, Hagerstown, p. 2, 1974.

2. McDonald, C. J., Kelly, A. P.: Textbook of Black-Related Diseases. McGraw-Hill, New York, p. 554, 1975.

3. Thatcher, R. W., Petit, T. H.: Gonorrheal conjunctivitis. J. A. M. A. 215:1494, 1971.

4. Ackerman, A. B., et al: Gonococcemia and its cutaneous manifestations. Arch. Dermatol. 91:227, 1965.

5. Abul-Nassar, H., et al: Cutaneous manifestations of gonococcemia. A review of 14 cases. Arch. Int. Med. 112: 731, 1963.

6. Ackerman, A. B.: Hemorrhagic bullae in gonococcemia. New Eng. J. Med. 282:793, 1970.

7. Kahn, G., Danielson, D.: Septic gonococcal dermatitis: Demonstration of gonococci and gonococcal antigens in skin lesions by immunofluorescence. Arch. Dermatol. 99: 421, 1969.

8. Keiser, H., et al: Clinical forms of gonococcal arthritis. New Eng. J. Med. 279:234, 1968.

9. Fitz-Hugh, T.: Acute gonococcic perihepatitis: A new syndrome of right upper quadrant abdominal pain in young women. Rev. Gastroenterol. 3:125, 1936.

10. Kimball, M. W., Knee, S.: Gonococcal perihepatitis in a male. The Fitz-Hugh-Curtis syndrome. New Eng. J. Med. 283:1082, 1970.

11. Shapiro, E., et al: Electrocardiographic changes in acute gonococcal arthritis and myocarditis simulating acute rheumatic polyarthritis. Am. J. Med. Sci. 217:300, 1949.

12. Hare, M. J.: Comparative assessment of microbiological methods for the diagnosis of gonorrhea in women. Brit. J. Ven. Dis. 50:437, 1974.

13. Koransky, J. R. , Scales, R. W. , Kraus, S. S. J. : Bacterial hemagglutination by Neisseria gonorrhoeae. Infec. Immun. 12:495, 1975.

14. Judd, R. C. , Koostra, W. L. : Gonococcal ribosome as skin test antigen. II. Precision of the method, attempts to identify the ribosomal antigen, and correlation with the macrophage migration inhibition test. Brit. J. Vener. Dis. 52:28, 1976.

15. Kraus, S. J. , Glassmann, L. H. : Scanning electron microscope study of Neisseria gonorrhoeae. Appl. Microbiol. 27:584, 1974.

## 42: SYPHILIS
by A. Paul Kelly

No better definition of syphilis exists than that of Stokes' in 1945.[1] A paraphrase of his statement is as follows: "Syphilis is an infectious disease due to <u>Treponema pallidum</u>, of great chronicity; systemic from the outset, capable of involving practically every structure of the body in its course; distinguished by florid manifestations on the one hand and years of completely asymptomatic latency on the other; able to simulate many diseases in the fields of medicine and surgery; transmissible to offspring in man; transmissible to certain laboratory animals; and treatable to the point of presumptive cure. "

Syphilis is usually divided into four clinical stages: primary, secondary, latent and late. Primary and secondary stages are considered as early syphilis. Congenital syphilis is also divided into stages similar to those of acquired syphilis. Since congenital syphilis is acquired <u>in utero</u> through fetal circulation, there is no primary stage.

### ETIOLOGY

The causative organism of syphilis is <u>Treponema (T. ) pallidum</u>, a thin, thread-like spiral organism which is a member of the order Spirochaetales and the family Treponemataceae.

<u>T. pallidum</u> is an actively mobile spirochete, 6 to 16 $\mu$ long, $0.25\mu$ wide and twisted in a corkscrew pattern. The organism has between 6 and 14 coils, and its movement is characterized by three elements: A corkscrew-like rotation on its own axis; undulation of the center with relatively fixed ends; and a movement of propulsion in the direction of its own axis. It causes disease by local destruction; it has no demonstrable toxin. It is quickly killed by exposure to cold or drying within a few minutes. It has never been cultured in artificial media.

### CLINICAL MANIFESTATIONS

PRIMARY SYPHILIS (Fig. 61): The initial clinical lesion of syphilis is the chancre. Chancres are solitary lesions, but multiple lesions can occur. They appear as small, eroded, painless papules, firm and indurated. Although eroded or ulcerated, they produce no discharge unless secondarily infected. Chancres vary from a few millimeters in diameter to one

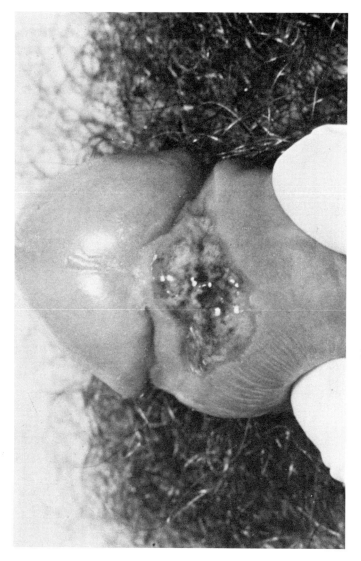

FIG. 61: Primary chancre, syphilis.

or two centimeters. They occur on a genital site, although extragenital sites, such as the mouth, the anus and the nipple are not uncommon. Extragenital lesions are often painful. Regional lymph nodes usually become enlarged, especially on penile lesions, where there is bilateral inguinal lymphadenopathy.

The chancre may appear anywhere from 10 to 90 days (an average of 21 days) following exposure. It occurs at the site of treponemal invasion - the skin, or mucous membrane. Prior to the appearance of the chancre, no other lesions or symptoms may occur. However, the patient's blood may contain spirochetes and is infectious. An occasional patient may become listless, run a slight fever and lose weight during the incubation period. Without treatment, the chancre heals within three to eight weeks.

Any genital lesion should be considered as chancre until ruled out by dark-field examination and other serologic tests for syphilis. Diseases which are most often confused with primary syphilis are: chancroid, where the lesions are multiple, soft and painful; herpes simplex, where the lesions are usually numerous, grouped and painful; lymphogranuloma venereum, where the primary lesion is a rarely seen papulo-vesicular lesion; and granuloma inguinale, which is also painless, but without any significant inguinal lymphadenopathy.

SECONDARY SYPHILIS: Six weeks to six months after the appearance of the chancre, secondary manifestations of syphilis may appear. It is possible that one may have the primary chancre when secondary lesions appear. It is due to the myriad constitutional and cutaneous signs and symptoms in the secondary stage that syphilis has received the label of the "great imitator". The secondary stage also probably prompted the famous quotation by Sir William Osler, "He who knows syphilis knows medicine". Although constitutional symptoms may be present, the diagnosis of secondary syphilis is mainly entertained because of cutaneous manifestations. The cutaneous lesions are non-pruritic, and symmetrical in distribution. In Caucasians, they are dull red to copper-colored, whereas in Blacks, or those with dark skin, they are hyperpigmented, often violaceous in color. Cutaneous eruptions usually persist for months if untreated, but they are often present for only a few weeks. Types of skin lesions include: macular lesions, especially of the palms and soles (Fig. 62), papular lesions from 2 to 6 mm. in diameter and annular or plaque-like lesions, which are especially common on the faces of Blacks,

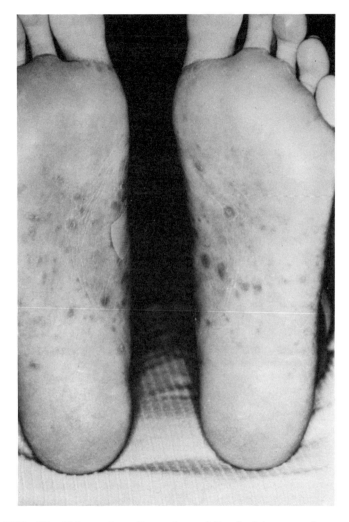

FIG. 62: Skin rash on the soles of the feet in secondary
         syphilis. These spots were light coffee-brown
         in color. They resemble Janeway's lesions
         (see Fig. 53).

and so-called "nickle and dime" syphilis (Fig. 63). Papules
in the anal-genital region may become large, flat, verrucous
and moist; they are then called chondylomata lata. Sometimes
skin lesions resemble psoriasis, so-called psoriasiform syphilis (Fig. 64). Ulcerating lesions in secondary syphilis are very
rare and occur only in severe cases, so-called lues maligna.

Lesions may appear on any of the mucous membranes, especially on the mouth, pharynx and anal canal. The mucus patch
is usually an oval area covered by grayish tissue and surrounded
by a dull, red halo. The lesion is highly infectious and may
account for mouth-to-mouth transmission of syphilis. It is
painless unless secondarily infected.

Generalized lymphadenopathy is common in secondary syphilis, especially the epitrochlear, occipital and inguinal nodes.
Vesicular bullous lesions are found only in congenital syphilis.

There is a characteristic "moth-eaten" alopecia of the scalp,
especially of the occipital area, and there may be a loss of the
lateral third of the eyebrows.

Constitutional symptoms of secondary syphilis include enlargement of the spleen and liver, sometimes with jaundice. Nephrosis may occur in secondary syphilis and is thought to represent an immune complex disease, since on immunofluorescent
microscopy, a positive IgG and complement are found along
the glomerular basement membrane. Acute iritis may be the
first and only symptom in some patients. There may be hoarseness and chronic sore throat. Acute arthritis may develop
along with bone pain, which is worse at night. Other constitutional symptoms include headaches, arthralgia, fever and a
variety of vague organ-specific complaints.

The maculopapular lesions of syphilis must be distinguished
from the lesions of pityriasis rosea (PR). In PR, the lesions
are usually pruritic and often are preceded a week or two by
the "Herald patch". Drug eruptions, like syphilis, are widely
varied in their presentation. They are usually pruritic and
do not involve the palms or soles. The fissured, split papules
which often occur at the angles of the mouth in secondary syphilis may mimic perleche, associated with cheilitis, oral candidiasis or hypovitaminosis.

The central nervous system can be involved during the secondary stage of syphilis, giving rise to an acute type of syphilitic meningitis. Also, there may be occasional cranial nerve

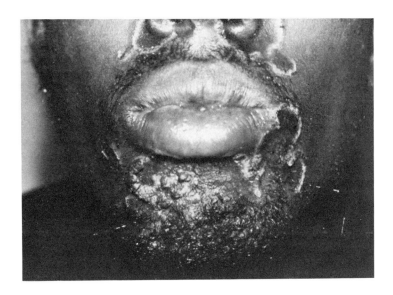

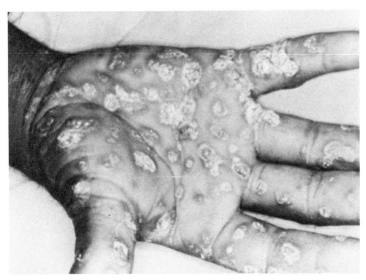

FIG. 63: Gyrate painless cutaneous lesions on the face and the palm of the hand in a case of secondary syphilis. Treponema were found in these lesions under dark-ground illumination.

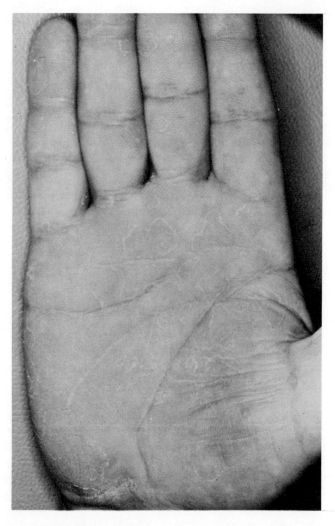

FIG. 64: Exfoliation of the skin of the palm due to secondary syphilis.

palsies, transverse myelitis or thrombosis of the cerebral or
spinal arteries.

LATENT SYPHILIS: After clinical remission of secondary
syphilis, the disease enters the latent stage. The diagnosis of
latency is based upon the absence of clinical signs or symptoms, a negative spinal fluid serologic test for syphilis (STS)
and a positive serum STS. The latent stage is divided into early
latent (up to two years following infection) and late latent (beyond two years) phases. Since the lesions of secondary syphilis occasionally reappear during the first part of latency, it
sometimes is difficult to clearly demarcate the two. As the
period of latency increases, the chances of transmitting the
infection decrease. After infection has persisted for more than
four years, it is seldom, if ever, communicable, except in
the case of a pregnant woman who, if untreated, may transmit
syphilis to her unborn fetus, regardless of the duration of her
disease.

LATE SYPHILIS: After the disappearance of the early manifestations in untreated or inadequately treated patients, there
follows a period of apparent good health; for the life of the patient, or, in approximately one-third of them, the disease advances to the late (formerly called tertiary) stage. Late manifestations may occur anywhere from three to thirty years following the primary infection.

Gumma is the most distinctive and characteristic lesion of late
syphilis. Almost any organ may be involved, but the most common sites of the gumma are the skin, bone and liver. Skin and/
or mucous membrane lesions may be solitary or multiple. The
characteristic picture is that of arciform borders surrounding
punched-out ulcers. The lesions are painless, destructive,
chronic and heal centrally while extending centrifugally. Gummas of the mucous membrane may eventually cause destruction of nasal septum cartilage, leading to a saddle-nose defect; perforation of the soft palate; or thickening of the tongue,
which may either ulcerate or become cancerous. Patients with
active gummas or typical scars caused by gummas usually have
negative STS tests. The most frequent locations for gummas
are the shins of the legs, forehead, nose, sternum, supraclavicular regions and the lips. Non-ulcerated gummas must
be distinguished from sarcoidosis, sporotrichosis, malignant
tumor and glanders. Scrofuloderma, blastomycosis and tuberculosis verrucosa cutis must be ruled out when ulcerated gummas are present. The gumma is often a midline lesion. It may
have to be distinguished from a midline granuloma, a locally
malignant disease.

LATE BONE AND JOINT SYPHILIS: Several of the late luetic bone lesions are necrotic. This results in the exostosis secondary to periostitis which makes the shins, the clavicles, the sternum and cranial bones nodular. Luetic arthritis is usually monoarticular. It is a gummatous thickening of the synovial membrane and joint capsule. It is characterized by triple displacement (Charcot's joint), a result of destructive painless arthritis (see Fig. 90, page 468). It affects the large joints, especially the hip and the knee. It can be secondary to tabetic changes in the spinal cord. Charcot's joint can result from syringomyelia and medullary tumor of the spinal cord.

CARDIOVASCULAR SYPHILIS: Cardiovascular syphilis occurs in approximately 10% of all untreated patients. Aortitis is the basic lesion, although other great vessels and the myocardium itself may be affected. Long-standing aortitis may be calcified. Further damage may lead to debilitation of the aortic ring and cause aortic insufficiency or saccular aneurysms of the thoracic aorta (Fig. 65). Left ventricular hypertrophy and congestive heart failure may develop. Non-treponemal serology (pages 357, 358) is positive in about three-quarters of the patients with cardiovascular syphilis, and a slightly higher percentage is noted when the treponemal STS is used.

NEUROSYPHILIS: Involvement of the central nervous system may be parenchymatous, asymptomatic or meningovascular.

Parenchymatous neurosyphilis presents as either paresis or tabes dorsalis. In paresis, personality changes may range from minor to frankly psychotic. Impairment of intellectual function and memory are the earliest changes. These may be followed by belligerent behavior, outbursts of temper, errors in judgment and other changes indicative of intellectual deterioration. Focal neurological signs, such as tremor, aphasia and pupillary changes may also be present. STS for syphilis is positive during this phase.

Tabes dorsalis is caused by parenchymatous involvement of the posterior column of the spinal cord. Men seem to be affected more than women. There are a myriad of symptoms, with pain in the leg the earliest manifestation. This pain may be severe and lancinating; so-called "lightening pains". Other symptoms include impairment of bladder function, impotency, ataxia, bowel control impairment, decreased vision, and even

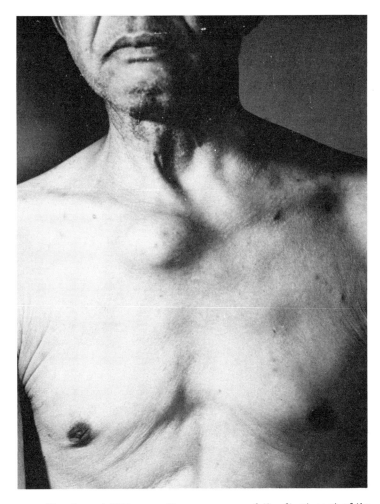

FIG. 65: A syphilitic, aortic aneurysm of the first part of the
aortic arch may erode the sternum and ribs and appear as a pulsating mass at the right upper sternal
border.

optic atrophy leading to complete blindness. There may be abdominal crisis characterized by attacks of severe pain, anorexia and vomiting. These attacks may last for several hours
or days and then end abruptly. One of the most diagnostic
abnormalities is the Argyll-Robertson pupil, which will react to accommodation and convergence, but sluggishly or
not at all to light. The signs and symptoms of paresis
and tabes dorsalis may coexist and produce the so-called
tabo-paresis.

CONGENITAL SYPHILIS: Syphilis of the child is seldom acquired. Thus, practically all cases of syphilis in children are
congenital, and result from transmission of the Treponema
across the placenta to the fetus. There have been a few rare
cases reported where syphilis is acquired intrapartum, when
the child passes through the birth canal of a mother who has
primary syphilitic lesion acquired in late pregnancy. In congenital syphilis, a true primary lesion per se is absent, because the infection is similar to that of transfusion syphilis or
"syphilis d'emblee". Transplacental transmission of the Treponema does not take place before the sixteenth to eighteenth week
of gestation, therefore, it is imperative that all pregnant females have an STS during the early weeks of pregnancy so that
adequate treatment will prevent infection of the fetus. Primary
congenital syphilis is divided into early signs and symptoms
and late signs and symptoms.

The early stage of congenital syphilis is characterized by
signs and symptoms that appear before age two. Usually,
the earlier the onset, the poorer the prognosis. Following
are some early signs of congenital syphilis.

1) Cutaneous lesions: Skin lesions often seen in the third
   or fourth week after birth, may be seen up to the third
   month. Generalized maculopapular or papulosquamous
   lesions are frequent. Characteristically the plantar and
   palmar bullae may be teeming with spirochetes. The
   face is usually pinched and drawn and the skin has dirty
   brown or waxy white hue.

2) Mucous membrane lesions: A heavy mucoid discharge,
   known as the "snuffles", is often found on the mucous membranes of the nose and pharynx. This discharge is often
   teeming with spirochetes.

3) <u>Bone:</u> Oseous involvement may present as osteomyelitis, osteochondritis or osteoperiostitis, demonstrated by x-ray examination (see Chapter 57).  Only 10% to 15% of them will show clinical signs of bone involvement.  Pain caused by movement of these limbs often causes pseudoparalysis. Whether treated or not, osseous symptomatology resolves within a year.

4) <u>Anemia:</u>  A self-limiting hemolytic anemia is usually present.

5) <u>Hepatosplenomegaly:</u>  This may be present in 60% to 70% of the cases and may be associated with low-grade icterus due to extensive scarring of the liver, called <u>hepar lobatum</u> (Figs. 66, 67).

6) <u>Central nervous system:</u>  Although approximately 50% may have abnormal cerebrospinal fluid findings, only about 5% will develop neurologic abnormalities.  There may be meningeal irritation, convulsions, retardation, and, rarely, extensive meningovascular involvement leading to hydrocephalus.

Other manifestations of early congenital syphilis include marasmus, failure to thrive and lymphadenopathy.

LATE CONGENITAL SYPHILIS:  This is defined as congenital syphilis which has persisted beyond two years of age[2].  In about 60%, the disease is latent with no manifestations other than a reactive serologic test for syphilis.  The signs of late congenital syphilis are:

1) <u>Interstitial keratitis:</u>  This usually appears near puberty and although initially unilateral, usually becomes bilateral. Vascularization leads to a ground glass appearance of the cornea.  Symptoms include pain, photophobia, lacrimation and blurred vision.  Corneal opacities may cause blindness.

2) <u>Hutchinson's teeth:</u>  Pear-shaped and notched upper incisors of the second dentition develop, causing the teeth to be more widely spaced. Radiographic examination of the unerupted teeth will permit the diagnosis to be made while the primary set of teeth is still present.

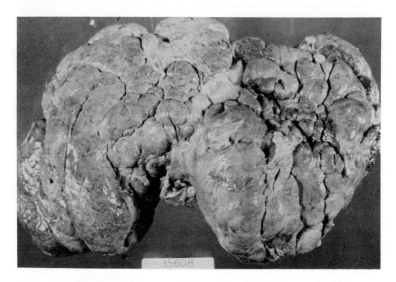

FIG. 66: Hepar lobatum. Syphilitic cirrhosis showing the liver
to be broken into many coarse lobules by depressed
scars that extend into the liver substance.

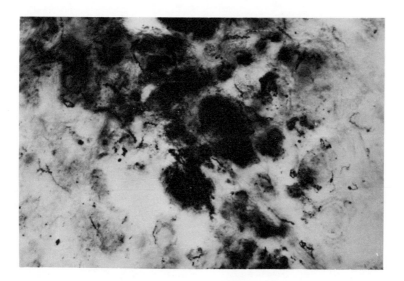

FIG. 67: Spirochetes in the liver. The organisms are seen as
small, slender spirals.

3) Mulberry or moon molars: The initial molars often show improper development of the cusps.

4) Eighth nerve deafness: Deafness is bilateral and usually has its onset at puberty, but this is sometimes delayed until middle age.

5) Neurosyphilis: Essentially the same manifestations as those seen in acquired neurosyphilis are found, although tabes dorsalis is less common and paresis is more common.

6) Bone involvement: Any part of the skeletal system may be involved, but the most characteristic stigmata are saber shins, frontal bossing, perforation of the hard palate, "tennis racket thumbs" (the fifth finger sign), thickening of the sternoclavicular joint (Higouminakis' sign) and saddle nose.

7) Cutaneous involvement: Perioral scars (Parrot's rhagades), cracks or fissures about the mouth or nose may result from syphilitic rhinitis. Gummas, as is true with acquired syphilis, may involve any portion of the skin or the organ system.

8) Cardiovascular lesions: These are rare in the tertiary stage of congenital syphilis.

9) Clutton's joints: This is a painless, hydrarthrosis of the knee joint, although occasionally the elbow or other joints may be involved.

10) Hutchinson's triad: This, composed of interstitial keratitis, eighth nerve deafness, and Clutton's joints, is the main sign of late congenital syphilis. Since these three signs do not respond to penicillin therapy, but improve or clear with corticosteroids, it seems probable that they are some kind of hypersensitivity or autoimmune reaction.

Since syphilis is the great imitator of many diseases, the clinical history and laboratory evaluation are very important. There are two types of serologic tests:

1. NON-TREPONEMAL OR REAGIN TESTS: These tests detect antibody-like substances called reagin, found in the serum of the infected patient. The first category of reaginic or reagin tests is the flocculation test - these tests

produce a reaction in which a suspension of antibody particles, when added to serum, plasma or spinal fluid containing antibodies will form small, usually visible clumps
or floccules. These tests are the VDRL (Veneral Disease
Research Laboratory), Kline, Kahn, Hinton and Mazzini.
The VDRL test is the most widely used.

Complement-fixation test involves bringing together an active component, an antigen and its antibody under proper
temperature and time conditions. These include the Kolmer
and the Wassermann test.

A third type of non-treponemal test is the agglutination test,
which was developed for rapid screening of large numbers
of patients. Two examples of such tests are the rapid plasma reagin (RPR), and the unheated serum reagin (USR) tests.

The reagin tests should be reported quantitatively; that is,
the serum or spinal fluid is diluted in geometrical progression. The titer is expressed as the highest dilution in which
the test is fully reactive. Thus, reactive 1:32 means that
a positive result was obtained in dilutions up to 1:32 and
negative reaction in dilutions of 1:64 and higher.

Most reagin tests become positive one week after the chancre appears; thus, it takes three to four weeks after a person acquires syphilis before these tests are positive. If
primary syphilis is adequately treated, the reaginic tests
revert to negative within six to twelve months, whereas in
secondary syphilis, 80% to 90% of the patients revert to
seronegativity within twelve to eighteen months. The remaining patients in secondary stage and those who reach
latency, usually have the reaginic test remain at a low titer
for the rest of their lives; they are considered serofast. All
patients should have titers on their serology, because this
is the only way one can determine if they have been rein-
fected, relapsed, or continued to remain seropositive. A
patient who has gone from 1:64 to 1:4 after treatment and
a year later returns with a titer of 1:64 would be considered to have reinfection, whereas one who goes from a titer
of 1:4 to 1:16 would be considered to remain stable. That
is, any reaginic test with more than a two-tube change is
considered significant.

Reaginic tests will be reactive in other treponematoses,
such as pinta and yaws. Acute false-positive tests may be
caused by narcotic addiction, viral infection, pregnancy,

aging, heroin addiction, and any acute bacterial infection, especially malaria. Chronic false-positive serology may be produced by lupus erythematosus or any other hyper-gammaglobulinemia disease process.

2. TREPONEMAL ANTIGEN TESTS: These tests are based on the fact that T. pallidum produces specific treponemal immobilizing antibodies in syphilitic patients, which have the specific ability to immobilize virulent Treponema pallidum in vitro. These tests make use of viable or non-viable virulent T. pallidum or chemical fractions derived from antibody to T. pallidum, or chemical fractions derived from non-virulent Reiter treponemae as antigen.

The Reiter protein complement-fixation (RPCF) test: This test uses the protein fraction of the non-pathogenic strain for T. pallidum. It is more specific than the non-treponemal tests, however, it is not as sensitive as the TPI or FTA (see below) tests. It is positive in only two-thirds to three-quarters of the patients with primary syphilis and in less than 50% of those with late syphilis.

Treponema pallidum immobilization test (TPI): Although time-consuming, expensive and technically difficult, this test is the standard by which all treponemal antigen tests are judged. It involves using a living Nichol's strain of T. pallidum from testicular syphilomas of rabbits. The treponemae are examined on the dark-field microscopy, and then the patient's serum and complement are added. If the majority of the spirochetes are immobilized, the test is positive, or if they remain mobile, the test is negative. Since the TPI test becomes reactive later in early syphilis, it is seldom used to diagnose primary syphilis, and only 50% to 75% of those with secondary syphilis will have a positive test. However, in late lues, 90% will have a positive TPI.

Fluorescent treponemal antibody-absorption (FTA-ABS) test: Here the patient's serum is overlaid on a slide on which killed T. pallidum organisms have been fixed, and fluorescein tagged anti-human globulin is applied. If anti-bodies are present, they will be bound to the treponemae, causing them to fluoresce under ultraviolet light. The reactivity may become positive before the chancre is present in primary syphilis. Eighty to ninety per cent of patients with primary syphilis will get a positive reaction. Once reactive, it usually remains active, despite adequate therpay, for years and sometimes for the duration of the patient's life. Occasionally, biologically false-positive tests may be due to hypergammaglobulinemic states, such as lupus erythematosus, but they are never more than 2+.

There have been two adaptations to the FTA-ABS test using monospecific IgM antiserum, the FTA-ABS IgM early warning test for syphilis and for congenital syphilis. Since the IgM humeral response seems to be the earliest response to T. pallidum, it was thought that this test would be either more specific or become reactive earlier. However, studies have not revealed any increased sensitivity or earlier detection of infection with the use of this test. [3] On the other hand, in congenital syphilis, since IgM does not normally cross the placenta, a positive FTA-ABS IgM in an infant indicates active syphilitic infection of the newborn. False-positive results with the FTA-ABS IgM test have been reported in normal infants, but occur in less than 10% of them. The major drawback of the FTA-ABS IgM test for neonatal congenital syphilis lies in its insensitivity, especially in the delayed onset type of congenital syphilis where its false-negative rate may exceed 35%. [4] Thus, while the FTA-ABS IgM test for congenital syphilis may be useful as a confirmatory test, it should not be used as a screening procedure.

A new development in serologic diagnosis of syphilis has been the hemagglutination test developed by Rathlev. [5] Since its introduction, there have been many modifications of this procedure. Overall, these tests are less costly and easier to perform than other treponemal tests and have the capability of automation and mass screening. They seem to be most useful in the diagnosis of ocular syphilis. With the exception of primary syphilis, where they are less sensitive, they have essentially the same sensitivity as the FTA-ABS test. The TPHA (Treponema pallidum hemagglutination) test appears to possess the characteristics of both a screening and a verification test. It is simple to perform, can be quantitative, is reproducible and has a wide spectrum of reactivity in different stages of syphilis. Its specificity and sensitivity are comparable to those of the FTA-ABS and the TPI test. These tests are of special value in the diagnosis of latent, late and congenital syphilis, but they are not suitable for the diagnosis of early congenital syphilis. They may be useful in the evaluation of problem cases. [6,7]

SPINAL FLUID EXAMINATION: Examination of the cerebrospinal fluid should be a routine procedure in almost every case
of syphilis, especially in those suspected of having late or neurosyphilis. Primary or early secondary syphilis that has been
adequately treated will not have spinal fluid involvement. However, a spinal fluid examination should be done one year after
treatment. If this is negative, then no further spinal fluid examinations are needed. A spinal fluid examination should always be performed before treating those with latent or late
syphilis. If the examination is negative, further examinations
need not be performed, because invasion of the cerebrospinal
system occurs during the first two years of infection. If the
initial cerebrospinal fluid examination is positive, then there
should be repeated examinations annually until the likelihood
of reactivation has been ruled out. In late syphilis, when the
spinal fluid is positive, repeated examinations should be performed every six months for three years after treatment. The
spinal fluid should be examined for the following:

1) Cell count: A cell count of over four lymphocytes is abnormal.

2) Total protein: In active neurosyphilis, spinal fluid protein
   is always elevated; positivity varies according to laboratory, but a protein of more than 40 mg.% is usually abnormal.

3) Non-treponemal antigen test: A positive VDRL test of CSF
   is indicative of central nervous system syphilis. False-
   positive reactions are rare. After treatment of active neurosyphilis, the cell count diminishes first, then the protein, and finally the titers for VDRL.

In obtaining cerebrospinal fluid, one should always avoid a
bloody tap, because a small amount of seropositive blood may
produce a seropositive CSF and red cells may be mistaken for
white cells, thereby causing an erroneous white count.

PATHOLOGY

The fundamental pathologic changes in syphilis are:

1) swelling and proliferation of the endothelial cells, and

2) a predominantly perivascular infiltrate composed of lym-
   phoid cells and many plasma cells

In tertiary syphilis, one usually finds, in addition, a granulomatous infiltrate of epithelioid and giant cells, often with necrosis in the center of the granulomas. [8]

## REFERENCES

1. Stokes, J. H. , Beerman, II. , Ingraham, N. R. : Mòdern
   Clinical Syphilology. W. B. Saunders, Philadelphia, p. 1,
   1945.

2. Brown, W. J. , et al: Syphilis: A synopsis. Health Service
   Publication No. 1660, January, 1968.

3. Kaufman, R. E. , Freeley, J. C. , Reynolds, G. H. : Early
   warning test for syphilis. Lancet 1:163, 1974.

4. Kaufman, R. E. , Olansky, D. C. , Weisner, P. J. : The FTA-
   ABS (IgM) test for neonatal congenital syphilis: A critical
   review. J. Am. Vener. Dis. Assoc. 1:79, 1974.

5. Rathlev, T. : Haemagglutination test utilizing antigens from
   pathogenic and apathogenic Treponema pallidum. W.H.O. ,
   B. D. T. -R. E. S. 77:65, 1965.

6. Shore, R. N. : Hemagglutination tests and related advances
   in serodiagnosis of syphilis. Arch. Dermatol. 109:854,
   1974.

7. Young, H. , Henrichsen, C. , Robertson, D. H. H. : Treponema pallidum hemagglutination test as screening procedure
   for diagnosis of syphilis. Brit. J. of Venereal Disease 550:
   341, October, 1974.

8. Lever, W. F. , Lever, G. S. : Histopathology of the Skin.
   J. B. Lippincott, Philadelphia, p. 298, 1975.

43: LYMPHOGRANULOMA VENEREUM
by A. Paul Kelly

Lymphogranuloma venereum (LGV) is caused by the Chlamydia organism Miyagawanella lymphogranulomatosis. It does not affect the animals. It is contracted through intimate sexual contact. The prevalence of LGV is unknown. The highest incidence occurs in the West Indies, Africa, South India, South America and Indonesia. In the United States, it has varied from as high as nearly 3,000 cases a year, reported in 1944, to as low as 350 during 1970.

## CLINICAL MANIFESTATIONS

The incubation period is usually three to twenty-one days, after which the primary lesion appears; sometimes it may be as long as three months.

PRIMARY LESION (Fig. 68): The primary lesion is either a solitary papule or vesicle which may rupture, leaving a small, shallow, grayish ulcer surrounded by a peripheral rim of erythema. The edge of the ulcer is well-demarcated but not indurated. It is often painless and non-tender, and therefore may go unnoticed. In women, the primary lesions occur on the vaginal wall, the cervix, the labia or within the urethra, whereas in men, and in women having genital-rectal contact, it can be found in the anal region. The primary lesions often heal within a week even without treatment. On occasion, systemic manifestations, such as fever, headache, pneumonia or myalgias and light sensitivity may be present.

LYMPHADENOPATHY: Ten to thirty days after the appearance of the primary lesion, the regional lymph nodes begin to enlarge unilaterally and occasionally, bilaterally. Initially, they are firm, discrete, movable and slightly tender; they later become inflamed and matted together, adherent to the adjacent tissue (climactic bubo). They subsequently form a single, large, tender and a fluctuant mass. Among those with lighter pigment of the skin, the area overlying the enlarged node assumes a violaceous hue, whereas in dark skin, it may appear "dusky". In more than half of the patients reaching the late stage, the enlarged nodes suppurate, leaving a tender, fluctuant mass. If this fluctuant mass goes untreated and ruptures, sinus tracts form and perforate, discharging a seropurulent exudate through the skin. When untreated, the discharge may continue for weeks

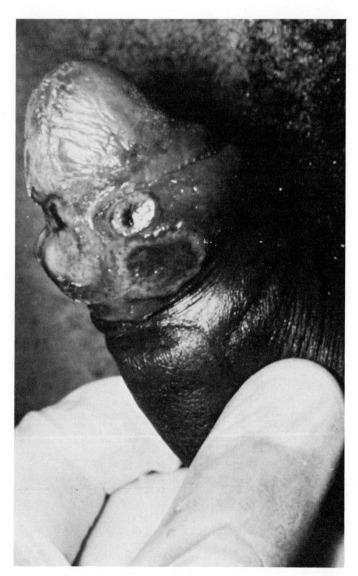

FIG. 68: Primary lesion in lymphogranuloma venereum.

or months. Eventually, it heals, leaving behind a thick, puckered and retracted scar. [1]

Systemic manifestations at this stage include fever, conjunctivitis, arthritis (especially the digits, wrists, ankles, and shoulders), stiff neck, chills, anorexia, generalized lymphadenopathy, muscle pains, epistaxis, and bronchitis. Hepatosplenomegaly has also been observed. Various hypersensitive-like skin eruptions, including scarlatiniform rash, urticaria, erythema multiforme, erythema nodosum and gyrate erythemas have been noted. These findings should be looked for in women suspected of having LGV.

When LGV begins as proctitis, mucosanguineous rectal discharge, tenesmus, constipation, diarrhea and rectal pain may be present.

TERTIARY DISEASE: The tertiary disease may present months to years after the secondary lesions. It is characterized by thick, hypertrophic or keloid-like scars over the healed inguinal sites in men, occasionally complicated by elephantiasis and/or plastic induration of the penis and the scrotum. In women, the tertiary lesions are characterized by:

1) Secondary involvement of the rectal wall, resulting in rectal stricture (the rectal syndrome)
2) Perirectal and perianal abscesses
3) Fistulous tracts around the rectum
4) Rectovaginal, vesicovaginal fistulae
5) Elephantiasis of the genitalia with chronic ulcerations and scarring (the genital syndrome or esthiomene), and
6) Lobulated polypoid and pedunculated growths around the anus (the anal syndrome).

The anorectal strictures may be missed if rectal examination is not performed.

## COMPLICATIONS

In rare cases, pneumonitis and meningoencephalitis may be found. In addition to the strictures and the elephantiasis mentioned above, Parinaud's conjunctivitis with subsequent keratitis and loss of vision has been described. Squamous cell carcinomas of the vulva, anus, rectum, bladder and penis may supervene in cases of chronic infections.

## DIAGNOSIS

LABORATORY FINDINGS: Anemia and leukopenia are late manifestations. Hepatosplenomegaly and generalized lymphadenopathy may be found in such cases. When the lymph nodes suppurate, leukocytosis of 7,000 to 20,000 cells per cu. mm. with
a slight monocytosis may occur. The sedimentation rates may
be elevated. During the disseminated stage, the organism may
be recovered from the blood, spinal fluid or from material obtained by liver and splenic biopsy. Other findings include:

1) Elevated total serum proteins with a reversal of the albumin-
globulin ratio. The increase is usually due to elevation of
the alpha-II and gamma globulin. Nearly three-quarters of
them may have elevation in the serum IgA. Changes in the
A/G ratio may be used as an indirect gauge to assess the
disease activity; therapy may restore to normal.

2) Elevated SGOT, SGPT, bilirubin and LDH activity may occur, suggesting severe liver impairment.

3) Complement-fixation test (CFT): The complement-fixation
test becomes positive within a month after the initial infection. Early in the course of the disease, in both symptomatic and asymptomatic patients, the CFT titers of 1:40
to 1:60 occur. Later stages may produce titers as high as
1:640 in most instances. A four fold or greater increase
in the titer is diagnostic. The CFT often becomes positive
before the Frei test and will remain positive as long as the
infection permits. Patients with tertiary disease, even when
thought to be adequately treated, may continue to show circulating complement-fixation antibodies. In such cases, a
gradual reduction in titers may indicate eradication of the
infection.

4) The Frei test: It has been used for years in the diagnosis
of LGV. However, its reliability is now in question because
of false-negative and false-positive reactions. The skin test
material is commercially known as Lygranum C.F. (Squibb).

It is performed by injecting 0.1 ml. of antigen and 0.1 ml.
of control material at two different sites intradermally. An
infiltrated papule measuring 5 mm. or greater appearing
within 48 to 96 hours after injection is considered positive
if the control papule measures 5 mm. or smaller. Allergy
to eggs may also produce a false-positive reaction without
adequate control. The positive reaction remains visible and

palpable for one to two weeks. In some instances, the skin reaction is so severe as to lead to ulceration; but it is un- related to the severity of the infection. The test becomes positive from one to six weeks after the onset of the ade- nitis. A negative Frei test should therefore be repeated at a later date. Repeated testing does not increase or inten- sify cutaneous sensitization. The test, once positive, will remain so for the rest of life. When LGV is adequately treated early, it may eventually become negative. The Frei test, like the CFT, is not species-specific, unless per- formed with acid-extract material. Therefore, active or inactive infections with the Bedsonia group of organisms can produce a positive test. On many occasions, the Frei test and the CFT do not correlate. In such instances, the diagnosis is based on clinical grounds alone.

5) Microimmunofluorescence test and the counterimmunoelec- trophoresis analysis: These are some of the newer tests for Chlamydia organisms.

6) Cultures: The Chlamydiae (Bedsoniae) can be cultured on yolk sac of embryonated eggs, in mouse brain and in tissue culture. There are different serotypes, of which serotypes in group A and occasionally group B have been implicated in the etiology of LGV.

The serological test was devised by Wang and Grayson. [2] Hobson [3] and Philip, et al [4] have improved and redefined the microfluorescence technique. Recently, Caldwell and Kuo [5] have described a method for making the serologic diagnosis of LGV by counterimmunoelectrophoresis, using Chlamydia trachomatis protein antigen.

## PATHOLOGY

There are no characteristic tissue changes in the lesions of lymphogranuloma venereum. Late stage disease is character- ized by central caseation necrosis, which resembles that of tuberculosis and tertiary syphilis. As the disease progresses, marked proliferation of fibrous tissue occurs in the capsule of the lymph node, and then spreads to involve the adjacent lym- phatic and soft tissue. Histopathologically, the stellate abscesses must be differentiated from those seen in "cat scratch" disease.

## DIFFERENTIAL DIAGNOSIS

LGV must be differentiated from other venereal diseases, such as granuloma inguinale, syphilis, chancroid, and from tularemia, cat scratch disease, tuberculosis, plague, and carcinoma of the genital-rectal area. However, one must remember that the presence of active lymphogranuloma venereum does not exclude the presence of coexisting venereal disease and/or squamous cell carcinoma.

## REFERENCES

1. McDonald, C. J., Kelly, A. P.: Lymphogranuloma Venereum. Current Diagnosis 4. W. B. Saunders, Philadelphia, p. 11, 1974.

2. Wang, S. P., Grayson, J. T.: Immunologic relationship between genital TRIC, lymphogranuloma venereum, and related organisms in a new microtiter indirect immunofluorescence test. Am. J. Opthalmol. 70:367, 1970.

3. Hobson, D., et al: Simplified method for diagnosis of genital and ocular infections with Chlamydia. Lancet II:555, 1974.

4. Philip, R. N., et al: Fluorescent antibody responses to chlamydial infection in patients with lymphogranuloma venereum and urethritis. J. of Immunol. 112:2126, 1974.

5. Caldwell, H. D., Kuo, C. C.: Serologic diagnosis of lymphogranuloma venereum by counterimmunoelectrophoresis with a Chlamydia trachomatis protein antigen. J. of Immunol. 118:442, 1977.

## 44: GRANULOMA INGUINALE
by A. Paul Kelly

SYNONYMS: Donovanosis, granuloma venereum, granuloma donovani, sclerosing granuloma, infective granuloma, ulcerating granuloma of the pudenda, granuloma genitoinguinale, granuloma contagiosa, chronic venereal sores, serpiginous ulcer.

Granuloma inguinale is a chronic ulcerative disease usually affecting the skin over the inguinal area and the genitalia. It is primarily a disease of the skin and mucous membranes. It is generally regarded as a venereal disease of low contagiousness. The causative organism is Calymmatobacterium granulomatis (1 to 2 x 0.6 to $0.8\mu$), a gram-negative bacillus, known as the "Donovan body". The disease is prevalent in the tropics and subtropics, especially in India, East Indies, the Caribbean, and some parts of Africa. In the United States, there was a steady decline from 2,611 cases in 1949 to 88 in 1972. [1]

### CLINICAL FEATURES

The exact incubation period is unknown, but seems to vary from three days to six months, the average being two to six weeks. It is predominantly a disease of men between 20 and 40 years old.

GENITAL LESIONS: The initial lesions usually begin as a solitary, painless, often pruritic papule, vesicle or a small nodule on the skin or mucous membranes. Nearly 90% of these lesions occur on the genitalia. Most patients refer to the initial lesion as a "lump" and, because of its insidious nature, seldom consult a physician for diagnosis or therapy at that stage. It soon sloughs, forming a shallow, well-demarcated ulcer with a base of friable granulation tissue. The entire lesion is comparable to a red, angry-looking pomegranate seed. A rolled edge of granulation tissue forms the centrifugally advancing border. Often, while one border of the ulcer is healing, the other advances. Several weeks later, satellite lesions may develop (apparently caused by auto-inoculation) and coalesce with the initial lesion.

EXTRAGENITAL LESIONS: The extragenital lesions may occur in the inguinal areas. Occasionally, they are found in the mouth and on the face, probably due to auto-inoculation or by direct oro-genital contact. These lesions may arrest spontaneously or spread slowly in the warm, moist, intertriginous areas. The final appearance of the inguinal region resembles the wing of a bird. When treatment is inadequate or delayed, they may last for months or years. They can get infected, bleed, or scar, obstructing the lymphatic system and causing elephantiasis. Superinfection with fusospirochetal organisms can produce painful, non-healing ulcers covered with foul-smelling exudate, often mistaken for anaerobic infections (Fig 69).

Papillomatous vegetative lesions may appear fungiform, cicatricial, nodular, hypertrophic and elephantiasic. They may resemble elephantiasis, although there is no lymphangiectasis. The nodular lesions in the groin can be confused with ruptured buboes of lymphogranuloma venereum. In inguinal granuloma, as its name implies, there is exuberant granulation tissue, "proud flesh". When it heals, it may leave behind keloids and hypopigmentation.

Lymphadenopathy is seldom present unless secondary infection supervenes. These larger and deeper granulomatous lesions are usually tender.

Rectovaginal and vesicovaginal fistulae may occur, but rectal strictures, as found in lymphogranuloma venereum, are rare.

The period of communicability is unknown, but may last until treated for an indefinite period. Hematogenous spread is rare but can occur to the liver, lungs, bone and other viscera.

## LABORATORY FINDINGS

DONOVAN BODY (DB): The laboratory diagnosis of granuloma inguinale depends upon the demonstration of DB in the large mononuclear cells of the granulation tissue. The organisms are gram-negative, rod-shaped bodies found either individually or in clusters. [2] They have chromatin masses at either end, giving a "closed safety pin" or bipolar appearance. Mature bacilli may have well-developed capsules. The bacteria can be intra- or extracellular. Calymmatobacteria resemble Klebsiella on Gram's stain, and capsular antigenic resemblance has been demonstrated.

1) Scrapings: The DB is best identified by scrapings of the granulation tissue from the surface of a clean lesion or, if infected, from the deeper part. They can be obtained with a curette or other sharp instrument. The tissue is then crushed between two glass slides; air-dried and stained with Giemsa's,

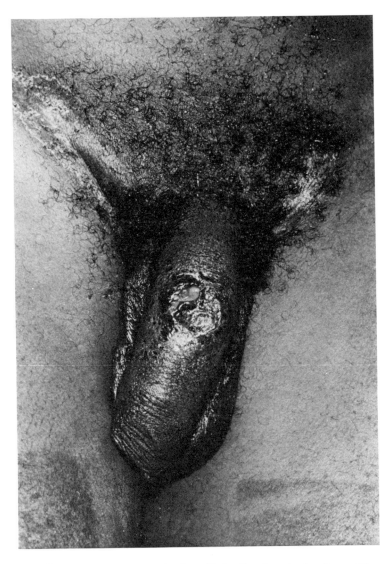

FIG. 69: Granuloma inguinale. Note the inguinal adenopathy.
The penile ulcer with purulent discharge was mistaken for fusospirochaetal infection. No anaerobes were
cultured. Both the inguinal node aspirate and the ulcer
were positive for Calymmatobacterium granulomatis,
generally known as "Donovan body".

Wright's, Warthin-Starry, or 1% pinacyanole stain. If Giemsa's stain is used, the slides should first be fixed in methyl alcohol. With Giemsa's stain, Donovan bodies appear bright red. With Wright's stain, they are purple structures surrounded by a pink-staining ovoid capsule. With the Warthin-Starry stain, the capsule stains black; and with the pinacyanole stain, they have pink capsules and blue-black inclusions. Multiple scrapings should be examined for DB before being declared negative, especially if the scraping is taken from an old lesion.

2) Biopsy: A biopsy is imperative if the scrapings are negative or when squamous cell carcinoma is suspected. Microscopically, in cases of inguinal granuloma, one may find marked acanthosis, plasma cells, histiocytes, lymphocytes, and occasionally microabscesses. The parasitized histiocyte may show DB with hematoxylin and eosin stain, but it is better appreciated with other stains discussed earlier. There are three other diseases that can show parasitized histiocytes. They are rhinoscleroma, histoplasmosis and leishmaniasis. However, of the four, only granuloma inguinale organisms are less than $2\mu$ in size.

Alternately, the tissue can be plastic-embedded, sectioned and stained by the polychrome method of Ghidoni.[3] With this method, the DB are well demonstrated in both early lesions and delayed cases where there may be tremendous secondary infection.

BACTERIAL CULTURES: The bacillus cannot be isolated from the lesions by ordinary bacterial culture methods. It can be cultivated in embryonated eggs or embryonic yolk medium. Subcultures can be propagated on meat infusion agar. A low oxidation-reduction potential is needed for optimum growth, which can be achieved by adding thioglycolate to the culture slants.

INTRADERMAL TEST: An intradermal test, using an antigen prepared from egg yolk cultures, has been used. Although a negative test may rule out granuloma inguinale, numerous false-positives can result. Serum complement-fixation test is unreliable in early lesions.

## DIFFERENTIAL DIAGNOSIS

Granuloma inguinale should be differentiated from other venereal diseases, such as syphilis, chancroid and lymphogranuloma venereum. It should also be differentiated from lupus vulgaris and squamous cell carcinoma. Inguinal granuloma may coexist with other venereal diseases. It can also be found in association with cancer.

## REFERENCES

1. Dodson, R. F. , et al: Donovanosis: A morphologic study. J. Invest. Dermatol. 62:611, 1974.

2. Kelly, A. P. , McDonald, C. J.: Granuloma Inguinale in Conn, H. F. , Conn, R. B.: Current Diagnosis 4. W.B. Saunders, Philadelphia, p. 181, 1974.

3. Ghidoni, J. J. , et al: A new multicolored staining procedure for one micron sections of epoxy embedments. Electron Microscopy Soc. Am. Proc. 29:240, 1968.

## 45: CHANCROID
### by A. Paul Kelly

Chancroid (soft chancre, ulcus molle, Ducrey's infection) is an acute, localized, infectious, ulcerative, venereal disease caused by <u>Haemophilus ducreyi</u>, a short, plump, gram-negative bacillus. It is auto-inoculable, and is characterized by tender ulcerations, usually on the genitalia, and is often accompanied by suppurative regional adenopathy. The incidence is low, but widespread, and it seems to be encountered mainly in the tropical areas of the Far East, Africa, and South America. Its incidence is lower in the United States and other temperate regions. Although chancroid is transmitted by sexual contact, it appears to be rare in females.

## CLINICAL MANIFESTATIONS

The <u>incubation period</u> is usually two to three days, but it may be as short as twelve hours (if an abrasion is present at the site of contact), or it may be as long as seven days.

Chancroid starts with a painless macule or small papule which rapidly develops into a vesicopustule with surrounding erythema. [1] This soon ruptures, forming a sharply circumscribed, small ulceration with an erythematous base. The patient usually attributes these lesions to trauma or a "hair cut" during intercourse. New lesions may form around or near the initial ulceration, or on skin in apposition to the initial lesion. Ulcers are usually painful and tender to touch, but soft and non-indurated. This finding contrasts with the hard, indurated and painless chancre of secondary syphilis. The ulcer usually enlarges rapidly, and the edges become irregular, ragged and undermined. The base is covered with a purulent, dirty yellowish or grayish exudate, and it bleeds easily with minimal manipulation. In men, the most common location for ulcers is the preputial orifice, internal surface of the prepuce, frenulum, penile shaft, and anal orifice. In women, they are found on the labia, clitoris, fourchette, vestibule, anus and cervix. Extragenital ulcers may occur on the abdomen, thighs, fingers, lips, breast and the tongue. However, they are rare.

## LYMPHADENOPATHY

Fever and pain may precede the enlargement of the inguinal nodes. Lymphadenopathy may not occur for several days after the appearance of the ulcers. Sometimes, there may be no adenopathy until after the ulcerations heal. The initial adenopathy is often unilateral and begins close to the pubic symphysis, but may be bilateral. These nodes may be later matted together and tender, but within a few days, become soft and fluctuant, forming the characteristic "chancroidal bubo". If untreated, the bubo may regress by absorption, but usually it forms an abscess which may ulcerate through the skin and form a single draining fistula, in contrast to lymphogranuloma venereum (LGV), which forms several fistulae. Also, in contrast to syphilis, chancroids may be accompanied by a cord-like lymphangitis along the shaft of the penis, originating from the primary site. The skin overlying the buboes may be erythematous, but, unlike LGV, it never becomes edematous or thickened. There is no relationship between the severity of the ulceration and inguinal lymphadenopathy; small ulcers can produce large buboes, and large ulcers may be attended with minimal lymphadenopathy, if any.

## DIAGNOSIS

SMEAR: The diagnosis is best made by the composite of the clinical features described above; however, smears taken from the base of the ulcer or from bubo aspirate will show short, gram-negative bacilli, which appear in small clusters, like "schools of fish".

Before taking a smear from an ulcer, the yellowish or grayish material should be removed from the ulcer with a tongue blade or number 15 scalpel blade; then the material for smear should be taken from the borders of the ulcer. The slide is then heat-fixed and stained with Gram's, Wright's or Unna-Pappenheim's stain. There is also the Barrit modification of the Unna-Pappenheim stain, where the organism stains bright red and the pus cells blue-green. The smears are positive in only about one-third to one-half of the cases.

For labs so equipped, Haemophilus ducreyi may be identified in smears by fluorescent antibody examination. [2]

AUTO-INOCULATION: It may be impossible to demonstrate Ducrey's bacilli when there is secondary infection. Therefore, in the past, one took advantage of the easy transmissibility of the organism by disinfecting the abdominal or arm skin, scarifying the area, then rubbing in the pus from a chancroid ulcer. The area is covered with a watch glass held in place by a bandage and, if positive, a papulopustule developed within 24 to 72 hours. Ducrey's bacilli are easily demonstrated in these lesions. If not treated, the papulopustule caused by the inoculation will soon change into a typical ulceration. However, I have neither used this method nor do I advocate it because of a high percentage of false-negative tests and due to possible medical-legal implications.

CULTURE: Culture of Haemophilus ducreyi requires special media containing defibrinated rabbit's blood, dextrose, cystine, and beef infusion agar. The temperature should be kept between 28° to 32°C. in a moist environment. A positive culture shows clear, dewdrop-like colonies in approximately 48 hours. The yield is much higher from pus obtained from an unruptured, rather than from a ruptured bubo.

SKIN TEST: One of the most reliable methods for proving the diagnosis of chancroid is Borchardt's and Hoke's method[3] of inoculating the patient's heat inactivated serum with exudate from a thoroughly cleansed ulceration. After 48 hours, parallel rows of H. ducreyi organisms are seen on Gram's stain.

BIOPSY: The chancroid ulcer presents characteristic granulomatous reaction with three zones of inflammation. A surface zone of neutrophils, fibrin, red cells and necrotic tissue; an edematous zone, with many proliferating endothelial cells and granulation tissue; and a deep zone, of a dense infiltration of plasma cells and lymphocytes.

## COMPLICATIONS

The most common complication is suppuration of inguinal lymph nodes. Prepuce lesions may lead to both phymosis and paraphymosis. Urethral fistulae may occur, as can destructive phagadenic ulceration and mutilation of the genitalia from secondary fusospirochetal infection.[4]

## CONCOMITANT DISEASES

Concurrent infection can occur with other venereal diseases. To rule these out, some physicians employ a therapeutic test or oral sulfonamide. Sulfonamides in a dose of 1 mg. four times a day are effective in treating chancroid, but will not mask the diagnosis of syphilis, i.e., do not interfere with a potentially positive VDRL or dark-field examination. Furthermore, when a chancroid ulcer is made cleaner with sulfonamide therapy, it is much easier to visualize the Treponemae by dark-field examination.

## DIFFERENTIAL DIAGNOSIS

The main differential problems have been discussed previously, but other conditions which have to be considered in addition to syphilis and LGV are herpes simplex of the genitalia, scabies, trauma, mixed drug eruptions, and Behcet's syndrome.

## REFERENCES

1. Heyman, A. , Beeson, P. B. , Sheldon, W. H. : Diagnosis of chancroid. J. A. M. A. 129:935, 1945.

2. Decon, W. E. , et al: Fluorescent antibodies for detection of the gonococcus in women. Public Health Report 75:125, 1960.

3. Borchardt, K. A. , Hoke, A. W. : Simplified laboratory technique for the diagnosis of chancroid. Arch. Dermatol. 102: 188, 1970.

4. Storey, G. : Clinical manifestations of chancroid. Brit. J. Urology 42:738, 1970.

## 46: ENDEMIC SYPHILIS (BEJEL)
### by H. Thadepalli

Endemic syphilis (bejel) is caused by <u>Treponema (T.) pallidum,</u> or an organism indistinguishable from <u>T. pallidum</u> that causes syphilis. Bejel is transmitted by body contact, by fomites and perhaps flies; it is not a venereal disease. Unlike yaws, which is found in wetland areas, bejel is found in dry lands, like the deserts of Iran and Iraq. The primary lesion begins during childhood, and is often long gone prior to the onset of the secondary lesions. The secondary and tertiary stages of endemic syphilis are similar to venereal syphilis. In bejel, mucocutaneous lesions, condylomae and gummae occur, just as in syphilis. It seems that as civilization progressed from the rural to urban style, mankind steadily traded the old lamp bejel, the non-venereal form of syphilis, for the new lamp, venereal syphilis. The areas where bejel was once endemic are now rapidly yielding place to venereal syphilis.

### DIAGNOSIS

Endemic and venereal syphilis are clinically and bacteriologically indistinguishable.

### PINTA

Pinta, in Spanish, means spotted or mottled appearance; it is caused by <u>Treponema (T.) carateum</u>, of size 12 to 18μ, which can be stained by silver impregnation or Giemsa stain. It is distributed along the banks of the rivers in the coastal areas of the tropical Americas.

### CLINICAL FEATURES

The incidence is high among children below the age of three. It is not congenitally transmitted. The <u>first stage</u> of the disease is characterized by an itchy papule associated with hyperchromic patches, often starting after seven to twenty days of incubation. The <u>second stage</u> of the disease begins nearly five to twelve months later, which is characterized by scaly lesions. The <u>third stage</u> of the disease is characterized by achromic or pigmentary spots, erythematous keratodermatitis. It is this stage of the disease that gives the mottled and painted or spotted appearance for which the disease is called "pinta". Cardiovascular manifestations are rare but have been reported from Cuba.

## DIAGNOSIS

T. carateum has not been cultivated in vitro. It can be inoculated and cultivated in vivo in champanzees.

## YAWS

Yaws is a non-venereally transmitted disease caused by Treponema (T.) pertenue. T. pertenue is of size 8 to 16 x $0.2\mu$ , non-cultivable in vitro, and has 8 to 16 spirals. Like other non-venereal treponemal infections of man, it is a fast-disappearing disease with very small foci left in tropical Africa, the tropical Americas, Sri Lanka, India, Haiti and Jamaica. The last case of yaws I saw was in 1963 in an itinerant hill tribesman, in Araku Valley in India. This disease has since disappeared and the villages vacated by yaws are now being occupied by syphilis.

## DIAGNOSIS

1) Clinical features: After an incubation period of three to four weeks, a primary lesion appears as a large ulcer (Madra buba) on the exposed parts of the body, such as legs and hands, which enlarges to the size of 1 to 7 cm. in diameter, associated with regional lymphadenopathy.

The secondary lesions are characterized by generalized furfuraceous desquamation. The satellite lesions later coalesce to form minute papules. The lesions of yaws are insensitive to pain. Over a period of a few months, the lesions in yaws clear themselves, often leaving behind depigmented spots. When yaws involve the feet, they cause coarse skin and multiple tiny nodules, resembling the bottom of the crab, and hence are called "crab yaws". The tertiary lesion of yaws is characterized by gummatous lesions of the skin and bones.

Yaws can destroy the nasal bones and hard palate and produce a ghastly caricature resembling the leonine facies of leprosy. Loss of nasal bones leads to muffled voice and is called "gangosa".

In children, ivory hard lesions may be produced, arising from both maxillae appearing like a horn in front of the face, obstructing the vision. Such a lesion is called "goundou".

Extensive peritonitis, osteitis, epiphysitis and painful nodules can occur on the long bones ("boomerang legs"). Juxta-
articular nodules of yaws may resemble syphilis.

2) Biopsy of the lesions characteristically reveals no perivascular cuffing or endarteritis, the hallmark of syphilis.

3) Rabbit inoculation: T. pertenue, when injected subcutaneously, causes no local lesion in rabbits.

4) Culture: There are no good in vitro media available.

5) Dark ground: The tissue sections may be stained by silver
impregnation technique for the spirochetes. Abrade the surface of the lesion with a blade, clean the blood with a dry
gauze; when the serum is oozing, apply a cover slip to the
surface and pick up the exudate, invert it onto a microscope slide and examine for spirochetes under dark-ground
illumination.

## DIFFERENTIAL

It is extremely difficult to differentiate yaws from syphilis unless the lesions are characteristic and present in the extragenital regions of the body.

## TREATMENT

Penicillin is the drug of choice. All skin and bone lesions show
prompt healing with a single injection of long-acting penicillin.

47:  DERMATOLOGIC DIAGNOSTIC PROCEDURES
by A.  Paul Kelly

Some of the most helpful diagnostic procedures of a cutaneous infectious process are discussed in this chapter.

## SKIN BIOPSY

A skin biopsy, for light or electron microscopic study, is an invaluable aid in the diagnosis of bullous and granulomatous infectious diseases, but less helpful for many common infectious processes.  The choice of biopsy site depends on the nature of the eruption.  If the cutaneous eruption is diffuse, then the site that can most readily bear a small scar, and at the same time display typical lesions, is the most desirable.  For acute eruptions and vesicular bullous lesions, an entire small early lesion should be removed.  For large granulomatous lesions, a specimen from the periphery of the lesion, including an edge of normal skin and the radius of the lesion should be removed.  The area to be biopsied depends on the size of the lesion and the age of the patient.

Biopsies of cutaneous lesions can be performed by either scalpel or with a dermal punch.  The scalpel requires suturing, whereas a dermal punch does not.  If no sutures are used, healing takes place rapidly, and the danger from secondary infection is minimal.  Selection of a biopsy site is of the utmost importance.  In granulomatous disease, a mature or fully developed lesion yields the most histopathologic information.  For vesicular or bullous lesions, the first stage or a newly forming stage are the most desirable to biopsy.  For histopathologic examination, a 2 to 4 mm. punch biopsy is preferable, for it permits an adequate amount of tissue for examination.  When the clinical appearance is variable, more than one biopsy is desirable.  The biopsy specimen should be deep enough to include all of the dermal tissue, as well as some of the subcutaneous fat.  Excisional biopsies require suturing. After biopsy, the specimen should be placed in a bottle containing 10% aqueous buffered formaldehyde and submitted for histopathologic examination, supplying adequate clinical details.  Additional biopsies may be taken for bacterial and fungal cultures.

A 2 to 3 mm. biopsy specimen is usually sufficient for electron microscopic studies. The specimen should be supported on a hard surface and divided vertically through the dermis and epidermis into small pieces, using a sharp single-edged razor blade. The pieces are then placed in 3% buffered glutaraldehyde solution and stored in a refrigerator at 4°C, or shipped to the laboratory, where the specimen will be dehydrated and post-fixed in osmium tetroxide. Tissue for electron microscopic examination should not be frozen because cellular detail will be destroyed.

The most common stain used in microscopic tissue examination is hematoxylin and eosin, but Giemsa stain may be used for leishmaniasis; the Fite stain is used for acid-fast bacilli; the PAS (periodic acid Schiff) stain to identify both deep and superficial fungi. Fungi may also be identified with the Gridley methenamine silver stain. It is important to advise the pathologist of the differential diagnoses under consideration so that appropriate stains may be used.

## POTASSIUM HYDROXIDE PREPARATION FOR DEMONSTRATION OF FUNGI

Potassium hydroxide (KOH) is used to identify superficial fungi on microscopic examination. The area in question should be cleaned with alcohol and then scraped with a number 15 Bard-Parker blade or the edge of a glass slide. The scrapings should then be placed on a microscopic slide. One to two drops of 20% KOH are added to the scrapings, and the debris is mixed to make a suspension. A cover slip is then applied, and the slide is gently heated over an alcohol burner until a bubble or two is noticed under the cover slip. The cover slip is then pressed tightly on the slide, and the preparation is examined microscopically with a medium power objective, with a condenser turned down to its lowest position. Fungal elements appear as linear segmented structures crossing the cell borders. Spores appear as rounded or budding lesions. India ink stain and lactol phenol blue preparations are also helpful in outlining fungal elements.

Another method for ascertaining if fungi are present in cutaneous lesions is culture. Cultures to rule out fungi are obtained by scraping the lesion with either a glass slide or a Bard-Parker blade, and placing the scrapings on some type of agar for identification. Sabouraud's medium is the culture medium that is most frequently used. Candida usually grows quickly in two to five days, whereas most superficial and deep mycoses take one to two weeks to demonstrate a characteristic growth. If there is heavy bacterial contamination, scraping should be cultured on mycosal agar (a combination of Sabouraud's medium with antibiotics) to avoid bacterial overgrowth.

Another form of diagnosis used in dermatology is the Tzanck smear. This is especially useful in Herpes simplex and Herpes zoster. The vesicles or bullae are unroofed, the base is scraped, and the scraping placed on a glass slide. The glass slide is immediately placed in 90% alcohol, and sent to cytology for a Papanicolau smear. After the slide is stained, it is examined for giant cells and inclusion bodies, which are characteristic of Herpes virus infections. Ballooning degeneration of epidermal cells is also noted in viral infections.

## DERMATOPHYTE TEST MEDIUM (DTM)

Since fungal cultures may take one to two weeks for identification, pending culture results, many physicians use a color-indicator test. In this case, the scales are planted on DTM. However, identification of the fungi is made by certain characteristic color differences in the growth patterns for pathogenic and non-pathogenic fungi.

## DARK-FIELD EXAMINATION

This test is used to detect Treponema (T.) pallidum in syphilitic lesions. T. pallidum is hard to identify by histopathological examination. A dark-field condenser that blocks out central rays of light and re-aligns the peripheral light rays to focus on the object is used for this study. The lesion is question may be cleaned and abraded with a piece of gauze to allow a serous discharge, but not vigorously enough to cause bleeding. A drop or two of the serum is placed on a glass slide; a cover slip is added, and immediately it is looked at under the dark-field scope. If the dark-field examination is positive, one will see whitish or silvery spirochetal-like organisms moving back and forth in a sort of spiral corkscrew motion. The spirochete of syphilis resembles the non-syphilitic spirochete found in the genitalia and oral mucosa; therefore, some expertise is required to distinguish the pathologic from non-pathologic spirochetes.

## WOOD'S LIGHT EXAMINATION

The Wood's lamp is helpful in the diagnosis and delineation of many fungal diseases. The instrument is a mercury lamp fitted with a filter, which emits most of its light at the 360° Angstrom wavelength. Certain fungi and bacteria have specific immuno-fluorescence, that is, tinea capitis usually has a greenish-blue fluorescence, whereas erythrasma has a coral red fluorescence.

## FLUORESCENT MICROSCOPY

This is useful in the diagnosis of superficial fungi. Not only the presence of fungi, but also their morphology, is vividly demonstrated with this method. At present it is not generally available in all laboratories.

## 48: SUPERFICIAL FUNGAL INFECTIONS
by A. Paul Kelly

The major obstacle in diagnosing superficial fungal infections is the reluctance of most physicians to perform either KOH or a proper fungal culture of the suspected lesion.

### TINEA PEDIS

Tinea pedis, known as ringworm of the feet and athlete's foot, is the most common fungus disease. Unlike most other forms, which are more prevalent in the young, tinea pedis is rare before puberty. It is estimated that over one-half of the world's adult population will have athlete's foot at some time during their lives. Most cases are caused by Trichophyton rubrum, Trichophyton mentagrophytes or Epidermophyton floccosum. Susceptibility to this disease is mainly environmental, rather than racial. The skin lesions caused by tinea are of three types: vesiculobullous, interdigital and scaling or hyperkeratotic. Under certain conditions, one variety may blend into another.

Most of the vesicular bullous lesions are caused by Trichophyton mentagrophytes. These lesions are usually extremely pruritic, and they sometimes have a violaceous hue. When the dermatosis is recurrent, it is usually associated with vesicles on the hand, known as an id or dermatophytid reaction. Trichophyton rubrum usually produces scaly hyperkeratotic or interdigital lesions. On occasion it may produce a pronounced scaling of the entire sole, giving a "moccasin" appearance. When found on the soles in the region of the toes, accompanied by scaling and vesiculation, it is usually due to Epidermophyton floccosum.

The clinical diagnosis is easily confirmed by KOH examination and/or fungus culture. With the exception of fungus elements demonstrated by special stains, no specific changes are seen on histopathological examination. Tinea pedis must be differentiated from psoriasis, contact dermatitis, dyshidrosis, secondary syphilis, erythrasma, candidiasis, pyodermias and arsenical keratosis.

The course of tinea pedis is determined by the type of infection. The rubrum type, with dry, scaly lesions, is often present for years as a chronic problem with an occasional burst of inflammatory activity; whereas the acute vesicular type, caused by mentagrophytes, may be severe and disabling, but it is self-limiting after a few weeks.

Other complications of tinea pedis include pyoderma, cellulitis, lymphangitis and lymphadenopathy.

### TINEA CORPORIS (tinea circinata, tinea glabrosa, ringworm of the body)

Tinea corporis is caused by various species of Trichophyton, Epidermophyton and Microsporum, and includes all ringworm infections involving areas other than the scalp, groin, hands, feet and beard. The disease is usually acquired from animals. Tinea corporis is found world-wide but appears to be more common in tropical and temperate climates. There is no sexual or racial predilection. Children are affected more than adults. Studies of United States troops in Vietnam by Allen and Taplin[1] show that Black infantrymen with environmental exposure identical to Whites had only slightly lower incidence of fungal skin disease, but the difference was not statistically significant. On the other hand, zoophilic Trichophyton mentagrophytes tinea corporis was a common cause of highly symptomatic lesions in Blacks and Whites, but in Blacks, these lesions appeared as areas of psoriasiform scaling and hyperpigmentation, rather than as erythematous inflammatory lesions.

The most common clinical manifestation of tinea corporis is the annular or circinate erythematous, papulosquamous lesion. The border is elevated, scaling and vesicular, while the central portion is usually clear or slightly scaly with little or no evidence of inflammation. The lesions may be single or multiple. In addition, lesions of tinea corporis may be pustular, eczematous, or granulomatous, and may be found in various configurations. Symptoms may include pruritus, burning and pain. The diagnosis of tinea corporis is most often easily made by KOH examination and/or fungus culture of the involved skin. Wood's light examination of involved hairs, particularly of the eyebrows, may reveal fluorescence when Microsporum canis and auduoini are the causative organisms. Psoriasis, pityriasis rosea, secondary syphilis, nummular eczema, seborrheic dermatitis, granuloma annulare, mycosis fungoides, tinea versicolor, lupus erythematosus and contact dermatitis are among the many dermatoses that should be included in the differential diagnosis of tinea corporis. The acute type of tinea corporis may clear spontaneously in three to six weeks, whereas the chronic plaque type may persist for months to years, even after seemingly adequate therapy.

## TINEA CAPITIS (ringworm of the scalp, "tetter", Microsporum capitis, favus)

Tinea capitis is a fungal infection of the scalp and hair caused by species of Microsporum and Trichophyton. It occurs primarily in schoolchildren and rarely in infants or adults. In children, the lesions usually clear at puberty and are more common in boys than in girls. When adults are infected, women have a higher incidence than men. There are five classical forms of tinea capitis:

1) The non-inflammatory human, or epidemic type (gray patch ringworm): This form of tinea capitis is caused by Microsporum audouini and is acquired by direct person-to-person transmission or by way of fomites (hats, hairbrushes, washcloths, combs, theater seats, etc.). Animals are seldom infected with this organism. Clinically, the non-inflammatory type presents as scaling, patchy alopecia and dull, broken hairs ("gray patch"). Most often, this type occurs on the occipital and nuchal areas, although the rest of the scalp, plus the eyebrows and eyelashes, may be involved.

2) Inflammatory or animal type: The causative organism is usually Microsporum canis, also called M. lanosum or M. felineum, although Microsporum gypseum sometimes causes similar lesions. This type is most often contracted through direct contact with an infected animal, usually a pet cat or dog. Epidemics do not occur and person-to-person transmission is rare. The initial clinical manifestation, localized scaliness of the scalp, is seldom recognized. A slightly pruritic, erythematous, papulovesicular area with hair protruding from the papules and vesicles is usually the first clinical manifestation noted by both the patient and physician. [2] Involved hairs are usually broken off 1 to 2 mm. from the scalp, but in some lesions, there is complete hair loss. The central portion of the lesion is raised and the borders are inflamed.

3) Kerion formation: This type is very inflammatory and usually consists of follicular pustules, a boggy eczematous area, or an indolent abscess. If extensive, the kerion may be accompanied by fever, lymphadenopathy, and other toxic symptoms. Also, papular, vesicular, or lichenoid eruptions may appear on the trunk or on the extremities. Kerions usually heal with scarring.

4) Black dot tinea: This type of tinea is caused by Trichophyton tonsurans and Trichophyton violaceum. It is characterized by multiple bald patches on the scalp, with hair
broken off at, or below, the surface of the scalp. The affected area ranges from minimal inflammation to kerion-
like lesions, resulting in atrophy and alopecia.

5) Favus (honeycomb ringworm): Favus is a chronic fungal
infection caused by Trichophyton schoenleini, or, at times,
Trichophyton violaceum or Microsporum gypseum. It is
usually limited to the scalp, where it produces characteristic honey-colored, cup-shaped crust (scutula) which has
a distinctive "mousy" odor. Favus may also affect the gla-
brous skin and the nails (brittle, thickened and encrusted
under the free margins). It is frequent among the Bantu in
South Africa, where it is called witkop (white head).

Diagnosis of tinea capitis may be accomplished by any of the
following methods:

   a) Wood's lamp fluorescence
   b) KOH examination
   c) Biopsy, or
   d) Fungus culture

The following mnemonic is helpful in remembering which fungi
show fluorescence with Wood's lamp examination: "sometimes
all canis do not fluoresce" = Trichophyton schoenleini, Microsporum auduoini, Microsporum canis, Microsporum distortum,
Trichophyton nanum  and Trichophyton ferrugineum.

When taking material for KOH preparation of fungus culture, it
is imperative that hairs from the involved areas be examined,
because scales may not contain fungi. Highly inflammatory lesions, such as a kerion, seldom have fluorescent hairs. For
this reason, Wood's light examination is neither useful in inflammatory Microsporum gypseum infections, nor is the light
of significant value in Trichophyton infections with tonsurans
and violaceum, which have a non-distinct fluorescence. Trichophyton tonsurans infections, however, sometimes have a distinct silvery fluorescence, especially in infections having the
circular pattern of alopecia. Occasionally, extensive T. tonsurans infections are seen in which most of the scalp lights up.

### TINEA CRURIS

SYNONYMS: Ringworm of the groin, tinea inguinalis, dhobie
itch, "jockey itch", eczema marginatum. Tinea cruris is an

acute or chronic infection of the groin and its environs caused by various species of Trichophyton and Epidermophyton. Trichophyton rubrum, Trichophyton mentagrophytes and Epidermophyton floccosum are the most common offenders. Tinea cruris is common in males but rare in females. The infection is more prevalent and symptomatic in an environment of increased temperature and high humidity. Tight-fitting underwear, tight-fitting pants, athletic supporters, jockey shorts and other clothing which prevent the evaporation of perspiration in the groin predispose to the infection. It is aggravated by obesity, sweating and friction. Transmission may take place secondary to sharing towels, athletic equipment or undergarments.

Lesions caused by Epidermophyton floccosum are characterized by well-marginated, elevated, papular, scaly patches or plaques of dermatitis with active, sometimes vesicular, borders. There is only minimal central flaring. Usually, the lesions are bilateral, and they may be either symmetrical or asymmetrical. A brownish discoloration often overlies the inflammatory lesions. It may extend distally to the thighs, posteriorly to the sacrum and anteriorly to the scrotum and suprapubic area. With Trichophyton rubrum, the clinical manifestations are similar, but contiguous spread is greater, often extending proximally to the waist or distally to the knees, and is usually more symmetrical (Fig. 70). Trichophyton mentagrophytes infection is more inflammatory and characterized by scaly, circinate plaque, with pustules in the hair-bearing areas.

As with other superficial fungal infections, the clinical diagnosis can be confirmed by KOH examination, fungus culture, or by histological examination of PAS stain sections. Even though the clinical characteristics may be classical, the following must be ruled out: erythrasma, seborrheic dermatitis, candidiasis, psoriasis, lichen simplex chronicus, pemphigus vegetans and contact dermatitis.

## TINEA MANUS

Tinea manus refers to dermatophyte infection on the volar surface of the hand and fingers, whereas fungal infection on the dorsum of the hand is considered to be a form of tinea corporis. It occurs less frequently than tinea pedis and usually develops only when the feet are infected. Most often, two feet and one hand are involved in the infection, but why one hand is spared is not known.

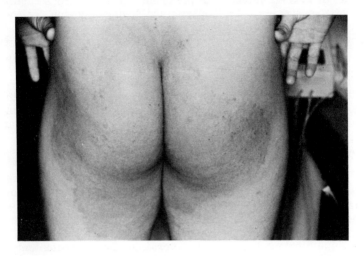

FIG. 70: Tinea cruris lesion.

Dry, scaly, erythematous plaques are the most common lesions, although eczematous, vesicular and interdigital lesions are sometimes noticed. Trichophyton rubrum is the most common etiologic agent. The diagnostic procedures and differential diagnosis are essentially the same as those in tinea pedis.

When there is ringworm infection of either the hands or feet, there is often concomitant fungal involvement of the nails (onychomycosis), tinea unguium. Onychomycosis usually starts at the tip of the nail and involves the subungual area. The nail gradually becomes yellowish, brittle and separated from the nail bed by subungual keratosis.

TINEA BARBAE (ringworm of the beard, tinea sycosis, barber's itch, trichophytosis barbae)

Tinea barbae is an uncommon dermatophytosis of the beard and mustache which is mainly derived from animal sources. Trichophyton verrucosum, Trichophyton mentagrophytes, Trichophyton violaceum and Trichophyton schoenleini are the most common etiologic agents. The disease only affects adult males and occurs most often in farmers and cattle raisers. There are two clinical types of tinea barbae: deep, nodular and suppurative; and superficial crusted areas of folliculitis with partial alopecia. The deep type develops slowly and produces boggy indurated kerion-like areas with abscesses. Purulent material can be expressed from these lesions by application of minimal pressure. Hairs in the involved areas are either loose or absent. The superficial type produces a mild, pustular-like folliculitis at the border with broken-off hairs. There is scaling of the central area. Clinically, they resemble the lesions of tinea corporis. In both types, the lesions are usually limited to one side of the face, and the upper lip is seldom involved.

Direct KOH examination of the hair and/or hair culture is all that is necessary to confirm the clinical diagnosis. Histopathological sections of the involved area usually demonstrate fungi in the hair follicles, with the exception of infections due to Trichophyton tonsurans or Trichophyton verrucosum, where the fungi may not be present. If present in the hair follicles, the fungi are found both within and around the hair. They descend in the hair to a line about 30 millimicrons distal to the zone of keratinization. There are no fungi in the dermis, but a perifollicular infiltrate of varying intensity may be present. The infiltrate is most pronounced in those with kerion-like lesions. If special stains, like PAS and Hotchkiss-McManus are used, the fungi may be seen not only on and in the hair, but also occasionally on the epidermal surface.

Clinically, sycosis vulgaris, a bacterial folliculitis, is the most difficult disease to rule out. Contact dermatitis, seborrheic dermatitis, iododerma, bromoderma, pustular syphilis, anthrax and actinomycosis must also be differentiated from tinea barbae. In Black patients, tinea barbae is often mistaken for pseudofolliculitis barbae.

TINEA VERSICOLOR (pityriasis versicolor, tinea flava, liver spots, chromophytosis, dermatomycosis, furfuracea, hodi-potsy, achromia parasitica)

CLINICAL MANIFESTATIONS: Lesions of tinea versicolor usually occur on the upper back, posterior neck and upper chest (Fig. 71). The face, areas below the waist, or skin distal to the elbow are seldom involved, although the dermatosis may occasionally be generalized, especially in those on high doses of corticosteroids, those who are malnourished and those with a type of genetic susceptibility, which seems to favor both the spread and occurrence of tinea versicolor. The clinical hallmark is a furfuraceous (dandruff-like) scale which is easily scraped off with a fingernail. These scales cover hypo- or hyperpigmented annular macules, patches, papules or plaques. Sometimes, the lesions become confluent and form

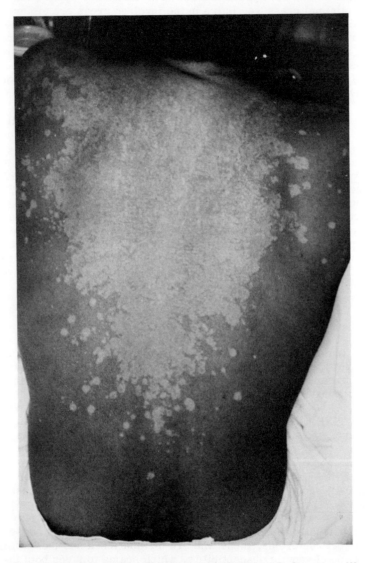

FIG. 71: Tinea versicolor. Note the depigmented areas with centrifugal distribution. For some reason, it is common among heroin addicts, and also among washermen (dhobie) who wash in the rivers of South India. It is one of the most common fungal infections of the skin all over the world.

large circinate patches. Except for occasional pruritus, the patient's concern for tinea versicolor is primarily cosmetic.

Viewed under Wood's light, a yellowish or light green fluorescence is noted in the involved area. This procedure is extremely important because it enables the physician to determine pretherapy involvement and allows for the evaluation of therapeutic success.

Diagnosis is best made by scraping several lesions with a number 15 scalpel blade or glass slide and placing the scrapings on a glass slide, adding 1 or 2 drops of 10% potassium hydroxide solution and placing a cover slip on top of the scrapings and solution. The slide should not be heated because the causative organisms of tinea versicolor, Pityrosporon obiculare or Malassezia furfur, are very fragile and often fragment with the slightest increase in temperature. The KOH preparation, when viewed under the microscope, usually shows either small, curved, segmented hyphae and/or spores in grape-like clusters; the so-called spaghetti and meatball picture.

If the lesions of tinea versicolor are divided into two types, one of which forms large scaly plaques (patchy type), and the other which consists of small, pea-sized papules or macules (disseminated type), a different microscopic picture will be seen in each. There are more spores seen in the disseminated type, and this type also has hyphae that tend to be arranged radially around the pilosebaceous orifice. Those situated near the orifice are positioned vertically to it. Hyphal elements are also frequently seen in areas adjacent to the lesion, where numerous spores are also found. In the center of the lesion, the hyphae are predominant and there are relatively few spores.

Along with the conventional scraping and KOH examination, the ease of diagnosis and the frequency of positive diagnosis can often be increased by the use of an ink blue stain. The ink is of value in that it is stable in KOH. Other methods include stripping the stratum corneum with scotch tape and staining the strippings with methylene blue. In those people who are very fastidious and bathe often, hyphae and spores are often difficult to demonstrate with microscopic examination.

The scales from tinea versicolor do not grow on Sabouraud's agar or on most standard mycologic agar unless the agar is covered with olive oil or some type of similar lipid. However, since the diagnosis is so readily made by way of KOH examination, culture diagnosis is not important.

Histologic sections from tinea versicolor lesions demonstrate hyphae and yeast-like cells in the superficial stratum corneum, often in great abundance. There is usually minimal inflammatory change.

Electron microscopic examination of tinea versicolor lesions demonstrates melanocytes, which produce less melanin, and structurally altered melanosomes, in addition to exhibiting cytologic changes, ranging from mitochondrial vacuolization to frank degeneration. Epidermal reaction to the infection is manifested by mitotic Langerhan's cells.

The differential diagnosis of tinea versicolor may include vitiligo, tinea corporis, pityriasis rosea, post-inflammatory hypo- or hyperpigmentation, secondary syphilis, seborrheic dermatitis, pinta, erythrasma, erythema dyschromicum perstans and pityriasis alba.

## REFERENCES

1. Allen, A. M. , Taplin, D. : Epidemic Trichophyton mentagrophytes infections in servicemen: Source of infection, role of environment, host factors, and susceptibility. J. A. M. A. 226:864, 1973.

2. McDonald, C. J. , Kelly, A. P. : Dermatology and Venereology. In Textbook of Black-Related Diseases by Williams, R. A. McGraw-Hill, New York, p. 526, 1975.

49: IMPETIGO

by A. Paul Kelly

## DEFINITION (Impetigo contagiosa)

Impetigo is an acute superficial contagious bacterial infection of the skin caused by group A beta-hemolytic Streptococci and/ or coagulase-positive Staphylococcus aureus. The incidence varies according to season, being higher in the latter part of the summer. Crowded living conditions, warm climate, malnutrition, poor hygiene and limited access to medical care contribute to an increased incidence of impetigo. Also, insect bites and other skin injuries are additional factors favoring impetigo.

In 60% to 70% of impetigo cases, both Streptococcus and Staphylococcus are cultured, but in 20% to 30% of the cases, streptococci alone and in 10%, staphylococci alone are cultured. Streptococci are cultured more often from the early stage lesions than staphylococci. [1]

In impetigo, staphylococcal organisms are thought to occur as secondary, rather than primary, invaders. Phage type 71 organisms produce a bacteriocidin which is cidal to group A beta-hemolytic streptococci. Thus, it is probable that in late infections, the bacteriocidin kills off all the streptococci, thereby leaving only the invading staphylococci as the resident bacterial population.

## CLINICAL MANIFESTATIONS

Impetigo begins as a small erythematous macule and rapidly develops into a fragile vesicopustule with erythematous borders. These break and exude an oozing sticky fluid. In this stage, the lesions are usually very pruritic. Soon, golden-yellow (honey-colored) "stuck on" crust begins to form and enlarge peripherally, as well as spreading by satellite lesions. The initial lesions may appear anywhere on the body, but are usually adjacent to the nose or mouth and lower extremities. Depending on the severity, the lesions may spread widely or remain localized. Regional adenopathy and fever may be present. The high contagiousness of impetigo is borne out by the frequency with which members of the same family are afflicted.

## COMPLICATIONS

Streptococcal impetigo may be antecedent to acute glomerulonephritis. Hall has reported a 1% incidence of glomerulonephritis in 150 consecutive cases of impetigo,[2] whereas as many as one-third of the patients with acute glomerulonephritis give a recent history of impetigo. Younger children have the highest incidence. The renal complications may be silent and discovered on routine urinalysis or may result in a stormy course with edema and hematuria. Respiratory tract infections with streptococci also occur in many patients with impetigo, but seldom result in clinical complications.

## DIAGNOSIS

All patients suspected of having impetigo should have a Gram's stain of a vesiculopustular lesion, culture for typing and sensitivity, a complete blood count and a urinalysis to rule out glomerulonephritis. The presence of honey-colored "stuck on" crusts, pustular lesions and family members or playmates with similar lesions suggests the diagnosis of impetigo.

## LABORATORY FINDINGS

Gram-positive organisms are found in the untreated lesions. Streptococci reveal ovoid gram-positive cocci in chain configuration; whereas gram-stained staphylococcal organisms usually demonstrate densely-stained gram-positive cocci, some within leukocytes or surrounded by them. They are usually single, but may occur in pairs or chains. Most of the staphylococci in impetigo are phage group II, type 71, whereas streptococci usually fall into one of four T antigen agglutination patterns: T49; 8/25/Imp. 19; 5/27/44; and 3/13/B 3264. In contrast to those streptococci isolated from respiratory infections, these serotypes are difficult to type with M antiserum.

ASO titers are seldom elevated in impetigo, except with secondary glomerulonephritis, where either the ASO or anti-DNAase B titers are elevated 100% of the time.[3]

## HISTOPATHOLOGY

Subcorneal neutrophil-filled vesicles or bullae characterize impetigo. They are unilocular, and may have a few acantholytic cells. The epidermis underlying the vesicles and bullae is usually spongiotic with exocytosis of neutrophils. The papillary dermis is infiltrated with neutrophils and lymphocytes. After the bullae rupture, a crust composed of serous exudate, in which are enmeshed bacteria and polymorphs, covers the remaining epidermis. It is impossible to differentiate impetigo histologically from subcorneal pustular dermatosis.

## DIFFERENTIAL DIAGNOSIS

Clinically, subcorneal pustular dermatosis may resemble impetigo. However, absence of bacteria on Gram's stain, and lack of improvement with antibiotic therapy, excludes this diagnosis. The Tzanck smear may be used for the rapid diagnosis of herpes simplex or varicella, which may initially resemble impetigo. The satellite pustules of Candida albicans may resemble impetigo, but potassium hydroxide (KOH) examination will demonstrate spores and/or mycelia in such lesions.

## REFERENCES

1.  Dajani, A. S. , et al: Natural history of impetigo. II. Etiologic agents and bacterial interactions. J. Clin. Invest. 51: 2863, 1972.

2.  Hall, W. D. , et al: Studies in children with impetigo. Bacteriology, serology and incidence of glomerulonephritis. Am. J. Dis. Child. 125:800, 1973.

3.  Dillon, H. C. , Reeves, M. S. , Maxted, W. R. : Acute glomerulonephritis following skin infections due to streptococci of M-type 2. Lancet 1:554, 1968.

## 50: ERYSIPELAS
### by A. Paul Kelly

Erysipelas is an acute cellulitis of the skin and subcutaneous tissue caused by group A beta-hemolytic Streptococcus infection, although an occasional case can be caused by pneumococci. [1] Rarely, Staphylococcus aureus may be the cause. It occurs most frequently in infants, very young children, elderly patients and in those with debilitating illnesses. It also seems to be more frequent with chronic lymphedema and/or chronic cutaneous ulcerations.

## CLINICAL MANIFESTATIONS

Erysipelas is characterized by a localized plaque with erythema, warmth, edema, and a raised indurated border. The plaque spreads peripherally for several days at a rate of approximately 2 to 10 cm. per day. [2] The maximum size is usually 12 cm., although occasionally, lesions attain a diameter of up to 25 and 30 cm. A characteristic feature is the palpable advancing edge of the enlarging plaque. In severe cases, vesicles and bullae may be seen as well as local gangrene.

The face is the most frequent area of involvement, except in infants, where periumbilical lesions may predominate. Any cutaneous site may be involved. The hairline seems to act as a barrier against expansion of facial lesions, although sometimes, in severe cases, the whole scalp may be tender, painful, boggy and edematous.

The lesion usually reaches maximum size in less than a week, but takes several weeks to resolve. During resolution, desquamation is common, and when the scalp is involved, permanent hair loss may occur.

## SYSTEMIC MANIFESTATIONS

Prodromal symptoms include malaise, chills, fever, headache, vomiting and sometimes joint pain. These symptoms usually get worse during the first few days of the cutaneous lesion. During healing, the lesion often changes colors from the initial erythematous lesion to a violaceous color, to brown, and then yellowish-brown before fading completely. These color changes usually take place over a two- to three-week period.

## LABORATORY FINDINGS

The white count is usually 20,000/cu. mm. or more with 80% to 95% polymorphonuclear leukocytes being present. The ASO titer becomes elevated in seven to ten days. Superficial skin cultures are negative, whereas aspirates from the advancing border usually yield streptococci. Streptococci may also be found in the pharynx and in the blood.

## HISTOPATHOLOGY

The dermis shows marked edema and dilatation of the lymphatics and capillaries. There is a diffuse infiltrate, composed chiefly of neutrophils. The infiltrate extends throughout the dermis and occasionally into the subcutaneous fat. It shows a loose arrangement around the dilated blood and lymph vessels. If sections are stained with Giemsa's or Gram's stain, streptococci may be found distributed in the tissue. In chronic recurrent erysipelas, there may be marked fibrosis of the vesicles of the dermis and subcutaneous tissues, even leading to complete or partial occlusion.

## COMPLICATIONS

1) Recurrent infections may lead to lymphedema; a special type of lymphedema of the lips is called macrochilia
2) Vascular accidents due to emboli
3) Acute glomerulonephritis
4) Serous inflammation of the meninges, leading to convulsions
5) Septicemia

## ERYSIPELOID

Erysipeloid is a disorder which clinically resembles erysipelas, but is due to a gram-positive organism, Erysipelothrix suis (swine erysipelas). The lesions are usually found on the hands and are generally acquired as an occupational hazard among persons who handle fish and meat. It starts as a violaceous area which slowly spreads to involve most of the hand. The general symptoms are mild as compared with erysipelas, and the disease is self-limiting.

## DIFFERENTIAL DIAGNOSIS

Lymphangitis, cellulitis and phlebitis are usually less erythematous and do not have a sharp advancing border.

## REFERENCES

1. Milstein, P. , Gleckman, R. : Pneumococcic erysipelas: A unique case in an adult.   Am. J. Med. 59:293, 1975.

2. Fekety, F.R.:  Erysipelas in Clinical Dermatology by Demis, D.J., Dobson, H.L., McGuire, J. (Eds.) Harper and Row, Hagerstown, p. 1, 1976.

## 51: ERYTHRASMA
### by A. Paul Kelly

### DEFINITION

Erythrasma is a superficial bacterial infection of the skin caused by Corynebacterium minutissimum. It is more common in persons living in tropical and subtropical climates, although many people in temperate climates have asymptomatic intertriginous erythrasma infection. The incidence is higher in diabetics and in those with debilitating diseases.

### CLINICAL MANIFESTATIONS

Clinically, erythrasma is characterized by well-demarcated, dry, brownish, finely scaling patches of the intertriginous areas, especially the axillae, groin and toe webs. The patches are irregular in shape, and enlarge slowly. They are asymptomatic. Occasionally, a widespread plaque form may appear. Middle-aged Black females in tropical climates, diabetics, and those with debilitating diseases have a greater propensity for the generalized type.

### DIAGNOSIS

Diagnosis is best made with a Wood's lamp. The involved areas show a coral red fluorescence due to the presence of porphyrins in the stratum corneum. These porphyrins are produced by the bacteria. It is best to examine the patients in a dark room with a Wood's lamp of more than 75-watt output, because some of the lamps with smaller wattage may fail to demonstrate fluorescence in the presence of erythrasma. Also, fluorescence is diminished after bathing, especially if anti-bacterial soaps are used.

### LABORATORY FINDINGS

Gram's stain examination of fluorescent scales contains gram-positive filaments, single diphtheroid forms, and chains of diphtheroids. The filaments predominate in dry areas, while diphtheroid forms predominate in moist areas.

C. minutissimum can be cultured on several culture media, especially 6% sheep blood and brain heart infusion agar.[1] However, the slightest raised, smooth, grayish-white colony cannot be differentiated from other species of Corynebacterium.

A better method for obtaining positive cultures is to use homogenates from porphyrin-fluorescent scales on Sarkany's modification of tissue culture medium. [2] After 24- and 48-hour periods, the plates are exposed to Wood's light to elicit the presence of red fluorescent porphyrins. The presence of phenol red in the medium may interfere with the red fluorescence, particularly in the presence of acid-producing organisms, such as staphylococci.

The characteristics which differentiate C. minutissimum from other skin Corynebacteria are as follows: it does not have a strong odor, does not require oleate for growth, is non-hemolytic and it produces abundant diffusable porphyrins on Sarkany's modified 199 medium. [3]

## HISTOPATHOLOGY

Epidermal change consists of hypergranulosis, vacuolated cells in the granular layer and upper stratum malpighii, mild acanthosis, focal atrophy and, on occasion, elongated rete ridges. There may be mild to moderate inflammation of the papillary dermis. Incontinence of pigment may be present. The organisms appear blue in sections stained with hematoxylin and eosin.

## HISTOCHEMISTRY

Rod-like organisms, filaments and coccoid forms of C. minutissimum are demonstrated by various stains. In most colonies, rod-like organisms and coccoid forms predominate. Filaments, when present, are more common at the periphery of the bacterial colonies. The organisms are PAS-positive and diastase-resistant.

## DIFFERENTIAL DIAGNOSIS

Erythrasma must be differentiated from superficial fungal infections, candidiasis, contact dermatitis, intertrigo and seborrheic dermatitis. Generalized erythrasma may clinically resemble tinea versicolor and psoriasis. In Blacks, discoid lupus erythematosus must be ruled out.

## REFERENCES

1. Sarkany, I., Taplin, D., Blank, H.: The etiology and treatment of erythrasma. J. Invest. Dermatol. 37:382, 1961.

2. Sarkany, I., Taplin, D., Blank, H.: Organisms causing erythrasma. Lancet 2:304, 1962.

3. Sarkany, I., Taplin, D., Blank, H.: Incidence and bacteriology of erythrasma. Arch. Derm. 85:578, 1967.

## 52: ECTHYMA
### by A. Paul Kelly

## DEFINITION

Ecthyma is a deep ulcerative type of impetigo. It is considered a "dirt" disease caused by minute trauma in poor hygienic conditions.

## CLINICAL MANIFESTATIONS

Skin lesions begin as pustules or bullae which rapidly break down, enlarge, and become ulcerated (Fig. 72). The ulcers are covered with a dark brown to yellow adherent crust which, when removed, yields a saucer-shaped purulent ulcer with raised erythematous borders. Lesions range from 1 to 3 cm. in diameter and in most cases, only a few are present. They usually occur on the legs, although the arms and buttocks may be involved. The lesions usually heal in a few weeks, with slight scarring and hyperpigmentation of the border. New lesions may develop by auto-inoculation. Subjective symptoms are those of any other infectious process: heat, pain and adenopathy.

## COMPLICATIONS

In temperate climates, there seems to be a direct relationship between the incidence of ecthymatous skin lesions and acute glomerulonephritis.

## DIAGNOSIS

Ecthyma is essentially impetigo with deeper lesions and ulcerations. It is caused by beta-hemolytic streptococci, although coagulase-positive staphylococci may invade the lesions secondarily. Thus, in addition to the characteristic clinical findings, diagnosis is best made by Gram's stain and bacterial culture.

## HISTOPATHOLOGY

The histopathologic picture of ecthyma is not specific. Usually, one observes an ulcer with neutrophils in the serous exudate, as well as in the dermis.

## DIFFERENTIAL DIAGNOSIS

Lesions of impetigo are smaller and do not ulcerate. Folliculitis, cutaneous diphtheria and erythema induratum must also be ruled out.

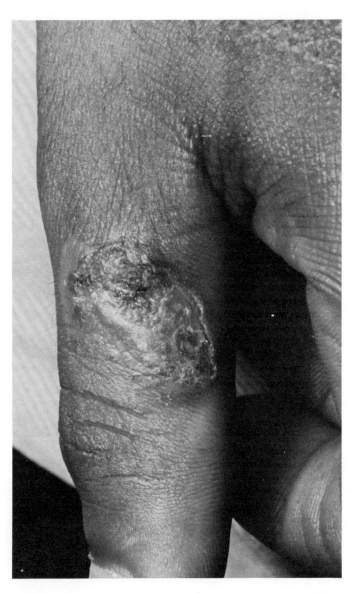

FIG. 72: A secondary lesion of ecthyma showing a piled-up crust overlying a superficial erosion.

## 53: SYCOSIS VULGARIS
by A. Paul Kelly

Sycosis vulgaris (SV) is a chronic bacterial folliculitis and peri-
folliculitis of the beard area (sycosis barbae). It is found almost exclusively in men, especially those with a heavy beard
or mustache. It seems to occur more often in warm, humid
environments. SV may develop any time after puberty, but is
usually found in the fourth and fifth decades. It is seen more
commonly in persons with curly or kinky hair, particularly
in Blacks. Shaving and ingrown hairs seem to precipitate the
process.

The primary lesion is an edematous, follicular papule or pustule pierced by a hair. These lesions tend to coalesce and form
edematous plaques covered by a yellowish crust. The plaque
may involve a single facial area or may involve the entire
bearded region. The initial papules and pustules are often preceded by eczematous patches that itch and burn. Chronic lesions show thinning of the hairs and cicatrization of the involved
areas. Marginal blepharitis with conjunctivitis is common in
severe cases. Occasionally, a destructive process develops,
which spreads peripherally and leaves permanent scars. This
process resembles lupus erythematosus and has been given the
name, "sycosis lupoides". Other variants of SV include folliculitis decalvans, which affects the scalp, causing permanent
hair loss, and acne keloidalis, which involves the posterior
neck and lower scalp, forming keloidal-like lesions.

The etiologic agent is usually Staphylococcus aureus, although
other bacteria have been isolated in the lesions.

The diagnosis is usually made from the direct smears of the
pustular lesions and by bacterial cultures.

Histologic sections usually show a follicular and perifollicular
inflammatory infiltrate, penetrating deeply into the dermis.
Lymphocytes, plasma cells and histiocytes are also present.
The sebaceous glands are usually destroyed while the hair follicles remain intact. Perifollicular scarring may take place,
but alopecia is seldom permanent.

SV must be differentiated from fungus infections of the beard
area, lupus vulgaris, lupus erythematosus and contact dermatitis of the face.

### 54: SCABIES
by A. Paul Kelly

Scabies is known by the colloquial names "the itch", "gale", "milbee", and "psora". It is caused by the itch mite, Sarcoptes scabiei var. hominis. It is world-wide in distribution and seems to be present as an epidemic about every 25 years.

## ACARUS SCABIEI

Scabies results from the itch mite, Sarcoptes scabiei, which thrives on human skin. The adult female is less than one-third of a millimeter long, while its consort is one-third to one-half its size. The mite has eight legs, with suckers on the two anterior pads and long bristle-like projections on the posterior pads. The cephalothorax lies between the first and second set of anterior legs. Besides size, the male differs from the female by having suckers on one pair of its hind legs. Mellanby,[1] who wrote the classic work on scabies, states that the female may burrow beneath the surface layer in 20 minutes. It begins to lay eggs within 48 hours after mating and continues to lay eggs throughout its life (four to five weeks). Three to four eggs are deposited daily and if the rate of burrowing is slow, about 1 mm. daily, the eggs are found close together; whereas those mites that move faster (5 mm. per day), lay their eggs farther apart. The eggs hatch after three or four days and, due to the normal process of skin desquamation and turnover, the newly-hatched larvae are on or near the skin surface. The female larva burrows beneath the surface and remains there for three to four days, giving rise to the first nymph stage. A second and third moult takes place, giving rise to the eight-legged adult non-fertilized female. The male goes through a similar cycle, except that after the first stage nymph, it emerges as an adult male, there being no second stage.[2] The male Acarus dies after mating and the female starts to burrow; thus, continuing the life cycle.

## CLINICAL MANIFESTATIONS

The cardinal symptom of scabies is itching, which is worse at night. The lesions are symmetrical and the sites of predilection are the genitalia, the flexor surface of the wrist, the umbilicus, the extensor surface of the elbows and knees, interdigital folds, anterior axillary folds, areola of the nipples, and buttocks. The face and back are seldom involved. In infants and young children, the eruption may be generalized, especially involving the palms and soles.

The pathognomonic lesion is the burrow, which usually appears as a grayish-black wavy or zigzag line, ranging from 1 to 20 cm. long. At the point of entry, there may be a few tiny scales. At the closed end, the resting place of the female, there is usually an erythematous or flesh-colored papule or vesicle. Vesicles seem to occur more often in children than in adults. Unfortunately, due to the extreme pruritus, these patients scratch their skin so much that the vesicles and burrows are obliterated.

Another characteristic feature is pinpoint excoriations at the site of previous papules and vesicles. In infants and children, there are characteristic pustules on the palms and soles. Crusts may be present and due to secondary infection from excoriations, there may be lesions of impetigo, ecthyma, and eczema. Urticarial lesions, thought to be secondary to an allergy to the mite, may also be present.

The generalized pruritus in scabies begins after the patient develops a hypersensitivity to the mite and its products. This usually takes from four to six weeks after the initial invasion of the mite, during which time the female may have laid 30 or more eggs. Thus, patients are able to transmit the disease long before any symptoms are manifested.

## NORWEGIAN SCABIES

This is a somewhat rare variant of scabies, where there are hundreds to thousands of mites on a given patient at any one time. This is in contradistinction to regular scabies, where there are usually only six to twelve mites present at any one time in a lesion, even though there may be generalized pruritus and dermatitis. Norwegian scabies is characterized clinically by thick, psoriasiform-like scales and crusts. There is marked palmar and subungual hyperkeratosis. Even the face and scalp are covered with thick, crusted, exudative lesions. Despite the overwhelming parasitic infestation and hyperkeratosis, there is minimal or no pruritus.

## PERSISTENT NODULES

One complication which is being seen with increased frequency in patients with scabies is the presence of pruritic nodular lesions, which persist after the patient receives adequate therapy. These nodules are usually skin-colored, brownish-red, or brown. They are firm, non-tender, appear infiltrated, discrete and measure 1 to 2 cm. in diameter. The mite, larvae and eggs cannot be recovered in these lesions.

## DIAGNOSIS

The diagnosis of scabies is confirmed by scraping the base of a burrow, vesicle or papule with a scalpel blade. The scraping, along with the top of the vesicle or burrow, is placed on a glass slide. A drop or two of water is applied and a cover slip placed on the debris. Water or oil is used rather than potassium hydroxide (KOH), because the keratin of the mite could be digested by the KOH. More than one scraping should be done, and one should look for the mite, larvae, eggs, feces, or any combination of the four.

## HISTOPATHOLOGY

The histologic findings in papular, vesicular, nodular and Norwegian variants of scabies have in common a superficial and deep perivascular mixed inflammatory cell infiltrate of lymphocytes, histiocytes, and numerous eosinophils. [3] A spongiotic vesicle occurs in the papulovesicular type, a dense cellular infiltrate in the nodular type, and a hyperkeratotic psoriasiform dermatitis in the Norwegian type. Eggs, larvae and adult mites are abundant in the cornified layer of Norwegian scabies and are practically never found in biopsy specimens from lesions of nodular scabies, and are discovered only episodically in papulovesicular lesions. [3]

## DIFFERENTIAL DIAGNOSIS

The differential diagnosis of scabies should include pediculosis corporis, pediculosis pubis, impetigo contagiosa, ecthyma, animal scabies, chickenpox, seborrheic dermatitis and atopic eczema.

## REFERENCES

1. Mellanby, K.: Scabies. Oxford University Press, Fairlawn, p. 9, 1943.

2. Heilesen, V.: Studies on Acarus scabiei and scabies. Acta. Dermato. Vener. 26:Supplement 14; 1, 1946.

3. Fernandez, N., Torres, A., Ackerman, V.A.: Pathologic findings in human scabies. Arch. Dermatol. 113:320, 1977.

55: LEPROSY (HANSEN'S DISEASE)
by A. Paul Kelly

Leprosy is a chronic, systemic, infectious, granulomatous disease of man caused by the acid-fast bacillus, Mycobacterium (M.) leprae. The lepra bacillus has a special predilection for the skin, mucous membranes of the upper respiratory tract, peripheral nerves, eyes and bones. Leprosy covers a myriad of clinical, histopathological and immunologic manifestations, the hallmarks of which are cutaneous anesthesia, hypopigmentation and cutaneous infiltrates. It is worldwide in distribution, with the highest incidence being in equatorial Africa, southern Asia and Central America. It is estimated that more than 20 million people have leprosy. There are less than 3,000 registered cases in the United States, and most of them are found in Hawaii, southern California, southeast Texas and Louisiana. There is no special racial predilection, although among Caucasians and Orientals, leprosy seems to progress to a more serious disseminated form.

## CLINICAL MANIFESTATIONS

In lepromatous leprosy, males outnumber females by two to one, whereas in tuberculoid leprosy, it is one to one. The incubation, or "latent" period of leprosy, varies, ranging from less than one year to ten or fifteen years, averaging three to five years. Leprosy is insidious in onset. Early signs and symptoms are usually absent. In most patients, the first clinical manifestation of leprosy is a single skin lesion, or sometimes, a few skin lesions. This is usually the first and the only symptom, but in a few, the disease progresses. The first lesion(s) may be located anywhere on the body. The lesions on the trunk are just as common as those on the extremities or the head. There is a considerable degree of regional variation in the distribution. The lesions on the nose, ear, elbow, knee and/or foot are almost always more than one in number. In a majority of the patients, the initial lesion is followed by one or more successive crops of new lesions. These new lesions, unlike the first lesion, occur mainly on the periphery. [1]

There are four characteristic forms of leprosy (Table 27), [3] for immunologic purposes, the five-numbered Ridley and Jopling [2] system is used. The four characteristic forms of leprosy are:

1) Lepromatous leprosy (LL)    3) Indeterminate leprosy
2) Tuberculoid leprosy (TL)    4) Borderline or dimorphous leprosy (BD)

TABLE 27: CHARACTERISTICS OF THE VARIOUS FORMS OF LEPROSY

| FEATURES | TUBERCULOID LEPROSY | BORDERLINE LEPROSY | INDETERMINATE LEPROSY | LEPROMATOUS LEPROSY |
|---|---|---|---|---|
| No. of lesions | One or very few | More than a few | Single or several | Many |
| Anesthesia | Always in lesions | Varying in degree | Equivocal | A later event |
| Biopsy | Langhans' giant cells; epithelioid cells; scattered lymphocytes; partial or complete destruction of dermal nerve bundles | Elements of both tuberculoid and lepromatous change; perineural as well as intraneural inflammation | Mild, non-specific, chronic infiltrate with perineural localization; occasional acid-fast rod within nerves | Heavily populated with macrophages filled with acid-fast bacilli; many organisms in nerve bundles but very little inflammation |
| Bacteriologic examination | Usually negative | Usually positive | Usually negative | Strongly positive |
| Lepromin reaction | Always positive | Variable, depending on which end of spectrum | Usually negative | Always negative |
| Neuritis | Limited to one or two nerves; usually acute | Often widespread; both acute and chronic | None to mild | Slow and insidious; symmetric and often widespread |

| Other Involvements | None | None or infrequent | None | Mucous membranes of mouth and upper respiratory tract; cornea, sclera, iris and ciliary body; small bones of hands and feet; testicles; liver |
|---|---|---|---|---|
| Prognosis | Excellent except for permanent nerve damage | Guarded; nerve damage usually severe; may become lepromatous | Usually good | Poor to fairly good depending on stage at which treatment was started |
| Usual length of treatment | 1 to 2 years | 3 to 5 years | 2 to 3 years | 5 to 10 years; maintenance dose for life |
| Reactional sites | Localized to skin and nerves | Limited to skin and nerves, but often with widespread involvement | None | Involving skin, nerves, mucous membranes of upper respiratory tract and eyes |
| Systemic dissemination of M. leprae | None | Questionable | None | Throughout reticuloendothelial system |

## TUBERCULOID LEPROSY (TL)

TL usually runs a chronic course, has a positive lepromin reaction, and bacilli are scanty in the skin. It is considered only
minimally infectious. TL is limited to the skin and peripheral
nerves  Cutaneous lesions consist of pale macules and patches,
plus raised annular plaques. The skin lesions of TL are of three
types:

1) Tuberculoid minor lesions: These are usually hypopigmented
with sharply defined erythematous borders and varying degrees of infiltration, which may be uniform or present a
characteristic "cobblestone" appearance. They are seldom
symmetrical. The superficial cutaneous nerves supplying
an area of skin are often enlarged and tender. Tactile and
pain sensations may be lost in these lesions.

2) Tuberculoid major lesions: As the name suggests, these
lesions are much larger than minor lesions. Also, the major
types of lesions tend to invade the so-called "immune" areas;
the axillae, eyelids, vertebral column and palms.

3) Macular lesions: Maculo-anesthetic, or pre-tuberculoid lesions, have the following characteristics:

   a) They are large and hypopigmented.
   b) They are few in number, from one to four lesions.
   c) They are asymmetrical in distribution on the outer as-
      pect of the extremities, face, scapulae and buttocks.
   d) The edges are well-demarcated.
   e) There is a slight loss of tactile and heat sensation.

METHACHOLINE TEST: All tuberculoid lesions are characteristically anhidrotic. This is of special importance in the
diagnosis of tuberculoid leprosy and the basis of the methacholine sweat test. It consists of injecting 0.1 ml. of 1% solution
of methacholine chloride (mecholyl) intradermally. Two injections are made; one in the involved skin and the other on uninvolved normal skin for control, after the skin has been painted
with a solution of 2% iodine and 10% castor oil in absolute alcohol. Powdered starch is then dusted over the two test areas.
If there is sweating, the starch granules will turn blue by the
interaction of iodine and sweat. However, in tuberculoid leprosy, the denervated cutaneous sweat glands will be inactive,
thus producing no bluish discoloration.

## BORDERLINE (dimorphous) TYPE

This type ranges from the tuberculoid-like lesions on one end of the spectrum to the lepromatous lesions on the other. At one extreme, it may present as erythematous, edematous, dome-shaped nodules resembling lepromatous leprosy. On the other hand, it may start as a solitary lesion, usually on the outer aspect of the thigh, in the region of the anterior femoral cutaneous nerve. The early lesion is hypopigmented, with ill-defined anesthetic borders. The surface is rough and frequently scaly. There may be central healing. Within a few months, multiple macules form all over the body symmetrically distributed, like lepromatous leprosy. When these lesions are small, the skin sensation may be intact. Lepromin reaction is variable in dimorphous leprosy.

## INDETERMINATE TYPE

Indeterminate leprosy represents those cases in which the lesions have not yet shown definite characteristics to enable one to determine whether further development will be toward lepromatous, tuberculoid or dimorphous leprosy. The indeterminate lesion is usually single, although sometimes three or four lesions are present. The most common sites are the forehead, buttocks, scapulae, face and outer aspects of the extremities. Confirmation of the diagnosis of leprosy in these lesions is usually based on the presence of anesthesia and/or the presence of bacilli. The bacilli are few in number and the lepromin test is usually negative.

## LEPROMATOUS LEPROSY

This is the most severe form of leprosy, thought to be due to anergy; therefore, the lepromin reaction is consistently negative. A variety of cutaneous lesions may be seen in the form of nodules, papules, macules and diffuse infiltrations, and they contain abundant numbers of lepra bacilli. They often reveal Virchow cells (macrophages with numerous bacilli and fat droplets) on biopsy. LL is highly infectious and runs a rapid course.

1) Macular lesions are usually multiple, small and symmetrical with indistinct borders with intact skin sensation and sweating. In sunlight, they appear like erythematous spots.

2) Diffuse lepromatous lesions result from a gradual coalescing of numerous vague macular lesions. The skin appears shiny. The eyebrows often show thinning and loss of hair, especially

the lateral third. It should be remembered that loss of eyebrows is a late sign of LL.

3) Grossly infiltrated lesions are merely a more advanced stage of macular LL. These lesions are often erythematous, hyperpigmented and soft with borders that merge into the surrounding skin.

4) Nodular lesions result from the progressive deterioration of the macular, diffuse or infiltrated forms of LL. In the early stage, nodules appear initially on the ears (Fig. 73). Later, they may appear anywhere on the body (Figs. 74,75) and are most often seen on the buttocks and the elbows, fingers and over the joints. Sometimes, they may be on the genitals. Initially, most of the nodules are not adherent to the skin, but later they become fixed and may ulcerate.

## NEURITIC PICTURE

In all forms of leprosy, in addition to visible cutaneous lesions, there may be signs of general neural involvement. Residual neural signs may remain long after the bacilli have disappeared from the skin. Types of neural involvement are:

1) Lepromatous; slow and symmetrical
2) Tuberculoid (maculo-anesthetic); severe, sudden, asymmetrical
3) Borderline; more rapid than lepromatous and symmetrical
4) Indeterminate; slight, symmetrical

In primary neuritic leprosy, or "pure neural" leprosy, as opposed to secondary, the disease manifests itself by neural signs without any clinical evidence of cutaneous involvement. This is a rather uncommon variety of leprosy. Anesthesia is usually confined to the extremities, especially to the areas enervated by the peroneal and ulnar nerves. Often, a "glove and stocking" type of anesthesia is present. Loss of sensation usually disappears in the following order.

1) Thermal
2) Tactile
3) Pain
4) Pressure

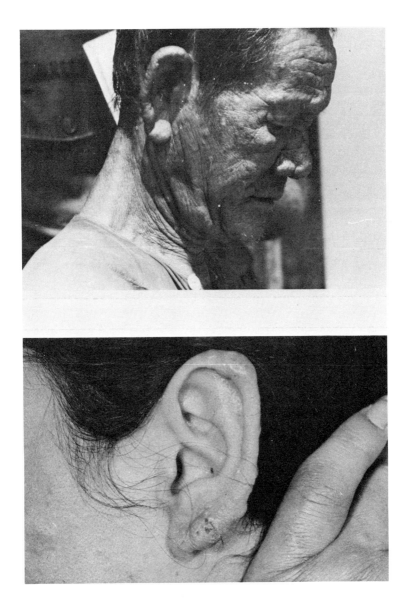

FIG. 73: Typical leonine facies in lepromatous leprosy in a
Vietnamese. Note the nodular lesions on the ears of
a Mexican male. This patient also developed Lucio
phenomenon (see Fig. 74).

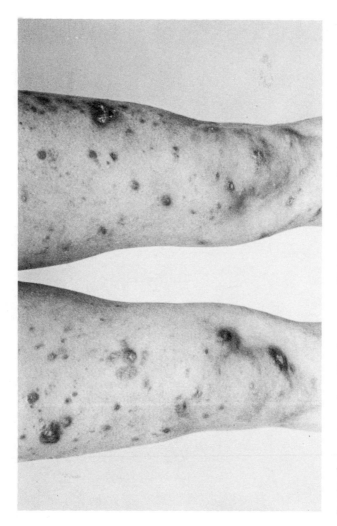

FIG. 74: Lucio phenomenon in a Mexican man. Note the polygonal lesions with ulcerations. Acid-fast bacilli, in clumps, were demonstrated in these lesions (see Fig. 75).

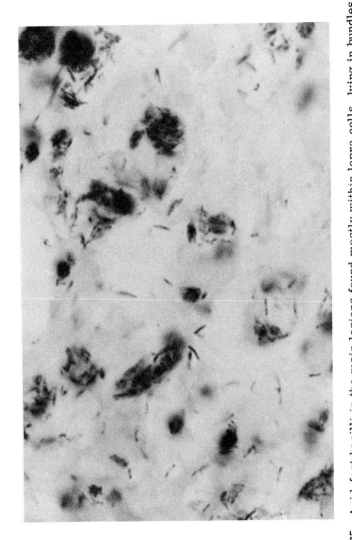

FIG. 75: Acid-fast bacilli in the main lesions found mostly within lepra cells, lying in bundles or in degenerated clumps, called "globi".

Nerve enlargement of the ulnar, peroneal and great auricular nerve is often present with or without pain and tenderness. In time, the nerve will become fibrous and smaller. Deep pain, joint sense and deep reflexes remain intact. The skin changes that result from anesthesia are xerosis, ulceration and trauma. Ulnar and common peroneal nerve involvement may lead to the characteristic wasting of the muscles supplied by these nerves, resulting in "claw hand" (Fig. 76) and "foot drop" respectively.

EYE INVOLVEMENT: This can be due to direct invasion of the cornea and conjunctiva by M. leprae or secondary to facial nerve palsy. Ocular involvement can occur in more than 50% of patients with lepromatous leprosy. The structures most commonly involved are the sclera, cornea, iris and ciliary body. Both a deep and superficial keratitis may result from corneal involvement. Occasionally, nodules may develop on the cornea. Iridocyclitis can be acute, causing glaucoma, or slow, with remissions and exacerbations. Chronic iritis may lead to anterior and posterior synechiae, leading to a fixed, irregular pupil. Facial nerve palsy may lead to ptosis and exposure keratitis. As in congenital syphilis, leprosy can cause interstitial keratitis. The optic nerve and tear duct involvement are rare.

MUCOUS MEMBRANE INVOLVEMENT OF THE NASAL MUCOSA: This may cause ulceration and destruction of the nasal cartilage and bone, resulting in a complete collapse of the nose. There may be laryngeal obstruction, causing a husky voice, or, if severe, it may rarely cause complete obstruction, requiring tracheotomy.

BONE AND JOINT LESIONS: Bone changes are uncommon. Most of the bone and joint changes result from sensory nerve loss. The terminal phalanges and other short bones of the hands and feet may become pointed and spindle-shaped, and fracture at multiple sites (see Fig. 76).

KIDNEY INVOLVEMENT: Non-specific nephrosclerosis with uremia, hypertension, anemia and pyelonephritis is often a terminal event. Lepromatous leprosy may be complicated by amyloidosis of the kidneys with progressive deterioration. In the U.S., secondary amyloidosis occurs in 45% to 55% of the cases of lepromatous leprosy. [4] It is also more common in patients with erythema nodosum leprosum. [5]

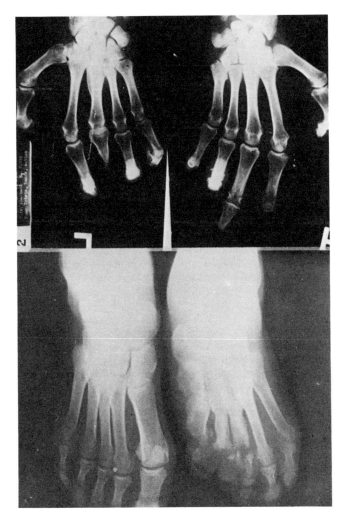

FIG. 76: Neurotrophic arthritis in leprosy. Note the deformed and auto-amputated fingers and toes, osteomyelitis of the metatarsal bones with multiple fractures. (Courtesy of John Campbell, M. D. , Charles R. Drew Postgraduate Medical School, Los Angeles, California)

GONADS: The testicles are often involved in lepromatous leprosy (LL), whereas the ovaries are usually spared. Severe orchitis can occur in exacerbations of LL.[6] More commonly, it is a chronic and indolent orchitis.[7] In end stages, they atrophy.[8]

OTHER AREAS OF INVOLVEMENT: Gynecomastia can occur in approximately 10% of those with LL during the third decade of life. Besides the cosmetic and psychological stress, local tenderness is often distressing.

## REACTIONAL STATES

The clinical course of leprosy is often punctuated by periods of crisis. Three major reactional syndromes can occur:

1) Erythema nodosum: This is a common complication of LL, especially among those who are being treated with sulfones. The patient develops numerous inflamed, subcutaneous nodules which usually subside within a week. These nodules may be accompanied by fever. An acute exudative polyarthritis may occur in association with erythema nodosum.[9] The clinical manifestations simulate the acute phase of rheumatoid arthritis, affecting the metacarpal, phalangeal and proximal interphalangeal joints. Unlike rheumatoid arthritis, the arthritic symptoms are temporary and resolve with resolution of the erythema nodosum. The rheumatoid factor may be positive in 60% of these patients. However, the biopsy of the synovial membrane in leprosy may show fibrin with numerous polymorphs, but in rheumatoid arthritis, plasma cell infiltration predominates.

2) Lucio phenomenon: The "Lucio" phenomenon, or erythema necroticans, is a rare but distinctive cutaneous eruption that characterizes the lepra reaction seen in patients with diffuse LL. It seems to occur mainly in patients from Mexico, Costa Rica and other Central American countries. It occurs only in patients who have had diffuse nodular LL for at least two to four years. Lucio described the lesions as having a typical evolution. At first, the lesion is pinkish, ill-defined and painful, and sometimes it is infiltrated. A few days later, it shows a darker center which does not disappear under pressure. The center soon approaches the surface and there forms a small, thin, dry, brown scale which eventually drops off, leaving behind an insignificant scar. In larger lesions, there is a dark, flaccid blister which bursts, leaving a deep ulceration with jagged edges,

surrounded by an inflammatory zone. In addition, particularly on the legs, there are secondary pyodermas associated with chronic cellulitis, which complicate the condition.

Since the original description, such changes as icthiotic skin, loss of body hair, telangiectasis of the face and trunk, destructive rhinitis, arthralgia, asthma, hepatosplenomegaly and fever have been added to this reaction. These lesions heal within two to four weeks. Patients develop a severe local reaction to the lepromin skin test (the Medina-Ramirez reaction), which occurs in four to six hours and persists for several days.

3) <u>Lepra reaction</u>: The lepra reaction in lepromatous leprosy may present the following picture:

    (a) Extension of old lesions and development of new ones in the skin and subcutaneous tissues
    (b) Erythema nodosum
    (c) Erythema multiforme
    (d) Erysipeloid reactions
    (e) Chills, fever, malaise, myalgia and arthralgia
    (f) Neuritis
    (g) Iritis
    (h) Visceral manifestations, including nephrosis, nephritis, orchitis, pleuritis and hepatosplenomegaly

The reaction varies from mild to severe and may last from a few days to even years.

LEPROMIN TEST: The lepromin test consists of intradermal injection of 0.1 cc. of lepromin (an autoclaved suspension of human tissue, containing lepra bacilli obtained from lepromatous nodules). There are two classes of lepromin reactions:

1) <u>The Fernandez reaction</u> is similar to the Mantoux tuberculosis test. The erythema and induration develop within 24 to 48 hours and may remain for 3 to 5 days. Histologically, it is due to an outpouring of fluid from the vessels, causing induration and infiltration with lymphocytes around the capillaries and perineural sheets of the dermis.

2) <u>The Mitsuda reaction</u> is a delayed reaction. It often appears within three weeks and is of greatest intensity at the fourth week, usually subsiding later within a week or two. Histologically, this nodule consists of epithelioid follicles and lymphocytes, frequently accompanied by giant cells. There

may be necrosis and abscess formation at the center of the reaction. The test is of value to distinguish between various types of leprosy. It is invariably positive in the tuberculoid type and negative in lepromatous and borderline leprosy. It may be either positive or negative in indeterminate leprosy. This test has no diagnostic value. False-positive reactions can occur in patients who have no leprosy. If positive in the absence of any cutaneous lesions, it shows a good resistance to the disease.

TISSUE SMEAR: This is most often taken from an ear lesion. The lesion in question should be cleaned thoroughly with alcohol, dried, and then the lesion should be squeezed between the thumb and forefinger, maintaining pressure while making an incision to 2 to 3 mm. depth in the skin. The sides of the incision should be scraped with a scalpel blade to obtain serous and cellular material, which is then spread on a slide, air dried and placed in 10% formalin for 15 minutes. The slide is then rinsed in tap water and stained with Ziehl-Neelsen carbolfuchsin for 20 minutes. Then rinse with acid alcohol for one minute, followed by tap water rinsing. The slide is then counterstained in alkaline methylene blue for 10 seconds, rinsed in tap water, air-dried and placed under the microscope for examination for acid-fast bacilli.

HISTAMINE TEST: This test is used to diagnose cutaneous nerve damage. A drop of 1:1,000 solution of histamine diphosphate is put on the skin of the involved area and another on clinically normal area. A pinprick is then made through each drop. A wheal will form at each punctured site, but the red flair will not develop around the wheal in an area of cutaneous nerve damage.

NASAL SMEARS: These may be positive in 37% of early LL; 86% of established LL and in 100% of patients with late lepromatous leprosy. [10] If the patient has a nasal discharge, it is less traumatic to wipe the interior of the nasal cavity with a cotton applicator, smear this material on a glass slide and stain with the Ziehl-Neelsen technique. The only situations in which a nasal smear could have an advantage over a specimen of nasal discharge are:

1) in very temporary places, where an early nasal infection has not yet reached the stage of producing an exudate

2) in patients whose nasal discharge has dried up as a result of chemotherapy

3) in late stages, when gross secondary infection, especially atrophic rhinitis, prevents one from obtaining an adequate specimen

BIOPSY OF THE SCROTAL SAC: Scrotal sac biopsies demonstrate a higher yield of bacteria than routine skin and nasal smears, or even multiple skin smears or skin biopsies. [11] Since the larger nerves are in the deeper part of the dartos muscle, a piece of the muscle should be obtained with a sharp scissors. Acid-fast bacilli may be searched for by histologic methods. Alternatively, the material can be homogenated and the homogenate then placed on a glass slide and stained for acid-fast bacilli.

HUMORAL RESPONSES IN LEPROSY: Increased levels of IgG, IgA and IgM are frequently found in lepromatous leprosy and erythema nodosum leprosum. Also, deficient T-cell function has been postulated as being present in leprosy. A marked elevation in the frequency of HL-A14 antigen has been reported in leprosy patients. [12] Phenotype HL-A14 was found in 35% of the 17 Mitsuda-negative patients and in only 7% of the 13 Mitsuda-positive patients.

SPOT TEST FOR IDENTIFICATION OF MYCOBACTERIUM LEPRAE: One of the newest diagnostic tests for leprosy, and one which has great promise for rapid screening, is the dopa method. [13] It consists of incubating a drop of bacterial suspension with a drop of dopa (3,4-dihydroxyphenylalanine) solution on a slide. Those bacterial suspensions with M. leprae present will oxidize dopa to melanin.

HISTOPATHOLOGY

Tuberculoid leprosy: This type consists of epithelioid cells and a few lepra bacilli. Lepra bacilli may be altogether absent. The advancing borders of the lesion may at times demonstrate a few bacilli.

Lepromatous leprosy: Histiocytes, lymphocytes, plasma cells, and fibroblasts predominate in the lesion. The so-called "lepra" or Virchow cells, large foamy histiocytes, are often present. Unlike TL, large numbers of bacilli are found lying freely and in globi within the lepra cells.

Borderline leprosy: This shows a wide range of histologic change, depending on which type of leprosy it resembles.

Indeterminate leprosy: A non-specific inflammatory infiltrate containing lymphocytes, histiocytes and plasma cells is arranged around cutaneous appendages. Only a few, if any, lepra bacilli are seen.

## DIFFERENTIAL DIAGNOSIS

1) Hypopigmented macular lesions: Rule out vitiligo, tinea versicolor, pinta, pityriasis alba, morphea, post-inflammatory hypopigmentation and lichen sclerosus et atrophicus.

2) Nodular lesions: Mycosis fungoides, leishmaniasis, neurofibromatosis, Kaposi's sarcoma, sarcoidosis, xanthomatosis, and lymphoma cutis must be ruled out.

3) Annular plaque-type lesions: Rule out tinea corporis, granuloma annulare, sarcoid and lichen planus.

4) Papular lesions: Rule out sarcoidosis, syphilis, leishmaniasis and disseminated granuloma annulare.

## REFERENCES

1. Leiker, D. L.: On the mode of transmission of Mycobacterium leprae. Leprosy Review 48:12, 1977.

2. Ridley, D. S., Jopling, W. H.: Classification of leprosy according to immunity: A five-group system. Int. J. Lepr. 34:255, 1966.

3. Gass, H., Arnold, H. L.: Clinical Dermatology, in Demis, Crounse, Dobson, McGuire. Clinical Dermatology. Harper & Row, Hagerstown, p. 16, 1976.

4. Grabstald, H., Swan, L. L.: Genital urinary lesions in leprosy. J.A.M.A. 149:1287, 1952.

5. Shuttleworth, J. S., Ross, S. R.: Secondary amyloidosis in leprosy. Ann. Int. Med. 45:23, 1956.

6. Tilak, C. T.: Acute epididymo-orchitis in lepromatous leprosy. Lepr. Rev. 39:31, 1968.

7. Davey, T. F., Schenk, R. R.: Endocrines in Leprosy, in Cochrane, R. G., Davey, T. F. Leprosy in Theory and Practice, 2nd Edition. Williams and Wilkins, Baltimore, p. 190, 1964.

8. Pardo-Castello, V.: Leprosy, in Gradwohl, R. D. Clinical Tropical Medicine. C. V. Mosby, St. Louis, p. 586, 1951.

9. Karat, S., et al: Acute exudative arthritis in leprosy. Brit. Med. J. 3:770, 1967.

10. Cochrane, R. G.: A Practical Textbook of Leprosy. Oxford University Press, London, p. 104, 1947.

11. Pandya, N. J., Antia, N. H.: The value of scrotal biopsy in leprosy. Lepr. Rev. 45:145, 1974.

12. Kreisler, M. et al: HL-A antigens in leprosy. Tissue Antigens 4:197, 1974.

13. Prabkhakaran, K.: A rapid identification test for Mycobacterium leprae. Int. J. Lepr. 41:121, 1973.

### 56: CUTANEOUS MANIFESTATIONS OF INFECTIOUS DISEASES
by A. Paul Kelly

Non-specific cutaneous manifestations may occur in infectious diseases (Table 28). They may be due to the organism itself, secondary invasion by another pathogen, elaboration of a toxin, a hypersensitivity reaction, or may be secondary to medication used for therapy of the infectious disease.

## ERYTHEMA MULTIFORME

Erythema multiforme (EM) represents a cutaneous reaction pattern, the hallmark of which is the so-called "iris" or "target" lesion. The cutaneous lesions may be macular, papular, nodular, petechial or bullous. The areas most often involved are the dorsum of the hands and feet, palms, soles, and mucous membranes. Lesions usually occur suddenly, without prodromal symptoms. The process is usually self-limiting and may be recurrent. It affects people of all ages, although the severe forms occur more often in adolescents and young adults. There is no sexual or racial predilection. There seems to be an increased incidence during the spring and fall, and the lesions usually last from two to four weeks. No antibodies are demonstrable from the serum, and the skin does not show any identifiable immunofluorescent pattern. The etiology is extremely varied.

Bacterial infections, e.g., pneumonia, tuberculosis, typhoid fever; viral infections, e.g., measles, mumps, Asian flu, vaccinations, hypersensitivity to herpes simplex virus; mycotic infections, e.g., histoplasmosis, coccidioidomycosis, blastomycosis; protozoan infections and drugs, especially penicillin and sulfonamide (used to treat infectious diseases) seem to cause EM. There is a severe form of erythema multiforme which involves the skin and mucous membranes, known as Stevens-Johnson syndrome. It is manifested by vesicular bullous lesions located anywhere on the body. The bullae are tense and surrounded by an erythematous base. Vesicular bullous lesions may be present on the mucous membranes of the mouth, conjunctivae, vagina, nares, urethral meatus, and anorectal junction. Only the scalp seems to be spared.

Skin lesions are usually preceded by general malaise and fever. Bullous lesions of the mucous membrane are rapidly denuded and present as bleeding, crusted ulcerations. Five to

## TABLE 28: OUTLINE OF CUTANEOUS LESIONS IN CERTAIN COMMON INFECTIOUS DISEASES

I. MACULES OR PAPULES

A. Viral exanthems
B. Secondary syphilis
C. Rickettsial diseases
D. Scarlet fever

II. PUSTULES

A. Impetigo
B. Ecthyma
C. Sycosis vulgaris
D. Follicular impetigo of Bockhart

III. VESICLES OR BULLAE

A. Rickettsial pox
B. Varicella
C. Herpes simplex
D. Herpes zoster
E. Variola
F. Enteroviruses, such as ECHO and Coxsackie

IV. PLAQUES AND PAPULES

A. Tinea versicolor
B. Tinea corporis
C. Syphilis
D. Erythrasma
E. Tinea cruris

V. GRANULOMATOUS PLAQUES

A. Tuberculosis
B. Leprosy
C. Leishmaniasis
D. Deep mycoses, such as blastomycosis and coccidioidomycosis

VI. ULCERS

A. Syphilis
B. Chancroid
C. Granuloma inguinale
D. Tertiary syphilis
E. Lymphogranuloma venereum
F. Ecthyma
G. Deep mycosis

VII. PURPURA

A. Meningococcemia
B. Gonococcemia
C. Pseudomonas bacteremia
D. Subacute bacterial endocarditis
E. Rocky Mountain spotted fever
F. Epidemic typhus
G. Enterovirus infections

fifteen per cent of such cases may be fatal. The rest of the patients usually experience cutaneous clearing in one to four weeks, but mucous membrane lesions may persist for months.

Several other bullous disorders must be ruled out. They are: bullous pemphigoid, pemphigus vulgaris, dermatitis herpetiformis, toxic epidermal necrolysis, Reiter's disease and bullous contact or photo-contact dermatitis.

## TOXIC EPIDERMAL NECROLYSIS

Toxic epidermal necrolysis (TEN, Lyell's syndrome, epidermal lysis necroticans) is a toxic necrotic erythema of the skin, so severe that the skin looks as if it has been scalded. There seem to be two basic forms - the childhood and adult types. In children, the separation of the epidermis is in the upper Malpighian layer, whereas in adults, it is characterized by separation of skin above the basal layer. The onset is abrupt with the eruption of clear urticarial plaques and bullae. The bullae are usually surrounded by a ring of erythema. These lesions may be accompanied by malaise, fatigue, diarrhea and fever. In contradistinction to the bullae of erythema multiforme, the bullae for TEN are flaccid and often peel off in large sheets, leaving a wall of erythematous base, making the skin look as if it had been scalded.

In children, the process is usually caused by Staphylococcus aureus, group 2, phage type 71, and in adults it may be caused by the antibiotics used to treat infectious diseases; the most common offenders being penicillin, sulfonamides, tetracycline, dapsone and nitrofurantoin.

## PRURITUS

Pruritus, or itching, is the most common cutaneous symptom of almost all cutaneous diseases, yet the most perplexing. It is a subjective or sensory problem of unknown etiology which produces an objective or motor response (scratch, rub, prick, etc. ). Cutaneous lesions may be present, but there is often an essential pruritus, itching without skin lesions. The itch sensation may be present on the entire skin, conjunctivae and genital mucosa, whereas it is absent from the oral mucosa. There is tremendous individual variation in the occurrence, location, duration, severity and response to therapy.

Many infectious diseases may be accompanied by pruritus, but most often, instead of the disease causing the pruritus, the precipitating factor is usually the medication used to treat the disease, the most frequent offenders being penicillin and sulfonamides.

## ERYTHEMA ANNULARE CENTRIFUGUM

Erythema annulare centrifugum (EAC) presents as either a solitary papule or multiple small erythematous papules which enlarge slowly or rapidly (six to eight centimeters in two weeks). They enlarge by clearing centrally and advancing peripherally, thereby creating lesions of various morphologies: annular, cercinate, gyrate, serpiginous or festooned. The outer advancing edge is an abruptly sloping, erythematous, cord-like wheal. The inner edge is gradually sloping and is usually the site of post-inflammatory response. Its color may range from yellow to dark brown, and there is occasionally slight scaling and rarely crusting. Sometimes tiny vesicles are found on the border. EAC lesions may vary from 1 to 50 cm. in diameter, with an active border ranging from 2 mm. to 2 cm. wide. New lesions usually continue to appear one after another, or in waves; thus the patient is seldom free of cutaneous symptoms. There are no characteristic laboratory findings, except an occasional increase in eosinophils. The exact etiology is unknown, but it seems to be associated more with Candida albicans, hydroxychloroquine therapy, chloroquine sulfate therapy and influenza.

In rheumatic fever, a special form of this disease, erythema annulare rheumaticum, is often present. These lesions usually appear on the trunk and extensor surfaces of the extremities. The process is short-lived, and most of the centrifugal spread occurs at the height of disease activity.

Clinical differential diagnosis includes tinea corporis, lupus erythematosus, chronic urticaria, erythema multiforme, parapsoriasis en plaque, mycosis fungoides, syphilis and sarcoidosis.

## PURPURA

Purpura refers to the red-brown or purplish discoloration of the skin due to extravasation of blood into the skin or mucous membranes. There are several types of purpura.

1) Petechiae: Superficial, round, macular, hemorrhagic lesions up to 3 mm. in diameter;

2) <u>Ecchymoses</u>: Known by laymen as black and blue marks, which are larger and deeper, flat, hemorrhagic lesions;

3) <u>Hematomas</u>: These are localized collections of extravasated blood into the tissue of sufficient size to produce a palpable swelling in the skin.

Purpura may be distinguished from erythema by finger pressure or diascopy, which fails to blanch lesions of the former. Also, in purpura, extravasated blood is usually broken down into various other pigments within two to three weeks. This accounts for the characteristic color changes of resolving purpuric lesions to blue, green, orange, brown and tan. Purpura may be further divided into inflammatory and non-inflammatory types. Characteristically, the non-inflammatory type produces flat, non-palpable lesions, whereas the inflammatory type of purpura produces palpable lesions. Non-inflammatory purpuric lesions are found in stasis dermatitis, viral exanthemas, viral enanthemas, scarlet fever and amyloidosis. Palpable, inflammatory-type purpura is seen in meningococcemia and gonococcemia.

## ERYTHEMA

This term refers to a localized or generalized reddish color of the skin due to a transient dilatation of the superficial blood vessels. Localized erythema is found in cellulitis, lymphangitis and erysipelas. A special type of localized erythema, palmar erythema, may be found in pulmonary tuberculosis. Generalized erythema may be a manifestation of scabies, leprosy, or secondary syphilis.

## URTICARIA

Urticaria (hives, nettle rash) is a transient vascular reaction characterized by pruritic erythematous wheals in various configurations, which range from a few millimeters to 10 to 15 cm. in diameter. It may be localized or generalized. It may occur with tonsilitis, cholecystitis, gastrointestinal parasites, rheumatic fever, serum hepatitis and with many chronic infections.

## ERYTHEMA NODOSUM

Erythema nodosum is thought to be a form of either erythema multiforme or urticaria, which is characterized by painful nodules in the lower dermis and subcutaneous tissue. The nodules may be generalized, but are usually located on the shins. They are most often bilateral, well-circumscribed, tender nodules, 1 to 5 cm. in diameter. The lesions usually persist from three to six weeks and do not ulcerate. When involuting, they all go through a spectrum of color changes as seen in an ecchymotic lesion. A small percentage of patients will have recurrent attacks months to years after the initial bout. It seems to occur more often in the spring and fall. Sixty to ninety percent of those affected are female, and most patients are between the ages of 20 and 30, although any age group may be affected.

In children, streptococcal and other upper respiratory infections are the most common etiologic agents. Primary tuberculosis is another frequent cause in children, whereas in adults, sarcoidosis and streptococcal respiratory infections are the most common causes. Other diseases associated with erythema nodosum are coccidioidomycosis, histoplasmosis, North American blastomycosis, lymphogranuloma venereum, cat scratch disease, psittacosis, and American leishmaniasis.

### 57: GAS GANGRENE AND CLOSTRIDIAL INFECTIONS
by H. Thadepalli

Gas gangrene is characterized by the death of a part of the body caused by gas-producing bacteria. A mere demonstration of gas in a dead tissue does not make the diagnosis of gas gangrene; collection of free air in the tissues can occur due to other causes, such as injected air from extraneous sources, application of certain salts, like magnesium, hydrogen peroxide, or mere drainage of an abscess, generally followed by nature's tendency to fill this empty space with fluid or air. Gas gangrene is caused by a variety of clostridial organisms and others. The classical malady, clostridial gas gangrene, will be described first, followed by others, discussed under differential diagnosis. Clostridial infections can present as:

A) Gas gangrene
B) Uterine infection, or
C) Septicemia

### CLOSTRIDIAL GAS GANGRENE

This is a disease of wars, earthquakes and accidents, when massive tissue necrosis can occur along with wound contamination. The following categories should be recognized separately - wound contamination, clostridial cellulitis and clostridial myonecrosis. As McLennan described in his classic monograph, "Clostridial wound infections are not bacteriological entities; they are clinical concepts".[1]

CLOSTRIDIAL WOUND CONTAMINATION: Simple contamination of the wound with Clostridia is common. Almost all open wounds, even when recuperating, are colonized by Clostridia. Absence of local infection distinguishes contamination from infection. Therefore, mere demonstration of Clostridia in a wound is not diagnostic of clostridial infection.

CLOSTRIDIAL CELLULITIS: Most postoperative and post-traumatic clostridial infections of the wound fit this category. Clostridial cellulitis is a form of heavy clostridial infection of the ischemic and necrotic tissue. The muscle tissue, however, is intact. There may be no pain, edema or general toxemia. The gas is confined to the superficial (sometimes deep) tissue spaces and the wound, but not the muscle. The skin is not discolored.

CLOSTRIDIAL MYONECROSIS: Myonecrosis is the most dreaded of all clostridial infections. It should be distinguished, without a doubt, from other less serious local clostridial infections, because no less than complete and extensive resection of the necrotic muscles and amputation are required if there is myonecrosis. In myonecrosis, Clostridia affect the intact muscle. There may be no history of local trauma. It may begin with clostridial wound contamination. Less than 1% of such colonized wounds ever lead to myonecrosis. The proximal parts of the limbs, girdle, shoulder, buttocks and thighs, where there is a great muscle mass, are affected frequently.

The incubation period may vary, depending on the species of Clostridia involved. It is usually twelve to twenty-four hours in cases of infections caused by Clostridium (C.) perfringens, although in some cases, gangrene may begin within three hours after trauma.

Pain is the characteristic initial feature of this disease, often severe enough to make one suspect vascular catastrophe for no good reason. Later, the pain progressively worsens.

Local swelling due to edema and hemorrhagic exudate may develop within the next few hours. Myonecrosis is often accompanied by systemic toxicity, such as tachycardia and fever, generally around 100° to 101°F. but rarely above. Gas may not be demonstrable at this early stage of the disease.

Pathetic mental changes are common, described as the most profound distressing terror of death, persisting to the end, with clear mental alacrity.

Gas is now manifest by four to five hours after the onset of gangrene. Often, there is more destruction of the muscle than the amount of gas that can be palpated.

The skin color gradually changes from red to gray, blue, black and finally, when far advanced, to greenish-purple.

Unlike uterine infections, clostridial myonecrosis rarely produces jaundice (see pages 438, 440).

CLINICAL DIAGNOSIS:

Clostridium perfringens infections have a short incubation period (12 to 24 hours). The pain is the heralding symptom; the exudate is blood-tinged. There are often signs of systemic

toxicity evidenced by tachycardia and fever. The bubbles of gas
appear within a few hours. There is little change in superficial
color. Jaundice, hemoglobinuria and hemoglobulinemia are rare.
Often, the extent of muscle involvement is greater than in the
adjacent skin.

Clostridium novyi infections have a long incubation period, often four to six (5.25) days. A sense of heaviness of the affected
limb precedes pain by eight hours. Once gangrene begins, it
progresses rapidly. Gas production is not an obvious feature
of C. novyi infection; it may be altogether absent. Skin changes
are rare. The systemic toxicity is out of proportion to the local
infection. The onset of delirium spells imminent death.

Clostridium septicum infections have an incubation period of
one to three days. The clinical picture is akin to C. perfringens
infection, but high fevers above 102°F. may occur.

Clostridium histolyticum infections are rare. It is highly sensitive to oxygen, compared to other Clostridia; therefore, it
is hard to culture.

Clostridium bifermentans infections resemble C. novyi infections.

Clostridium fallax infections are rare.

BACTERIOLOGY: The following are considered to be the histotoxic Clostridia in man:

| | |
|---|---|
| Clostridium (C.) perfringens | C. sordellii |
| C. novyi A | C. haemolyticum |
| C. novyi B | C. chauvoei |
| C. septicum | C. difficile |
| C. histolyticum | C. carnis |
| C. bifermentans | C. sphenoides |
| C. fallax | |

LABORATORY FEATURES:

C. perfringens is recognized as the characteristic thick gram-
positive rod with rounded ends and almost total absence of
spores when found in the tissues, and sometimes even in the
laboratory. It produces hemolytic colonies on blood agar plates
due to the production of B hemolysin (Nagler reaction), and
pearly white zones of opacities on egg yolk agar plates (due to
lecithinase production) and stormy fermentation of litmus milk.

Both motile and non-motile forms of C. perfringens occur in nature. Clostridia possess several enzymes, such as hyaluronidase, coagulase, leukocidin, deoxyribonuclease and fibrinolysin, the necessary paraphernalia that can cause tissue lysis, and death.

Clostridium novyi often shows spores when obtained from the fresh tissue. It is a highly fastidious, motile and non-capsulated organism. Like C. histolyticum, it is difficult to grow, because it is highly sensitive even to traces of oxygen. C. septicum often shows subterminal spores in the tissues. Because of its swarming nature, it is hard to separate from other associated bacteria. C. histolyticum is a pure non-vegetarian. Unlike other histotoxic Clostridia mentioned, it does not ferment carbohydrates, but it readily splits gelatin and meat. C. bifermentans resembles C. perfringens; it rarely forms spores in the tissues. For further details, the reader is referred to books devoted to this purpose.[1,2]

Gram's stain: A Gram's stain of the wound is extremely helpful. Pus cells need not be present to diagnose Clostridia infection; they are often absent. Clostridia are thick, gram-positive rods often void of spores in the tissues. Spores can be rarely demonstrated even after thorough searching of the gram-stained slide. Demonstration of Clostridia on Gram's stain alone does not mean clostridial gangrene; physical signs of infection are also required.

Blood culture: The blood cultures are often negative in clostridial wound and muscle infections. Clostridial septicemia can occur in other conditions (see page 440).

Serology: This has a limited place in the identification of Clostridia.

SURGICAL DIAGNOSIS:

Diagnosis of myonecrosis can be made with certainty only at surgery. The dead muscle does not contract when stimulated with a tissue forceps at surgery. Instead, it just peels off. The associated stench is an unmistakable clue of anaerobic infection. Complete and thorough excision of all infected muscles is imperative to achieve cure. Anything less will result in further myonecrosis and death.

RADIOLOGY:

The gas bubbles are seen early on the roentgenogram, before they can be felt by palpation or a subcutaneous crepitus. Roentgenogram of the soft tissue may show air bubbles (Fig. 77). Demonstration of gas does not diagnose gas gangrene. It can sometimes be seen secondary to surgical drainage

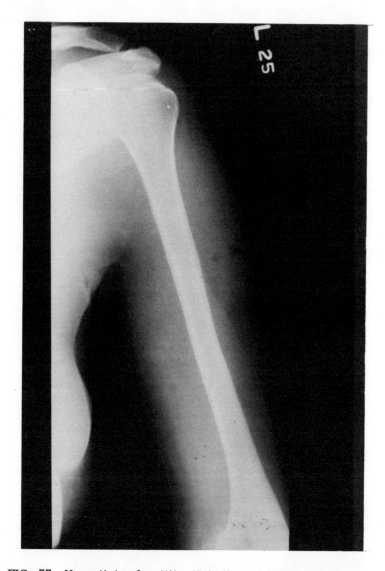

FIG. 77: Necrotizing fasciitis. Note the gas bubbles in the subcutaneous tissue. Cultures of pus revealed Peptostreptococcus parvulus and Eubacterium lentum. Same
organisms were also isolated in two separate sets
of blood cultures. (Reproduced with the permission
of West. J. Med. 130:200-204, 1979)

of pus. Fluid collection in the tissues as a result of fractures can be mistaken for gas gangrene. Gas in the tissues can also be due to certain aerobic and anaerobic bacteria other than Clostridia.

## DIFFERENTIAL DIAGNOSIS

Streptococcal myonecrosis can be clinically indistinguishable. The local tissue reaction is more severe in streptococcal myonecrosis than clostridial myonecrosis, and the fever is also higher, 102°F. or above. The incubation period is somewhat longer (three to four days), although rapid onset of streptococcal myonecrosis is not unknown. It can be produced by a variety of streptococci, notably, Streptococcus pyogenes and anaerobic streptococci (Peptostreptococcus and Peptococcus) and β hemolytic Streptococcus. Gas is also produced by Staphylococcus aureus and Escherichia coli. [3]

On Gram's stain, the cocci are seen in chains. Abundant numbers of pus cells is frequently present. It is difficult to distinguish streptococcal from clostridial myonecrosis without obtaining a small piece of the muscle. Streptococci do not invade the muscle.

Necrotizing fasciitis: This is a form of rapidly spreading gangrene caused by streptococci either alone or, most often, due to bacterial synergism, i.e., coliforms, enterococci, other streptococci, Bacteroides, diphtheroids, Proteus, staphylococci, and sometimes Clostridia. The adjacent skin may be involved. Gas formation is not a characteristic feature of this disease, but the muscle is seldom affected.

Progressive bacterial gangrene, also called Meleney's gangrene, can be secondary to underlying disease. It is a synergistic infection, caused by non-hemolytic microaerophilic Streptococcus and Staphylococcus. Several other bacterial synergies have been proposed; they include Proteus and Staphylococcus epidermidis; coliforms and Pseudomonas aeruginosa. [4]

Fournier's gangrene characteristically affects the scrotum and penis. It is a rapidly spreading, devastating infection of the perineum. One of our patients initially seen in the emergency room for scrotal swelling was mistaken to have mumps because the skin was then unaffected. Within a few hours after hospitalization, the skin over the peno-scrotal junction turned blue and within the next eight to ten hours, the entire scrotum and both inguinal areas turned gangrenous. A Gram's stain obtained from the subcutaneous areas revealed a variety of bacteria. There was no gas in the soft tissues by roentgenogram. He underwent extensive debridement of the skin over the scrotum and both inguinal areas (Fig. 78). On culture, he yielded two aerobes, Enterobacter hafniae and Enterococcus, and five anaerobes, Bacteroides fragilis ss. ovatus, Fusobacterium varium, Peptostreptococcus anaerobius, Peptococcus asaccharolyticus and Bacteroides melaninogenicus ss. asaccharolyticus. A variety of bacterial combinations are reported with this disease.

Acute non-clostridial crepitant cellulitis is a rapidly spreading emphysematous infection involving the skin and subcutaneous epifascial planes, accompanied by severe toxemia. The fever may be as high as $103^{\circ}$ to $107^{\circ}$F., associated with leukocytosis. Like Fournier's gangrene, it is often a polymicrobial infection. [6] Diabetes mellitus is a frequent predisposing cause.

Gas gangrene in diabetes mellitus: Staphylococcus aureus and Escherichia coli are the predominant organisms in gas gangrene secondary to diabetes mellitus. Gangrene of the amputated stump of the limbs is usually due to E. coli. Gram's stains of these lesions often provide enough clues to start appropriate antibiotic therapy. Demonstration of a gram-negative bacillus is likely to be E. coli; gram-positive cocci, S. aureus; and mixed flora are due to anaerobic infection.

## CLOSTRIDIAL UTERINE INFECTIONS

Clostridia rarely involve the non-gravid uterus. Shock, toxemia, sepsis, hemolysis, jaundice, oliguria and azotemia are common with postabortal and puerperal clostridial infection of the uterus. Most of these drastic clinical effects are produced by the $\alpha$ toxin of C. perfringens. However, the amount of detectable toxin within the bloodstream, if any, is negligible. It is, therefore, presumed that the adverse effects could be caused by "fixed" toxin to the tissues.

Gas may be demonstrated in the uterus by plain roentgenogram (physometra). Physometra can be caused by C. perfringens, C. septicum, anaerobic streptococci and, rarely, Bacteroides group of organisms.

BACTERIOLOGY:

Clostridia are not normal flora of the cervix during pregnancy. In 150 patients studied during the third trimester, labor and

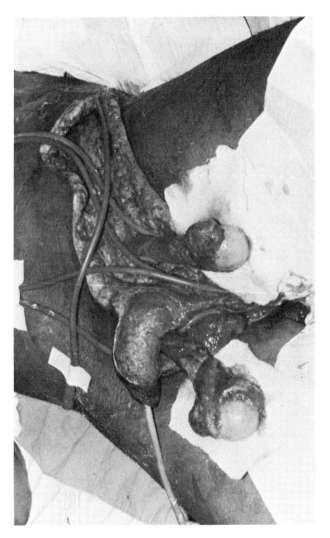

FIG. 78: Fournier's gangrene. See text for clinical details and culture results. (Photo courtesy of Drs. N. and K. Datta and Dr. N. Zinner)

the third day of puerperium, we have isolated Clostridia in 1% of the normal subjects. [7] Like clostridial wound infection, the cervix perhaps colonizes with Clostridia prior to the production of clostridial pyometritis.

Clostridia are almost always found in Gram's stain of the cervical smear of clostridial endomyometritis. Clostridial septicemia is a common accompaniment of clostridial uterine infections, but a positive blood culture is not diagnostic of Clostridia infection.

## CLOSTRIDIAL SEPTICEMIA

Nearly 2% to 3% of all positive blood cultures in our hospital are due to Clostridia. Nearly 70 species of Clostridia have been named. I am told that twice that many beg for a taxonomic status, and are simply called Clostridia species. Most Clostridia produce butyric acid and isobutyric acid as by-products.

After C. perfringens, C. ramosum is the most common Clostridia isolated in man. The role of C. ramosum in human disease is unknown.

Clostridial septicemia is a non-specific diagnosis. We have found Clostridia in cases of intra-abdominal abscess, empyema, pelvic abscess, and prostatic infections. [8] In one case, C. perfringens was isolated with meningococcus in the blood; others had Streptococcus pneumoniae and some had coliforms. Nearly 30% to 40% of the patients with clostridial septicemia also had other organisms in the blood.

A somewhat characteristic syndrome found in a group of patients was alcoholism, pneumonia, liver disease and clostridial septicemia. I have encountered several such patients in my practice. Their clinical outcome is often benign.

### TREATMENT OF CLOSTRIDIAL INFECTIONS

SURGERY: Extensive and complete debridement of necrotic muscle tissue is imperative for clostridial myonecrosis, or else all other therapeutic modalities are bound to fail.

Hysterectomy is required in cases of postabortal or puerperal clostridial endomyometritis.

ANTIBIOTICS: They are of doubtful value. Many prefer penicillin and consider it as the drug of choice. We have used clindamycin or carbenicillin.[9]

ANTISERUM: Gas gangrene antiserum has no place, if any, in the treatment of gas gangrene. I have never used it.

HYPERBARIC OXYGEN: The value of hyperbaric oxygen in the treatment of gas gangrene is a subject of great controversy. Some have claimed success.[10] I am still unconvinced about its efficacy in the treatment of gas gangrene; it may be tried for whatever it is worth.

## REFERENCES

1. McLennan, J. D.: The histotoxic clostridial infections of man. Bacteriol. Reviews 26:177, 1962.

2. Holdeman, L. V., Moore, W. E. C. (Eds.): Anaerobe Laboratory Manual, third edition. Virginia Polytechnic Institute Anaerobe Laboratory, State University, Blacksburg, 1975.

3. Bessman, A., Wagner, W.: Nonclostridial gas gangrene. J. A. M. A. 233:958, 1975.

4. Ledingham, I. McA., Tehrani, M. A.: Diagnosis, clinical course and treatment of acute dermal gangrene. Brit. J. Surg. 62:364, 1975.

5. Himal, H. S., McLean, A. P. H., Duff, J. H.: Gas gangrene of the scrotum and perineum. Surg. Gynec. and Obstet. 139:176, 1974.

6. Altmeier, W. A., Culbertson, W. R.: Acute nonclostridial crepitant cellulitis. Surg. Gynec. and Obstet. 87:206, 1948.

7. Thadepalli, H., et al: Cyclic changes in cervical flora. Proceedings of Amer. Soc. Microbiol., 1977.

8. Gorbach, S. L., Thadepalli, H.: Isolation of Clostridium in human infections: Evaluation of 114 cases. J. Inf. Dis. 131:581, 1975.

9. Thadepalli, H. , Huang, J. T.: Treatment of anaerobic infections: Carbenicillin alone compared with clindamycin and gentamicin. Current Ther. Res. 22:549-555, 1977.

10. Brummelkamp, W.H. , Boerama, I. , Hoogendyk, J.: Treatment of clostridial infections with hyperbaric oxygen drenching: A report on 24 cases. Lancet 1:235, 1963.

SECTION G: BONE AND JOINT INFECTIONS


58: OSTEOMYELITIS
by David W. Webb


Osteomyelitis can be caused by a wide variety of bacteria and fungi. Table 29 summarizes the sources for osteomyelitis.

| TABLE 29: PATHOGENESIS OF OSTEOMYELITIS |
| --- |

**HEMATOGENOUS - 20%**

Skin infection
Pneumonia
Urinary infection
Gastrointestinal infection

**CONTIGUOUS FOCUS OF INFECTION - 50%**

Surgery
Decubitus ulcer
Sinusitis

**PERIPHERAL VASCULAR DISEASE - 30%**

Diabetes mellitus
Vasculitis

Table 30 summarizes the varieties of microorganisms involved. [1] Staphylococcus aureus is the most common bacterium. Although Streptococcus pyogenes and Streptococcus pneumoniae were once frequent causes of osteomyelitis, their incidence has decreased in recent years. Gram-negative bacteria are more important causes of osteomyelitis today. Anaerobic bacteria infrequently involve the bone, although their presence may have been overlooked because of inadequate culture techniques. Brucella and Nocardia are rare causes of osteomyelitis. Such normally non-invasive bacteria as Staphylococcus epidermidis and diphtheroids may also cause osteomyelitis when a foreign body, like prosthesis, is in place. Treponema pallidum is a rare cause of osteomyelitis, but it is still prevalent in the developing nations. Mycobacterium tuberculosis and the typical Mycobacteria are important causes of osteomyelitis. Finally,

444/ Bone and Joint Infections

## TABLE 30: MICROBIOLOGY OF OSTEOMYELITIS*

| | |
|---|---|
| STAPHYLOCOCCUS AUREUS | 70% |
| S. EPIDERMIDIS | < 1 |
| STREPTOCOCCUS PYOGENES | 3 |
| S. PNEUMONIAE | < 1 |

GRAM-NEGATIVE FACULTATIVE 25

Pseudomonas
Serratia
Klebsiella
E. coli
Salmonella
Arizona

ANAEROBIC BACTERIA          2

Bacteroides
Peptococci
Peptostreptococci
Fusobacteria
Actinomyces

OTHER BACTERIA          < 1

Brucella
Nocardia

OTHERS

Mycobacterium tuberculosis
Atypical Mycobacteria
Treponema pallidum
Cryptococcus
Coccidioides
Blastomyces
Candida
Aspergillus
Histoplasma

* Approximate percentages calculated on the basis of various
publications. [1,5]

various fungi, like coccidioidomycosis and blastomycosis can also cause osteomyelitis.

## BONES INVOLVED

Fig. 79 shows the bones most commonly involved in hematogenous osteomyelitis in all age groups combined. It can be seen that the long bones of the lower extremity are most frequently involved. Although vertebrae are involved in only 15% of the cases, overall, this figure would be much higher if only adults were considered. Vertebral osteomyelitis commonly occurs in the lumbar (45%) and thoracic (40%) areas, cervical in 10% and sacral in 5%. Multiple bone involvement may occur in 5% of the cases of osteomyelitis.

## CLINICAL FEATURES

A. MODE OF ONSET: The initial episode of bacterial osteomyelitis is usually acute and associated with signs of systemic infection, such as chills and fever, in addition to localized pain and signs of inflammation. On the other hand, recurrent or chronic osteomyelitis usually presents insidiously with vague pain as the only manifestation. Constitutional symptoms are rare.

Subacute osteomyelitis (Brodie's abscess) represents a subperiosteal collection of pus that may follow acute osteomyelitis (Fig. 80). This may persist for years with only minimal symptoms. At times, this classification may not hold; acute exacerbations of chronic osteomyelitis may occur. Acute osteomyelitis in adults may be indolent without such systemic toxicity.

B. AGE DIFFERENCES: Osteomyelitis is seen most commonly in children under 12 and in adults over the age of 50. During the first year of life, osteomyelitis frequently spreads to the adjacent joint and the patient may present with a septic arthritis. From the age of one year to puberty, contiguous spread of infection to the joint capsule is rare, but infection can spread to the subperiosteum, forming an abscess. This abscess may rupture into the subcutaneous tissue, and such patients may present with a soft tissue abscess. In adults, periosteal abscess is less common, but infection can again spread to the adjacent joint.

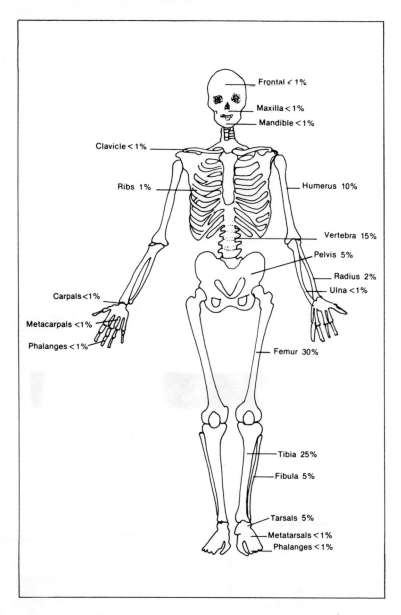

FIG. 79: Osteomyelitis. Incidence of osteomyelitis at various sites. Nearly 75% of the cases involve the femur, vertebrae, tibia and fibula. [1,5]

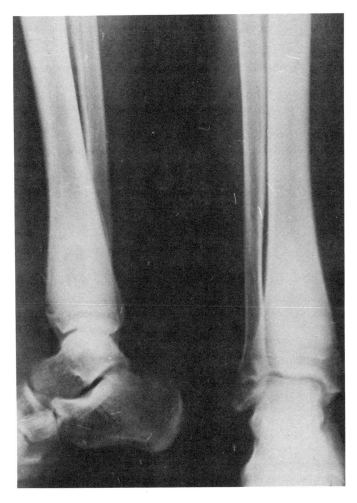

FIG. 80: Brodie's abscess of the tibia. (Courtesy of John
Campbell, M. D. , Charles R. Drew Postgraduate
Medical School, Los Angeles, California)

In children, osteomyelitis usually involves the long bones, whereas vertebral involvement is more common in adults. Children are more likely to have constitutional symptoms, such as fever and chills.

## SYMPTOMS

A. SYSTEMIC:

1) Fever: Fever is present in almost all cases of acute hematogenous osteomyelitis seen in children. The fever is high and associated with chills. The patient appears toxic. The fever and associated symptoms begin abruptly, and the patient can often state exactly when his illness began. In adults with acute hematogenous osteomyelitis, the onset may be less abrupt and the fever lower or absent entirely. Fever is often absent in cases of vertebral or mandibular osteomyelitis. Fever is usually low-grade or absent in patients with osteomyelitis due to a contiguous focus of infection or peripheral vascular disease. In chronic osteomyelitis, fever is usually absent unless there is an acute exacerbation. Some patients may have a continuous or intermittent low-grade fever. Fever in fungal or tuberculous osteomyelitis is usually low-grade and not associated with signs of toxicity, unless the osteomyelitis occurs as part of disseminated infection.

2) Weight loss: Mild weight loss (less than 10% of body weight) is frequently reported in cases of acute osteomyelitis. Weight loss is less common in chronic osteomyelitis, but when present, may be more severe.

3) Malaise: Most patients with acute osteomyelitis experience malaise; this is less common in chronic osteomyelitis.

B. LOCAL:

1) Pain: Pain and tenderness are the most prominent findings in osteomyelitis. Pain is an early symptom. At first, it is diffuse and then later becomes localized to the site of infection. The pain is very severe in acute hematogenous osteomyelitis and is described as a boring, excruciating pain. Movement or touch aggravates the pain. Pain in vertebral osteomyelitis may be quite severe and localized to one vertebral body, or may be

dull, poorly localized and made worse by straining. Point
tenderness of the involved vertebra is usually present.
The pain of chronic osteomyelitis is usually dull and
less severe. Pain may be absent in diabetics with osteomyelitis of one of the small bones of the foot, due to the
presence of a peripheral neuropathy. Because pain is
such a characteristic finding, whenever localized bone
pain is present, osteomyelitis must be ruled out.

2) Inflammation: In acute hematogenous osteomyelitis,
local signs of inflammation may be present. Swelling
of the involved area will be seen in about 50% of the
cases. The involved area will feel warm in 30% of the
cases. Erythema is present in about 20% of cases. In
chronic osteomyelitis, swelling is seen in about 30% of
cases, but heat and erythema are rare. Fluctuation is
not commonly seen, except in children when a subperiosteal abscess forms; such fluctuation develops slowly
and is not seen early in the disease.

3) Limitation of motion: Limitation of motion is due to pain
in most instances. It is present in about 30% of cases
of acute hematogenous osteomyelitis; it is less common
in chronic osteomyelitis. Children may present with a
"pseudoparalysis" of an extremity, due to their unwill-
ingness to move the bone due to pain.

4) Draining sinus: Chronic osteomyelitis may be complicated by sinus formation with drainage of purulent material to the skin surface. These sinuses may be single
or multiple and are seen in about 50% of the cases of
chronic osteomyelitis. Draining sinuses may also complicate osteomyelitis caused by tuberculous or fungal
infection. Tuberculosis of the ribs characteristically
produces draining sinuses of the chest wall. Actinomyces
may also cause such draining sinuses (see Figs. 27,28,
pages 172 and 173). Acute hematogenous osteomyelitis
is uncommonly associated with sinus formation, unless
the infection is allowed to progress untreated. These
sinuses may form anywhere over the involved area; there
is no regularity in their location. [2]

5) Joint effusion: A sterile "sympathetic" effusion may
form in a nearby joint. This is seen in 5% to 10% of the
cases of acute hematogenous osteomyelitis. Less commonly, a septic purulent arthritis may form due to contiguous spread of the infection.

DIAGNOSIS

A. DIAGNOSTIC PROCEDURES:

1) Blood tests: Certain tests should be ordered in all cases
of suspected osteomyelitis. A complete blood count and
differential should be done. In acute hematogenous osteomyelitis, the white blood cell count is usually elevated and there is a shift of granulocytes "to the left"
(more immature forms). The erythrocyte sedimentation
rate (ESR) is usually elevated. However, these tests
may be normal in some cases of acute osteomyelitis
and, therefore, a normal value does not rule out osteomyelitis. In chronic osteomyelitis, the ESR is usually
elevated, but the white blood cell count is usually normal. In tuberculous or fungal osteomyelitis, the ESR is
elevated in about 50% of the cases, but the white blood
cell count is often normal. Anemia may be present in
acute or chronic osteomyelitis, but is not a characteristic feature. A calcium, phosphorus and alkaline phosphatase should always be obtained; they are usually normal in osteomyelitis, but may be abnormal in cases of
metastatic or metabolic bone disease. A serologic test
for syphilis should always be obtained.

2) Skin tests: A PPD test for tuberculosis should be placed
in all cases of osteomyelitis.

3) X-rays: Plain roentgenographs should be obtained in all
cases of suspected osteomyelitis. It must be appreciated
that such x-rays can be normal early in the course of
osteomyelitis and may lag behind the disease process
by several weeks. Nearby soft tissue swelling is the first
x-ray sign of osteomyelitis and usually appears within
the first week of infection. Such swelling represents
edema of the muscles, fascia and subcutaneous tissue,
and is not specific for osteomyelitis, but may be seen
in cellulitis or any soft tissue infection. Subperiosteal
elevation is a sign of underlying pus and may occur after two weeks of infection. Layers of new bone may be
laid down around the periosteum, giving the first radiographic sign of the involucrum. A lytic lesion represents
bony destruction and is a classic sign of osteomyelitis,
but this may not appear on the x-ray for two to three
weeks, as about two-thirds of the density of bone must
be lost for it to be seen. An oval area of rarefaction in
the metaphysis is usually the first sign of such a lesion.

Later, sequestra may be seen on the x-ray (Fig. 81).
Sequestra are of normal density, in contrast to the
rarefied bone, which usually surrounds them.

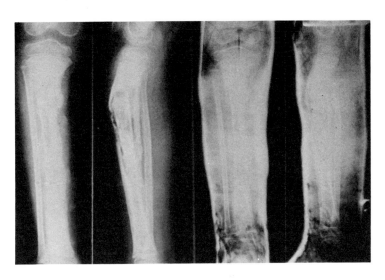

FIG. 81: Osteomyelitis with sequestrum formation and fracture
of tibia (left); same in a cast (right). (Courtesy of John
Campbell, M. D. , Charles R. Drew Postgraduate Medical School, Los Angeles, California)

In vertebral osteomyelitis, similar x-ray findings occur. Usually two adjacent vertebral bodies are involved. Narrowing of the intervertebral disc space is
usually the first abnormality to appear; later, osteolytic lesions appear in the vertebra. A soft tissue swelling around a vertebral body may be seen on the x-ray
and represents a paravertebral abscess. In cases of
metastatic carcinoma of the spine, usually only one
vertebra is involved and the disc space is intact. Therefore, the involvement of adjacent vertebral bodies is
a key finding, suggesting vertebral osteomyelitis. In
evaluating patients with suspected osteomyelitis, tomo-
grams of the involved vertebra are often helpful.
It must be emphasized that x-ray findings are not
entirely specific for osteomyelitis and may be seen
also in cases of tumor or metabolic disease of the bone.

Positive x-rays demand further work-up to define the nature of the lesion. Conversely, negative x-rays do not rule out osteomyelitis.

4) Sinogram: A sinogram may be helpful in cases of chronic or acute osteomyelitis complicated by sinus formation. Radiopaque dye is injected into the sinus and films taken. In this way, collections of pus can be identified in such sinus tracts.

5) Bone scan: Radionuclide scanning has brought a new dimension to the diagnosis of osteomyelitis. Many bone scanning nuclides, such as isotopes of strontium, calcium and phosphorus have been tried, but technetium-99m diphosphonate has been found to be most satisfactory. This material is a highly specific bone-seeking nuclide which yields an excellent image of the skeleton. The material is given intravenously, and then whole body scanning is done with a scintillation camera. Increased uptake of the isotope occurs in diseased bone and can be seen as a "hot" area on scan (Figs. 82-85). This increased uptake is non-specific and is seen in areas of primary and secondary tumor, metabolic disease, fractures, aseptic necrosis and infection. The increased uptake that is seen in osteomyelitis depends on new bone formation, the osteoblastic reaction that occurs around the osteolytic lesion. Therefore, such scans may not be positive early in infection (see Fig. 83) before new bone formation begins, although it is claimed these scans may often be positive 24 hours after symptoms begin. [3] Because bone scans are non-specific, their usefulness is somewhat limited. Their main use lies in the fact that they may be positive before any signs of osteomyelitis can be seen on the x-ray. A bone scan is helpful in separating osteomyelitis from soft tissue infection. Although increased uptake may be seen in cellulitis on scans done immediately after injection, delayed scans will be normal in cellulitis and abnormal in osteomyelitis. In general, a bone scan should be done in any patient with suspected osteomyelitis when the x-ray is non-diagnostic. If positive, the patient needs further work-up to define the etiology of the bone disease present. If negative and osteomyelitis is still suspected, either a repeat bone scan in 72 hours or a gallium scan should be done.

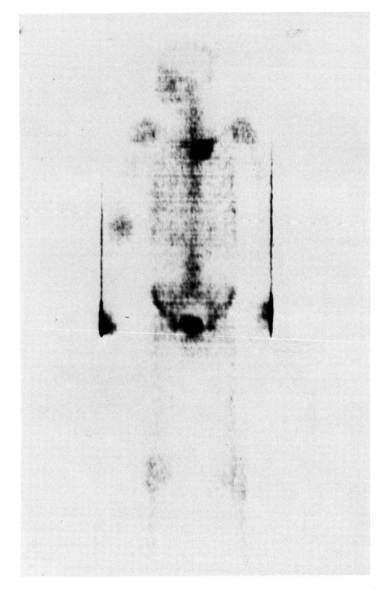

FIG. 82: Bone scan with Tc-99m diphosphonate (anterior view) showing osteomyelitis of the left sternoclavicular joint (see Fig. 87 for plain x-ray).

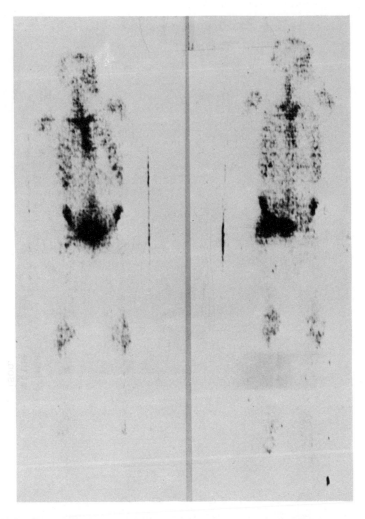

FIG. 83: Bone scan. This patient complained of right hip pain, for which she was evaluated and clinically suspected of having arthritis. Bone scan done at that time (10/19/76) is shown on the left, which was normal. The roentgenogram of the hip joint was also normal. However, since the symptoms worsened during the next month (11/20/76), the bone scan was repeated (shown on the right), which showed increased uptake in the right hip.

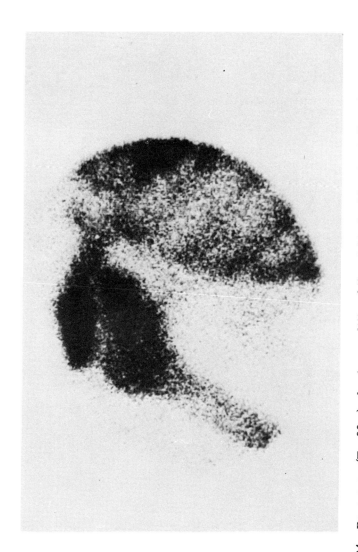

FIG. 84: Bone scan (Tc-99m) of osteomyelitis of the right shoulder due to Pseudomonas aeruginosa. Mark the intense uptake shown at the acromioclavicular joint, the site of infection. Fig. 85 shows left shoulder for comparison.

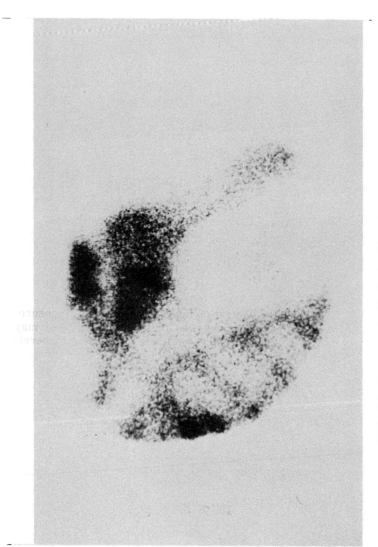

FIG. 85: Bone scan of left shoulder for comparison.

6) Gallium scan: Scanning with gallium-67 may be a more sensitive diagnostic procedure than scanning with technetium. Gallium-67 localizes in inflammatory cells and, therefore, increased uptake will be seen early in cases of osteomyelitis as soon as inflammation is present. Gallium-67 scans may, therefore, be positive early in infection, before either x-rays or bone scans are positive. Unfortunately, this test has several drawbacks. It is usually necessary to wait 48 hours after injecting the material before scanning is carried out. Also, the test will not separate cellulitis from osteomyelitis.

7) Myelography: A myelogram is indicated in cases of vertebral osteomyelitis in which an epidural abscess is suspected (see section on Complications). The technique involves injecting Pantopaque or a similar contrast medium into the subarachnoid space to permit visualization of an intraspinal lesion. It should not be done in patients who have had a recent lumbar puncture, as the contrast media may leak outside the subarachnoid space. The site of puncture depends on symptomatology. Puncture should not be carried out through the involved segment, or pus might be pushed from the extradural to the subarachnoid space. Whenever myelography is done, the needle should be advanced slowly, and repeated aspiration must be carried out to ensure an area of pus has not been entered. Myelography may safely be carried out at the lumbar, thoracic or cervical areas, depending on where the lesion is to be visualized. After Pantopaque is injected into the subarachnoid space, films are taken and areas of obstruction and areas of nerve compression are easily seen. The procedure is easiest under fluoroscopic guidance.

Pantopaque may also be injected directly into the cisterna magna. This approach is favored by some when epidural abscess is suspected, as the subdural space can be entered at a site away from the suspected abscess. A spinal needle is inserted in the midline between the occipital protuberance and the upper margin of the spine of $C_2$ and directed slightly cephalad. When the subarachnoid space is entered, cerebrospinal fluid is withdrawn and Pantopaque injected. Recently, the lateral cervical approach has come into increasing use because of its safety and ease, compared to the cisternal route. [4] Indications are the same as for cisternal puncture, except that $C_1$-$C_2$ space is not well seen. The site of the puncture is between the laminar pillars of $C_1$ and $C_2$. The tip of the needle is aimed at the anterior third of the bony spinal canal under fluoroscopic guidance.

8) <u>Cultures</u>: Whenever osteomyelitis is suspected, appropriate cultures must be taken:

(a) <u>Blood cultures</u>: Three sets of blood cultures drawn over a period of several hours must be taken in all cases. The highest yield is in acute hematogenous osteomyelitis, when the blood cultures will be positive in 10% to 40% of the cases.

(b) <u>Cultures of distant sites of infection</u>: Whenever another source of infection is present or suspected, appropriate cultures must be taken. A urine culture should be obtained in all cases of vertebral osteomyelitis. If a carbuncle or other site of infection is present, it should be cultured. Transtracheal aspiration should be performed on patients with pneumonia.

(c) <u>Cultures of the local site of infection</u>: In any case of known or suspected osteomyelitis, a culture of the involved site is mandatory. Various procedures are available for obtaining such material, and they will be discussed separately. Such cultures should be obtained as soon as possible in cases of suspected osteomyelitis. It is not necessary to wait for results of scans if the diagnosis is clinically evident.

(d) <u>Swab culture</u>: When an open wound is present, or there is a sinus tract leading to the skin, a swab of the drainage may be obtained for culture. In obtaining such a swab, it is important to avoid contamination of the specimen with normal body flora. The surrounding skin should be cleaned with isopropyl alcohol before the sample is taken. If several such swabs are taken, the accuracy of this technique approaches that of bone biopsy, although in rare cases, such drainage will not reflect the bacteria that is present deep in the infection.

9) Needle aspiration: Needle aspiration is easily performed on superficial bones, such as the tibia. The overlying skin should be scrubbed with soap and then dis-
infected with an iodine solution. The area is then infiltrated with a local anesthetic, such as 1% lidocaine.
A large-bore needle (14-gauge) should be introduced
into the point of maximum tenderness and aspiration
carried out with a syringe. It is best to try to obtain
material from deeply within the bone. If no material
can be aspirated, 0.5 ml. of sterile water or saline
(not bacteriostatic) should be injected into the area and
aspiration carried out again. At times, the cortex may
be thickened and the needle will not penetrate the bone;
if this occurs, bone biopsy is necessary.

10) Needle biopsy: Needle biopsy of bone has the advantage
of providing material for histological examination, as
well as culture. The procedure is easy to do on vertebrae and is probably the procedure of choice in evaluating vertebral lesions of unknown cause. It is safe to do
on the lower four cervical, lower four thoracic and all
lumbar vertebrae. In addition, this procedure can be
done on other bones and should be done if needle aspiration does not yield a diagnosis. A Craig trephine needle is suitable for this procedure. Vertebral biopsy is
best done under fluoroscopic guidance with the patient
prone on the x-ray table. The needle is inserted firmly
into the involved bone and pushed inward until it comes
in contact with bone. The needle is then withdrawn and
the trephine removed to withdraw tissue. A good core
of bone can be obtained in this way.

11) Open biopsy: Open biopsy should be done when the involved area is not accessible to aspiration or needle
biopsy, or when material so obtained is not diagnostic.
As the upper cervical and thoracic vertebrae are not
safely biopsied by needle, this procedure is ideal for
obtaining tissue from these areas. Open biopsy has
the advantage of obtaining a large amount of bone for
histologic examination. The surgeon can directly visualize the area and obtain material from the center of
infection.

B. PROCESSING OF THE SPECIMEN:

1) Aspirate: The specimen should be divided into separate
portions and the following studies done:

(a) Gram's stain: This should be done promptly. If bacteria are seen, their staining reaction and morphology may make early diagnosis possible.

(b) Ziehl-Neelsen stain: This should always be done to diagnose tuberculous infection and is helpful if positive. A negative stain does not rule out tuberculosis.

(c) KOH preparation: Both mycelial and yeast forms may be seen, so this should be done in all cases where fungal osteomyelitis is a possibility.

2) Culture:

(a) Aerobic: The material should be plated on aerobic media.

(b) Anaerobic: The material should be placed in an anaerobic container and taken to the laboratory promptly for anaerobic culturing.

(c) Tuberculous: This should be done routinely.

(d) Fungal: This should be done routinely.

3) Tissue: If tissue is obtained by biopsy, all of the above studies should be done on the tissue, as well as the following stains:

(a) Hematoxylin and eosin (H&E): This will enable a pathologic diagnosis. Signs of acute or chronic inflammation may be seen. Granulomas may be seen in cases of tuberculous or fungal osteomyelitis.

(b) Periodic Acid-Schiff (PAS) stain: This stain is especially helpful in identifying fungal elements.

(c) Methenamine silver: This stain is also helpful in identifying fungal elements.

## COMPLICATIONS

A. INFECTIOUS ARTHRITIS: As previously discussed, septic arthritis may complicate osteomyelitis due to contiguous spread of infection. The most frequently involved joints are the hip, shoulder or knee, although any joint may be involved. [5]

B. PATHOLOGIC FRACTURE: Bones weakened by osteomyelitis are prone to fracture, although this occurs in less
than 1% of cases. In osteomyelitis of the femur or humer-
us, separation of the epiphysis may occur, resulting in
loss of growth potential.

C. SPINAL EPIDURAL ABSCESS: Vertebral osteomyelitis
may result in epidural abscess due to posterior spread of
the infection. Such patients may present with rapidly evolv-
ing neurologic signs. Back pain occurs first, which is dull,
constant and well localized. It is made worse by motion
of the spine. Radicular symptoms may appear next and are
often bilateral. Pain and sensory loss in the distribution
of the involved nerve appears. This may be followed by
weakness, which can quickly progress to paralysis.[6] Spastic weakness and loss of vibratory and position sense occur early, while disturbances of bowel and bladder control occur late. Neurologic symptoms in a patient with
vertebral osteomyelitis could also be caused by sudden
collapse of a vertebral body with nerve root compression.
Neurologic signs in a patient with vertebral osteomyelitis
constitute a medical emergency, and myelography should
be done promptly.

D. RETROPHARYNGEAL ABSCESS: Cervical osteomyelitis
may be complicated by a retropharyngeal abscess as a result of anterior spread of the infection. Symptoms are pain
and the sensation of a "lump" in the throat. Airway obstruction may develop.

E. MEDIASTINITIS: This is a rare complication of thoracic
vertebral osteomyelitis and results from anterior spread
of the infection. Such patients appear acutely ill with dyspnea, cough and chest pain.

F. ABDOMINAL ABSCESS: Rarely, anterior spread of infection from a lumbar osteomyelitis will lead to subphrenic
or retroperitoneal abscess.

G. PSOAS ABSCESS: Abscess of the psoas muscle may result from direct extension from a lumbosacral osteomyelitis (not commonly due to Mycobacterium tuberculosis).
A mass may often be felt in the inguinal area or by rectal
exam. The patient typically lies with his thigh flexed to
prevent pressure on the lumbar nerve, which lies within
the psoas sheath. X-rays will show widening of the psoas
muscle.

H. AMYLOIDOSIS: Secondary amyloidosis may complicate chronic osteomyelitis of many years duration. This is rare.

I. NEOPLASM: Epidermoid carcinoma may occur in a fistulous tract in chronic osteomyelitis. A fungating mass is often palpable, but the carcinoma may be deep in the fistulous tract and may only be discovered by biopsy.

## SPECIFIC CAUSES

STAPHYLOCOCCAL OSTEOMYELITIS: Staphylococcus aureus remains the leading cause of osteomyelitis today, although it is less commonly seen now than in the past. S. aureus can gain access to the bone either by hematogenous route or by direct extension from a contiguous focus of infection. Hematogenous spread usually occurs from a skin or soft tissue infection (such as a faruncle or carbuncle). Often, such infections may seem insignificant. Most cases are seen in children below the age of 12. Often, history of seemingly minor trauma to the involved area may be present before a sign of infection occurs (Fig. 86). This history may be obtained in about one-third of the cases. Most children with S. aureus osteomyelitis appear acutely ill with chills and high fever. In adults, symptoms may be less pronounced. S. aureus osteomyelitis may occur in "mainline" drug addicts and in patients on chronic hemodialysis who may have infected access sites. Patients with acute bacterial endocarditis due to S. aureus may develop metastatic osteomyelitis as a complication. S. aureus is also the most frequent cause of post-operative osteomyelitis. This may occur in patients who have had craniotomy or open heart surgery (where the sternum is split), and in those with recently plated fractures; and, in particular, after internal fixation of hip fractures. Whereas S. aureus usually is the sole pathogen in cases of hematogenous osteomyelitis, it is commonly found in association with other bacteria in cases of osteomyelitis due to a contiguous focus of infection.

PNEUMOCOCCAL OSTEOMYELITIS: Although common in the pre-antibiotic era, pneumococcal osteomyelitis is rare today. Hematogenous seeding to the bone from a pneumonia is the mechanism of such infections. Less commonly, hematogenous spread from a non-pulmonary source, such as an otitis media, may occur. In children, one of the long tubular bones is usually involved, whereas in adults, one of the vertebrae is usually involved. Pain in the involved bone usually arises after the pneumonia has become apparent. Spread of infection to a contiguous joint frequently occurs. Early treatment of pneumonia with antibiotics has made this infection rare today.

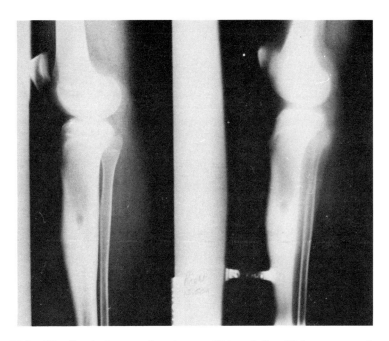

FIG. 86: Staphylococcal osteomyelitis of the tibia, proven by
culture of the fluoroscopically guided needle biopsy.
Blood cultures were negative.

GRAM-NEGATIVE OSTEOMYELITIS: In recent years, the incidence of osteomyelitis caused by gram-negative aerobic bacteria has been increasing. Currently, Pseudomonas aeruginosa
is the organism most commonly associated with gram-negative
osteomyelitis (Fig. 87). Salmonella osteomyelitis will be discussed separately. Hematogenous gram-negative osteomyelitis
is seen in "mainline" drug addicts and patients on chronic hemodialysis. Vertebral involvement is most common and the
infection is usually due to Pseudomonas or Serratia. The pelvic venous plexus drains the urinary bladder, prostate, uterus
and other pelvic tissues. When any of these areas become infected, the infection can spread into the lumbar vein, to the
vertebral bodies of the lumbosacral spine. This is an important mechanism in the pathogenesis of gram-negative vertebral osteomyelitis in patients with urinary tract infection. The
most common pathogens are Klebsiella, E. coli, Enterobacter
and Pseudomonas. Gram-negative bacteria may also reach
bone by direct extension from an adjacent focus of infection.

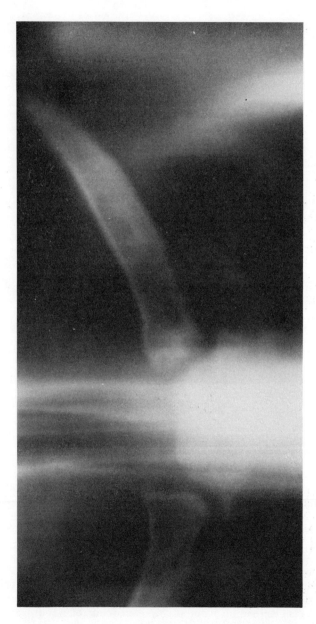

FIG. 87: A 32-year-old heroin addict admitted with left sternoclavicular pain and swelling, but no fever. Aspirate of the left sternoclavicular joint grew Pseudomonas aeruginosa (see Fig. 82 for bone scan of the same patient).

Puncture wounds of the foot, especially in children, may be complicated in two to three weeks by osteomyelitis due to Pseudomonas. [7] Bites of animals (usually cats) may be complicated by osteomyelitis due to Pasteurella multocida, a pleomorphic gram-negative coccobacillus. [8] Human bites may be complicated by osteomyelitis due to Eikenella corrodens, [9] a fastidious gram-negative bacillus. Gram-negative bacteria are frequent causes of post-operative osteomyelitis, often occurring as part of a mixed infection with S. aureus. Gram-negative bacteria are often found in association with anaerobic bacteria in osteomyelitis of the mandible due to a tooth infection, and in osteomyelitis of the sacrum due to a decubitus ulcer in the sacral area. Osteomyelitis caused by gram-negative bacteria tends to be a more indolent infection than osteomyelitis caused by S. aureus.[10] High fever, rigors and a toxic state are unusual. Pain and tenderness of the involved area are often the only symptoms. Draining sinuses are common and may occur early. Gram-negative osteomyelitis cannot be diagnosed on clinical grounds, and cultural proof is necessary.

ANAEROBIC OSTEOMYELITIS: Osteomyelitis due to nonsporulating anaerobic bacteria is relatively rare. Anaerobes can affect the vertebrae or the long bones. Osteomyelitis of the mandible is frequently a mixed infection, involving both aerobic and anaerobic bacteria. It usually occurs at a site of previous trauma or near infected and carious teeth. Actinomyces israelii is a common isolate from such infections, either alone or with "other bacteria" (see page 167). Osteomyelitis of the frontal bone, secondary to chronic sinusitis, may occur. Pott's puffy tumor, osteomyelitis of the frontal bone characterized by doughy edema of the forehead, osteomyelitis secondary to bony penetration of a decubitus ulcer, and osteomyelitis due to peripheral vascular disease are other examples of osteomyelitis caused by anaerobic bacteria.

The most common anaerobes seen in osteomyelitis are Bacteroides melaninogenicus, Bacteroides fragilis, Peptostreptococcus, Peptococcus and Fusobacterium.[11] Usually, more than one organism can be cultured from the site, and often aerobic bacteria are present as well. Thus, one of the most helpful clues to anaerobic infection is the presence of more than one morphologic type of organism on Gram's stain. Certain clinical features may also suggest anaerobic infection. Foul-smelling pus and soft tissue gas, when present, suggest anaerobic infection. Such signs are also present in infections caused by coliforms. Tissue necrosis and gangrene may occur often.

Diagnosis will be missed unless anaerobic cultures are done routinely on all specimens obtained from patients with osteomyelitis.

SYPHILIS OF BONE:  Treponema pallidum may affect the bone at any of the stages of syphilis. [12] Due to modern antibiotic therapy, skeletal lesions are now rare in early syphilis (primary or secondary).  In early syphilis, a periostitis is the most common skeletal lesion.  The tibia, sternum, skull and ribs are most commonly involved.  Pain over the involved area is common; it may be mild or severe and gets worse at night.  Fever may be present.  X-rays show thickening of the periosteum, which may be mistaken for bacterial osteomyelitis (Fig. 88, 89). Rarely, the infection may go on to produce bone destruction and syphilitic osteomyelitis.

Bone involvement is more frequent in late syphilis.  Periostitis is frequent.  Gummas may develop in the bone; the long bones are most frequently involved.  Extensive, painless destruction of the femoral head can cause triple displacement of the hip joint (Charcot's joint - Fig. 90).  Local pain and tenderness occur, but constitutional symptoms are rare.  Syphilitic osteomyelitis may occur in proximity to an intramedullary gumma. X-rays usually show an osteolytic lesion with thickening of the periosteum; such lesions are often mistaken for bacterial osteomyelitis.  Saber tibia and increased density of bones may be noted in congenital syphilis (Fig. 91).

Diagnosis of syphilis is serologic (see Chapter 42). When a bone lesion is present in a patient with syphilis, it may be necessary to do a bone biopsy if the lesion does not resolve rapidly after penicillin is given.

TUBERCULOSIS OF THE BONE:  Skeletal tuberculosis is almost always secondary to pulmonary tuberculosis, although the latter is not always discernible.  It usually presents with local pain, limitation of movement, night sweats and fever, and occasionally, weight loss.

In the United States and England, skeletal tuberculosis may have acute and toxic onset among imigrants, whereas among the natives, it often has an indolent onset.  The clinical signs and symptoms often precede the radiologic and the scintigraphic changes by five to six months.

The vertebral column is most frequently involved (Fig. 92), followed by the large joints, such as the hip (Fig. 93) and the knee.

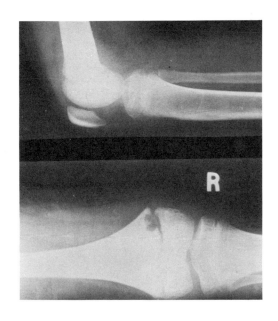

FIG. 89: Osteitis due to syphilis. Note the punched lesion on the femur and the periosteal thickening of the radius. (Courtesy of John Campbell, M.D., Charles R. Drew Postgraduate Medical School, Los Angeles, California)

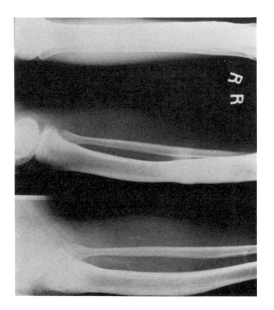

FIG. 88: Syphilitic osteomyelitis of the tibia. Note the marked periosteal thickening and outward curving of the tibia (saber tibia).

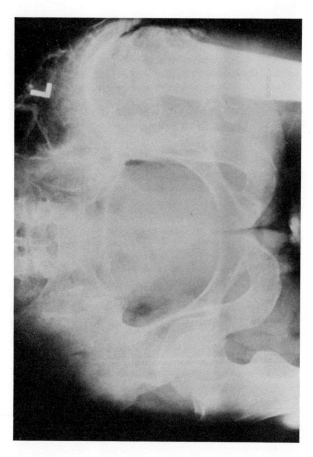

FIG. 90: Charcot joint of the left hip. Note the gross destruction of the head of femur, bony fragments in the joint capsule and displacement of the femur up, anteriorly and outward (triple displacement), without pain. (Courtesy of John Campbell, M.D., Charles R. Drew Postgraduate Medical School, Los Angeles, California)

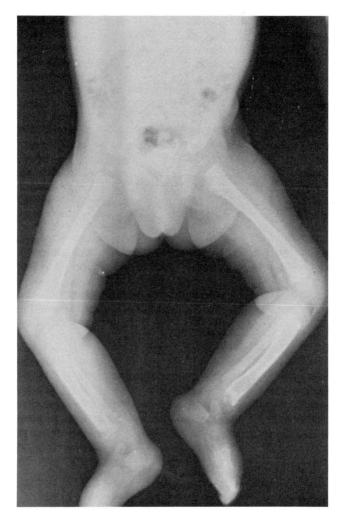

FIG. 91: Congenital syphilis.  Note the saber tibia, increased density of the bones.

The rib involvement is infrequent. The skull is rarely affected. Chronic low back pain is the most constant symptom of vertebral osteomyelitis. An unfortunate victim may present with paraplegia or nerve root compression secondary to cord compression by a cold abscess or granulomatous tissue (Fig. 94). On occasion, it can be due to thrombosis of the anterior spinal artery (endarteritis), when paraplegia may be acute in onset. Local tenderness of the spine and gibbous formation may be present. The cold abscess (Fig. 95) may be felt as a mass in the groin, nape of the neck, back, mass on the chest roentgenogram, or intra-abdominal mass. When it occurs in the deeper portions of the neck, the trachea and the esophagus might be displaced.

In children, the large joints, such as the hip and knee, are the most frequently affected. A sudden onset of pain in any of these major joints, preceded by even trivial trauma, should arouse the suspicion of tuberculosis. If it is associated with fever and chills, swelling and inability to move the joint, tuberculous arthritis is the most likely diagnosis, and every effort should be made to obtain proper cultures. Initially, tuberculous arthritis is clinically indistinguishable from other forms of septic arthritis.

Tuberculous dactylitis may present as rheumatoid arthritis. In tuberculous dactylitis, the fingers are extremely tender and fusiform in shape, with swelling at the mid-interphalangeal joint (Fig. 96). Tuberculosis may mimic the carpal tunnel syndrome by involving the tendinous sheets and the ligaments of the hand.

Investigations: Rarefaction of the bones, demineralization and destruction are characteristic of tuberculosis infection (Figs. 97, 98). It might occur in any bone in the body that is involved. A plain roentgenogram may reveal destruction of the vertebrae, the intervertebral joint and the intervertebral discs, with consequential narrowing of the joints and spaces, and wedging of the vertebrae. The intervertebral discs are rarely involved by the metastatic deposits and sickle cell disease, which distinguishes tuberculous spondylitis. The vertebral cold abscess may be mistaken for an aneurysm of the aorta by plain chest roentgenogram.

The supraclavicular masses, due to tuberculous lymphadenitis, may be mistaken for Hodgkin's disease. The iliac fossa abscess has been frequently mistaken for other abscesses and even for a hernial sac.

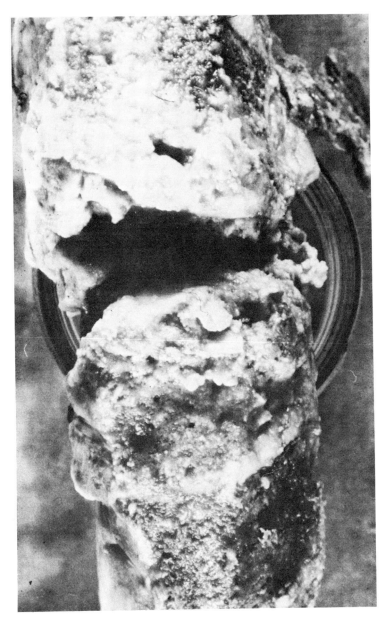

FIG. 92: Pott's disease of the spine.

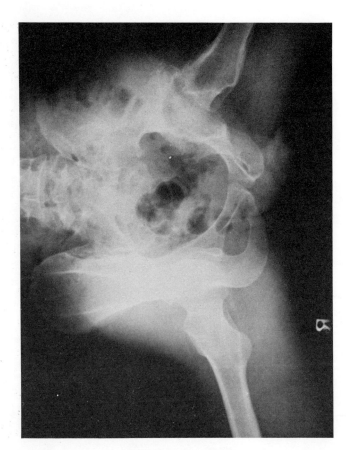

FIG. 93: Tuberculosis of the left hip and sacroiliac joint. Note the destruction of acetabulum and the head of the femur on the left.

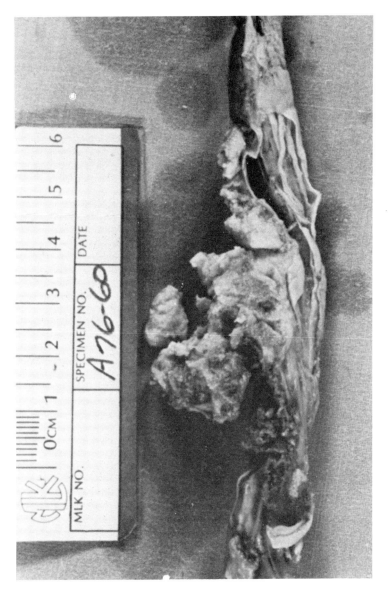

FIG. 94: Compression of the spinal cord by tuberculous caseous
material from vertebrae. The patient had paraplegia.

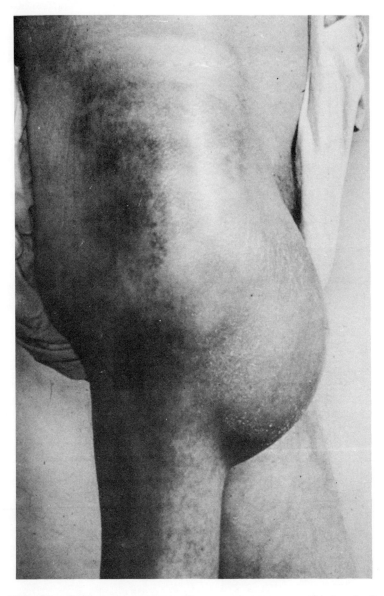

FIG. 95: Cold abscess presenting as a tumor over the front of the right thigh in a case of tuberculous osteomyelitis of the vertebrae.

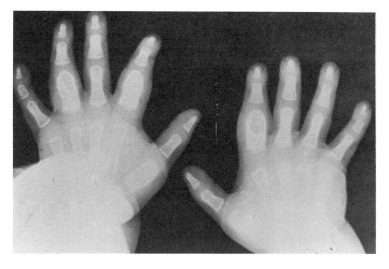

FIG. 96: Tuberculous dactylitis of the proximal phalanges of both hands in a child. Note the periosteal thickening and the lytic lesions in both hands.

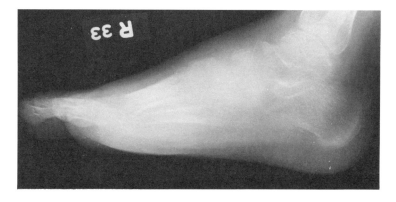

FIG. 97: Tuberculous osteomyelitis of the right tarsal bones. Note the evidence of rarefaction. Mycobacterium tuberculosis was isolated from the ankle joint needle aspirate.

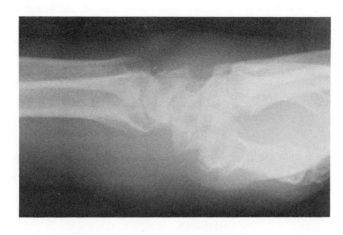

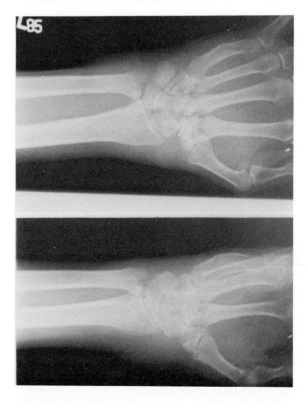

FIG. 98: Tuberculosis of the carpal bones. M. tuberculosis was cultured from the synovial fluid. Synovial biopsy was compatible with tuberculosis (posterior anterior and lateral views).

The diagnosis can be established by aspiration, biopsy of bone or by open surgical dissection. Sputum cultures are rarely positive unless the patient has concomitant pulmonary tuberculosis. The PPD skin test may be positive in only 30% to 40% of the patients.

Skeletal tuberculosis is most frequently caused by Mycobacterium tuberculosis and rarely, by atypical Mycobacteria.

Treatment: Bone tuberculosis, including Pott's disease of the spine, can be cured by ambulatory medical therapy. Surgical debridement, bone grafting and spika application with or without immobilization of the spine and hospitalization are unnecessary. INH and ethambutol are sufficient to treat skeletal tuberculosis; a third drug may be added if resistance is suspected.

FUNGAL OSTEOMYELITIS: Osteomyelitis can be caused by several of the fungi. Such infections are usually indolent and not associated with constitutional symptoms. These infections are seen more frequently in patients who are immunosuppressed.

Cryptococcus neoformans may rarely infect bone. The usual portal of entry is the lung, with hematogenous spread to the bone. Even more rare is primary infection of bone without involvement of other organs; this occurs as a result of direct inoculation of the organism in the bone. Swelling and pain of the involved area are usually present for months before the diagnosis is made. Often, a mass attached to underlying bone can be felt. Multiple bones are usually involved, although in rare cases, only one bone may be infected. Vertebrae, pelvis and ribs are most commonly involved. [13] Infection often spreads to the adjacent joint.

Coccidioides immitis invades the bone in about 20% of the cases of disseminated infection. Spread to a nearby joint frequently occurs. The bone lesions are usually multiple and have a predisposition for cancellous bone, especially bony prominences. Ribs, vertebral bodies and small bones of the hands and feet are usually involved. [14] The portal of entry is the lung, with hematogenous spread to bone. Osteomyelitis may be part of generalized dissemination, or may become apparent years after a primary infection, and represent reactivation of a latent focus.

Candida rarely invades the bone as part of disseminated infection. This infection occurs most frequently in "mainline" drug addicts and in patients predisposed to Candida infection by long courses of antibiotics, gastrointestinal surgery or central venous catheterization. The spine is the most common site for candida osteomyelitis.[15] Symptoms are insidious and may occur only months after an apparently benign candidemia. Signs of disseminated Candida infection may be present, such as eye or skin lesions (see Chapter 28).

Blastomyces dermatitidis may involve the bone; the lung is the portal of entry with hematogenous spread to the bone, either to cause symptoms immediately as part of disseminated disease, or years later, due to reactivation. Vertebrae, ribs and tibia are most often involved. Extension to a nearby joint frequently occurs. Skin involvement is common and there may be chronic draining disease.

Aspergillus species may involve bone as part of disseminated infection. Such patients are usually immunosuppressed with signs of Aspergillus infection elsewhere.

Histoplasma - although Histoplasma capsulatum may invade the bone marrow, involvement of the bone cortex is very rare and therefore, osteomyelitis is not a characteristic feature of histoplasmosis. On the other hand, Histoplasma duboisii, which causes African histoplasmosis, frequently produces multiple osteolytic lesions.

OSTEOMYELITIS IN DRUG ADDICTS: Osteomyelitis is a recently recognized complication of "mainline" drug abuse. [16] Hematogenous seeding in the bone may occur in these addicts who continually introduce unsterile material directly into their veins. Occasional cases are due to a contiguous source of infection, such as a needle fragment embedded in adjacent soft tissue. Hematogenous osteomyelitis in a drug addict often occurs in the spine or pelvis; long bone involvement is rare. Most infections are due to gram-negative bacteria; Pseudomonas is the most common organism involved (see Figs. 82-85, 87). Less commonly, such infections are due to S. aureus. A few cases due to Candida have been reported. Clinically, such patients do not appear very ill; their only complaint is localized pain and tenderness. Systemic symptoms are unusual. Fever, if present, is low-grade and the white blood cell count may be normal. The erythrocyte sedimentation rate is increased. Any drug addict who complains of back pain must be investigated for possible osteomyelitis. Although most drug addicts with osteomyelitis do not have endocarditis, it should be considered, as occasionally a septic embolus to the bone may arise from an infected heart valve.

HEMOGLOBINOPATHIES AND OSTEOMYELITIS: Patients with sickle cell disease have a special propensity for developing hematogenous osteomyelitis due to Salmonella (S.) species (usually S. cholerae-suis, S. paratyphi B, or S. typhimurium). In patients with sickle cell disease, about 90% of cases of osteomyelitis are due to Salmonella species, whereas such organisms account for less than 1% of the cases of osteomyelitis seen in patients who do not have a hemoglobinopathy. Salmonella osteomyelitis is also seen, with increased frequency, in other patients with hemoglobinopathies where chronic hemolysis occurs. The reason for this is not completely understood, but it appears that it is related to the decreased macrophage function found in such patients due to engorgement of cells of the reticuloendothelial system with pigment. Salmonella osteomyelitis may occur several months or even years after an apparent attack of Salmonella gastroenteritis. The initial attack may even be asymptomatic. It is theorized that hematogenous spread to the bone occurs during such an infection and then reactivates at a later date. Salmonella osteomyelitis is rarely associated with gastrointestinal complaints. Multiple bones are often involved in Salmonella osteomyelitis, most often the long and short tubular bones. The resultant pain may be hard to distinguish from sickle cell crisis, and scans may not be able to differentiate between the two. Therefore, all patients with sickle cell crisis should have blood cultures drawn, and if symptoms persist, bone aspirate or biopsy is indicated. Additionally, it has been reported that patients with hemoglobinopathies are also prone to develop osteomyelitis from other enterobacteriaceae, such as Shigella and Arizona species.

FOREIGN BODY OSTEOMYELITIS: Osteomyelitis may complicate bone surgery, especially if a foreign body is left in place. Prosthetic hip or knee replacement may be followed by osteomyelitis weeks or months later. [17] If prophylactic antibiotics are used at the time of surgery, several years may elapse before infection becomes apparent. The course is usually indolent, and increased pain in the involved area is the only symptom. The patient may give history of having had pain in the hip since surgery and having been unable to use it for weight bearing. Examination often reveals no sign of local inflammation. If present, fever is usually low-grade. Staphylococcus aureus is the predominant organism causing such infections; however, streptococci, gram-negative bacilli and even such normally non-invasive organisms as Staphylococcus epidermidis and diphtheroids may produce infection about a prosthesis. Cure of such infections usually involves removal of the prosthesis, as well as appropriate antibiotic therapy.

Fracture of the femur is often treated with an intramedullary nail. Early or late osteomyelitis may complicate such procedures. Multiple trauma, an open fracture and delay in surgery all lead to an increased incidence of infection.[18] The same organisms that cause prosthetic joint osteomyelitis are usually involved. Treatment involves prolonged antibiotic administration; the nail itself should not be removed, as non-union of the fracture and spread of the infection will result. Other fractures treated with metal plates may also be complicated by osteomyelitis; such metalware should not be removed until union of the fracture has taken place.

## TREATMENT

Treatment of osteomyelitis depends on the organism involved. Therefore, osteomyelitis should never be treated blindly until all cultures have been taken. In acute hematogenous osteomyelitis, early treatment is desirable if progression to chronic osteomyelitis is to be prevented. Therefore, antibiotics should be started as soon as cultures have been taken, based on the most likely etiologic agent (as determined by Gram's stain and clinical features). Treatment for four to six weeks with parenteral therapy (preferably a bactericidal agent) is optimal. The choice of drugs will depend on sensitivity tests.

Chronic osteomyelitis usually requires surgery for cure; all sequestra must be removed by saucerization. Parenteral antibiotics should be given for four weeks after such surgery and then continued by mouth for several months thereafter.

## REFERENCES

1. Waldrogel, F. A. , Medhoff, G. , Swartz, M. N. : Osteomyelitis: A review of clinical features, therapeutic considerations and unusual aspects. New Eng. J. Med. 282:198-206, 260-266, 316-322, 1970.

2. Steindler, A. : Osteomyelitis. Postgraduate Lectures on Orthopedic Diagnosis and Indications 3:167, 1952.

3. Handmaker, H. , Leonards, R. : Bone scan in inflammatory osseous disease. Seminar Nucl. Med. 6:95, 1976.

4. Shapiro, R. : Myelography. Year Book Medical Publishers, Chicago, 1975.

5. McHenry, M. C. , et al: Hematogenous osteomyelitis: A changing disease. Cleveland Clinic Quarterly 42:125, 1975.

6. Baker, A. S. , et al: Spinal epidural abscess. New Eng. J. Med. 293:463, 1975.

7. Brand, R. A. , Black, H. : Pseudomonas osteomyelitis following puncture wounds in children. J. Bone and Joint Surg. 56-A:1637, 1974.

8. Bell, O. B. , Marks, M. I. , Eickhoff, T. C. : Pasteurella multocida arthritis and osteomyelitis. J. A. M. A. 210:343, 1969.

9. Johnson, S. M. , Pankey, G. A. : Eikenella corrodens osteomyelitis, arthritis and cellulitis of the hand. South. Med. J. 69:535, 1976.

10. Meyers, B. R. , et al: Clinical patterns of osteomyelitis due to gram-negative bacteria. Arch. Int. Med. 131:228, 1973.

11. Meyer, R. , Finegold, S. : Anaerobic infections: Diagnosis and treatment. South. Med. J. 69:1178, 1976.

12. Dismukes, W. E. , et al: Destructive bone disease in early syphilis. J. A. M. A. 236:2646, 1976.

13. Chleboun, J. , Nade, S. : Skeletal cryptococcosis. J. Bone and Joint Surg. 59-A:509, 1977.

14. Bisla, B. S. , Taber, T. H. : Coccidioidomycosis of bone and joints. Clinical Orthopedics 121:196, 1976.

15. Edwards, J. E. , et al: Hematogenous Candida osteomyelitis. Am. J. Med. 59:89, 1975.

16. Holzman, R. S. , Bishko, F. : Osteomyelitis in heroin addicts. Ann. Int. Med. 75:693, 1971.

17. Wilson, P. O. , et al: The problem of infection in endoprosthetic surgery of the hip joint. Clinical Orthopedics 96:213, 1973.

18. Kovacs, A. J. , Richard, L. B. , Miller, J. : Infection complicating intramedullary nailing of the fractured femur. Clinical Orthopedics 96:266, 1973.

## 59: INFECTIOUS ARTHRITIS
by David W. Webb

### INTRODUCTION

Infectious arthritis is invasion of the synovial membrane with extension into the joint space. The infection can be bacterial, tuberculous, fungal or viral.

### PATHOGENESIS

There are three mechanisms whereby bacteria may reach the synovial membrane (Table 31). In hematogenous infectious arthritis, the microorganisms reach the joint via the bloodstream from a distant site of infection. This is the most common form of infectious arthritis. This can be a genital or urinary tract infection, pneumonia, meningitis, otitis media or skin or soft tissue infection. Rarely, acute endocarditis may lead to a septic arthritis as a result of high grade bacteremia. Infectious arthritis can also occur via direct extension from an adjacent bone or soft tissue infection. In children under one year and in adults, an osteomyelitis may spread to the adjacent joint. A gastrointestinal or genitourinary infection may spread directly to the hip by the retroperitoneal route and along the psoas muscle or through the sciatic notch. Finally, bacteria may gain access to the joint space directly, as by trauma, surgery or arthrocentesis.

### JOINTS INVOLVED

Any joint of the body can be involved by infectious arthritis. The infection is monoarticular in 80% of the cases and polyarticular in 20%. Bacterial arthritis most commonly involves the large joints, such as the hip, knee, shoulder, elbow and wrist. Small joints, such as the interphalangeals, are less commonly involved. Joint involvement in tuberculous, fungal and viral disease will be discussed separately.

### ETIOLOGY (Table 32)

Staphylococcus aureus is the most common cause of infectious arthritis, although gram-negative bacteria (E. coli, Proteus, Pseudomonas, Serratia and Salmonella) have recently increased in their incidence. In recent years, Streptococcus pyogenes and Streptococcus pneumoniae have been seen less commonly as a cause. Neonates are at special risk of arthritis due to

## TABLE 31: PATHOGENESIS OF INFECTIOUS ARTHRITIS

A. HEMATOGENOUS SPREAD FROM DISTANT INFECTION

Genital infection
Urinary tract infection
Pneumonia
Meningitis
Otitis media
Skin, soft tissue infection

B. EXTENSION FROM CONTIGUOUS INFECTION

Osteomyelitis
Skin, soft tissue infection
Gastrointestinal infection
Genitourinary infection

C. DIRECT INOCULATION INTO JOINT

Trauma
Surgery
Arthrocentesis

### TABLE 32: ETIOLOGY

| | |
|---|---|
| Staphylococcus aureus | 45% |
| Neisseria gonorrhoeae | 20%* |
| Streptococcus pyogenes | 10% |
| Streptococcus pneumoniae | 6% |
| Gram-negative | 12%** |
| Haemophilus influenzae | 5%*** |
| Neisseria meningitidis | < 1% |
| Anaerobic bacteria | < 1% |
| Treponema pallidum | < 1% |
| Brucella | < 1% |
| Chlamydiae | < 1% |

OTHERS: Fungal (Coccidioides, Blastomyces, Cryptococcus, Candida, Sporotrichum); Tuberculous (Mycobacterium tuberculosis and atypical Mycobacteria); Viral (Hepatitis B, rubella, mumps)

* Incidence much higher in sexually active, especially females
** Incidence much higher in neonates and the elderly
*** Incidence much higher age 6 months to 5 years

gram-negative enteric bacteria. Arthritis due to Haemophilus influenzae is the most common between six months and five years. In the sexually active female, Neisseria gonorrhoeae has become the most common cause for arthritis. Neisseria meningitidis, Brucella and Nocardia are infrequent causes for arthritis. Anaerobic bactoria have only rarely been implicated in the etiology of arthritis. Treponema pallidum rarely invades the joint space.

Tuberculous arthritis may be caused by Mycobacterium tuberculosis as well as the atypical Mycobacteria. Fungi that cause joint involvement include Cryptococcus, Coccidioides, Sporotrichum, Blastomyces and Candida. Of the viruses, rubella and hepatitis B virus are the most common causes.

## CLINICAL FEATURES

HOST FACTORS: Certain patients are predisposed towards developing infectious arthritis: 1

1) Prior arthritis in the affected joint; Arthritis of any type may predispose patients to develop infectious arthritis, although most commonly it is seen in patients with rheumatoid arthritis of long duration.

2) Heroin addiction: Intravenous drug abuse serves to introduce bacteria directly into the bloodstream.

3) Impaired host defenses: Those with diabetes mellitus, malignancy, cirrhosis of the liver and those receiving steroids or other immunosuppressive agents are at special risk.

## SIGNS AND SYMPTOMS

Classical manifestations of infectious arthritis are pain, stiffness and inflammation of the affected joint. The pain is aggravated by the slightest movement of the joint, so the patient often holds the joint immobile. The joint is exquisitely tender to the touch. Signs of inflammation are usually present; the joint is swollen, erythematous and warm to the touch. Such signs may be absent in patients receiving steroids or other immunosuppressive agents. An effusion may or may not be detectable, but soft tissue swelling will always be present. Signs of tenosynovitis are rare, except in gonococcal arthritis. Deep joints, such as the shoulders and hips, may show no outward signs of inflammation because of the overlying musculature. Pain on rotation may be the only sign. Whenever a patient presents with complaints referred to one joint, all of his joints must be carefully examined for any swelling, tenderness or limitation of motion.

Systemic manifestations of infection, such as fever and chills, are often present, although they may be absent in tuberculous or fungal infection.

The signs of infectious arthritis are not specific and can be mimicked by non-infectious forms of arthritis, where active inflammation of the synovium is taking place, such as rheumatoid arthritis and gout. Patients with rheumatoid arthritis classically present with a symmetrical polyarticular arthritis, but at times monoarticular symptoms may predominate. Such patients may also have fever (although chills are unusual), so clinical differentiation from infectious arthritis can be very difficult.

## DIAGNOSIS

BLOOD TEST: A complete blood count should always be done. The white blood cell count will be elevated, and there will be a shift of the granulocytes to the left in most cases of bacterial arthritis. The white cell count is normal in most cases of tuberculous and fungal arthritis. The erythrocyte sedimentation rate is usually elevated. Both leukocytosis and elevated erythrocyte sedimentation rate can also occur in cases of non-infectious inflammatory arthritis.

Other causes of arthritis should be ruled out by obtaining appropriate studies. Tests for antinuclear antibodies and rheumatoid factor should be done. The uric acid should be measured. A VDRL should be done and, if positive, a fluorescent treponemal antibody absorption test should be done because of the high incidence of biologically false reagin tests in patients with arthritis. The antistreptolysin-O titer should be measured if rheumatic fever is being considered. If Reiter's syndrome is being considered, histocompatibility testing should be done for the HLA-B27 antigen, which is present in most cases.

SKIN TEST: A PPD should be placed on all patients with arthritis of unknown etiology.

ROENTGENOGRAMS: Whenever signs of arthritis are present, an x-ray should be taken of the involved joint. Such radiologic examination of the involved joint is helpful but not diagnostic. Surrounding soft tissue swelling and distention of the joint space are early clues and are followed much later by destruction of the joint space with loss of subchondral bone. These x-ray findings are non-specific and similar findings may be seen in other types of inflammatory arthritis.

BONE SCAN: Technetium-99m bone scanning is described in Chapter 58. Such scans show increased uptake in cases of infectious arthritis and usually become positive during the first week of infection, before x-ray findings are seen. Unfortunately, the test is not specific, and increased uptake may also be seen in most cases of inflammatory arthritis (rheumatoid arthritis, gout, etc.) as well as non-inflammatory arthritis (trauma, degenerative joint disease). A positive bone scan indicates that an abnormality of the joint is present and that further diagnostic tests are indicated.

GALLIUM SCAN: Scanning with gallium-67 has been described in Chapter 58. These scans may be positive very early in the course of infection, sometimes long before any changes can be noted in the x-ray and bone scan. However, it is not specific and will be positive in any arthritis with active inflammation such as gout, rheumatoid arthritis, and early osteoarthritis.

ARTHROCENTESIS: The only means of reliably establishing the diagnosis of infectious arthritis is by arthrocentesis, and this should be done in all patients in whom infection is suspected. Arthrocentesis should be done as part of the initial work-up; results of blood tests and scans should not be waited for.

Arthrocentesis involves insertion of a needle into the joint space and the removal of synovial fluid for examination. Strict aseptic technique must always be observed, lest infection be introduced into the joint. Arthrocentesis is not recommended if there is overlying cellulitis on the joint.

The knee is one of the most accessible sites for arthrocentesis. The procedure is carried out with the patient lying flat with the knee extended. The skin is infiltrated with a local anesthetic, such as 1% lidocaine, and a 19-gauge needle is inserted medially into the space behind the patella (Fig. 99). Fluid is then aspirated via a large syringe; it is desirable to evacuate all fluid from the joint.

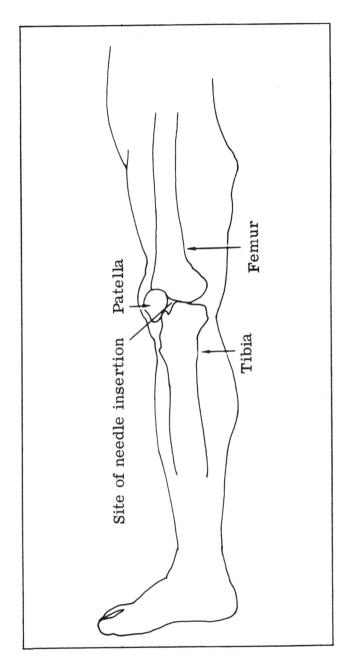

FIG. 99: Anatomy of the knee joint, depicting the site for needle insertion for joint aspiration.

SYNOVIAL FLUID ANALYSIS:  The following tests should be performed on all samples of synovial fluid [2] (Table 33):

1) Gross inspection:  The fluid is usually turbid in infectious arthritis.  Turbid fluid will also be found in other causes of inflammatory joint disease, such as gout and rheumatoid arthritis.  Normally, and in cases of degenerative or traumatic arthritis, the fluid is clear and straw-colored.

2) Viscosity:  Dripping a few drops of joint fluid from a syringe normally produces a sticky strand over 6 cm. long.  This will be decreased in inflammatory arthritis.

3) Mucin clot:  This is basically another test for viscosity.  The fluid is centrifuged and a few drops of the supernatant are added to a beaker containing 20 ml. of 5% acetic acid.  Normally, a tight rope-like clot will form in one minute.  Mucin clot formation is poor in inflammatory joint disease.

4) Fibrin clot:  Normal joint fluid does not clot when allowed to stand in a test tube for one hour.  However, in inflammatory joint disease, a fibrin clot will form.

5) Glucose:  A simultaneous blood glucose should also be measured.  Normal joint fluid has a glucose about 90% of blood glucose.  In inflammatory joint disease, the glucose is usually less than 60% of blood glucose.  In infectious arthritis, the synovial glucose may be extremely low.

6) Cell count and differential:  A total white cell count and differential must always be done.  Normally, less than 200 cells, mostly mononuclear, are present.  In bacterial arthritis, very high counts may be seen, usually with more than 80% polymorphonuclear.  In rheumatoid arthritis and gout, high counts may also be seen, with a predominance of polymorphs.  In general, the higher the cell count, the more likely the arthritis is bacterial.  In tuberculous or fungal arthritis, less cells are usually seen and there is usually a predominance of mononuclear cells, although in some cases, up to 90% may be polymorphs.  In viral arthritis, the cell counts are low and mostly mononuclear.

7) Polarizing microscope:  Anticoagulated joint fluid should be examined under the polarizing microscope for the appearance of crystals, indicative of gout or pseudogout.

TABLE 33: SYNOVIAL FLUID ANALYSIS

| | Normal | Trauma/ Degenerative | Inflammatory Arthritis | Bacterial Infection | Tuberculous and Fungal Infection |
|---|---|---|---|---|---|
| Appearance | Straw | Straw or hemorrhagic | Turbid | Turbid, purulent | Turbid |
| Viscosity | High | High | Low | Low | Low |
| Mucin Clot | Good | Good | Poor | Poor | Poor |
| Fibrin Clot | None | Small | Large | Large | Large |
| Glucose | Normal | Normal | Low | Very low | Very low |
| Cells (WBC) | <200 | Usually <2,000 | Usually 1,000 to 70,000 | Usually 5,000 to 300,000 | Usually 10,000 to 25,000 |
| Per cent Polymorphs | <25 | <25 | >50 | >75 | Usually<50 (may be high) |

8) <u>Complement</u>: Normal joint fluid complement is low as compared to serum complement. In arthritis, the joint fluid complement may be high. However, in active rheumatoid arthritis and occasionally in infectious arthritis, the joint fluid complement may be very low. In hepatitis B viral arthritis, the joint fluid complement is characteristically low. Joint fluid complement is normal in gout.

9) <u>Stains</u>: Both a Gram's stain and Ziehl-Neelsen stain should be done. In bacterial arthritis, the Gram's stain will be positive in 75% of the cases and in tuberculous arthritis, the Ziehl-Neelsen smear will be positive in 19% of the cases.

10) <u>Cultures</u>: Aerobic, anaerobic, tuberculous and fungal cultures should be done. At the bedside, fluid should be plated on Thayer-Martin media if gonococcal arthritis is a possibility.

The following two tests are not generally available, but may be helpful in making an early diagnosis:

11) <u>Counterimmunoelectrophoresis</u>: This is a test for small amounts of capsular antigen of specific bacteria. It appears to be a promising new technique that can identify specific bacteria in joint fluid in a matter of hours.

12) NBT test: The nitroblue tetrazolium test measures the ability of white cells to phagocytize NBT; increased numbers of NBT positive cells are seen in the joint fluid of patients with pyogenic arthritis, but not in patients with rheumatoid arthritis or gout.[3]

SYNOVIAL BIOPSY: A synovial biopsy is usually not needed to diagnose acute bacterial arthritis. However, this procedure is very helpful in cases in which synovial fluid analysis and culture have not yielded a diagnosis, and whenever tuberculous or fungal arthritis is suspected. This procedure can now be done percutaneously by means of the Parker-Pearson needle.[4] The technique is the same as described for arthrocentesis, except that after joint fluid is removed for study, the trochar of the Parker-Pearson needle is inserted into the joint space and several biopsies taken by means of a hooked biopsy needle, which is inserted through the trochar. With this technique, open synovial biopsy should not be required, except in cases where

repeated needle biopsy does not yield a diagnosis. Open synovial biopsy involves surgical synovectomy; a large amount of
tissue can be obtained for study. A needle biopsy is less invasive and is preferable in most cases.

The sample of tissue is examined histologically (for granulomas, etc.) and cultured in the same manner as described in
Chapter 58, the section on bone biopsy.

CULTURES OF OTHER SITES: Three sets of blood cultures
should be obtained in all cases before antibiotics are started.
Nearly a third of the patients with bacterial arthritis will have
positive blood cultures. Cultures of other infected sites should
be taken, i.e., skin, sputum, urine, cerebrospinal fluid or
stool, if symptoms referrable to these areas are present.
Cervical, urethral, rectal and pharyngeal cultures for gonococcus should be taken in all sexually active persons, even if
no specific symptoms are present.  These specimens should
be plated on Thayer-Martin media immediately.

## SPECIFIC ETIOLOGIC AGENTS

STAPHYLOCOCCAL ARTHRITIS: Overall, Staphylococcus
aureus is the most common cause of infectious arthritis. Most
cases are due to hematogenous spread from a distant focus of
infection. The primary infection is usually a skin or soft tissue infection, although any infection may serve as the source.
Staphylococcal endocarditis may be complicated by infectious
arthritis. Intravenous drug addicts may develop infectious arthritis due to indirect injection of bacteria into their bloodstream.
The onset of illness is usually abrupt with constitutional symptoms, such as chills and fever, being prominent. The infected
joint is painful and signs of inflammation are conspicuous. The
larger joints are most frequently involved, although any joint
may be involved. About 15% of the cases are polyarticular.

GONOCOCCAL ARTHRITIS: Arthritis due to Neisseria gonorrhoeae is seen most often in females (80% of cases). It is most
often associated with asymptomatic endocervical, rectal or
pharyngeal infection. It occurs more frequently during menses
or pregnancy. Gonococcal arthritis occurs in two syndromes.[5]
The first syndrome which is associated with gonococcal bacteremia begins with fever, chills and a polyarthritis, which may
be migratory. It often involves the wrist, elbow, knees and ankles. Tenosynovitis, when it occurs, is a characteristic, but
not invariable, feature. Skin lesions are a common accompaniment; they are usually located on the distal areas of the

extremities. These lesions are often few in number and seldom as prodigious as in meningococcemia. They may appear as macules, papules, vesicles or bullae. They usually begin as papules and later become pustules with a necrotic center.

The second syndrome is seen as a monoarticular "septic" arthritis in which one joint develops pain and signs of inflammation. Skin lesions are not characteristic of this syndrome. These two syndromes represent the two ends of a clinical spectrum; intermediate forms can occur. Gonococcal arthritis may begin with the signs and symptoms of the first syndrome and end in the second, as described.

It is important to always suspect gonococcal arthritis when joint symptoms occur in a sexually active patient, especially a female. Culture of the endocervix, pharynx, rectum and, in the male, the urethra, must be taken. Blood cultures are often positive in the polyarticular stage, although joint fluid cultures are often negative. In the monoarticular stage, blood cultures may be negative, but the joint fluid cultures are often positive. Although the skin lesions may seem to be an obvious source to recover the gonococcus, they are rarely positive.

GRAM-NEGATIVE ARTHRITIS: In recent years, there has been an increased incidence of infectious arthritis due to gram-negative bacteria, such as E. coli, Serratia, Pseudomonas, Klebsiella, Proteus and Salmonella. About two-thirds of patients with gram-negative arthritis have some underlying condition predisposing them to such infection. Gram-negative arthritis is common in neonates. Patients with malignancy, diabetes mellitus, sickle cell disease, heroin addiction, and those with pre-existing joint disease, usually long-standing rheumatoid arthritis, are at special risk. Most cases are due to hematogenous spread from a distant focus of infection, such as the urinary tract or, less commonly, a pulmonary, skin or gastrointestinal tract infection. Direct introduction of the organism into the joint space, as may occur in trauma, surgery or arthrocentesis may result in arthritis. Gram-negative arthritis is almost always monoarticular, usually involving the knee or, less commonly, the hip or shoulder.[6]

Clinical findings of gram-negative arthritis are not distinctive. Most patients have fever and about half have chills. Leukocytosis is usual, except in patients receiving immunosuppressive drugs. Pain and inflammation of the involved joint are usually prominent, although signs of inflammation may be absent in patients on immunosuppressive drugs.

Diagnosis depends on culturing the involved organism from the synovial fluid. Pseudomonas is most frequently isolated from the patients with malignancy and from drug addicts. Salmonella is most commonly seen in patients with sickle cell anemia.

PNEUMOCOCCAL ARTHRITIS: Streptococcus pneumoniae accounts for about 6% of all cases of infectious arthritis. Hematogenous spread to the joint from a primary pneumonia is the usual cause, although occasional cases are secondary to hematogenous spread from an extrapulmonary source. Only 0.3% of pneumonias are complicated by infectious arthritis. [7] Pneumococcal arthritis may also arise from direct extension of a pneumococcal osteomyelitis into the joint. So-called cryptogenic pneumococcal arthritis arises without a discernible pneumococcal infection elsewhere in the body.

ANAEROBIC ARTHRITIS: Infectious arthritis due to anaerobic bacteria is rare but may be underestimated, because of inadequate anaerobic culture techniques. Immunosuppressed patients and those with underlying joint disease are especially predisposed to anaerobic arthritis. Most cases are hematogenous from a primary pulmonary infection. Larger joints, such as the hip and knee, are usually involved, although the sternoclavicular and sacroiliac joints seem predisposed to anaerobic arthritis. Clinical clues are foul-smelling joint fluid and gas in the joint space. Diagnosis may be established by anaerobic cultures of the synovial fluid. Most reported cases have been due to Fusobacterium necrophorum,[8] although Bacteroides species, Peptococci and Peptostreptococci may also be involved.

MENINGOCOCCAL ARTHRITIS: Neisseria meningitidis infection may involve the joints. Suppurative infection of one or more joints may occur in meningeal infection or in meningococcemia. A polyarticular immune complex arthritis may occur during treatment of meningitis. Furthermore, a chronic or recurrent meningococcemia may manifest as episodic fever and chills with arthralgias. A maculopapular rash is present in many of the cases.

SYPHILITIC ARTHRITIS: Modern antibiotic therapy has caused a decreased incidence of syphilitic arthritis. Syphilitic arthritis may be a manifestation of congenital, secondary or tertiary infection. Most cases are congenital; direct invasion of the synovium by Treponema pallidum is uncommon. [9] Acute osteochondritis usually occurs in the first few weeks of life and involves the shoulder. The shoulder is painful and swollen, resulting in so-called Parrot's pseudoparalysis of the arm. Clutton's joints occur during puberty and are swollen, tender knees inflamed by a synovitis.

Secondary syphilis may be complicated by a migratory polyarthritis. Tertiary syphilis may be complicated by gummas of the synovium. Charcot's joints (see Fig. 90, page 469) are joints damaged by wear and tear due to a neuropathy, and do not represent infection of the joint by Treponema pallidum.

TUBERCULOUS ARTHRITIS:  Tuberculous arthritis differs from other bacterial arthritis in that it is insidious in onset.  The patient may have no fever, at worst, slight discomfort of the joint on motion and minimal swelling of the joint.  As a rule, tuberculosis involves only one joint, usually the knee, wrist or hip.  Other joints such as the elbow, shoulder and small joints of the hands and feet are less commonly involved.[10]  The patient often attributes the joint pain to a recent minor trauma and may even impress the physician that such is the case.  Much less than one-half of the patients may have obvious pulmonary tuberculosis. Granulomas may be seen on the chest roentgenogram.  A small number may have tuberculosis of the genitourinary tract or lymph nodes.  Some may have no other evidence of tuberculosis other than joint involvement.  Tuberculous arthritis may represent reactivation of a latent infection in the joints. Bacillemia which occurs in primary tuberculosis may seed the joint and remain dormant for years, only to reactivate when host defenses are suppressed.

Arthrocentesis and synovial biopsy should be carried out in all suspected cases.  Acid-fast smears of the joint fluid will be positive in 19% of cases, and culture of the fluid will be positive in about 80% of cases.  The biopsy specimen will show caseating granulomas in 94%, and culture of the synovium will be positive in 94% of cases.[11]  It is important that cultures be done to differentiate atypical Mycobacteria that may produce arthritis from Mycobacterium tuberculosis.

FUNGAL ARTHRITIS: Fungal arthritis often presents as a chronic, indolent infection, like tuberculous arthritis. Coccidioides, Blastomyces, Cryptococcus, Candida, Sporotrichum and, less commonly, Histoplasma and Aspergillus may all invade the joint.

Coccidioides immitis: A mono- or polyarticular arthritis
occurs with erythema nodosum in primary coccidioidomycosis
as a manifestation of "valley fever", which is temporary and
leaves no residual damage. Alternatively, a joint may be directly invaded by the fungus, as occurs in disseminated coccidioidomycosis (see Figs. 145, 146, pages 796 and 797). Osteomyelitis of an adjacent long bone is often present, although isolated joint involvement may also occur.[12] A single joint is
usually involved, most commonly the knee. Arthritis can occur
without obvious pulmonary involvement. Such patients have no
fever, and pain is the only symptom. Roentgenograms and joint
fluid examinations are not characteristic. Diagnosis depends on
synovial biopsy and culturing Coccidioides from the tissue. Cultures of the synovial fluid are less likely to yield the fungus.[13]

Blastomyces dermatitidis: Blastomycosis may be complicated
by hematogenous spread to the joint space. Arthritis may also
occur secondary to direct extension from an adjacent osteomyelitis. The larger joints of the lower extremities are most
commonly involved.[14] Evidence of pulmonary infection is usually apparent; most patients also have evidence of skin involvement. When arthritis occurs in such a setting, the diagnosis
will usually be apparent. The fungus can usually be cultured
from the joint fluid. Synovial biopsy is indicated only when the
diagnosis cannot otherwise be made.

Cryptococcus neoformans: Cryptococcal infection of a joint
is usually secondary to a contiguous osteomyelitis (see Chapter
58, pages 443-481).

Candida: Candida arthritis often occurs in association with
disseminated candidiasis. It may present as a delayed manifestation of transient candidemia, for example, from an infected CVP line and no other signs of Candida infection may
be apparent at that time. Candida arthritis is often polyarticular, affecting the larger joints of the lower extremities.[15]
Most of those patients are debilitated by either a significant
underlying disease or by immunosuppressive therapy. Clinical features are joint pain and swelling; local signs of inflammation are rare. Joint fluid examination often shows
a predominance of polymorphonuclear leukocytes, in contrast to the lymphocytic response usually seen in other types
of fungal arthritis. The organism can usually be cultured
from the joint fluid, making synovial biopsy unnecessary in
most cases.

Sporotrichum schenckii: This organism may gain access to the joint either by contiguous spread from a cutaneous infection, or by hematogenous spread in disseminated infection. Elderly patients are most often infected; disseminated infection is more common in immunosuppressed patients. Chronic pain and swelling of the joint are usually the only symptoms. Fever is rare. The most commonly involved joints are the knee, ankle, wrist and elbow. In disseminated disease, multiple joints may be involved. Diagnosis is made by synovial biopsy and culture of the tissue. Open biopsy may be necessary, as experience with needle biopsy in this disease is limited. [16]

Histoplasma capsulatum: Rarely, an allergic type polyarthritis may be seen as a manifestation of primary histoplasmosis.[17] Actually, invasion of the joint by Histoplasma is rare. [18]

Aspergillus: Disseminated aspergillosis may be complicated by infection of the joint. Such patients are usually immunosuppressed and have signs of Aspergillus infection elsewhere.

VIRAL ARTHRITIS: Hepatitis B infection is occasionally associated with a serum sickness type polyarticular arthritis due to circulating immune complexes; such complexes fix complement, and the serum and joint fluid complement are characteristically low. The arthritis is usually symmetrical and may be migratory. Both small and large joints may be involved. A variety of skin lesions, such as urticaria, petechiae and maculopapular eruptions may also occur concomitantly with arthritis. This arthritis usually appears before the onset of jaundice, and vanishes within a week, leaving behind no residual joint damage.

Rubella is accompanied by a polyarticular arthritis in about 20% of the cases. This occurs more commonly in females. The arthritis usually appears after the rash. It is symmetrical and polyarticular, commonly involving the small joints of the hands, the knees and the wrists. The arthritis resolves within one to two weeks, leaving no residual damage.

Mumps rarely causes an arthritis. This arthritis is more common in older males and involves the large joints. Parotid enlargement is present in most, but not all, cases. The arthritis lasts from two days to three months and leaves no residual damage. [19]

Other viruses that have rarely been associated with arthritis include smallpox, rubeola, varicella, influenza and enteroviruses. [20] Two arboviruses seen only in Africa cause a syndrome characterized by fever, arthritis and a morbilliform rash. These are Chikungyunya and O'nyong-nyong diseases.

## UNUSUAL CAUSES OF ARTHRITIS

Chlamydiae may rarely cause arthritis. Both psittacosis and lymphogranuloma venereum may be associated with a polyarthritis. [20] Both Chlamydiae and Mycoplasma have been suspected of causing Reiter's syndrome, but this has never been proved. It is known that Mycoplasma pneumoniae infections may be associated with a migratory polyarticular arthritis involving the larger joints. No residual damage to the joints results. [21]

Brucella infection may be accompanied by a transient polyarthritis. Several months after the acute infection, pain and stillness of a single joint (usually hip or sacroiliac) may occur. This represents a true infectious arthritis. Spondylitis also occurs commonly in these patients.

Leptospirosis and rat bite fever can be complicated by a polyarthritis. The course of such patients is dominated by other manifestations of their infection.

Nocardia are rare causes of arthritis, usually as a part of disseminated infection.

## THERAPY

Infectious arthritis due to bacteria requires both antibiotic treatment and drainage for cure. Bactericidal antibiotics should be given parenterally in full doses based on the sensitivity testing of the involved organism. Usually, treatment is continued for four weeks; two weeks is usually adequate for gonococcal infection. Drainage of the involved joint is carried out by daily aspiration of the joint; the joint should be tapped dry. Open surgical drainage of the hip is usually indicated because of the difficulty in repeated aspiration of this joint. In addition, open drainage may be needed if the infection is more than four to seven days old at the time arthrocentesis is first performed. It is controversial whether intra-articular injection of antibiotics is indicated.

Tuberculous arthritis can be medically treated, usually with two drug therapy, although some physicians prefer "triple therapy" until sensitivity results are available.

Fungal arthritis can be very difficult to treat. Amphotericin B is the drug of choice when the joint is actually invaded by the fungus. Surgical debridement is often necessary.

## REFERENCES

1. Goldenberg, D. L. , Cohen, A. S.: Acute infectious arthritis. Am. J. Med. 60:369, 1976.

2. Davidson, J. , Henry, J. B.: Todd-Sanford Clinical Diagnosis, 15th Edition. W. B. Saunders, Philadelphia, 1974.

3. Gupta, R. C. , Steigerwood, J. C.: Nitroblue tetrazolium test in the diagnosis of pyogenic arthritis. Ann. Int. Med. 80:723, 1974.

4. Schumacher, H. R. , Kulka, J. P.: Needle biopsy of the synovial membrane - experience with the Parker-Pearson technic. New Eng. J. Med. 286:416, 1972.

5. Holmes, K. K. , Counts, G. W. , Beaty, H. N.: Disseminated gonococcal infection. Ann. Int. Med. 74:979, 1971.

6. Goldenberg, D.L. , et al.: Acute arthritis caused by gram-negative bacilli: A clinical characterization. Medicine 53: 197, 1974.

7. Jaffe, H. L.: Metabolic, Degenerative and Inflammatory Diseases of Bones and Joints. Lea and Febiger, Philadelphia, 1972.

8. Ziment, I. , David, A. , Finegold, S. M.: Joint infection by anaerobic bacteria: A case report and review of the literature. Arthritis Rheum. 12:627, 1969.

9. Rodnan, G. P. , McEwen, C. , Wallace, S. L.: Primer on the Rheumatic Diseases. The Arthritis Foundation, New York, 1973.

10. Berney, S. , Goldstein, M. , Bishko, F.: Clinical and diagnostic features of tuberculous arthritis. Am. J. Med. 53: 36, 1972.

11. Wallace, R. , Cohen, A. S.: Tuberculous arthritis: A report of two cases with review of biopsy and synovial fluid findings. Am. J. Med. 61:277, 1976.

12. Bayer, A. S. , et al. : Unusual syndromes of coccidioido-
    mycosis: Diagnostic and therapeutic considerations. Med-
    icine 55:131, 1976.

13. Greenman, R. , et al. : Coccidioidal synovitis of the knee.
    Arch. Int. Med. 135:526, 1975.

14. Fountain, F. F. : Acute blastomycotic arthritis. Arch. Int.
    Med. 132:684, 1973.

15. Murray, H. W. , Fialk, M. A. , Roberts, R. B. : Candida
    arthritis. A manifestation of disseminated candidiasis.
    Am. J. Med. 60:587, 1976.

16. Crout, J. E. , Brewer, N. S. , Tompkins, R. B. : Sporo-
    trichosis arthritis. Ann. Int. Med. 86:294, 1977.

17. Class, R. N. : Histoplasmosis presenting as acute poly-
    arthritis. New Eng. J. Med. 287:1133, 1972.

18. Vanek, J. V. , and Schwarz, J. : The gamut of histoplas-
    mosis. Am. J. Med. 50:89, 1971.

19. Smith, L. H. , Wilkes, R. M. : Arthritis caused by viruses.
    Medical Staff Conference, University of California, San
    Francisco. California Med. 119:38, 1973.

20. Smith, J. W. , Sanford, J. P. : Viral arthritis. Ann. Int.
    Med. 67:651, 1967.

21. Murray, H. W. , et al. : The protean manifestations of My-
    coplasma pneumoniae infection in adults. Am. J. Med. 58:
    229, 1975.

# SECTION H: INFECTIONS OF THE LYMPHATIC SYSTEM

## 60: ANTHRAX
by H. Thadepalli

Anthrax is caused by <u>Bacillus anthracis</u>, a spore-forming, non-motile, gram-positive aerobic organism of size 3 to $7\mu$ x $1\mu$. They are found in pairs or chains with a centrally located elliptoid spore.

## CLINICAL FEATURES

Anthrax starts with a small, pimple-sized cutaneous lesion of 3 to 5 mm. in size, which, in a day or two, becomes surrounded by several satellite vesicles. It later turns bluish to dark color before it ulcerates within a day or two. The incubation period is less than seven days. The cutaneous ulcer caused by anthrax is characteristically black in color [anthracos = black (Greek)] and it almost never suppurates. [1] The ulcer itself is rarely larger than one-half to one inch in diameter, but the surrounding inflammatory reaction may vary from two to three inches. In severe cases, it may spread all over the trunk, the limbs and the scrotum. In spite of the severity of the surrounding inflammation, the ulcer remains relatively painless. Regional lymph nodes are often enlarged.

Fever (101° to 102° F.) and chills, occasionally rigors, malaise, anorexia, nausea and vomiting are some of its accompanying symptoms. The majority of patients are asymptomatic.

## PULMONARY ANTHRAX

This is caused by inhalation of the spores, resulting in a severe fulminating form of pneumonia resembling the post-viral staphylococcal pneumonia with mediastinitis or pleural effusions. Pulmonary anthrax is fatal in most cases within two to three days.

## OCCUPATION

Anthrax is a disease of herbivorous animals, i.e., cattle, goats, sheep and the like. It is not a disease of dogs and cats. The disease is acquired by exposure to the infected animals or their products, such as bone and fish meal, hides, handcrafts, rugs, bongo drums, etc. [2]. Imported yarn was also implicated.

## DIAGNOSIS

This is established by the demonstration of the thick gram-positive bacilli central-spore-bearing (literally the "big black bacillus") from the serous exudates of the ulcer, and by culture. The eschar should be removed from the top of the ulcer, and smears for Gram's stain are obtained from the base of the ulcer. Blood cultures may also be positive.

## TREATMENT

Penicillin is the treatment of choice; two million units, administered intravenously every six hours for five days. [3] Administration of a single dose of two million units eradicates the organism from the cutaneous ulcers in five to six hours. Rough handling and surgical intervention should be avoided. Anthrax antitoxin has no place in the therapy. Steroids are of debatable value.

## REFERENCES

1. Christie, A. B.: Infectious Diseases. E&S Livingstone Ltd., London, 1969.

2. Lamb, R.: Anthrax. Brit. Med. J. 1:157, 1973.

3. Ronaghy, H. A., et al.: Penicillin therapy of human cutaneous anthrax. Current Therapeutic Research 14:721, 1972.

## 61: BARTONELLOSIS
## by H. Thadepalli

Bartonellosis may present in one of the two clinical forms:

A) Oroya fever
B) Verruca peruviana

A) OROYA FEVER: This is characterized by macrocytic hypochromic anemia, associated with a somewhat irregular fever, occasionally rising to 100° to 101°F. During the late stages, the patient may develop body pains and hepatosplenomegaly. Untreated Oroya fever is highly fatal; nearly 50% of the patients die in two to four weeks.

B) VERRUCA PERUVIANA: This is a cutaneous form of bartonellosis which might occur either by itself or as an end stage of Oroya fever. It begins two or three weeks after the subsidence of Oroya fever. It is characterized by the verrucous lesions which look like multiple hemangiomas or nodular lesions in yaws, or like multiple neurofibromatosis. They are often miliary when they occur on the face; they can involve the skin of the extremities, and occasionally the buccal mucous membranes. The entire disease may run for two to three weeks. At the end, the skin lesions may drop off, leaving no scar.

Oroya fever and verruca peruviana are caused by the same organism; this was established by a medical student in Peru by the name of Carrion, after whom the disease is named.

### THE ORGANISM

Bartonella bacilliformis, a gram-negative, aerobic bacteria, of size $2\mu$ x $0.5\mu$, is an intra-erythrocytic organism which may look like a "V" or a "Y" because of the type of arrangement of these diplobacilla, either side by side, or in pairs, or one behind the other. On Giemsa stain, it shows a deep red or purplish granule, the rest of the organism staining somewhat bluish. It grows well within seven days at 28°C. on nutrient agar with 10% rabbit serum and 5% rabbit hemoglobin. It is transmitted by the sandfly called Lutzomyia verrucarum., which is native to Peru.

## DIAGNOSIS

Bartonellosis is a geographic disease limited exclusively to South America, occurring in the river valleys and canyons of Peru, Ecuador and Columbia at 800 to 3,000 meters above sea level.

1) Blood smears may show macrocytic, hypochromic anemia with intra-erythrocytic organisms and relative leukocytosis.

2) Cultures of the blood, and cultures from the verruca obtained from the verrucous lesions, are positive for the organism.

## DIFFERENTIAL

Carrion's disease should be differentiated from malaria and multiple neurofibromatosis by blood smears and by culture of the skin nodules.

## 62:  BRUCELLOSIS
by H.  Thadepalli

Brucella (Br. ) is a coccobacillary pleomorphic bacteria of size 0.6 to $1.5_\mu$ x 0.5 to $0.7\mu$. It is urease-, catalase-, nitrate- and oxidase-positive and citrate-negative. It does not ferment carbohydrates and may take nearly 21 days to grow. It causes undulant fever, a fever, as its name suggests, characterized by intermittent periods of remission and relapse, each lasting for a week or two. There are four species of clinical importance:

1) Br. melitensis (melita = honey island, now called Malta), a disease of the goats
2) Br. abortus, a disease causing abortions in cattle
3) Br. suis, a disease of the hog, and
4) Br. canis, a disease of the dog

The disease is acquired by close contact with the infected animals or their carcasses (as in the abattoirs), and by drinking raw milk or by inhalation. Brucellosis is not transmitted from man to man. It is reportable in the U. S. A. Brucellosis is pandemic in distribution. In the United States, it is endemic to the midwestern states (particularly Iowa) and California. [1] In Britain, Br. suis infection is rare, but Br. abortus infection is common.[2] In the United States, Br. suis is common in the midwest. In the Mediterranean countries, Br. melitensis is more common than others. [2] One may acquire this disease by ingesting imported dairy products. [2]

## CLINICAL FEATURES

More men than women are employed in abattoirs, hence, it is prevalent among men. Even though children drink a lot of milk, this disease is uncommon during childhood, but it is prevalent between 20 and 50 years of age.

Nearly 90% or more of the patients complain of malaise, fever and chills, with night sweats and weakness. Body aches, anorexia and weight loss are less common (50% to 60%). A third of the patients have headaches and cough. Bone and joint pains, orchitis and dyspnea may occur in nearly 10% of the patients. An average weight loss of 15 to 20 pounds is frequent. The incubation period is 6 to 21 days. Pain in the eyes on lateral movement and pain on movement of the temporomandibular joint, when present, are apparently characteristic.

Sleeplessness is the rule. The patient is bedridden because of weakness. He appears bright, alert and asymptomatic in the morning until noon, but around 2 to 4 p. m. , the fever spikes to 103⁰ to 104⁰F. Later, at night, 6 to 8 p. m. , the fever lyses with profuse sweating and drenching of the bedclothes. Most fevers due to abscess and endocarditis, etc. , rise in the evening (4 to 6 p. m. ) and lyse at midnight. The patient may have this fever for five to ten days, followed by a complete remission lasting for one to two weeks (60%). The mode of onset can be acute (40%) or subacute (60%).

When undiagnosed, it may run a chronic course and present with inanition. Physical examination may be otherwise entirely unremarkable. Lymphadenopathy may be found in 10% to 15%. Splenomegaly is an inconstant feature of brucellosis. During the acute phase of illness, for nearly three to four weeks the spleen is palpable (10%). When the fever runs a chronic course, the spleen is more frequently enlarged, but seldom massive.

Roentgenographic examination may reveal osteomyelitis of the spine with narrowing of the intervertebral spaces, sometimes destruction of the vertebrae. Most frequently, for some unknown reason, the fourth lumbar vertebra is involved. The chest roentgenogram may be suggestive of bronchitis. Pulmonary signs and symptoms are infrequent during the acute stage of the illness. About 1% to 3% may develop orchitis and epididymitis. In chronic cases, the gums may become spongy and bleed easily.

## DIAGNOSIS

Leukopenia, with relative lymphocytosis, anemia and increased erythrocytic sedimentation rate are common in chronic brucellosis.

1) Blood cultures: A positive blood culture is the only definitive proof of brucellosis. When brucellosis is suspected, the laboratory should be advised to hold the blood cultures for several weeks. Only 17% of the reported cases of brucellosis had positive cultures, and 83% were diagnosed by serology.

2) Brucellin skin test: This is unreliable. It may be positive in normal individuals.

3) Agglutination titer: A titer of 1:80 and 1:160 or above are considered abnormal but not diagnostic. A rising titer, with

a fourfold or more increase to 1:640 or 1:1280 suggests recent infection. Titers of >1:1000 are diagnostic of brucellosis. The agglutination titer for brucellosis may be falsely
increased due to:

(a) repeated skin testing for brucellosis in spite of adequate
therapy
(b) cholera vaccination
(c) tularemia, and
(d) anamnestic reaction

A rising agglutination titer for brucellosis, therefore, should
be interpreted on the basis of other evidences. Prozone phenomenon is a false-negative response due to antigen excess;
for this reason, the Brucella agglutination tests may be
falsely negative. Presence of 7S agglutinins indicates active infection. Increase in the IgG agglutinins, as measured
by the 2-mercaptoethanol test in a patient with symptoms,
is also considered to be suggestive of infection. Card agglutination* test is a rapid and relatively specific test for
brucellosis.

4) Complement-fixation test (CFT): This may be positive in
the acute stage of the disease. The standard agglutination
test is also positive when the CFT is positive. Most of the
successfully treated cases become CFT negative.

5) The radioimmunoassay: This is a radiolabelled antiglobu-
lin test labelled with I-125 antibody. [3] It is a very sensitive
diagnostic test. The reliability and the relative value of this
test in brucellosis is unknown. IgM, IgG and IgA Brucella
antibodies can be measured by this method.

## DIFFERENTIAL

Brucellosis should also be considered along with other diseases
in the differential from fevers of undetermined origin (see page
504), which include: miliary tuberculosis, Hodgkin's disease,
infectious mononucleosis, mumps, osteomyelitis due to other
bacteria, and typhoid fever.

## TREATMENT

Combined tetracycline, 500 mg. by mouth every six hours,
and streptomycin, 1,000 mg. intramuscularly per day for

* Brewer Diagnostic Kits, Brucellosis Card Test
Hynson, Westcott and Dunning, Inc.
Baltimore, Maryland

six weeks cured most cases. Brucellae abortus is an intracellular pathogen inaccessible to antibiotic therapy and, therefore, the need for the prolonged therapy. Single drug therapy
with either tetracycline or streptomycin is likely to fail and the
disease may relapse (30%), for which reason combined therapy
is preferred. Relapses are rare on tetracycline and streptomycin combined therapy. The relapse rate with cotrimoxazole
therapy[4] is close to 20% and therefore, it is not recommended.

## REFERENCES

1.  Buchanan, T. M. , et al. : Brucellosis in the United States,
    1960 - 1972. Part I,  II and III. Medicine 53:403, 1974.

2.  Williams, E. : Brucellosis. Brit. Med. J. 1:791, 1973.

3.  Pratt, D. , et al. : Radioimmunoassay of IgM, IgG and IgA
    Brucella antibody. Lancet 1:1075, 1977.

4.  Kontoyannis, P. A. , et al. : Cotrimoxazole in chronic bru-
    cellosis: A two-year follow-up study. Brit. Med. J. 2:480,
    1975.

## 63:  DIPHTHERIA
### by H. Thadepalli

Diphtheria (malignant quinsy) is a disease of childhood (below age twelve). Occasionally in epidemics, when six to seven dozen people are affected, nearly 20% of them are adults. Today, diphtheria is a disease of poverty, ignorance and malnutrition, be it due to natural or political disasters, or self-invited by alcoholic dereliction. [1] About two hundred cases are reported in the United States every year. No infectious disease is as thoroughly investigated and has as much already known about it as diphtheria. Yet, the mortality from this illness remains unchanged, from 10% to 15% for the past fifty years. [2] Man is the only host for diphtheria. It is a droplet infection.

It is caused by Corynebacterium (C.) diphtheriae, a gram-positive coccobacillary (Coryne = club-shaped, bacterion = rod) non-flagellated, non-spore-forming aerobic organism. It classically forms a membrane (diphtherion) at the oropharyngeal junction and on the infected skin. It measures 2 to $4\mu$ x 0.5 to $1\mu$. It grows well on tellurite medium, where it forms black colonies. C. diphtheriae, depending on the degree of blackness of the colonies on tellurite agar, is divided into three biotypes - gravis, which is black; intermediate, which is less black; and mitis, which is gray. The degree of the darkness of the colony (as believed in the past) is not tantamount to the severity of the disease it is apt to produce.  Mitis (small) can cause death, whereas the gravis (deathly) may remain as mere commensals of the throat in a carrier.  Maximum toxigenicity in one epidemic was due to mitis strains.[3]  It is a marvel of nature that a non-toxigenic strain of C. diphtheriae can transform itself into a toxigenic strain by the action of a certain phage called beta-phage.  This type of conversion is called lysogenic conversion. C. diphtheriae, for epidemiologic purposes, can be phage typed into 19 types.  Types I to III are mitis, types IV to VI are intermediate, VII is the non-virulent gravis, and VIII to XIX are virulent gravis strains.

### DIAGNOSIS

CLINICAL FEATURES:

Incubation period:  This is two to five days. The presenting symptoms are not ameliorated by prior immunization.

Age: It can affect any age, although those who are 15 years or younger may develop more serious infections. In one epidemic, 25% of the affected were adults. [4]

Sore throat and fever are the outstanding features found in nearly 85%, but often these symptoms are indolent in onset.

Nausea and dysphagia follow and can be severe in 25% of the cases. Other symptoms include headache (20%) and edema of the neck (20%).

Physical examination of the throat may reveal a true membrane formation which is somewhat dirty green or grayish, and the under-surface bleeds when the membrane is removed. In the case of a pseudomembrane, as found in cases of pharyngitis or infectious mononucleosis, the under-surface does not bleed. The breath smells like a necrotic tissue. A membrane may be found on the palate, the tonsils or the back of the pharynx, uvula or the soft palate. It can occasionally be found in the nose, larynx, vulva, vagina, cervix or penis. It is not a venereally transmitted disease.

The neck is swollen with anterior cervical lymphadenopathy. The normal line of the sternocleidomastoid disappears and the neck appears round and smooth like a "bull neck", also called "erasure edema". The whole neck is brawny to feel, but not necessarily tender.

Cutaneous diphtheria may appear as an ulcer, boils or abrasions on the skin. It can be caused by both toxigenic and non-toxigenic strains. [3] The latter was reported among the skid row derelicts. Skid row is an area of cheap saloons and flophouses frequented by vagrants and alcoholics. Apparently, the phrase "skid row" is a distortion derived from "skid road", a road adjacent to Puget Sound Bay in Seattle along which huge logs of wood were skidded from the hill close by into water during the days when logs were floated down the stream to the factories.

The white blood cell counts may or may not be increased. Most of the laboratory tests may be within normal limits. Protein-uria is uncommon.

The electrocardiogram may show ST-T wave abnormalities. First degree block is found in 15% to 20% of the patients.

Neurological manifestations, like palatal paralysis, may be found either during or after one or two weeks of the infectious episode. Sometimes they are delayed for four to six weeks. For this reason, the patients may have nasal regurgitation. Both the spoken words, and the liquids swallowed, tend to escape through the nose. Peripheral neuritis may occur in nearly 5% to 15% of these patients. The diphtheria toxin does cross the blood-brain barrier and it can rarely cause cranial nerve palsies. Most neurologic complications due to diphtheria reverse in two to four weeks.

LABORATORY FEATURES:

Throat swabs: Obtain at least two throat swabs from the site of infection. One may swab the membrane for this purpose. During a known epidemic of diphtheria, it is unnecessary to routinely remove the membrane to see if it is true or not. Gram's stain may show the characteristic organisms only in 50% of the cases. The yield by culture is close to 70% (30% will have negative throat swabs). Routine cultures may take two to three days, and treatment should never be withheld while waiting for positive cultures. Carey-Blair medium may be used for transport. In the laboratory, one of the swabs should be stained for Vincent's group of organisms (spirochaetes and Fusobacteria) and the other swab processed on tellurite medium and Loffler's slant. In addition, it should also be routinely plated on blood agar for the isolation of group A Streptococci. Group A Streptococci are frequently isolated along with C. diphtheriae (32%). [2]

A Gram's stain of the individual colonies may show the organisms arranged in palisades, resembling those of the Chinese letters.

The organism should be tested against antibiotics and examined for toxigenicity by Elek plate method. C. diphtheriae is generally susceptible to penicillin and erythromycin.

Blood cultures: Once the membrane is formed, the blood cultures are negative. Blood cultures may be positive before the membrane formation. C. diphtheriae, by itself, rarely invades the body.

Schick test: This test is useful to test the immune status of the patient and to test if vaccination is necessary. Further, the Schick test can be used to determine if the patient is allergic to the vaccine.

Inject 1/50 M. L. D. of toxin intradermally on the volar aspect of one forearm. For control, inject 0.1 ml. of 1:10 dilution of toxoid on the other. Inspect the sites at 36 and 120 hours for erythema, induration and necrosis.  The interpretation of the results follows:

| SKIN RESPONSE | | | | | |
|---|---|---|---|---|---|
| | Toxin | | Toxoid | | |
| Reaction | 36 hr. | 120 hr. | 36 hr. | 120 hr. | Interpretation |
| Positive | - | + | - | - | Non-immune and non-sensitive |
| Negative | - | - | - | '- | Sufficiently immune, non-sensitive |
| Pseudo | + | - | + | - | Immune, sensitive |
| Combined | + | + | + | - | Non-immune, sensitive |

(From Davis, B. D. , et al. : Microbiology, 2nd Edition. Harper & Row, Hagerstown, 1973, p. 689).

## DIFFERENTIAL

The following should be considered in the differential:

1) Infectious mononucleosis by the spot mono-test.

2) Streptococcal sore throat by throat cultures.

3) Scarlet fever is a rare disease among adults. I have not seen a case of scarlet fever in an adult during the past 15 years.

4) Mumps: The throat is rarely involved. Lymphocytosis predominates in mumps. The anterior cervical lymph nodes are not involved.

5) Vincent's angina: There is no unmistakable way of differentiating Vincent's angina from diphtheria, short of culture. They look and smell alike.

6) Quinsy or peritonsillar abscess: The peritonsillar area is swollen in both quinsy and diphtheria. Leukocytosis is very frequent with quinsy. The cell count in diphtheria may be normal or slightly increased.

7) Poliomyelitis: In diphtheria, both sensory and motor division are involved. In poliomyelitis, the sensory roots are infrequently involved.

8) Monilia: Candida infection of the throat also forms a pseudomembrane. Gram's stain the throat swab for evidences of budding yeast cells.

Hemorrhagic complications (DIC) of diphtheria carry a poor prognosis, but paralysis itself is not a poor prognostic sign; it is almost always reversible. Death may result in spite of early and liberal serum therapy.

## THERAPY

1) Penicillin (10 to 20 million units I. V. or I. M. /day) or erythromycin (500 mg. P. O. every six hours) or clindamycin (150 mg. every five hours) should be given. [5]

2) Serum therapy: About 40 to 80 thousand units of antitoxin on admission in saline may be administered I. V. by 100 to 200 ml. every 30 minutes. The patient should be examined for sensitivity by injecting 0.1 ml. of 1:100 dilution antitoxin. If sensitive, desensitization should be performed by serial dilutions of antitoxin. Reactions to serum therapy are frequent (20%). Nearly 50% of the throat cultures become negative within a day of serum therapy; 75% within the third and 100% within the fourth day. In one study of 3,000 cases, the mortality among those who received penicillin alone was 2.2% as compared with antitoxin alone (3.6%), and in combination (6-7%). This suggests that penicillin and antitoxin therapy, perhaps should not be combined. [6]

## REFERENCES

1. Heath, C. W. , Zusman, J. : An outbreak of diphtheria among skid row men. New Eng. J. Med. 267:809, 1962.

2. Brooks, G. F. , Bennett, J. V. , Feldman, R. A. : Diphtheria in the United States. J. Inf. Dis. 129:172, 1974.

3. Ayyagari, A. , Venugopalan, A. , Ray, S. N. : Studies on diphtheria infection in and around Delhi. J. Indian M. A. 63:328, 1975.

4. McCloskey, R. V. , et al. : The 1970 epidemic of diphtheria in San Antonio. Ann. Int. Med. 75:495, 1971.

5. McCloskey, R. V., et al. : Treatment of diphtheria carriers: Benzethine, penicillin, erythromycin and clindamycin. Ann. Int. Med. 81:788, 1974.

6. Romulus, C. J. , Gonzalez, H. R. : Estado actual del tratamiento de la difteria con penicilina exclusivamente. Bol. Hig. Epiden. Havana 3:77, 1965 (as quoted by Christie, A. B. : Infectious Diseases: Epidemiology and Clinical Practice. Livingstone, Edinburgh, 1969).

## 64: PLAGUE
### by H. Thadepalli

Yersinia (Y.) pestis is the causative organism of plague, a zoonotic disease that is transmitted from the rat or any other rodent to man by the flea called Xenopsylla cheopis. Approximately 1,500 cases are reported every year world-wide, and 10 to 15 cases per year within the United States; [1] it is a quarantinable disease. The plague can occur in any part of the world, but it is more prevalent in the tropics. An epizootic in rats often precedes an epidemic of human plague.

## CLINICAL MANIFESTATIONS

There are five clinical manifestations for plague:

1) Bubonic plague:[2] After an incubation period of two to three days, it starts with an abrupt onset of fever, chills and a painful bubo, often accompanied by intense headache and prostration. Fever may precede the onset of bubo and subside when the buboes appear.

   Anorexia, nausea, vomiting, abdominal pain, cough, chest pain and skin rash are relatively inconstant features, occurring in less than 25% of the patients. The femoral and inguinal lymph nodes are the most frequently involved (90%); the axillary, cervical and epitrochlea are involved less frequently (10% to 15%). The mortality is around 20%.

2) Pneumonic plague: Five per cent of the cases may present as pneumonia. Pneumonic form of plague can be secondary to bubonic plague, or, more frequently, secondary to inhalation. It is usually a fulminating infection with high fever, tachypnea and tachycardia, with or without the buboes. Severe prostration is common with the pneumonic form of plague. Cough and dyspnea are its outstanding features. It is fatal in 50% to 70% within one to five days after the onset. Pneumonic plague is highly contagious and transmittable from man to man.

3) Septicemic form: One per cent of the patients may have neither buboes nor pneumonia but may have positive blood cultures. They may have nausea, vomiting, and diarrhea, (sometimes bloody) resulting in death in two to three days.

4) Pestis minor: Some patients may have buboes due to plague without systemic toxic manifestations; they are frequently mistaken to have lymphadenopathy, due to other causes.

5) Asymptomatic:[3] A group of patients may be totally asymptomatic despite infection. In one study, 13% of the asymptomatic contacts had positive throat swabs for Yersinia pestis.

## DIAGNOSIS

Lymph node aspiration: Bubo aspirates for smear and culture are positive in nearly all cases. With the help of a 2 ml. syringe pre-filled with 0.2 ml. of saline and fitted with a 23-gauge needle, aspirate the contents of the bubo. A drop of the aspirate should be placed on a glass slide and air-dried, fixed with 5% methyl alcohol to kill the organisms and stained with methylene blue, Giemsa, or Gram's stain for the presence of "safety-pin"-shaped, gram-negative organisms. Carey-Blair medium can be used for transporting the specimens to the laboratory for culture.

Blood cultures: Nearly 50% of the patients will have positive cultures. No special media are required; the culture grows well in the routine media within 24 to 36 hours.

Blood smears: They can be stained with Giemsa and examined for the characteristic safety-pin-shaped bacteria. Positive peripheral blood smears indicate poor prognosis (50% mortality).

Limulus test: This may be positive but not diagnostic.

Sputum cultures: They may be positive for Y. pestis in the pneumonic form of plague.

Chest x-ray: Mediastinal lymphadenopathy, more frequent in children, can occur along with inguinal adenopathy.

Disseminated intravascular coagulation (DIC): This may occur secondary to Schwartzman reaction elicited by the endotoxin.

Guinea pig inoculation: When in doubt, guinea pig inoculation should be used with extreme caution, because the laboratory personnel can acquire plague from the animals.

Urine cultures: Urine cultures are positive in 20% to 30% of the patients.

Fecal cultures: They are seldom positive.

## BACTERIOLOGY

Yersinia pestis is a gram-negative, non-motile, non-spore-forming facultative coccobacillus of size 1.5 to 2.0 $\mu$ x 0.5 to 0.8$\mu$, which grows well on conventional media. It has the characteristic safety-pin-like appearance on simple stain. It should be differentiated from other organisms of the same group, such as Y. pseudotuberculosis and Y. enterocolitica (Table 34).

## TABLE 34: DIFFERENTIATING FEATURES OF YERSINIA (Y.) ORGANISMS PATHOGENIC IN MAN

| Test | Y. pestis | Y. pseudo-tuberculosis | Y. entero-colitica |
|---|---|---|---|
| Motility | 0 | + | + |
| Urease | 0 | + | + |
| Ornithine decarboxylation | 0 | 0 | + |
| Reduction of methylene blue | 0 | + | + |
| Lysis by plague phage | + | 0 | 0 |
| Pathogenicity for mice | + | 0 | 0 |

## DIFFERENTIAL

Early stages of plague can be mistaken for typhoid fever and typhus fever. Bubonic plague can be mistaken for tularaemia, lymphogranuloma venereum (LGV) and syphilis. The bubo due to plague, develops within hours to a day; whereas the bubo due to LGV may develop over a period of several days. A simple stain of the needle and aspirate is required for differentiation. Therapy should be promptly initiated when plague is suspected.

Other Yersinia infections include Y. multocida infection, which can be acquired by dog bite. Y. enterocolitica causes diarrhea. Y. pseudotuberculosis can also be acquired by animal bites, and it clinically resembles acute appendicitis. Y. pseudotuberculosis, as its name implies, can be mistaken for tuberculosis because it causes mesenteric lymphadenopathy.

## TREATMENT

Streptomycin is the drug of choice. The clinical response is usually prompt, within 12 to 24 hours. No satisfactory vaccine is yet available.

## REFERENCES

1.  Morbidity and Mortality: Plague - United States, 1976. U. S. Department of Health, Education and Welfare, Atlanta, May 13, 1977.

2.  Butler, T.: A clinical study of bubonic plague. Amer. J. Med. 53:268, 1972.

3.  Marshall, J. D., Quy, D. V., Gibson, F. L.: Asymptomatic pharyngeal plague infection in Vietnam. Am. J. Trop. Med. Hyg. 16:175, 1967.

## 65: RAT BITE FEVER
by H. Thadepalli

Rat bite fever is caused by two organisms; <u>Spirillum (S.)</u> minus and <u>Streptobacillus (Strept.)</u> moniliformis.

## THE ORGANISMS

<u>Spirillum minus</u> is a spirochete of the size 1.5 to $6\mu$ with three to four curves. It moves with flagellae, but, like other spirochetes, the body does not vibrate. It has not been cultured.

<u>Streptobacillus moniliformis</u> is a gram-negative bacillus which is easily cultivable. The bacilli are attached to each other like Streptococci.

## TRANSMISSION

<u>Strept. moniliformis</u> is a normal commensal of the mouth of the rodent, of the same species that transmits plague (see page 514). There are no insect vectors involved in the transmission of rat bite fever. It is called sodiku (so = rat, diku = poison) in Japan, where it is transmitted by the bite of the rat or any other rodent, including cats. <u>Strept. moniliformis</u> is also acquired by drinking contaminated milk. Such an epidemic was reported from Haverhill, Massachusetts, therefore nicknamed Haverhill fever (Table 35).

<u>S. minus</u> is found in the blood of the infected rat, but not in the saliva. In mice, it can be transmitted hereditarily.

## GEOGRAPHY

<u>S. minus</u> infections are reported mostly from Japan, and <u>Strept. moniliformis</u> is reported from the United States.

## CLINICAL FEATURES

<u>Fever:</u> This is a constant symptom, starting one to five days after the bite. The temperatures may range from $103^O$ to $105^O$F. It runs a course similar to relapsing fevers (see page 78); the fever lasts for three to four days, and it subsides by crisis with sweats, followed by an afebrile period of five to ten days.

TABLE 35: DIFFERENTIATING FEATURES IN THE
RAT BITE FEVERS

| CLINICAL FEATURE | RAT BITE FEVER | HAVERHILL FEVER |
|---|---|---|
| Causative agent | Spirillum minus | Streptobacillus moniliformis |
| Transmission | Rat bite | Rat bite or con-taminated milk |
| Geography | Mostly Japan | Mostly in the United States |
| Site of bite | Delayed healing | Heals promptly |
| Period of relapses of fever | Regular | Irregular |
| Lymphadenopathy | Frequent | Infrequent |
| Arthritis | Rare | Common |

Lymphadenopathy: This is frequent with S. minus infections; usually the regional lymph nodes are involved. The site of the bite may heal long before the lymphadenopathy begins. On occasion, the site of the bite may become tense and reddish during a bout of fever.

Exanthem: A purple papular exanthem may appear on the extremities and the chest immediately before or after the fever subsides.

Arthritis: This is common with Strept. moniliformis infections. It is rare with S. minus. The difference between the rat bite fever caused by S. minus and Haverhill fever are summarized in Table 35.

DIAGNOSIS

1) Eosinophilia with leukocytosis (15,000/cu. mm. ) is common, though not invariable.

2) <u>Animal inoculation</u>: Inoculate white mice or guinea pigs with the blood or lymph node extract of the patient. Within seven days after the inoculation, the organism can be recovered from the blood. The mice may live for months in spite of this infection.

3) In rabbits, <u>Proteus OXK</u> reaction may become positive when they are injected with <u>S. minus</u>. This reaction does not occur when man is infected with <u>S. minus</u>.

## TREATMENT

Penicillin is the drug of choice; if the patient is allergic to this drug, tetracycline may be used.

66: SICKLE CELL ANEMIA AND INFECTION
by H. Thadepalli

Infection does not necessarily precipitate crisis in sickle cell anemia (SCA). It is true that SCA patients are highly prone to certain infections, and nearly a fourth of them present with an infection. Among children with SCA, infection, but not crisis, is the most common cause for hospitalization and death.[1] In fact, crisis in SCA often occurs without an infection, and most infected SCA patients are not in crisis. Infections in SCA patients generally respond slowly to antibiotic therapy. Several hypotheses exist to explain the high incidence of infection in the "sicklers" — defective phagocytosis, relative asplenia, defective complement system, and lack of sufficient opsonins are some such explanations.

## MALARIA AND SCA PATIENTS

Those with sickle cell trait have markedly decreased susceptibility to malaria, especially for P. falciparum. The parasitized red cells often sickle because of the additional demand for oxygen from the parasite. The deformed cells with the parasite are later readily destroyed by the reticuloendothelial system, thus ensuring the resistance of the host to malaria. Had this been otherwise, malaria perhaps would have eradicated the sickle cell gene long ago. Hemoglobin C also offers similar protection against malaria.

## PNEUMOCOCCUS AND SCA

Pneumococcus is one of the most common causes for bacteremia in SCA. Whereas H. influenzae is the most common cause for meningitis among the non-SCA children, pneumococcus is the most common cause of meningitis among the SCA patients. Pneumococcal meningitis in SCA carriers is just as serious as among the non-SCA patients.

Pneumococcal pneumonia and septicemia should be considered in all cases of sickle cell crisis with lung infiltrate. It is uncertain whether these infiltrates result from pulmonary infection due to sickle cell crisis, or secondary to pneumococcal infection. Often, the diagnosis of bacterial pneumonia, made on the basis of sputum smears along in patients with sickle cell crisis, is at best purely presumptive.

## SALMONELLA OSTEOMYELITIS AND SCA

Osteomyelitis is more common among the SCA patients in all age groups. In times of crisis, the roentgenographic appearances of acute osteomyelitis and bone infarcts may be indistinguishable. In adults with SCA, osteomyelitis often presents in a chronic form. Whereas 80% of osteomyelitis among non-SCA are due to Staphylococcus aureus, nearly 60% of the cases of osteomyelitis in SCA patients are due to Salmonella group of organisms. Salmonella osteomyelitis among the non-SCA patients is rare; when it does occur, abnormalities of the hemoglobin should be suspected. The exact reason for the several hundred-fold special predilection of SCA patients for Salmonella osteomyelitis, instead of S. aureus or E. coli osteomyelitis, is unknown.

## URINARY TRACT INFECTIONS AND SCA

Pregnancy and childbirth in SCA greatly predispose to urinary tract infections. Pyelitis, pyelonephritis and perinephric abscess are common; rarely, severe papillary necrosis can also occur. Like in non-SCA patients, Escherichia coli, Klebsiella-Enterobacter infections are common. Staphylococcus aureus should also be considered among this group.

The precise incidence of viral and Mycoplasma infection among these patients is unknown. It is conceivable that they may receive greater blame than they actually deserve. Certain other infections, like tuberculosis, a companion of the poor in the urban ghetto, are no more frequent among the SCA patients than others.

## REFERENCE

1. Barrett-Connor, E. : Bacterial infection and sickle cell anemia. Medicine 50:97, 1971.

## 67: SPLENIC ABSCESS
by H. Thadepalli

The spleen protects us from pneumococcal, Herpes virus and Hemophilus influenza infections. Serious infections may develop after splenectomy for staging Hodgkin's disease.[1] "Incidental splenectomy" is a more frequent cause of infections than elective splenectomy.[2] Autosplenectomy in sickle cell disease predisposes to pneumococcal, septicemia, meningitis or endocarditis. Herpes zoster, in one study, occurred in five out of forty-seven splenectomized patients (10.6%) within a year; in most instances, it was of abrupt onset and ran a fulminating course, ending in death within six to twenty-four hours after the onset. Most of the post-splenectomy infections occur within the first two years. The precise role of the spleen in the prevention of infections is not well understood.

### CLINICAL FEATURES

Pain and tenderness over the left upper quadrant of the abdomen, with fever and leukocytosis, should suggest the possibility of splenic abscess. The spleen is not palpable in nearly two-thirds of the cases of splenic abscess and the liver-spleen scan may also be negative in one-half of them.

### PREDISPOSING CAUSES

The most common predisposing causes for splenic abscess are:

1) trauma
2) typhoid fever
3) diabetes mellitus
4) hemolytic anemia-like sickle cell anemia or thalassemia
5) infectious mononucleosis
6) endocarditis
7) alcoholism
8) lupus
9) perinephric abscess
10) malaria
11) relapsing fever
12) lung abscess
13) parasitic infections
14) drug addiction

Multiple abscess sites, including spleen, suggest a different primary focus elsewhere, such as the heart.

Depending on where the patient has been, the predisposing causes vary. For example, in Asia, malaria and typhoid fever are the most common predisposing causes for splenic abscess. In North America, drug addiction, endocarditis and trauma (motorcycle accidents) are the leading causes.[3]

Splenic abscess is a rare disease. It was found in 1 in 10,000 hospital admissions and 2 to 6 per 1,000 deaths.

## DIAGNOSIS

Diagnosis is made by the presence of left upper quadrant pain and tenderness, accompanied by leukocytosis in a patient with a history of one of the predisposing causes as listed above. A plain roentgenogram of the abdomen might show gas containing an abscess in the left upper quadrant, and is mistaken for the "stomach bubble" occasionally. In spite of strong clinical suspicion, one may miss splenic abscess even by exploratory laparotomy. Occasionally, thoracotomy may be performed for the mistaken diagnosis of left-sided empyema.

Since gallium citrate normally accumulates in the spleen, gallium scans are of little value in the diagnosis of splenic abscess. Instead, technetium (Tc-99m) sulphur colloid scans may be useful. Abscesses of sizes larger than 3 cm. may be recognized by Tc-99m scan. Splenic abscess, if not operated on in time, is fatal.

The role of ultrasound and angiography in the diagnosis of splenic abscess is not established. An avascular space in the spleen, demonstrated by splenic angiography, should raise the suspicion of a cyst or an abscess in the spleen. [4]

## BACTERIOLOGY

Gram-negative aerobic bacteria, coliforms, are the most common cause of splenic abscess. As mentioned, the prevalence of the organisms might vary from one country to another. Coliforms like Escherichia coli, Klebsiella ozaenae, Salmonella, Serratia, Enterobacter cloacae, Proteus morganii, and Pseudomonas are the frequent isolates in splenic abscess. Bacteroides fragilis, Streptococcus moniliformes, Nocardia and Salmonella group of organisms rarely are reported to cause splenic abscess. Nearly one-third of the pus cultures from the splenic abscess had bacteria on Gram's stain that later failed to grow. This suggests that suboptimal techniques could have been responsible for failure to isolate anaerobic bacteria.

## THERAPY

Therapy should include surgical drainage and antibiotic therapy. Whether a needle aspiration of the spleen would suffice, or a splenotomy (drainage) is preferable to a total splenectomy, is unknown. The available data suggests that splenectomy is the treatment of choice, because it is technically safe and defini-tive. Antibiotic therapy should be aimed against both aerobic gram-negative bacilli and the anaerobic organisms.

## REFERENCES

1. Ravry, M. , et al. : Serious infections after splenectomy for the staging of Hodgkin's disease. Ann. Int. Med. 77:11, 1972.

2. Chulay, J. D. , Lankerni, M. R. : Splenic abscess: Report of 10 cases and review of the literature. Am. J. Med. 61: 513, 1976.

3. Gadacz, T. , Way, L. , Dunphy, E. : Changing clinical spec-trum of splenic abscess. Ann. J. Surg. 128:182, 1974.

4. Jacobs, R. P. , et al. : Angiography of splenic abscess. Am. J. Roentgenol. Rad. Ther. and Nuc. Med. 122:419, 1974.

## 68: TULAREMIA
by H. Thadepalli

Tularemia is caused by the bacteria called Francisella (F.) tularensis, named after the late Edward Francis, who described this disease in man, and after the Tulare County in California, where it was discovered in rabbits. Tularemia is acquired by direct contact with infected rodents, or, as in plague, it can be transmitted by an insect vector. Man-to-man transmission is rare. Tularemia is rare south of the equator.

## BACTERIOLOGY

F. tularensis is an aerobic, non-motile, non-spore-forming, non-capsulated gram-negative bacillus of size 0.3 to 0.5 x 0.2 $\mu$m, which stains faintly bipolar with aniline dyes. Special media containing cystine or cysteine are required to cultivate this organism. It is penicillin-resistant, but highly susceptible to streptomycin. There are two varieties of F. tularensis. One variety, Jellison type A, ferments glycerol and is pathogenic to both man and the rabbit. A second variety, Jellison type B does not ferment glycerol and is pathogenic only to man but not to rabbits. Both varieties belong to a single serotype.

## MODE OF TRANSMISSION

Tularemia can be acquired by skinning infected animals without gloves. It can also be acquired by the flea, tick or louse. These insects can transmit the disease to man and from one animal to another. F. tularensis is the only known bacteria that is transmitted transovarially in the ticks. Tularemia is more prevalent during the spring and summer. The disease begins within two to seven days after the exposure.

## CLINICAL FEATURES

The disease usually begins three to four days after exposure to the infected rodents or ticks. A cutaneous ulcer associated with regional lymphadenopathy and fever and chills are its classic manifestations. Several clinical varieties of tularemia have been described. It can manifest in any of the following forms:

1) Ulceroglandular type is the most easily recognized form of this malady. It starts with a sudden onset of fever and chills, with a bleb at the site of inoculation that changes to an ulcer within 80 to 96 hours after the bite. It is soon followed by

regional lymphadenopathy. The lymph nodes are tender and enlarged to the size of 2 to 3 cm. They may later suppurate and ulcerate.

2) Glandular form alone can occur without the evidence of an ulcer. Nearly 60% may have no history or evidence of an insect bite. The associated lymphadenopathy can be regional or generalized.

3) Oculoglandular form is not very common. The portal of entry for oculoglandular form may be the conjunctiva; therefore, the regional lymph nodes, i.e., the pre-auricular and the cervical lymph nodes, are often palpable and tender. Conjunctivitis and blepharitis with corneal edema can occur.

4) Typhoidal form is also typified by generalized lymphadenopathy, but this form is heralded by nausea, vomiting and diarrhea. The portal of entry is presumably the mouth.

5) Pneumonic form manifests as lobar or segmental pneumonia. These patients are extremely ill and have dry hacking cough with high fevers.

The fever may be as high as 105°F. , usually running a septic course. The lymph nodes are hot and tender. They may become soft and often suppurate with caseating necrosis. The liver and spleen, when enlarged, are extremely tender. In spite of such severe systemic symptoms, the peripheral leukocyte count may be surprisingly normal.

## DIAGNOSIS

Diagnosis of Tularemia can be suspected on the basis of:

1) Clinical picture

2) History of exposure

3) Blood cultures: are often unrewarding.

4) Culture from the pustules or lymph node aspirates: These specimens should be directly inoculated onto the culture medium, and an aliquot should be stored in a small tube containing sterile nutrient broth at neutral pH and frozen for further reference.

5) Lymph nodes, if they are not ruptured: Inject 2 ml. of sterile saline and withdraw the material for culture. The lymph node biopsy specimens can be cultured directly.

528/ Infections of the Lymphatic System

6) Pharyngeal washes: These are relatively poor specimens for culturing F. tularensis.

7) Sputum and gastric aspirates: These, obtained early in the morning before the patient drinks water or brushes his teeth, are useful to culture. Penicillin, polymyxin B and cyclohexamide may be added to inhibit other bacteria in the clinical samples.

8) Animal inoculation: Guinea pigs may be inoculated intraperitoneally and examined three days later for the organisms. Death occurs in five to ten days.

9) Agglutination test: This becomes positive, as a rule, during the second week of the disease and reaches its maximum in four weeks. The titer varies from 1:160 to 1:5,000. Cross reactions with Brucella abortus are frequent in titers above 1:320.

10) Skin test antigen: This consists of a phenolized vaccine diluted to 1:1,000, and positive in 90% of the cases within the first seven days of exposure. It is not commercially available.

## DIFFERENTIAL

Tularemia is often confused with plague. Clinical differentiation is impossible. In a given patient, both diagnoses should be considered until one of them is confirmed. Soon after appropriate cultures are obtained, prompt therapy should be instituted. Histologically, tularemia can be confused with tuberculosis because of necrosis, giant cells and epithelioid cells. Diagnosis of tuberculosis is established by skin reaction to PPD and culture. Once the diagnosis of tularemia is suspected, treatment should be promptly initiated.

## THERAPY

F. tularensis is resistant to penicillin. Streptomycin is the drug of choice. Chloramphenicol or tetracycline can also be used in place of streptomycin.

SECTION I: DISTURBANCES IN BODY TEMPERATURE


69: ACCIDENTAL HYPOTHERMIA
by H. Thadepalli


Body temperature below 94°F. (34°C. ) is defined as hypothermia.[1] Accidental hypothermia is a common problem in cold
climates during the winter months. Among the civilians, alcoholism, drug addiction, mental illness and old age are some
of the predisposing causes. In Great Britain, nearly 2,000 elderly persons die of this condition each year. An estimated
2.5% of all acute admissions to London Medical Ward were due
to hypothermia.[2] Hypothermia is not an infectious disease, but
it is included here because most patients with accidental hypothermia have an underlying chronic pulmonary, or other infection, and the death toll is higher among them than among
those with hypothermia alone.

INVESTIGATIONS

The following investigations are helpful for recognizing high-risk
patients. In addition to routine biochemical investigations, these
procedures are recommended:

1) Rectal temperatures are adequate for monitoring. When the
   body temperature is found to be rapidly falling, the esophageal temperature should also be recorded.

2) Portable chest roentgenogram to exclude pulmonary infection.
   In case of a known lung lesion, mouth-to-mouth resuscitation
   should be discouraged. If the chest roentgenogram is clear and
   if cardiac arrest occurs, mere mouth-to-mouth resuscitation is adequate in most instances. Intubation should be
   deferred unless it is absolutely necessary.[3]

3) Sputum smears for acid-fast bacilli and cultures for M. tuberculosis and fungi.

4) Blood cultures should be obtained to detect the often associated septicemia.

5) <u>Transtracheal aspiration</u>, if indicated, should also be obtained for smears and cultures for <u>M. tuberculosis</u> and other bacteria.

6) <u>Stool</u> and <u>urine cultures</u> for Enterobacteriaceae organisms.

7) <u>Wound cultures</u>, if any open wounds are present.

## THERAPY

Therapy should not wait for culture results. Antibiotic therapy should be instituted along with the rewarming procedures. Large doses of penicillin or cephalosporin are satisfactory. Aminoglycosides should be avoided because of the high risk of acute tubular necrosis in patients with hypothermia.

## REFERENCES

1. Fruehan, A. D.: Accidental hypothermia. Arch. Int. Med. 106:218, 1960.

2. Prescott, L. F., Peard, M. C., Wallace, I. R.: Accidental hypothermia: A common condition. Br. Med. J. 2:1367, 1962.

3. Editorial: Severe accidental hypothermia. Lancet 1:237, 1972.

## 70: HEAT STROKE
### by H. Thadepalli

Heat stroke is due to a steep rise in body temperature, as a result of faulty body heat loss mechanisms, which occur with strenous physical effort in warm surroundings and the tropics, and heat wave in the subtropics. Heat stroke was the largest single cause of death in the Mecca pilgrimage during 1959-1960; 800 of 1 and 1/4 million pilgrims died; some had high fevers due to infections. The terms hyperthermia or hyperpyrexia are preferable to "heat stroke", but they were used for post-anesthetic reactions (malignant hyperthermia). The infectious disease specialist is often called to consult on all high fevers, whether or not they are due to an infectious agent.

### INVESTIGATIONS

Heat stroke is characterized by very high body temperature and profound bodily disturbances, including delirium, convulsions and partial or incomplete loss of consciousness. [1] Sensation of sweating is a cardinal feature of heat stroke. The skin is hot, but it can be either dry or moist. The popular belief that the skin is dry and hot in heat stroke, and moist and hot in malaria is incorrect. The heat stroke usually begins with an acute onset (91%) within a few seconds to a few hours. A small number of patients (9%) have insidious onset lasting for days.

Body temperature of 105°F. or above constitutes a medical emergency. The patient should be cooled rapidly and maintained below 100°F. Rectal temperatures are adequate for this purpose. The ordinary clinical thermometer records temperatures from 94° to 108°F. (normal body temperature, 98.6°F.). Special thermometers are needed to record temperatures above 108°F. Above 105°F., the body begins to gradually lose the thermoregulatory control.

Blood smears should be examined for malarial parasites in all endemic areas. If the patient is comatose and cerebral malaria is suspected, immediate therapy should be started. Blood cultures should be drawn and antibiotic therapy instituted to cover the suspected infection (not prophylactically). Gram-negative and staphylococcal pulmonary infections in the aged may also present as heat stroke. [2] Appropriate cultures should be obtained from all suspected sites of infection.

Meningitis can present and be mistaken for a heat stroke. Spinal fluid should be obtained for culture in all patients with mental symptoms. Chest roentgenograms should be obtained in all cases on admission. Interpretation of a pneumonic infiltrate could be due to pulmonary hemorrhage. Caution should be exercised in the interpretation of these films. Transtracheal aspirations may be somewhat risky in these patients because of the high incidence of associated bleeding tendency. Disseminated intravascular coagulation has been reported to be associated with heat stroke.

## THERAPY

This consists of rapid cooling and rehydration, and other symptomatic measures. If infection is suspected, antimicrobial therapy should be started only after appropriate cultures are obtained. Aminoglycosides should be avoided because of the high incidence of pre-renal azotemia found in association with heat stroke.

## REFERENCES

1. Editorial: Heat stroke. Lancet 2:31, 1968.

2. Levine, J. A.: Heat stroke in the aged. Amer. J. Med. 47: 251, 1969.

SECTION J: PARASITIC INFECTIONS

71: AMOEBIASIS
by H. Thadepalli

Amoebiasis is a disease caused by the protozoan parasite Entamoeba histolytica. Acute dysentery and liver abscess are the
two major manifestations of amoebic infection. Amoebiasis
is a disease of insanitation, not exclusively tropical. It
is transmitted by fecal-oral route, and certain outbreaks are
caused by food carriers. [1] Amoebic dysentery is a household
or a family infection. When one is infected, nearly 60% to 70%
of the household are also involved; children (below age 10) are
less frequently affected than adults.

The incubation period is seven to thirty days (occasionally as
long as thirty years). It is insidious in onset and runs a chronic
course with intermissions and relapses. In mild cases, the patient
complains of just a "nuisance diarrhea" which does not incapacitate
the patient, often called "walking diarrhea" or "dysentery".

## CLINICAL FEATURES

Abdominal pains and tenderness localized to the right lower
quadrant, simulating appendicitis, or tenderness in the epigastric region, simulating peptic ulcer, might be the presenting features.[2] Amoebic stools are often bulkier than the stools
in bacterial dysentery, averaging six to twelve stools per day,
often streaked with mucus and blood mixed with liquid feces. High
fevers are uncommon with amoebic dysentery per se. Presence
of high fever and greater frequency of stools, more than twelve
per day associated with tenesmus, should suggest the diagnosis
of bacillary dysentery (Table 36). On occasion, bacterial and
amoebic dysentery may coexist. If the dysentery is prolonged,
the patient loses weight and becomes emaciated.

## DIAGNOSIS

Seventy to eighty per cent of polymorphonuclear leukocytosis,
(10,000 to 12,000/cu. ml.) with shift to the left, is not uncommon. Untreated amoebic dysentery might subside, relapse or
become chronic or, on occasion, it can be fatal. The
liver may be enlarged and readily palpable in association with

## TABLE 36: DIAGNOSIS - AMOEBIC VS. BACILLARY

| AMOEBIC | BACILLARY |
| --- | --- |
| 1. Chronic or subacute "walking" dysentery and occasionally acute | Acute "lying down" dysentery |
| 2. Usually afebrile or $< 102^{\circ}F$ | Fever usually above $101^{\circ}F$ |
| 3. Liver may be enlarged, but spleen is seldom enlarged | Spleen may be enlarged, but the liver is not |
| 4. Thickening and tenderness over the sigmoid or all over the abdomen | Tenderness all over the abdomen |
| 5. Maximum 12 stools per day | No limit |
| 6. Bulky, malodorous, mixed with streaks of blood and mucus, "anchovy sauce" | Scanty, gelatinous, odorless |
| 7. Tenesmus is uncommon | Tenesmus is frequent |
| 8. Microscopy: Red cells, polymorphs, macrophage cells; large number of motile Entamoeba histolytica containing ingested red cells | Mostly red blood cells, polymorphs or mononuclear leukocytes, relatively scanty microorganisms |
| 9. Peripheral Leukocyte count: 10,000 to 12,000/ cu. mm.; seventy percenr or more polymorphs | Usually 12,000 to 22,000, with shift to the left |
| 10. Charcot-Leyden crystals present | No Charcot-Leyden crystals |
| 11. E. histolytica in stool and positive serum indirect hemagglutination test | Positive blood or stool culture for bacteria is confirmatory |

amoebic dysentery without a liver abscess. Occasionally, amoebic liver abscess is associated with amoebic dysentery. It is, therefore, difficult to distinguish amoebic hepatitis from liver abscess associated with dysentery. In amoebic hepatitis, the liver is enlarged and tender. The liver-spleen scan and Ga-67 scans are negative. Liver biopsy may show round-cell infiltration, but no pus and no amoebae. It resolves completely with chloroquine, metronidazole or emetine. It is unknown if amoebic hepatitis ever progresses to amoebic liver abscess. The patient is rarely jaundiced in amoebic liver abscess or in hepatitis.

Acute amoebic dysentery may be mistaken for acute appendicitis. Similarly, acute appendicitis might occur in association with amoebic dysentery. In such situations, it is safer to treat the patient for both amoebiasis and appendicitis. If the suspicion of appendicitis is strong, surgery is mandatory.

Clinical distinction between amoebic dysentery and bacillary dysentery might sometimes be difficult. In such situations, therapy may have to be directed against both and a fresh stool smear obtained for examination of vegetative forms of amoeba, in addition to several stool cultures (see Table 36).

Stool smears: Time spent in examining a freshly prepared stool smear for vegetative forms of amoeba is worth the effort. The specimen should be warm. Cold specimens yield negative results. Collect a specimen from a freshly passed stool on the tip of a match stick from an area containing large quantities of mucus and transfer to the top of a sterile slide; add a drop of normal saline, place a cover slip and examine for the typical motile forms of amoeba, putting forward pseudopodia. Erythrophagocytosis is the sine qua non of Entamoeba histolytica. The stool smears should also be stained with Lugol's iodine and re-examined. These parasites stain yellow. The vegetative forms of E. histolytica have a single nucleus and several ingested red blood corpuscles. They are about three times in size as compared to the red blood corpuscles. E. histolytica should be distinguished from the harmless commensals, E. coli, Iodamoeba buetschlii, Endolimax nana and Dientamoeba fragilis. Erythrophagocytosis is not a feature of the commensal Entamoebae. They can also be differentiated by looking for the cystic forms of amoeba. The cysts of E. histolytica have four nuclei; E. coli, eight and I. buetschlii has only two. It should be remembered that cystic forms of E. histolytica are rarely seen in acute amoebic dysentery. It is the cyst which is contagious, not the vegetative forms. Therefore, the non-cyst-passing acute amoebic dysentery patients need not be isolated. Charcot-Leyden crystals are common in the feces of amoebic dysentery. Their presence is, however, not diagnostic because they may be found in other situations as well. Charcot-Leyden crystals are derived from the eosinophils. They may be present in any situation, causing disintegration of eosinophils.

Sigmoidoscopic examination should be included in the work-up of all patients with dysentery. [3] Instrumentation in amoebic dysentery is painless. In bacillary dysentery, it is extremely painful and the patient may refuse this examination. The sigmoid colon may be hyperemic with several small yellow-colored ulcers. They may coalesce and form large flask-shaped craters. The mucous membrane in amoebic dysentery is compared to "pin-point craters", "pinpricks on a plasticine surface", "aerial photograph of bomb craters", "pig-skin appearance", "craters like Mount Fujiyama" of Japan, "sea anemone ulcers", and "scattered pits". [4] See Figs. 100-103, obtained from a patient who died of amoebic colitis. They can be touched and scraped without pain. The mucous membrane may be biopsied for examination of amoeba, by wet mount and by histologic examination. Large ulcers are rare. Aspiration of the mucus secretions might also provide a larger amount of specimen to examine for the parasite than a mere scraping. The vegetative forms of amoeba in these specimens can be seen readily without any special preparations.

The radiological appearances of amoebic colitis may be misleading. It may be mistaken for inflammatory bowel disease [5] and diagnosed as ulcerative colitis or Crohn's disease of the colon, because of the similarity in history and physical findings. The barium enema in amoebic colitis may show loss of haustrations and shortening of the colon, with loss of normal mucosal pattern, like ulcerative colitis. The cecum might be shortened and filled with inflammatory exudate, like Crohn's disease or carcinoma of the colon. Amoebic colitis may occur in a patient with carcinoma of the colon. Occasionally the colon might be irritable and appear very irregular and contracted with areas of stenosis. Rectal biopsies should be done to confirm the diagnosis. Amoebic colitis and ulcerative colitis may coexist in one patient.

The indirect hemagglutination (IHA) test for amoebiasis may be positive in nearly 80% to 90% of the cases. IHA therefore, should be included as an essential part of the evaluation of all patients with inflammatory bowel disease.

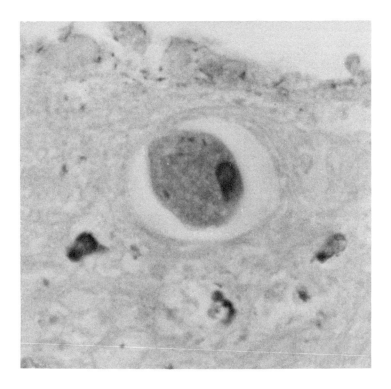

FIG. 100: Higher magnification of Entamoeba histolytica showing a finely granular cytoplasm and a single nucleus.

## CHRONIC AMOEBIASIS

Chronic amoebiasis is characterized by vague abdominal pain;
there is discomfort, occasional periodic diarrhea without fever
or other constitutional symptoms of infection. Physical examination may show an enlarged palpable and tender liver (amoebic hepatitis). The spleen is not palpable. Both vegetative forms
and cystic forms of Entamoeba histolytica may be seen in the
stool, and the bacterial cultures of the stools are negative.
Proctosigmoidoscopic examination and barium enema may show
no abnormality. They respond to anti-amoebic treatment. These
patients are sometimes misdiagnosed as having gastric ulcers,
duodenal ulcers, cholecystitis, acute or chronic cholelithiasis
and acute pancreatitis, etc. In endemic areas, amoebiasis
should be considered in all cases of suspected ulcer disease.

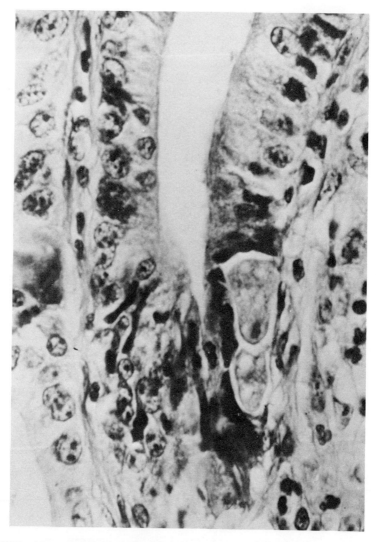

FIG. 101: <u>Entamoeba histolytica</u> present in the depth of a colonic gland and appearing as penetrating into the lamina propria. This patient died of acute amoebic colitis mistaken for toxic megacolon for which a colectomy was performed (see Figs. 100, 102-103 from the same patient).

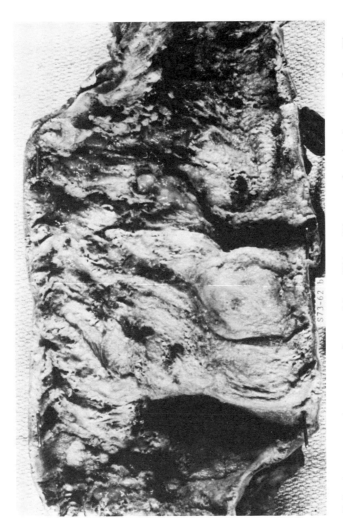

FIG. 102: Colonic mucosa in a case of amoebic colitis with secondary toxic megacolon. The mucosa appears friable, with extensive undermined ulceration.

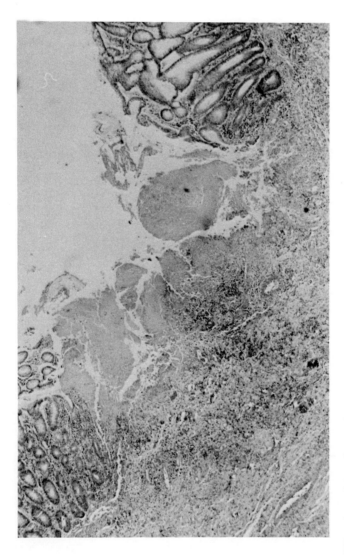

FIG. 103: Amoebic ulcer showing necrotic base with undermined margin and secondary inflammatory exudate at the base.

The patients may or may not lose weight, or, surprisingly, may gain weight because of their increased appetites. I saw some present with anasarca, occasionally; with coarse suffusion of the body; and with coarse dry skin. These patients may be mistaken for having myxedema.

It is a good practice to examine the stool of a patient diagnosed to have amoebic diarrhea routinely for other associated parasitic infections, as well as Ancylostoma duodenale, Ascaris lumbricoides and Giardia lamblia.

## AMOEBIC LIVER ABSCESS

Certain aspects of amoebic liver abscess are discussed in conjunction with pyogenic liver abscess. The precise incidence of associated liver abscess in amoebic dysentery is unknown. Amoebic liver abscess should be considered in the differential diagnosis of all subdiaphragmatic infections, especially if the patient is from highly endemic areas or has traveled to endemic areas.

It affects men more frequently than women, predominantly during the second and third decade of life. It is rare in childhood and old age. The youngest case I ever saw was five years old, and the oldest was 50 years old. Nearly 70% to 80% of the cases of amoebic liver abscess in the southern California area occur among the immigrants from Mexico.

By clinical examination alone, the amoebic liver abscess is difficult to distinguish from pyogenic liver abscess. In cases of amoebic liver abscess, the level of dullness in the right mid-scapular line is higher than that of the right mid-axillary line. This is due to atelectasis of the lower lobe of the right lung. In cases of non-amoebic pleural effusion, the level of dullness in the right mid-scapular line is lower than that of the right mid-axillary line. Shoulder pain, usually the right and occasionally the left, may occur if the disease affects the left lobe of the liver. There may be fullness of the subcostal margin, and the right intercostal spaces. The liver is usually palpable and tender. In my experience, the liver was not palpable in nearly 20%, although it was found enlarged by scintiscan procedures. The spleen is seldom enlarged in an amoebic liver abscess. There may be signs of pleural effusion on the right or left side. Amoebic liver abscess can rupture through the diaphragm into the lung and develop a hepato-bronchial fistula (Fig. 104).

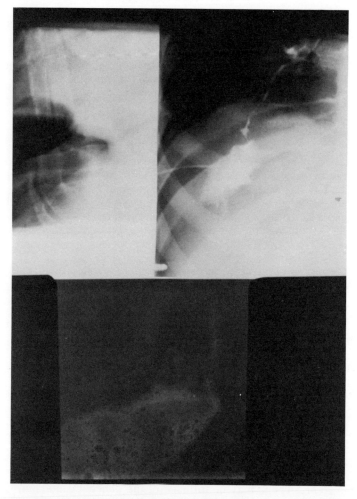

FIG. 104: A case of amoebic liver abscess with bronchial fistula; the upper left section shows air injected into
the abscess cavity after drainage of the pus. Contrast material, injected into the right lobe of the
liver, passed through the bronchial fistula into the
lung, (upper right corner). The patient coughed up
and complained of bitter taste in the mouth. See
the bottom portion of the picture showing the contrast material in the sputum.

LABORATORY

Leukocytosis and shift to the left are inconstant associated features of amoebiasis. The liver enzymes may or may not be elevated. Alkaline phosphatase is increased in most cases of amoebic liver abscess. Jaundice and increased bilirubin are rare in amoebic liver abscess.

The liver-spleen scan by Tc-99 colloid shows defective uptake in the liver (Fig. 105). The Ga-67 scintiscan may also show a defect in the liver with an area of increased uptake surrounding the defect (Fig. 106).

The ultrasound would confirm the cystic nature of the lesion (Fig. 107), and angiograms are seldom required.

When in doubt, and when amoebic liver abscess is suspected, IHA titers are confirmatory. This test is positive in nearly 99% of the cases.

Blood cultures are always negative in amoebic liver abscess. A positive blood culture with a scintiscan defect in the liver should suggest pyogenic liver abscess.

ASPIRATION OF PUS

When IHA titers cannot be obtained within a period of three days, the patient should be tentatively treated for amoebic liver abscess with metronidazole and liver abscess aspirated. I prefer to treat them for at least three days prior to needle aspiration. Acute amoebic liver abscesses, when untreated, tend to bleed on needle aspiration. After three days of therapy, the bleeding tendency markedly decreases. The liver size also decreases, liver becomes harder, and aspiration of pus is successful. It is sufficient if the diagnosis is established by IHA, physical examination and scintiscan procedures. Routine needle aspiration for amoebic liver abscess is unnecessary. Most patients respond to metronidazole therapy even without aspiration. Aspiration is indicated in cases of threatened rupture or unusually large-sized liver abscess in the left lobe threatening to rupture into the pericardium and cause pericardial tamponade and death.

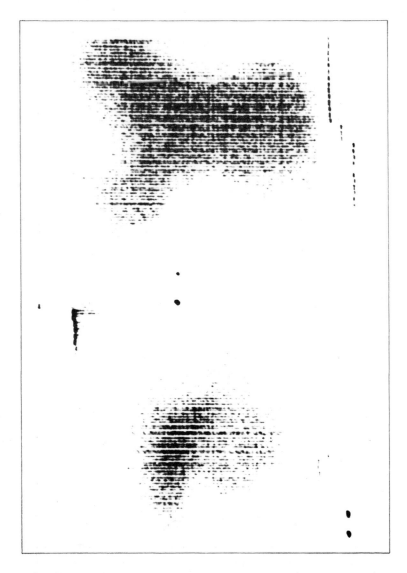

FIG. 105: Liver scan in a case of amoebic liver abscess of the
right lobe of the liver (above, anterior; below, left
lateral). Note the large focal defect in the right lobe
of the liver.

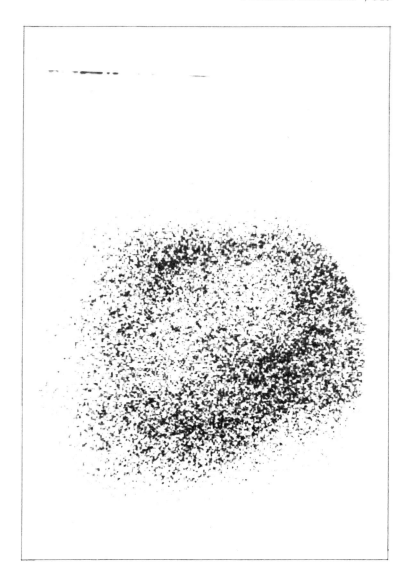

FIG. 106: Ga-67 scan in the same patient as in Fig. 105, done three days later, also shows the focal defect noted earlier, but in addition, there is a rim of increased activity noted around this focal defect. This is characteristic of amoebic liver abscess or a tumor with central necrosis.

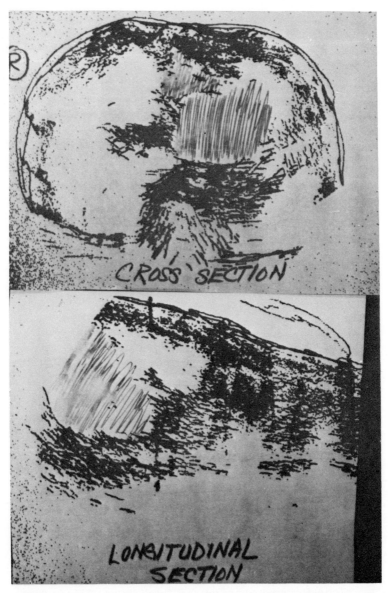

FIG. 107: Ultrasound of an amoebic liver abscess of the right
lobe, cross and longitudinal sections.

## THE AMOEBIC PUS

The amoebic pus is anchovy-sauce in color and it is bacteriologically sterile. Wright's stain of this pus may show a large number of eosinophils and leukocyte debris. We performed direct gas chromatography of amoebic liver abscess pus, and found lactic acid as the sole major product. [8]

## DIFFERENTIAL DIAGNOSIS

Amoebic liver abscesses are mistaken for right lower lobe pneumonia, tuberculous pleural effusion, Echinococcus cysts, pericardial effusion, tuberculosis, gumma of the liver, and tumors of the liver.

Tuberculosis and amoebic liver abscess might coexist. A young Korean studying dentistry in the U. S. was admitted for evaluation of a large right-sided pleural effusion. It was a serous effusion and had no bacteria on Gram's stain. A liver scan was done, which showed a large defect in the right lobe of the liver, and purulent anchovy-sauce color pus was aspirated from the liver. The IHA titer was positive. Following therapy for amoebiasis, the size of the liver decreased and the pleural effusion disappeared. Six weeks later, the culture of the pleural fluid grew 30,000 colonies of M. tuberculosis per milliliter. He was then treated with antituberculous chemotherapy. Another patient had some atypical lung infiltrates seen on chest roentgenogram. He had amoebic abscess of the left lobe of the liver. He recovered on metronidazole and needle aspiration of the liver abscess, but continued to have high fevers. Several sputa examinations later grew M. kansasii. A third patient was admitted with right upper lobe consolidation and cavitation, and had M. tuberculosis seen and cultured from the sputum. However, he had no liver enlargement, except that on the chest roentgenogram, the right dome of the diaphragm was found elevated with a globular configuration. The IHA titers were 1:2,400. He was treated with metronidazole and antituberculous therapy. These three cases prove that tuberculosis can coexist with another common infectious disease, amoebiasis. Hence, in patients with lung infiltrates found in association with liver abscess which fail to improve on anti-amoebic therapy, investigations should be made for the possible association of pulmonary tuberculosis.

## AMOEBIASIS CUTIS

Entamoeba histolytica can involve the skin adjacent to the infected areas, such as the skin around the anus and the skin
around a ruptured liver abscess. Amoeba can be readily demonstrated in the sections of tho skin or the scrapings obtained
from the marginal areas of the ulcers. In India, I saw three
cases of ulceration of the skin around the area of the sacrum,
coccyx and perineum in patients admitted with acute amoebic
dysentery. The scrapings from the margins of these lesions
showed vegetative forms of amoeba in all three patients. The
lesions healed with emetine treatment. Isolated skin involvement without dysentery is rare.

## PULMONARY AMOEBIASIS

Pulmonary amoebiasis secondary to liver involvement is common. Primary pulmonary amoebiasis without liver involvement is uncommon.

Female genital tract infections, such as amoebic granulomas
of the clitoris, of the vagina or of the cervix, are rare.

Serology: Although indirect hemagglutination test is an extremely
important diagnostic test of extra-intestinal amoebiasis, it may
occasionally be positive among those not suffering from amoebiasis. Once the IHA test becomes positive, it may remain so
for four to five years or longer. In Mexico, 5% to 7% of the
population had positive IHA reactions, including 3.9% of the
newborn. [6] This incidence might be even higher among the poorer
people of certain highly endemic areas.

Counterimmunoelectrophoresis (CIE), gel diffusion precipitation
tests (GPT) and latex fixation test (LF) are equally efficient alternatives to IHA titers in the diagnosis of extra-intestinal amoebiasis. CIE, LF and GPT are less sensitive, and might become negative much sooner than IHA.

Among the liver scans used were Ga-67 scan, I-131 rose bengal,
198 colloidal gold and 113 indium scans. Ga-67 appears to be
most efficient. In our experience, the gallium scan in conjunction with Tc-99 scan, in most cases, reliably differentiates the
pyogenic from amoebic liver abscess (see Figs. 105, 106).

# REFERENCES

1. Sexton, D. J. , et al. : Amoebiasis in a mental institution: Serological and epidemiologic studies. Amer. J. Epidemiol. 100:414, 1974.

2. Judy, K. L. : Amoebiasis presenting as an acute abdomen. Amer. J. Surg. 127:275, 1974.

3. Pittman, F. E. , Henninger, G. R. : Sigmoidoscopic and colonic mucosal biopsy findings in amebic colitis. Arch. Pathol. 97:155, 1974.

4. Manson-Bahr, P. : Manson's Tropical Diseases. Bailliere, Tindall & Cassell, London, 1966, pp. 417-436.

5. Tucker, P. C. , Webster, P. D. , Kilpatrick, Z. M. : Amebic colitis mistaken for inflammatory bowel disease. Arch. Int. Med. 135:681, 1975.

6. Lara, R. , et al. : Infecciones mixtas por e histolytica, shigella y otras bacterias enteropathogenas encontradas en ninos con diarrhea. Archivos de Invest. Medica 5:Suppl. 2, 515, 1974.

7. Miyamoto, A. T. , Thadepalli, H. , Mishkin, F. S. : Gallium images of amoebic liver abscess. New Eng. J. Med. 291: 1363, 1974.

8. Mandal, A. K. , Thadepalli, H. : Surgical aspects of amoebiasis and diagnostic clues. American Surgeon 44:564-570, 1978.

72: GIARDIASIS
by H. Thadepalli

Giardia lamblia is a parasite of the duodenum and small intestine. Man is the natural host and the only known reservoir of this parasite. Its prevalence in the United States ranges from 1% to 30%. Giardiasis rarely causes death, but can cause great discomfort. The diagnosis of this condition is not considered early enough to prevent the "suffering from investigations in a large number of cases".[1] In most referral cases, it may take six to seven weeks to reach the diagnosis. In one instance, a two-week infant underwent several investigations, such as withholding cow's milk, and a series of roentgenographic examinations for malabsorption; the diagnosis of giardiasis was not established until the child was about one year old.[2]

SYMPTOMS

Diarrhea, abdominal cramps, nausea and weakness associated with weight loss, abdominal distension, greasy stools, belching and vomiting are some of the common features of giardiasis. Fever is the least common symptom (Table 37).

TABLE 37: SYMPTOMS OF GIARDIASIS

| SYMPTOM | APPROXIMATE PERCENTAGE OF INCIDENCE |
| --- | --- |
| Diarrhea and fatigue | 90 |
| Anorexia and weight loss | 70 |
| Abdominal cramps | 70 |
| Nausea | 60 |
| Abdominal distention and flatulence | 60 |
| Greasy stools | 60 |
| Vomiting | 30 |
| Fever | 15 |

The most notable outbreaks of giardiasis within the United States occurred among the travelers who returned from Leningrad, Russia. Several small outbreaks resulted from contaminated water systems in a group of skiers in Aspen, Colorado; in a group of hikers on the mountains of Utah; and in Rome, New York.[3,4,5,7] Of these outbreaks, the diarrhea among the travelers to Leningrad, Russia received the widest publication. Giardiasis is an etiologic agent of the so-called travelers' diarrhea, with the exception that it occurs at the end of the tour, in contrast to the classical travelers' diarrhea, "turista", which occurs during the first few days of the visit. This giardiasis was therefore nicknamed as turista leningradista. Giardiasis should be considered in the differential diagnosis of all who present with abdominal distention, diarrhea and chronic loss of weight, and with stool cultures for bacteria which are negative. Children are more prone to develop this disease than adults.

## THE PARASITE

Examine the stools for the cysts of the parasite. The trophozoite forms of Giardia may be found in severe cases of diarrhea (Fig. 108). The trophozoite is a bilateral, symmetrical, pear-shaped organism 12 to 15 $\mu$ in length, with four pairs of flagella. It has two prominent nuclei with large central karyosomes. A sucking disc occupies the flat ventral surface through which it attaches to the intestine. It inhabits the duodenum and jejunum, propelling from place to place by the help of flagella. The trophozoites die outside the host. They encyst in the ileum and the large bowel. The cysts are then passed and can survive indefinitely under moist circumstances. By fecal-oral contamination, the cysts enter the stomach, where they are digested; in the duodenum, the cyst divides to form two trophozoites.

## DIAGNOSTIC PROCEDURES

Duodenal aspirates may be examined for the trophozoites. This test is successful 80% to 90% of the time.

Small intestine biopsy is a harmless procedure which can be done in the outpatient clinic within an hour or two, and from the biopsy specimen, a wet mucous smear can be obtained. This mucosal imprint can be examined for the parasite. Later, the duodenal tissue itself is stained with hematoxylin and eosin, and examined for the parasite.

The enterotest duodenal capsule is useful in the diagnosis of giardiasis. [6] The principle of this test involves passing a thread into the duodenum, which is then rapidly removed and smeared on the surface of a slide for the presence of trophozoites. The enterotest capsule is a gelatin capsule packed with a nylon yarn. It has a spherical lead weight which, when ingested, enters the duodenum. The free end of the thread is tied close to the nose. The patient washes the capsule down by swallowing gulps of

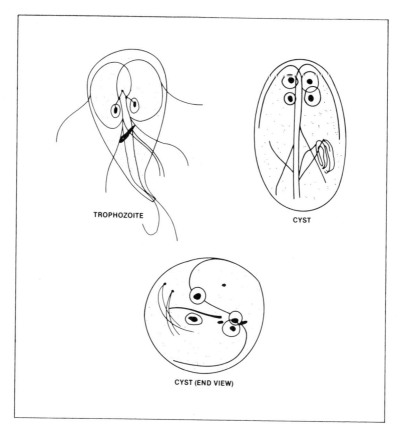

TROPHOZOITE

CYST

CYST (END VIEW)

FIG. 108: Giardia lamblia.

water. It then enters the duodenum and occasionally the upper part of the jejunum. In the stomach, the gelatin capsule dissolves, leaving the lead weight free, which easily passes through the pylorus. The line is then withdrawn with a fairly rapid, but gentle, pull. The surface of this thread may have bile-stained mucus, which is scraped off between the two fingers of a gloved hand and examined for parasites. This test can also be used for detecting other parasites, such as Strongyloides stercoralis, Clonorchis sinensis, Fasciola hepatica, Trichostrongylus orientalis, Isospora hominis and Ancylostoma duodenale. The expected percentage of success of each diagnostic test used for giardiasis is listed in Table 38.

TABLE 38: POSITIVE DIAGNOSTIC SOURCES IN GIARDIASIS

| SOURCE | EXPECTED PER CENT OF YIELD |
|---|---|
| Cysts in stools | 50 |
| Duodenal aspirate | 80 |
| Mucosal imprint | 90 |
| Biopsy of duodenum | 95 |
| Enterotest duodenal capsule | 95 |

## DIFFERENTIAL DIAGNOSIS

Giardiasis should be considered in the differential diagnosis of celiac disease and similar syndromes such as anorexia nervosa, chronic diarrhea, retarded growth, inanition and undiagnosed abdominal distention.

IgE deficiency, diabetes mellitus, and chronic pancreatitis are some of the predisposing factors for giardiasis.

The sedimentation rate is usually normal. The serum immunoglobulin E level may also be normal.

Eosinophilia is an inconstant feature; it might be either increased or normal.

The roentgenographic appearance of the small intestine is often normal, but sometimes in chronic giardiasis, certain abnormalities, such as the loss of villi, thickening of the mucosal folds and increased transit time, might occur. There is no serological test for giardiasis.

Fecal smears should be first examined under physiologic saline and later with one percent potassium iodide. These smears may also permanently stain with iron hematoxylin. A concentrated specimen might be fixed in formalin and ether and examined for the cyst. Giemsa's stain is excellent for the identification of the trophozoites of G. lamblia in the fecal smears and mucous smears of duodenal and jejunal aspirates.

Animal models for giardiasis are of epidemiologic interest. In one investigation, beagle dogs were fed with water suspected to be the source of the outbreak of giardiasis. The parasite was easily recovered from the stools later.

In summary, giardiasis should be considered in the differential diagnosis of all patients admitted for chronic malabsorption syndrome, chronic undiagnosed dyspepsia, unexplained diarrhea, and anyone having abdominal symptoms with history of travel to areas known to be endemic for giardiasis. It should also be remembered that, unlike many parasitic infections, giardiasis may be found along with other parasitic infections.

## REFERENCES

1. Eastham, E. J. , Douglas, A. P. , Watson, A. J. : Diagnosis of Giardia lamblia infection as a cause of diarrhoea. Lancet 2:950, 1976.

2. Burke, J. A.: Giardiasis in childhood. Amer. J. Dis. Child. 129:1304, 1975.

3. Center for Disease Control. Morbidity and Mortality Weekly Report. U. S. Department of Health, Education and Welfare, Atlanta, March 2, 1974.

4. News from the Center for Disease Control. J. Inf. Dis. 124: 235, 1971.

5. Thompson, R. G. , Karandikar, D. S. , Leek, J. : Giardiasis, an unusual cause of epidemic diarrhoea. Lancet 1:615, 1974.

6. Thomas, G. E. , Goldsmid, J. M. , Wicks, A. C. : Use of the enterotest duodenal capsule in the diagnosis of giardiasis: A preliminary study. S. A. Medical Journal 48:2219, 1974.

7. Brady, P. G. , Wolfe, J. C.: Waterborne giardiasis. Ann. Int. Med. 81:498, 1974.

## 73: TRICHOMONAS
### by H. Thadepalli

Trichomonas (T.) vaginalis, a flagellated, protozoan parasite of the vagina, causes nearly 20% to 40% of all cases of vaginitis. It is transmitted by coitus and also by fomites. In men, T. vaginalis can cause urethritis.

### THE PARASITE

It is a tetra-flagellated, motile protozoa with a prominent axostyle (Fig. 109). It does not survive in the pH (3.8 to 4.4) of the normal vagina. A pH of 4.5 or more is a prerequisite for this infestation. It resembles T. hominis, a non-pathogenic commensal of the large bowel, and T. tenax, the only flagellate found in association with gingival infections. They do not transform from one species to another. T. vaginalis is of size 10 to 30$\mu$. It can be cultured in egg yolk medium and the cysteine-peptone-liver-maltose (CPLM) medium.

### CLINICAL FEATURES

Nearly 70% of the women infected with T. vaginalis are asymptomatic. Although vulvovaginitis is the most common presenting feature of Trichomonas infestation, this disease accounts for only 40% of the cases of vulvovaginitis. Candida, Haemophilus vaginalis, Mycoplasma and Chlamydia account for the remaining 60%. Ten per cent of the cases present with acute manifestation. T. vaginalis infestation often (90%) presents as a chronic indolent infection. Nearly 30% of all patients with carcinoma of the cervix harbor T. vaginalis. It causes urethritis in men. Frequently, the women act as the reservoirs, while asymptomatic men act as the vectors.

### DIAGNOSIS

Wet mount preparation in saline, obtained directly from the vaginal canal, even without staining, is adequate for the diagnosis.

Papanicolaou smears, obtained for the study of exfoliative cytology, may show trichomonal forms.

In men with urethritis, urethral or prostatic massage smears are recommended.

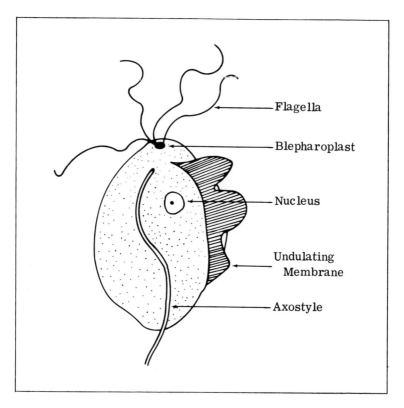

FIG. 109: <u>Trichomonas vaginalis</u>.

## TREATMENT

Metronidazole (Flagyl) is the drug of choice. Dose: 250 mg., three times a day, for ten days and 500 mg. vaginal suppository, once a day, for ten days. Alternatively, tinidazole, 1.4 to 1.8 grams/day may be administered in a single dose.

74: MALARIA
by H. Thadepalli

Malaria continues to be a major public health problem in Africa
and Southeast Asia. It is now posing greater challenges because of the development of resistance by the mosquito to in-
secticides, and the parasite developing resistance to chloro-
quin. In India, 75 million cases of malaria were recorded in
1947. It was brought down to 0.1 million in 1965 by DDT
spraying, but it has increased to a staggering $2\frac{1}{2}$ million cases
per year during 1974, due to development of resistance to DDT
by the anopheline mosquito.

Malaria is caused by a protozoan parasite of genus Plasmodium
(P.). It is characterized by periodic fever with chills, anemia,
and splenomegaly. Human malaria is caused by one of the following species of malarial parasites:

1) P. falciparum
2) P. vivax
3) P. malariae
4) P. ovale

P. malariae is not as common as P. falciparum and P. vivax,
and P. ovale is the least frequent of the four.

LIFE CYCLE:

A. SPOROGONY IN MOSQUITO: The mosquito ingests the male
(a microgametocyte) and the female (macrogametocyte) of
the parasite along with its human blood meal. The microgametocyte then divides and extrudes multiple motile flagellae
(exflagellation), one of which fertilizes the macrogametocyte to form a zygote, which, in turn, divides further into
sporozoa. This sexual cycle takes place in the foregut of
the mosquito. The sporozoa later migrate to the salivary
glands and get injected into the human host at the time of
the next blood meal by the mosquito.

B. SCHIZOGONY IN MAN: The sporozoa enter the reticuloendothelial cells where they multiply into merozoites, which enter
the blood stream and penetrate the erythrocytes. The merozoites are disc-like to start with, and later assume amoe-
boid form and acquire a brown pigment called hemozoin.
It later divides (asexually) into multicellular schizonts, which
rupture the erythrocyte, and each cell will then attack a
new erythrocyte. Some later become gametocytes, which,

when ingested, multiply in the mosquito. The pre-erythrocytic tissue phase in P. falciparum is temporary. Therefore, P. falciparum infection, by the time it manifests as a clinical attack, has only the erythrocytic phase. Once cured, therefore, true relapses are rare with P. falciparum infections.

Incubation period: This is nearly ten to fourteen days. It may vary for months, and even years.

## CLINICAL FEATURES

Fever periodicity varies. Tertian (third day) fever occurs every 48 hours in P. vivax (benign tertian) and P. falciparum (malignant tertian) infections. P. falciparum may also cause fevers in a somewhat shorter than 48-hour period when it is called subtertian. Quartan (fourth day) fevers occur every 72 hours with P. malariae infections. Quotidian (every day) fevers may be caused by all of the four species of parasites or in infections caused by two separate species of malarial parasite.

Prodromal symptoms, like body pains, irregular low-grade fever, asthenia, malaise and headaches may be present during the first week, after which, in most cases, the classic febrile paroxysms occur.

Each paroxysm starts with the cold, shivering stage, with rigors when the skin is cold, although the rectal temperature may be as high as 104°F. The patient covers himself with many blankets, yet is unable to warm himself, even on a hot day out in the sun. The cold stage may last for 15 to 30 minutes, followed by the hot stage, when the patient complains of hot sensation, rids himself of all blankets and even his clothing. The skin is now hot and dry. At this stage, he may complain of severe frontal headache. The hot stage lasts for about two to three hours, followed by the stage of sweating, when the patient sweats profusely and drenches the sheets within the next hour, and the temperature touches normal or subnormal. The patient may then feel excessively weak, but otherwise appears well.

The clinical attack of malaria is almost similar for all infections caused by all four species. Rigors are not common with P. falciparum.

The spleen is often palpable at the end of the first week. Malaria is the leading cause of splenomegaly in endemic zones. [5] It should enlarge at least twice its normal size to be palpable.

It can be palpated in children in the standing position. It can also be felt in the right lateral position of the patient, with the knees drawn in. Whereas massive enlargement of the spleen is easy to detect, smaller sizes may require more skillful examination. On deep inspection, a normal spleen moves to the left subcostal margin and hence, is not palpable.

The observer, while palpating the abdomen, should not try to grope for the spleen. Instead, on deep inspection, he should let the spleen move down to touch the examiner's fingertips, placed very lightly under the left subcostal margins. Massive enlargement of the spleen can be appreciated by inch-by-inch palpation from the right iliac crest to the left subcostal margin. I am amazed to find the frequency with which our postgraduate physicians miss the enlarged spleen by groping or kneading the abdomen for the spleen, instead of letting the spleen move down to hit one's fingers placed steadily on the abdomen.

OTHER CLINICAL MODES OF PRESENTATION: P. malariae may cause nephrotic syndrome in children and young adults and may be mistaken for post-streptococcal nephrotic syndrome. P. falciparum, appropriately titled malignant tertian, may cause drastic complications. The patient may present in a state of coma (cerebral malaria) with bizarre neurological manifestations like neck stiffness, convulsions, cranial nerve palsies or positive Babinski reflexes. The lumbar puncture is unrewarding. Malarial parasites are seldom found in the spinal fluid.

Fevers above 104°F. are not common with P. falciparum, but patients may present in a state of hyperpyrexia, mistaken for heat stroke. Malignant tertian malaria may manifest with fever and abdominal pain and may be mistaken for typhoid fever. Occasionally, the patient is jaundiced and mistaken for biliary cirrhosis. Dysenteric and choleraic forms of malaria have been described, but are not common.

Black water fever is a rare complication of malignant tertian malaria. Previous history of exposure to antimalarials, although not the cause, is frequently present. It is characterized by fever and rigors followed by hemolysis and hemoglobinuria. Various changes in the clinical picture are not uncommon. The urine is seldom black, as its name implies. It is usually dark brown in color. Brownish and granular casts may be present in the urine.

Death is a rare complication of P. vivax and P. malariae infections. The mortality rate is very high (20 to 40%) in cerebral and hyperpyrexial forms of P. falciparum infections and in black water fever.

## DIAGNOSIS

BLOOD SMEAR EXAMINATION: Several thin blood smears may be prepared and stained by Giemsa's method.

FIELD'S STAIN: The yield is higher with thick smears. The thick blood smears may be prepared in the following manner. Clean the surface of the finger with alcohol, dry and prick with a needle to bleed a drop; pick it up on the surface of a clean glass slide, and spread it over one square inch with a needle. Dry the smear and immerse it in solution A for a few seconds. Wash in water and dip in solution B for a few seconds. Wash the slide and dry in vertical position. Parasitemia is variable; hence, repeated blood smears should be examined.

While examining the thick film, count 100 white cells (or multiples of 100) and also count the malaria parasites seen in the same microscopic fields with the white cells. Calculate the parasites per cubic millimeter of blood as follows:

$$\frac{X \text{ (No. of parasites per cu. mm.)}}{\text{White cell count per cu. mm.}} = \frac{\text{No. of parasites counted in the same field with 100 white cells}}{\text{No. of white cells counted (100 in this case)}}$$

Example:

$$\frac{X}{4,000} = \frac{1,200}{100}$$

$$100X = 4,800,000$$

$$X = 48,000$$

The parasites are concentrated in the Field's stain; it requires some experience to interpret the smears correctly.

## THE PARASITE

DIFFERENTIATING FEATURES OF P. VIVAX AND P. FAL-
CIPARUM:

|  | P. vivax | P. falciparum |
|---|---|---|
| 1. Number of infected erythrocytes | 2% or less | 10% or more |
| 2. Number of parasites per erythrocyte | mostly one per cell | frequently two per cell (Fig. 110) |
| 3. Schizonts | larger than erythrocyte, usually present about 12 to 24 merozoites | smaller than erythrocyte, very scanty, up to 36 merozoites |
| 4. Trophozoite | large, signet ring shape with one chromatin dot | usually thin and small with one or two chromatin dots |
| 5. Size of erythrocyte | large size because P. vivax almost exclusively attacks the reticulocyte | normal size because P. falciparum invades the mature erythrocyte |
| 6. Pigment | yellowish brown pigment | present in heavy infections, dark brown or black |
| 7. Pigment in erythrocytes | fine stippling (Schuffner's dots) | coarse stippling (Maurer's dots) |
| 8. Gametocyte | round, larger than the red cell | sausage-shaped |
| 9. Relapse | frequent up to three years if untreated | relapses are rare |

P. ovale and P. malariae resemble P. vivax in peripheral blood
smears. The erythrocyte is frequently oval or fimbriated in P.
ovale infections, and band forms of the parasite are present in
P. ovale and P. malariae (Fig. 111). P. malariae, unlike P. vivax,

562/ Parasitic Infections

attacks the mature erythrocyte; hence, the size of the erythrocyte is usually normal.

Plasmodium is the commonest intra-erythrocytic pigmented
organism seen in man. Babesia is also an intra erythrocytic
organism rare in man (see page 590). Bartonella bacilliformis (causes oroya fever) is an intra-erythrocytic bacterium
endemic to Peru (see pages 502-503).

INDIRECT FLUORESCENT ANTIBODY (IFA) TITERS: IFA titers
are sensitive and specific. Nearly all patients with active malaria will have high antibody levels. A dilution titer of 256 or
greater indicates current or recent infection, while titers of
16 and 64 indicate more remote exposure to malaria. It is not
antigen-specific, but species-specific. A four fold increase
in the dilution of IFA suggests infection due to that species.
Babesia may cross react with IFA titers of Plasmodium. IFA
titers decrease following clinical recovery, although more than
50% may show detectable antibody titers at the end of one year.

EPINEPHRINE TEST: Injection of 0.5 ml. of 1:1000 epinephrine,
by causing peripheral vascular constriction and some splenic
contraction, increased the yield of the parasite in the peripheral blood smear. The results of this test are variable.

STERNAL PUNCTURE: Is useful to detect the parasites when
routine means are negative. In many cases of malaria, peripheral smears will show the parasite.

### DIFFERENTIAL DIAGNOSIS

The following are often mistaken for malaria or vice versa:

1) typhoid fever
2) tuberculosis
3) endocarditis
4) urinary tract
   infection
5) cholelithiasis
6) amoebiasis
7) dysentery
8) meningitis
9) Hodgkin's disease, or
   other malignancy
10) filariasis
11) relapsing fevers
12) brucellosis
13) trypanosomiasis
14) kala azar
15) dengue fever
16) pappataci (sand fly) fever

TRANSFUSION MALARIA: Donors exposed to P. vivax malaria
may have parasitemia for years and can transmit the infection
by blood transfusions. The parasite may live in the donated blood
for two to three weeks. Heroin and other drug addicts were

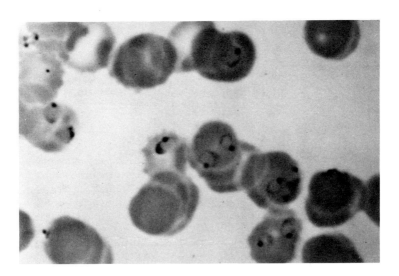

FIG. 110: <u>Plasmodium falciparum.</u> Note that there is more than one organism per cell, which is characteristic of this infection.

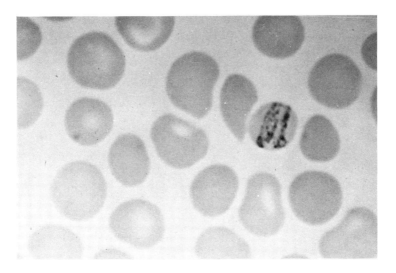

FIG. 111: Band forms of <u>Plasmodium malariae.</u> Note the corpuscle is not enlarged.

reported to have developed malaria by the usage of needle transfers.

RESISTANCE TO MALARIA: Persons with Fy Fy genotype, found predominantly in African and American blacks, are completely resistant to benign tertian (P. vivax) malaria. Also, persons with sickle cell hemoglobin and G-6PD deficiency are resistant to P. falciparum infections.

## TREATMENT

Certain strains of P. falciparum in South America and Asia have acquired resistance to chloroquine, amodiaquine and/or pyrimethamine. Most chloroquine-resistant malaria parasites are susceptible to quinine. Chloroquine resistance is alarming, but by no means common. Malaria can be prevented by the fullest regimen.

### CHART I: MALARIA CHEMOPROPHYLAXIS FOR TRAVELERS[4]

| Drug | Regimen |
|------|---------|
| Chloroquine phosphate | 500 mg. (300-mg. base) once weekly and continued for six weeks after last exposure in endemic area |
| PLUS | |
| Primaquine | 15-mg. base, daily for fourteen days after last exposure |

Travelers to areas with chloroquine-resistant malaria:

| Drug | Regimen |
|------|---------|
| Chloroquine-primaquine | Once weekly for duration of exposure and eight weeks after the last exposure |
| PLUS | |
| Dapsone | 25 mg. daily for duration of exposure and four weeks after last exposure |

TREATMENT OF A MALARIAL ATTACK: Chloroquine diphosphate, loading dose of 1000 mg. (600 mg. of base) followed by 500 mg. at six, twenty-four and forty-eight hours after the initial loading dose (total 2.5 grams or 1.5 grams of base). With the exception of P. falciparum infection, a gametocidal agent like primaquine or pamaquine ("pa" - father, "ma" - mother, "quine" for quinine) is administered after completion of chloroquine therapy in a dose of 15 mg. of base daily for fourteen days.

Chloroquine-resistant strains are susceptible to quinine administered in a dose of 650 mg. of quinine hydrochloride every eight hours for seven to ten days, followed by gametocidal therapy, as mentioned above.

There are several other alternative regimens available for resistant cases of malaria for which the reader is referred to the books on tropical medicine.[1,2,3]

## REFERENCES

1. Adams, A. R. D. and Maegraith, B. G.: Clinical Tropical Diseases, 6th Edition. Blackwell Scientific Publications, Oxford, 1976.

2. Hunter, G. W. , Schwartzwelder, J. C. , Clyde, D. F. : Tropical Medicine, 5th Edition. W. B. Saunders, Philadelphia, 1976.

3. Manson-Bahr, P.: Manson's Tropical Diseases. Bailliere, Tindall & Cassell, London, 1966.

4. Barrett-Connor, E.: Chemoprophylaxis of malaria for travelers. Ann. Int. Med. 81:219-224, 1974.

5. Butler, T. , et al. : Chronic splenomegaly in Vietnam. I. Evidence for malarial etiology. Amer. J. Trop. Med. & Hyg. 22:1-5, 1973.

## 75: TOXOPLASMOSIS
### by H. Thadepalli

Toxoplasmosis is a disease caused by an obligate intracellular (extra-erythrocytic) protozoan parasite called Toxoplasma gondii. Carnivorous animals, such as the domestic cat, [1] are its definitive hosts. The infection is acquired by ingestion of undercooked meat (mutton or beef) or contamination of food with the feces of the cat; or, it is transplacentally transmitted in utero, outside of which there is no human-to-human transmission. The adult trophozoite is crescent-shaped (Toxo) of size $3 \times 7 \mu m$, and can be stained with Wright's or Giemsa's stain. The cysts are larger - 10 to 100 $\mu m$ in size and stain with periodic acid Schiff stain. It can affect all warm-blooded animals and birds.

## CLINICAL FEATURES

It affects both vegetarians and non-vegetarians of both sexes and all ages anywhere in the world. Fifty per cent of the American people have been exposed to this disease, and nearly 3,000 babies are born each year exposed to toxoplasmosis. Although it is a common parasite, it is not often thought of in the differential diagnosis because in most cases, it causes no symptoms.

Usually, the disease is subclinical. In some patients, especially in children and in immunologically-compromised hosts, it can be symptomatic.

In adults, fever, lymphadenopathy, skin rash and hepatomegaly are some of its features. The majority of children born with this infection may remain clinically silent or manifest such occult changes as slow mental retardation, [2] progressive deafness, jaundice or hydrocephalus. However, 15% to 20% of the affected newborn may show extensive involvement with pneumonia, myocarditis, pericarditis, hepatitis, encephalitis or chorioretinitis.

Toxoplasmosis is a rare cause of death in young adults if there is no other predisposing cause.

It is a blessing that mothers previously affected by this disease, and those with antibodies to Toxoplasma, do not transmit the disease to the newborn. If the mother has no antibodies to Toxoplasma and develops infection during the first or second trimester, the newborn is likely to suffer from severe disease. If she develops infection during the third trimester, the disease tends to be subclinical and rarely fatal. [3] Toxoplasma may remain dormant in the endometrium of 10% to 12% of the affected mothers,[4] yet this guaranteed immunity from infection to the subsequent newborn remains an enigma. Toxoplasmosis does not cause infertility. [5]

Adult onset toxoplasmosis is clinically indistinguishable from infectious mononucleosis. The lymph nodes are enlarged, discrete and solitary, of size 1.5 to 2.0 cm. They do not suppurate or coalesce, but may remain enlarged for nearly 18 to 24 months. Lymphadenopathy occurs in acquired toxoplasmosis. Toxoplasmosis should be considered in the differential diagnosis of all cases of lymphadenopathy without splenomegaly. [6]

Maculopapular rash sparing the scalp, palms of the hands and the soles of the feet may occur with toxoplasmosis.

The spleen is often of normal size, even though the liver may be enlarged.

## DIAGNOSIS

1) Tissue diagnosis is the most important of all tests. A piece of the lymph node or liver biopsy may be homogenized with 0.9% saline and injected intraperitoneally into mice. The tissue sample should not be frozen or preserved in formalin, because both procedures kill the parasite. The peritoneal fluid ten days later may be aspirated and stained with methylene blue and examined for Toxoplasma. Human Toxoplasma is not lethal to the mice; therefore, they should be sacrificed after two or three weeks and the tissues examined for the protozoa. Giemsa's or Wright's stain may be employed for this purpose.

2) Sabin-Feldman dye test (DT): Toxoplasma, when exposed to the patient's serum (antibodies) becomes swollen and stains deep blue. The test result is expressed in terms of dilutions. The dye test is usually positive within 30 days after the infection. These titers later increase when repeated 2 to 3 weeks apart. A titer of 1:64 suggests previous infection, and 1:256 or more suggests recent infection. A four-fold increase in DT from 1:64 to 1:256, for example, strongly supports the diagnosis.

3) Indirect hemagglutination (IHA) test: Tannic acid-coated erythrocytes agglutinate when exposed to lysate from Toxoplasma. IHA test is positive after 10 to 30 days. A titer of 1:64 suggests previous infection, and 1:256 indicates recent infection. A rising titer, as in the case of DT, is diagnostic.

4) Complement-fixation test (CFT) is positive within 2 to 4 weeks after infection. The CFT appears after and disappears earlier than the dye test. A CFT titer of 1:4 suggests previous exposure to the disease, and a titer of 1:8 indicates recent infection. A two to four-fold increase in CFT is diagnostic of recent Toxoplasma infection.

5) Indirect fluorescent antibody (IFA) test is the most widely used test. IFA is as sensitive as DT. No live organisms are required to do this test. IFA is positive 30 days after the infection. A titer of 1:64 suggests previous infection, and 1:256 suggests recent infection. False-positive results may occur in patients with antinuclear antibody.

6) IgM-fluorescent antibody test [7] may be used to diagnose congenital toxoplasmosis. IgM antibody is specific for Toxoplasma and, if present in the newborn, it is diagnostic of toxoplasmosis. A negative IgM-fluorescent antibody test does not rule out this disease.

7) Radioimmunoassay (RIA): [8] Nearly 65% of the cases of toxoplasmosis can be diagnosed by RIA within an hour. Thirty-five per cent may require 24 hours. RIA is not yet as popular as DT, CFT or IFA.

8) Skin test for Toxoplasma is too sensitive to be of any value as a diagnostic tool.

## DIFFERENTIAL DIAGNOSIS

The following diseases should be considered in the differential diagnosis of toxoplasmosis:

1) Infectious mononucleosis: Paul-Bunnell test is always negative in toxoplasmosis.
2) Lymphoma, and
3) Leukemia by lymph node biopsy and bone marrow examination. A positive DT or CFT or IFA test with discrete follicular proliferation with plasma cell and eosinophil infiltration is characteristic of toxoplasmosis. It does occasionally occur as a complication of lymphoma.

4) The skin rash may be mistaken for Rocky Mountain spotted fever.
5) Typhus, or
6) Syphilis.

It can also be confused with other viral illnesses, such as:

7) Cytomegalovirus
8) Rubella, and
9) Herpes simplex encephalitis
10) Fungal, and
11) Tuberculous infections should be excluded by appropriate cultures.

Congenital toxoplasmosis may be mistaken for:

12) Erythroblastosis fetalis, and
13) Subdural hematoma.

Toxoplasma infection may coexist with Pneumocystis carinii infection, fungal or viral infections. Hence, diagnosis of one of these does not exclude the others.

## TREATMENT

The following drugs were tested and considered satisfactory:

1) pyrimethamine
2) sulfadiazine or trisulfapyridines
3) spiramycin

All of the above compounds are toxic. Close monitoring is necessary in all patients.

## REFERENCES

1. Krogstad, D. J., Juranek, D. D.: Toxoplasmosis: with comments on risk of infection from cats. Ann. Int. Med. 77: 773, 1972.

2. Terragna, A., et al.: Toxoplasmosi ed encefalopatie «minori» nel bambino. Minerva Pediatrica 26:328, 1974.

3. Desmonts, G., Couvreur, J.: Congenital toxoplasmosis: A prospective study of 378 pregnancies. New Eng. J. Med. 290:1110, 1974.

4. Remington, J. S. , Melton, M. , Jacobs, L. : Chronic Toxoplasma infection in the uterus. J. Lab. Clin. Med. 56:879,
1960.

5. Ganesh, K. , Chowdry, P. , Hingorani, V. : Toxoplasmosis
and infertility. Indian J. Med. Res. 62:1, 1974.

6. Dutta, J. K. , Prakash, O. : Toxoplasma antibodies in cases
of undiagnosed lymphadenopathy. J. Indian Med. Assoc. 63:
355, 1973.

7. Remington, J.S. , Desmonts, G. : Congenital toxoplasmosis:
Variability in the IgM-fluorescent antibody response and
some pitfalls in diagnosis. J. Pediat. 83:27, 1973.

8. Gehle, W. D. , Smith, K. O. , Fuccillo, D. A. : Radioimmunoassay for toxoplasmosis. Infection and Immunity 14:1253,
1976.

76: PNEUMOCYSTIS CARINII
by H. Thadepalli


Pneumocystis (P.) carinii is a protozoan parasite of the lung, infecting the debilitated [1] or the immunologically compromised host. [2] In spite of prompt and appropriate therapy, it carries a mortality of 40% to 50%.

The life history and the mode of transmission of P. carinii are unknown. It cannot be cultured on the laboratory media. It is of 5 to $12\mu$ in size and its cysts are arranged in clusters of 2 to 8.

## CLINICAL FEATURES

The most important predisposing causes include chronic malnutrition, leukemia, cancer, irradiation therapy, cadaver renal transplantation, and corticosteroid therapy. [2,3,4,5] It may have an insidious or abrupt onset. P. carinii infection commonly begins with cough, with the production of "slimy" sputum; progressively worsening dyspnea with peri-alar cyanosis and tachypnea (rate $\geqslant 40$/minute). Fever is not a common presenting symptom. On auscultation, in spite of areas of patchy pneumonitis seen in the chest roentgenogram, the lungs may be surprisingly clear. Often, one may hear crackling rales confined to both bases of the lung. Lymphocytosis, rarely above 20,000/ cu. mm., may occur. P. carinii infection of the lung can cause a syndrome akin to alveolo-capillary block. The chest roentgenogram may show:

1) Diffuse infiltrates 1 to 2 mm. in size with granular opacities in the lower lung fields and around the hilar regions, spreading from the center to the periphery, or
2) Bilateral multinodular opacities sparing the periphery of the lung, or
3) A picture quite similar to that of pulmonary edema.
4) The previous infiltrates are usually interstitial in character, but not alveolar.
5) Pleural effusion and mediastinal adenopathy are uncommon; when they are seen, one should consider an intrathoracic extension of the underlying disease.
6) Pneumothorax and pneumomediastinum are more frequent in children than in adults.

## DIAGNOSIS

P. carinii infection should be suspected in all immunoincom-
petent patients with lung infiltrates. A patient may have more
than one infection with P. carinii at a given time. Cytomegalovirus infection, Nocardia, tuberculosis, bacterial pneumonia,
Mycoplasma pneumoniae, Aspergillus infection and Cryptococcus infections may coexist with P. carinii infections. The diagnostic procedures include:

1) Sputum: Repeated sputa examinations are required - sputum
   smears are positive for P. carinii in less than 10% of the
   cases.

2) Pharyngeal and tracheal aspirates: These are also generally
   unrewarding (positive in less than 10% of the cases).

3) Transtracheal aspiration (TTA):   Percutaneous TTA is
   more rewarding than 1 and 2. It was found to be positive in
   13% of the 60 patients studied.   Of this, only one showed
   P. carinii in the sputum.[6]

4) Bronchial lavage:   By this method, large amounts of alveolar material can be obtained for examination. Bronchial
   lavage should be obtained when the sputum is negative.[7]

5) Endobronchial brush biopsy:   It is a useful method to obtain
   the alveolar material for the demonstration of the organisms.
   It is positive in a high percentage of cases.[5]

6) Transthoracic needle aspirate of the lung: Transthoracic
   needle aspirate, as opposed to lung biopsy, is a relatively
   benign procedure, and it is useful in the diagnosis of parenchymal diseases of the lung. Pneumothorax may occur in
   nearly 30% of cases, which is often reversible. Needle aspiration of the lung is useful in the diagnosis of P. carinii
   infections.

7) Lung biopsy:   For thoracotomy and lung biopsy with or without rib resection, general anesthesia is required. Pneumothorax and hemorrhage are the potential, but infrequent, complications associated with this procedure.[8]

Routine paraffin sections stained with hematoxylin and eosin
(H&E) are inadequate. Special staining procedures are required
to demonstrate the organisms:

(a) Gomori's methenamine silver nitrate stain is extremely useful. The ovoid crescent-shaped cysts stain black in the alveoli against a pale green background.

(b) Impression smears of the lung may be fixed and stained with Giemsa. The cytoplasma stains pale blue or colorless, with purple nucleus.

(c) Gram-Weigert stain may be used for smears and imprints. The initial part of the staining procedure is similar to that of routine Gram's stain. Instead of decolorizing with acid alcohol, decolorize with 50% aniline oil in xylene. Clumps of cysts, staining deep blue to purple against an eosinophilic matrix in the background, representing the alveolar exudate, may be seen. False-positives, due to fungi, and false-negatives do occur.

When a specimen of the lung is obtained for biopsy in suspected cases of P. carinii, it should be divided and processed for:

(a) Culture for aerobic and anaerobic bacteria
(b) Fungal cultures
(c) Viral cultures
(d) H&E stain
(e) Methenamine silver nitrate stain
(f) Imprints to be stained by silver nitrate or Gram-Weigert stain

Open lung biopsy is positive in 97% of cases, and silver nitrate stain is by far the most sensitive of all the stains mentioned.

8) Trans-bronchial lung biopsy:[9] This is also a useful procedure to establish the diagnosis when the sputum is negative.

One may use any of the previously mentioned procedures, but if P. carinii infection is suspected and if the patient can tolerate the procedure, open lung biopsy is preferred. The overall merits of other procedures are not as well established as the lung biopsy.

9) Complement-fixation test (CFT): The antigen obtained from the lung tissue infected with P. carinii, has been used for this purpose. CFT is less sensitive than the direct fluorescent test. P. carinii, found in Europe, seems to be antigenically different from those found in the U.S.A. The European antigen does not react with the American and vice versa.

10) <u>Direct fluorescent antibody test</u>: This appears to be a sensitive and reliable method. As in any other infection, increasing antibody titers are considered to be specific. The specificity of this test needs actual clinical evaluation.

## REFERENCES

1. Redman, J. C.: Pneumocystis carinii pneumonia in an adopted Vietnamese infant. J. A. M. A. 230:1561, 1974.

2. Burke, B. A., Good, R. A.: Pneumocystis carinii infections. Medicine 52:23, 1973.

3. Doak, P. B., et al.: Pneumocystis carinii pneumonia - Transplant lung. Quart. J. Med. 42:59, 1973.

4. Lau, W. K., Young, L. S., Remington, J. S.: Pneumocystis carinii pneumonia. Diagnosis by examination of pulmonary secretions. J. A. M. A. 236:2399, 1976.

5. Garre, M., et al.: Pneumopathies a Pneumocystis carinii apres transplantation renale - Diagnostic precoce par le brossage bronchique distal. La Nouvella Presse Medicale 8:393, 1975.

6. Lim, S. K., Eveland, W. C., Porter, R. J.: Direct fluorescent-antibody method for the diagnosis of Pneumocystis carinii pneumonitis from the sputa or tracheal aspirates from humans. Appl. Microbiol. 27:144, 1974.

7. Drew, W. L., et al.: Diagnosis of Pneumocystis carinii pneumonia by bronchopulmonary lavage. J.A.M.A. 230:713, 1974.

8. Rosen, P. P., Martin, N., Armstrong, D.: Pneumocystis carinii pneumonia. Diagnosis by lung biopsy. Amer. J. Med. 58:794, 1975.

9. Hodgekin, J. E., et al.: Diagnosis of Pneumocystis carinii pneumonia by transbronchoscopic lung biopsy. Chest 64:551, 1973.

# 77: TRYPANOSOMIASIS
by H. Thadepalli

Trypanosomes are protozoan flagellates, of which Trypanosoma (T.) gambiense, T. rhodesiense and T. cruzi are the impor- tant human pathogens. T. cruzi causes Chagas' disease, and it is confined to Central and South America. T. gambiense and T. rhodesiense are morphologically similar and both are confined to Africa. They cause sleeping sickness. The dis- ease caused by T. rhodesiense is somewhat more acute and rapidly fatal than T. gambiense (Table 39).

## CLINICAL FEATURES OF SLEEPING SICKNESS

Tumor at the site of bite (bite reaction): It is a firm and ten- der nodule, may ulcerate and persist for two to three weeks. The bite reaction may precede the clinical illness by two weeks to two years.

Fever and headache: The fever may subside in two to three weeks. Headache is usually worse and persists for weeks to months.

The eruption: They are usually annular erythematous areas which appear with fever, mostly on the trunk, which may fade in a few days. Scattered areas of transitory edema may appear on the face and limbs.

Lymphadenopathy: This may be the first and the most clear-cut manifestation. It is usually symmetrical. The cervical lymph nodes may be visibly enlarged (Winterbottom's sign) and per- sist for months or years.

Blood smears: They may show the parasite, scanty but fre- quent, persisting for several months during the illness.

Hepatosplenomegaly: This may occur.

Sleeping stage: This begins with lassitude, apathy and fatigue. Progressively, the patient is unable to concentrate and may fall asleep most of the time, usually during the day, but is eas- ily rousable for short periods to eat his food. He may finally become comatose.

Kerandel's sign:  Hyperaesthesia of the nerves may occur during the disease.  For instance, a slight tap over the ulnar nerve is followed by excruciating pain in that area of nerve supply after a slight delay.

## DIAGNOSIS

Blood:  Place a drop of blood on a slide with a cover slip.  The trypanosomes causing commotion among the red blood cells can be seen under the high power of the microscope.  Final identification is done by thin smears.  If no parasites are seen by this method, draw 9 cc's of blood into a 10 cc. syringe loaded with 1 cc. of 6% sodium citrate in 0.9% saline, and centrifuge at 1000 r. p. m. for 10 minutes to sediment the cells; pipette the supernatant into another tube and centrifuge at 2500 r. p. m. for 10 minutes, repeat pipetting the supernatant and centrifuge and examine the sediment as a wet film or dry smear. It may show the parasite in 39% of the cases.  The electric centrifuge should not exceed 3000 r. p. m.

The cerebrospinal fluid:  This may also be centrifuged like the blood and examined.

Gland juice:  Insert a medium-size needle into the lymph gland, massage gently and suction the material with a syringe.  Eject the needle contents onto a slide, examine fresh, air dry and stain with Giemsa and re-examine for the parasite.  It is positive in nearly 88% of the cases.

## CLINICAL FEATURES OF RHODESIENSE TRYPANOSOMIASIS

It differs from the classical gambiense infection in:

1) Visceral involvement is more obvious and the heart may be involved,

2) Lymphadenopathy is not an outstanding feature of rhodesiense infection, and

3) The meningoencephalitis process in rhodesiense is not as severe as in gambiense infection.

## CHAGAS' DISEASE (T. cruzi)

American trypanosomiasis (Chagas' disease) is caused by T. cruzi, which is found in the tissue cells but not in the blood.  The parasites are excreted in the feces of the reduviid bug during the bite and inoculated through the abrasion.  It is mostly a rural disease.

## CLINICAL FEATURES OF THE ACUTE DISEASE

Age:   It occurs in children from one to five years.
Incubation period is one to three weeks.

Fever:  The initial episode is accompanied by fever which may
last for several weeks, accompanied by tachypnea and tachycardia.

Chagoma:  This is a red, hot, firm mass which occurs at the
site of the bite within a few hours.  The face, around the eye
or the cheek, is the common site preferred by the reduviid bug
(kissing bug).  The swelling may persist for two to three months.

Regional lymphadenopathy: This is often found in association
with chagoma.

Romana's sign:  This is a unilateral edema of the eye and the
eyelids.  Lachrymal glands may also be involved and enlarged.

Epistaxis and convulsions: They are common in young children.

The liver and spleen:  They may become palpable but seldom
prominent.

Heart:  Cardiac dilatation, various forms of arrhythmias and
failure might occur.

Autonomic nervous system:  This may be paralyzed, resulting
in mega-esophagus and megacolon, and these may persist for
years.  Mal de Engasco (or suffocation disease) is a self-de-
scriptive term applied to this syndrome.  Abnormal dilatation
of other tubular organs (ureter, urinary bladder, duodenum and
stomach) may also occur, but less frequently.

## CLINICAL FEATURES OF SUBACUTE AND CHRONIC STAGE

The facial edema: This, due to chagoma reaction often has dis-
peared by this time.

Tachycardia and arrhythmias: They are common.

Cardiomyopathy, mega-esophagus and megacolon: They may
also occur in the chronic stage.

TABLE 39: DIAGNOSIS OF TRYPANOSOMIASIS

| Parasite | Disease Entity | Geographical Location | Insect Vector | Clinical Pattern | Diagnostic Sites |
|---|---|---|---|---|---|
| T. gambiense | Sleeping sickness; lymphadenopathy is frequent; usually runs a subacute and chronic course | Africa (15°N. - 20°S. ), North-western portion. Endemic to: Guinea Ghana Nigeria Gambia Sierra Leone Zaire | Glossina (G.) palpalis | Nodule at the site of bite; cervical lymph-adenopathy (Winterbottom's sign); hyper-aesthesia of nerves and sleeping stage | Fluid from the site of bite; gandular juice; blood smears; cerebrospinal fluid |
| T. rhodesiense (morphologi-cally similar to T. gambiense) | More acute form of sleeping sickness; rapidly fatal | Africa (5°N. - 20°S. ) Tanzania Uganda Zambia Rhodesia | G. morsitans | SAME          AS | ABOVE |

| | | | | | |
|---|---|---|---|---|---|
| T. cruzi | Chagas' disease | Central America South America Venezuela Brazil West Argentina Uruguay North Chile Peru Ecuador | Reduviid bug, Panstrongylus megistus and Triatoma infestans | Chagoma reaction (with regional lymphadenopathy); cardiac dilatation; mega-esophagus and megacolon | Blood smears in acute stage; lymph gland juice; blood cultures in N.N.N. medium; xenodiagnosis; Machado test |
| T. rangeli | Questionable pathogenicity | Same as Chagas' disease | Same as Chagas' disease | May be found along with T. cruzi infection but it does not produce intracellular forms | Blood smears |

## DIAGNOSIS

Blood: The trypanosomes may be found in the blood during the acute stage by direct examination of the fresh films. Identification of the parasite by Giemsa stain of the dry blood films is important. T. cruzi should be differentiated from T. rangeli, a non-pathogen, also found in areas endemic to Chagas' disease.

Lymph gland juice: This may contain the trypanosomes. They can be identified in African trypanosomiasis (see page 578). Lymph node biopsy may be examined for the leishmanoid forms, but it is usually unnecessary.

Blood cultures: They may be processed in the N. N. N. medium (page 586) for T. cruzi and examined after 21 days.

Cerebrospinal fluid: This may rarely show the parasite.

Xenodiagnosis: This may be made by allowing the uninfected reduviid bugs to feed on the suspect, and examine the feces of the insect after 30 to 60 days. At the end, sacrifice it and examine for the parasite. The controls are fed on T. rangeli instead and also processed in the same manner. Nearly 20% of chronic cases may be diagnosed in this fashion.

Mice: They are intraperitoneally injected with blood from the patient, and sacrificed at the end of 30 days, and the heart tissue is examined for the leishmanoid forms of the parasite.

Machado-Guerreiro test: This is a complement-fixation reaction, in which the antigen is a liver extract from an animal dead of Chagas' disease tested against the serum of the suspected case. It is positive in over 95% of the cases. Machado test may be weakly positive in leishmaniasis, but clinically, these two diseases are distinct enough to cause no confusion.

Intradermal test: A soluble protein antigen of 100 gamma per ml. obtained from the parasites is injected. The skin reaction is positive in chronic Chagas' disease. Cross reaction occurs with leishmaniasis, which is differentiated by the negative Montenegro reaction.

## 78: LEISHMANIASIS
by H. Thadepalli

Leishmaniasis is caused by the protozoa Leishmania (L.). It can present with one of the following clinical manifestations:

- A. Kala-azar
- B. Mucocutaneous leishmaniasis (espundia)
- C. Cutaneous leishmaniasis of the Old World
- D. Cutaneous leishmaniasis of the New World

A. Kala-azar is a visceral form of leishmaniasis caused by L. donovani. It is characterized by irregular fever of long duration, hepatosplenomegaly, anemia, neutropenia and emaciation associated with a disproportionate sense of well-being. It chiefly occurs in the Ganga-Brahmaputhra delta areas in India; the Mediterranean littoral, Fung and Upper Nile areas of Sudan and the West Coast of the Sahara; on the northern bank of the Yangtze river in China; and in some of the delta areas of the Amazon in Brazil; and in certain Latin American countries. It is transmitted from man to man by the female sandflies (Phlebotomus).

B. Mucocutaneous leishmaniasis [1] - also called "espundia", is caused by L. braziliensis, which is morphologically similar to L. donovani. It is characterized by the ulceronodular and verrucous lesions of the skin over the nose and mouth, destroying the skin, the adjacent mucous membranes and the underlying cartilages, often resulting in an unsightly and grotesque appearance. It occurs in Central and South America (except Chile and Argentina), east of the Andes at the mouth of the Amazon, and Southern Paraguay. It is transmitted from rodents to man by the sandflies.

C. Cutaneous leishmaniasis of the Old World is caused by L. tropica in three clinical forms:

1) Moist form: This is a self-limiting ulcerocutaneous lesion with scar formation. It is transmitted by the sandflies from the wild rodents. It occurs chiefly in rural areas.

2) Dry form: This is an exclusively cutaneous form of the disease leading to an often singular ulceronodular lesion, which also heals, but, slowly.

3) Lupoid form: As its name implies, it resembles lupus vulgaris, a slowly spreading ulcer with central healing areas and advancing margins.

D. Cutaneous leishmaniasis of the New World includes the following three categories:

1) Espundia (described under B): This is caused by L. braziliensis.

2) Leproid leishmaniasis (leishmaniasis tegumentaria diffusa): As its name implies, it is mistaken for leprosy, primarily a skin disease which spreads locally and causes pleomorphic, maculopapular erythematous lesions on the exposed parts of the body. It was described from Venezuela and Ethiopia. It is caused by L. braziliensis.

3) Chiclero ulcer: This is a self-limiting ulceronodular lesion occurring on the exposed parts of the body, mostly the legs, ears and the face. It is endemic to chicle (gum) forests of the Yucatan in Mexico, Belize and northern Guatemala. It is caused by L. mexicana. See Table 40 for differentiation of these clinical forms.

Kala-azar: In India, man is the only reservoir of the infection, and the insect vector is Phlebotomus argentipes. It occurs in young adults and older children. In the Mediterranean and Central and South America, where the children and infants are predominantly affected, the dog and the wild jackal are the reservoirs. In Africa, it affects the adolescents and young adults; the rodents are the reservoirs. The insect vector is the sandfly (Phlebotomus) except in Brazil, where it is the Lutzomyia.

Clinical picture: The patient appears ill but has a good appetite and a clean tongue and feels disproportionately well. The fever may be intermittent or remittent with a double or triple rise in temperature, i. e., early in the morning, noon and in the night up to 101° to 103°F. Leukopenia (neutropenia) is common. The spleen enlarges nearly an inch per month down to the iliac fossa. The liver also enlarges, but only to a moderate extent. Jaundice is a late and usually an ominous prognostic sign. Lymphadenopathy is not a feature of kala-azar (except in Sudan and China). Irritant cough is usually due to pulmonary involvement, although the roentgenograms may be normal. Hyperpigmentation of the skin frequently occurs during the illness, mainly over the abdomen and extremities (kala-azar = black disease). Untreated cases end in death within two to three years.

## TABLE 40: LEISHMANIASIS

| Name of the Disease | Kala-azar (Visceral Leishmaniasis) | Oriental Sore (Cutaneous Leishmaniasis) | Chiclero Ulcer | Espundia (Mucocutaneous Leishmaniasis) |
|---|---|---|---|---|
| Geography | India: Ganga and Brahmaputhra delta; Mediterranean littoral; Africa: Sudan and West Coast of Sahara; South American countries; China: Yangtze river area | India Middle East Mediterranean Africa Sudan Ethiopia | Mexico Belize Guatemala | Central and South America, except Chile |
| Leishmania Species | L. donovani | L. tropica | L. mexicana | L. braziliensis |
| Host | Man is the only reservoir in India; dogs and foxes in other places; rodents in South America | Man to man; also occurs in cats and dogs | Wild rodent | Wild rodent |

(Cont'd.)

Table 40 (Cont'd.)

| Name of the Disease | Kala-azar (Visceral Leishmaniasis) | Oriental Sore (Cutaneous Leishmaniasis) | Chiclero Ulcer | Espundia (Mucocutaneous Leishmaniasis) |
|---|---|---|---|---|
| Vector | Phlebotomus (P.) argentipes in all countries except Lutzomyia (L.) longipalpis in Brazil | P. papatasii | Lutzomyia | Lutzomyia |
| Age Group | Young adults and older children in India; infants in the Mediterranean | Children are frequently affected; adult male | Young adults and children; not infants | Young adults |
| Clinical Features | Double spike fevers every day, hepatosplenomegaly, anemia and neutropenia; response to pentavalent antimonials: Indian (good), Sudan (little) and East African (fair); | Papular or ulcerative lesions over the exposed parts of the body; formaldehyde test is negative; cultures positive on N. N. medium | "Tapir-nose", oreja de chicleros (gum-picker's ears) descriptive of this disease | Ulceronodular lesion - framboesiform lesions with regional lymphadenitis; parasites found in the tissue juice |

| | post-kala-azar dermal leishmaniasis: Indian (10%), Sudanese (30%) and East African (5%) | | | |
|---|---|---|---|---|
| Visceral Lesions | Always present | No | No | No |
| Cutaneous Lesions | Do not occur with Indian kala-azar; fairly common with Sudanese kala-azar | Primary | Primary | Primary |
| Spontaneous Cure | No | Yes | Yes (except ears) | No |
| Blood Smear | 60% positive in Indian kala-azar; rarely positive in Sudanese or East African kala-azar | Negative | Negative | Negative |
| Montenegro Test | Always negative; positive after cure | Positive | Positive | Positive |

Post-kala-azar dermal leishmaniasis, a curious eruption of nodular lesions and depigmented patches over the face and limbs, may occur following antimony treatment.

MUCOCUTANEOUS LEISHMANIASIS: This is a mutilating and disfiguring disease, usually seen in men working in forests, especially the gum (chicle) pickers in Paraguay, and Sao Paulo, Brazil. After several months, untreatable fungating and eroding ulcers occur in the nasal and oral regions. Often suffocating (espundia) lesions occur with regional lymphadenopathy.

CUTANEOUS LEISHMANIASIS: Synonyms are Delhi boil, tropical sore and oriental sore. The lesion starts as a minute itching papule, infiltrating the skin, which later forms a crust that later falls off, leaving behind an ulcer with a central horny spicule. Several daughter sores arise near the margins of this ulcer and may coalesce. The ulcers are either single or multiple and occur on the exposed parts of the body.

### DIAGNOSIS

Leishman-Donovan (L. D. ) bodies are typical of leishmaniasis (Fig. 112). They are small, roundish or ovoid organisms of size 2 to 4 microns in diameter. When stained with Leishman's or Giemsa's stain, they show two chromatin masses enclosed in a cytoplasm. In tissue sections, they resemble Histoplasma capsulatum in appearance.

(a) Blood smears: Examination of the buffy coat layer of the blood may show the intra-leukocytic L.D. bodies in 60% of the cases. This procedure, however, is laborious and time-consuming.

(b) Skin lesions: Clean the edge of the ulcer and run in a fine 21-gauge needle, or a glass pipette, through a puncture made in the skin to get beneath the ulcer and obtain serum (not blood). Stain the material with Leishman's or Giemsa's stain. Scrapings from the ulcers are seldom positive for L.D. bodies (except leproid leishmaniasis). L. D. bodies can be mistaken for Candida organisms. Leishmania can be cultured in N.N.N. medium (Novy, MacNeal and Nicolle's medium).

(c) Biopsy of the skin from the edge of the lesion: This may be useful. It should also be stained for acid-fast bacilli to exclude tuberculosis and leprosy.

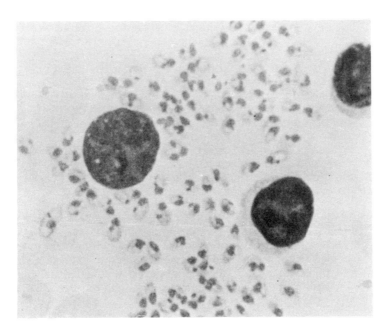

FIG. 112: Leishmaniasis. The organisms appear as round to oval bodies averaging two microns in diameter and having a central or peripheral nucleus.

(d) Splenic puncture:[2] Hold the edge of the spleen with the left hand and thrust an 18 or 20-gauge needle into the edge of the spleen, and allow it to remain until the pulp wells up into it. Lock the hub with the thumb and withdraw the needle. Blow out a small amount of it onto a slide, stain and use the remaining amount for culture. Routine syringe aspiration of the spleen in all suspected cases should be avoided. L. D. bodies are found in 90% of the cases by this method. Sternal puncture is preferable in early cases and in infants. Careless punctures can cause rupture of the spleen.

(e) Sternal puncture: The yield is 70% to 80%.

(f) Liver biopsy: The yield is 60%.

(g) Lymph node biopsy: This is also useful.

(h) <u>Blood culture</u>: Inoculate 0.25 ml. of blood directly into N. N. N. medium and cultivate at room temperature. Promastigotes stage of Leishmania can be found within 1 to 4 weeks in a majority of cases.

(i) <u>Formal gel test</u>: Draw 5 ml. of blood, let it stand for some time and transfer 1 ml. of serum into a 3"x $\frac{1}{2}$" test tube; and to this, add 1 drop of commercial formalin, shake and leave at room temperature. Also, use a control. Solidification with opacity (like the white of the egg) of the serum is diagnostic of kala-azar if the disease is of three to four months' duration. The formal gel test becomes negative six months after cure. Early cases may show only milkiness but no solidification. Formaldehyde test is negative in cutaneous and mucocutaneous leishmaniasis.

(j) <u>Complement-fixation test (CFT)</u>: CFT was developed using an antigen prepared from Kedrowsky's acid-fast bacillus. The test is positive in a majority of cases of kala-azar. It reverts to negative after treatment. Titers of 1:20 or higher are significant. Cross reactions occur with Chagas' disease and trypanosomiasis, but do not occur with tuberculosis or leprosy.

(k) <u>Leishmanin skin test or Montenegro reaction</u>:[1] This test is similar to the tuberculin (Mantoux) test. It consists of 0.1 to 0.2 ml. of antigen containing 5 to 10 million killed leptomonads, injected intradermally. It is negative in cases of active and untreated kala-azar. The skin test becomes positive after treatment with antimonials. It is also positive in cutaneous and mucocutaneous leishmaniasis. An area of 5 mm. induration, like a lead shot under the skin, is considered a positive reaction. The positive reaction may persist for some days. Many patients in endemic areas who never had the disease may have positive Montenegro reaction.

### DIFFERENTIAL DIAGNOSIS

Fevers, like tuberculosis, typhoid fever and endocarditis can be distinguished by the sense of well-being generally experienced by the leishmaniasis patient. The "double-hump" fever of leishmaniasis should be distinguished from the "dual-spike" Pel-Ebstein fever in Hodgkin's disease and the "saddle-back" fever pattern of Dengue. Syphilis, yaws and chronic fungal infections can be excluded by formal gel test, usually positive in chronic leishmaniasis. Leprosy can be excluded by demonstration of acid-fast bacilli. Diurnal fevers, a feature of leishmaniasis, are absent in malaria. Hepatomegaly due to bacterial or amoebic liver abscess can be differentiated by Ga-67 scans. Brucellosis is distinguishable by culture. In endemic areas, histoplasmosis should be distinguished from leishmaniasis by culture and special staining techniques. Reticulosis is differentiated by blood smears, bone marrow and liver biopsy. Leishmaniasis should also be differentiated from schistosomiasis and portal hypertension.

REFERENCES

1. Biagi, F.: Kala-azar. Tropical Medicine, 5th Edition. Hunter, G. W. , Swartzwelder, J. C. , Clyde, D. F. (Eds. ). W. B. Saunders, Philadelphia, Ch. 43, p. 415, 1975.

2. Manson-Bahr, P. E. C. : Leishmaniasis. Infectious Diseases. Hoeprich, P. D. (Ed. ). Harper & Row, New York, Ch. 126, p. 1127, 1977.

## 79: BABESIOSIS
### by H. Thadepalli

Babesiosis is caused by an intracytoplasmic protozoan parasite, called Babesia, which is usually found in animals. [2,3] It is transmitted to man by the hard-bodied (Ixodid) ticks. Babesiosis is a rare disease; only seven human cases were reported in the world literature until it was found to be endemic to Nantucket Island off the coast of Massachusetts, [1,3] where several additional cases were reported. On this island, babesiosis was also found among the various species of rodents. [3]

### CLINICAL FEATURES

Clinically, babesiosis is indistinguishable from malaria; in fact, malaria is the first diagnosis made in all cases of babesiosis. They may have fevers and shaking chills, drenching sweats, myalgias and anthralgias, accompanied by splenomegaly. The hemoglobin level may be low with increasing reticulocyte counts (3% to 5%).

### DIAGNOSIS

Diagnosis is established by demonstration of the parasite within the erythrocyte. Babesia strongly resemble Plasmodium falciparum, but they do not produce pigments like the malarial parasite. Diagnosis can be confirmed by inoculating hamsters and demonstrating the parasites in their blood smears. Fluorescent antibody test is used, but it can cross react with malarial parasites.

Splenectomy is the common, although not invariable predisposing cause of Babesia infections. Splenectomized patients carry relatively poor prognosis.

### THERAPY

A loading dose of chloroquine (1,500 mg.), followed by 500 mg. /day for two weeks, is usually effective. The response to chloroquine therapy may be delayed, and on occasion, the parasite may persist for four to six weeks. Recurrences are rare.

### REFERENCES

1. Ruebush, T. K. , II, et al. : Human babesiosis on Nantucket Island - Clinical features. Ann. Int. Med. 86:6, 1977.

2. Gorenflot, A. , Piette, M. , Marchand, A. : Babesioses animales et sante humaine. Premier cas de babesiose humaine observe en France. Re. Med. Vet. 152:289, 1976.

3. Healy, G. R. , Spielman, A. , Gleason, N. : Human babesiosis: Reservoir of infection on Nantucket Island. Science 192:479, 1976.

## 80: TRICHURIASIS
### by H. Thadepalli

Trichuriasis (whipworm infestation) is a cosmopolitan disease.
The adult female worm is 35 to 50 mm. (male is 35 to 45 mm.)
long and lays the characteristic barrel-shaped eggs of size 50
to 54 $\mu$ x 22 $\mu$ (Fig. 113). Abdominal pain (right lower quadrant)
associated with diarrhea is the common presenting picture.
Eosinophilia (30% to 40%) is frequent. Profuse diarrhea in children may lead to rectal prolapse. Diagnosis is established by
stool examination for the characteristic ova, and by proctoscopy.
It is essentially a parasite of the large bowel. At times, the entire mucosa of the colon may be found carpeted with these worms.

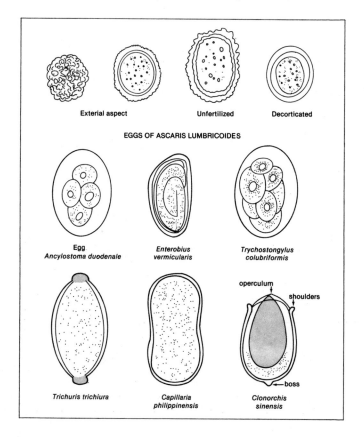

FIG. 113: Ova seen in stool (not to scale).

## 81: ENTEROBIASIS
by H. Thadepalli

Enterobius vermicularis or Oxyuris vermicularis is the parasite of pinworm infection (enterobiasis). It is cosmopolitan in
distribution. It is predominantly a disease of children. Under
overcrowded conditions, an entire family may be affected.

### THE PARASITE

The adult female measures nearly one centimeter. The eggs
are flattened on one side (planoconvex) of size 50 to 60 $\mu$m,
containing embryonated larvae (see Fig. 113, page 592). The
adult migrates to the anal canal and lays eggs. The infection
is transmitted by perianal scratching and autoingestion.

### CLINICAL FEATURES

Pruritus ani, worse during the night than during the day, is common. In children, it may cause loss of appetite and insomnia.
A cluster of the adult parasites, or their eggs, may occasionally cause appendicitis. In the tropics, I very frequently saw
the ova and the adult of this parasite in the histopathologic sections of the appendectomy specimens. Pruritus vulvae and vaginal discharge are not infrequent in children.

The diagnosis is established by demonstration of the eggs from
the perianal swabs. The stool specimens are less frequently
positive.

82: ASCARIASIS
by H. Thadepalli

Ascariasis is caused by the roundworm called <u>Ascaris lum-</u>
<u>bricoides,</u> which is a parasite of the jejunum. It is found where-
ever insanitation exists. The adult female measures nearly 9"
and the male about 7". Each female, whether fertilized or not,
produces nearly 2,000 eggs/gram of feces. It resembles the
ordinary earthworm in its appearance. When fertilized, the
the eggs have a mamillated coat (see Fig. 113, page 592).

## CLINICAL FEATURES

The eggs of ascaris may be found in a totally <u>asymptomatic</u>
individual. Children are frequently affected. Early invasive
phase is characterized by <u>bronchitis</u> and <u>pneumonia</u>, often associated with <u>eosinophilia,</u> when the clinical picture is indistinguishable from tropical eosinophilia (see page 618). The adult
worm has no device, such as a hook or a sucker, to attach itself to the bowel wall. Therefore, it may travel freely up and
down against peristalsis, and be vomited, coughed out or passed
through the nostril. It may, on occasion, block the bile duct or
pancreatic duct and cause <u>jaundice</u>, <u>cholecystitis</u> or <u>pancreati-</u>
<u>tis.</u> Massive deposits of eggs, or even the entire adult worm,
can enter the lumen of the appendix and cause appendicitis. <u>In-</u>
<u>testinal obstruction</u> is the most serious complication, caused
by a bunch of matted worms stuffing the small bowel like a sau-
sage.

## DIAGNOSIS

1) <u>Anemia</u> and <u>eosinophilia</u> are common.

2) The <u>eggs</u> (see Fig. 113, page 592) can be readily recognized
   in the unstained stool smears.

3) <u>Barium meal study</u> of the small and large bowel may show
   the parasites within the lumen of the bowel as linear radio-
   lucencies, or linear radiopacities, arranged in parallel when
   the worm ingests the barium (Fig. 114).

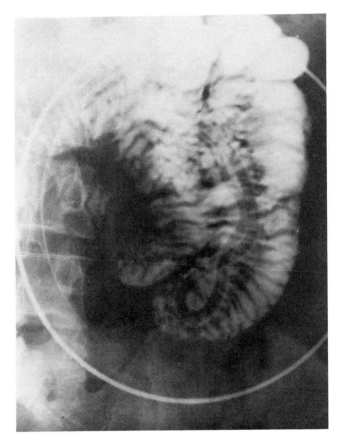

FIG. 114: Ascaris lumbricoides in the small bowel, observed during barium meal examination done
to rule out duodenal ulcer.

## 83: HOOKWORM DISEASE
### by H. Thadepalli

## THE PARASITE

The parasites that cause hookworm disease are called Ancylostoma duodenale and Necator americanus. They are predominantly the parasites of the jejunum, occasionally the duodenum, but rarely the large bowel. Both parasites produce a similar clinical picture. For the clinician, it is unimportant to differentiate these two species. The hookworm disease occurs in both tropical and subtropical parts of the world. It is an occupational disease of the coal miners and plantation workers, who may work barefooted. The adult parasite is nearly 1 cm. long. They are attached to the mucosa of the small bowel by a set of chitinous plates. Each worm, on an average day, may suck 1 ml. of blood per day, but wastes all erythrocytes and utilizes only the plasma. The eggs are nearly 50 to 70 $\mu$ m long (see Fig. 113, page 592). Each worm may pass several thousands of eggs per day. The eggs become larvae. The larvae penetrate the skin of the bare feet, where they may cause an intense sensation of itching, called "ground itch". The larvae then enter the retroperitoneal space and after moulting, they may migrate through the tracheobronchial system to the oropharynx and are swallowed back, finally, to settle in the jejunum. The worm then thrives on the blood (plasma).

## CLINICAL FEATURES AND DIAGNOSIS

1) Anemia is the outstanding feature of this disease, manifesting as extreme pallor. The tongue and the palpebral conjunctivae may be parchment-white in color. The hemoglobin may be as low as 2 grams % with a total erythrocyte count as low as 1.8 million/cu. mm. The peripheral blood smear may show iron deficiency anemia with or without the associated macrocytic anemia of $B_{12}$ and folic acid deficiency. The patient may also show signs of other vitamin deficiencies, such as angular stomatitis (riboflavin) and Bitot's spots in the eye (thiamine). The bone marrow is usually hypercellular. The Coombs' test may be negative. Eosinophilia, 10% to 30%, is frequent. The reticulocyte count may be normal. The liver and spleen are of normal size.

Hypoproteinemia (hypoalbuminemia) is frequent. Ancylostomiasis is one of the causes of protein-losing enteropathy. The albumin may be as low as 1.5 G. Congestive cardiac failure, hemic murmurs, hyperdynamic circulation and anasarca, pleural effusions and ascites may occur secondary to anemia and hypoproteinemia. Inanition is not a feature of ancylostomiasis. The patient with hookworm disease may appear to be chronically ill, but there is enough facial suffusion, often complemented with bilateral parotitis; sometimes mistaken for myxedema, nephrotic syndrome, and wet beriberi.

2) Dyspepsia, epigastric discomfort, hyperacidity or hypochlorhydria (histamine-fast) with or without demonstrable duodenal ulcers (by barium meal) are frequently present with ancylostomiasis. In endemic areas, therefore, surgery should not be performed on the gastrointestinal tract without examining the stool for parasites.

3) Stool examination: The characteristic ova can be easily seen in the wet mounts of the stool smears (see Fig. 113, page 592) in cases of anemia due to hookworm infestation. In endemic areas, stool examination for ova and parasites should be as routinely done as the bone marrow examination in all cases of anemia. Concentrated specimens by floatation techniques should be done in all cases of anemia in endemic areas. Since ancylostomiasis is a disease of insanitation, the stool specimens of these patients may contain an additional variety of ova and cysts of several other parasites. My motto in cases of parasitic infestation is "look for its brothers - if a stool specimen is positive for one, others are there to be found". The ova of Trichostrongylus orientalis can be mistaken for hookworm ova (see Fig. 113, page 592) but this parasite is far less prevalent than the hookworm.

The morbidity and mortality caused by ancylostomes in the tropics is formidable. Relegation of the stool examination to the novice can be a disastrous mistake. I cannot forget the tragedy of a 21-year-old woman in Guntur, India who gave birth to twins and died of congestive cardiac failure secondary to so-called iron and folic acid deficiency anemia. She was in the hospital for 18 days prior to her demise and had several sophisticated investigations, which included one cursory look at the stool smear on admission, and multiple blood transfusions for anemia. At autopsy, the entire length of the mucosa of the small bowel, from the second part of the duodenum to the ileum, was riddled with thousands of hookworms, dotted with myriads of punctate hemorrhagic spots. The mucosa itself was as smooth as the surface of a white bond paper. Surprisingly, the twins exhibited no signs of anemia.

## 84: STRONGYLOIDIASIS
by H. Thadepalli


This disease is caused by a nematode called Strongyloides (S.) stercoralis (threadworm), a parasite of the small bowel.

## THE PARASITE

The adult female is minute, measuring 2 mm. in length. It burrows into the mucosa of the duodenum and jejunum to lay eggs of size 50 to 60 $\mu$ long. The eggs are often embryonated; they soon hatch to produce larvae that may be encountered in the stool. Infection occurs either by direct penetration of the skin by this larvae from the soil or re-entry, either through the intestinal mucosa or through the perianal skin. Heavy worm burden can occur in certain diabetics or those on corticosteroid therapy, and the immunologically incompetent hosts. Like other nematodes, they also take a transcelomic trip before they settle down in the small bowel.

## CLINICAL FEATURES

The disease is characterized by epigastric pain (or discomfort) associated with eosinophilia (10% to 40%) due to mucosal invasion. Alcohol and food may worsen the abdominal pain and it may be mistaken for peptic ulcer.

Skin rash: Multiple blotchy areas of erythema, urticarial rash and other allergic skin reactions can periodically occur among these patients.

Watery, colicky diarrhea may also occur, for which reason it is nicknamed as Cochin-China diarrhea, although this disease is not confined to Cochin-China. It is a cosmopolitan parasite. Strongyloidiasis, when untreated, may last for decades.

## DIAGNOSIS

1) Consider strongyloidiasis in all cases of eosinophilia, even if the symptoms are absent. Motile rhabditiform larvae, measuring 200 to 250 $\mu$, may be found in the stool (expert advice is needed to differentiate these from hookworm larvae).

2) The formalin-ether technique and Harada-Mori tests may be used to recover the larvae in the laboratory. The larvae may be found only in 75% (will not be found 25% of the time).

3) Duodenal aspirate or enterotest (see page 551) may be used to detect the larvae in the duodenum.

4) Biopsy of the duodenal or jejunal mucosa may show the eggs, larvae and the adult parasites. Intestinal biopsies are often confirmatory.

5) Complement-fixation test for filariasis is often positive. This test may be used as a diagnostic tool in the non-filarial areas.

6) Barium swallow may show evidences for enteritis due to the parasite, such as thickening of the mucosa or deformity of the duodenal loop.

## 85: INTESTINAL CAPILLARIASIS
by H. Thadepalli

Intestinal capillariasis in man is a recently discovered disease, caused by Capillaria philippinensis. It is 10 times smaller (3 to 5 mm. ) than Trichuris trichiura, but its eggs are almost of the same size ($45_\mu$) as the other (see Fig. 113, page 592). The life cycle of this parasite is a subject for speculation. It is primarily a parasite of man, reported from the province of Ilocos Norte, Philippines and southern Thailand.

Borborygmi, epigastric discomfort, watery or sprue-like diarrhea with loss of electrolytes, protein, fats and carbohydrates, followed by muscle wasting are some of its features. If the disease is not recognized, it is fatal in 20% to 30%. All those with positive stools for the eggs of this parasite will manifest the disease at one time or another.

### DIAGNOSIS

Diagnosis is established by:

1) Demonstration of the characteristic eggs in the stool.

2) Small intestine biopsy revealing the ova and the worms embedded in the mucosa.

3) Clinical and radiologic features compatible with sprue-like syndrome. A skin test has been recently developed.

86: FILARIASIS
by H. Thadepalli


Filariasis is caused by a nematode (filariae) parasite of the
lymphatic system which discharges its embryos (microfilariae)
into the bloodstream. The two species of importance in man
are Wuchereria (W.) bancrofti and Brugia malayi. It is
transmitted by the female mosquitos of species Anopheles,
Culex, Mansonia and Aedes.

## GEOGRAPHY

In the western hemisphere, W. bancrofti is found in the West
Indies, Venezuela, Guineas and Brazil. In the eastern hemisphere, it is found in tropical Africa, India, China and in several Pacific Islands. The nocturnal form (microfilariae are found
only in the blood samples obtained at night) is the most common. The diurnal form (positive daytime blood sample
for microfilariae) occurs in the Fiji and other South Pacific
Islands.

## THE PARASITE

Brugia malayi, a nocturnal form of filariasis, is found in India,
Burma, Malaysia, Thailand, Vietnam, China, Taiwan, South
Korea and Japan, and its distribution, in some areas, may
overlap with W. bancrofti. The clinical pictures of both Ban-
croft's and Brug's filariasis are somewhat similar and, therefore, will be described together.

The adult parasites dwell in the lymphatic system. The females
are longer (8 to 10 cm.) than males (4 cm.). The microfilariae
seen in the blood smears are generally of size 2.5 to 3.0 mm.
long. The diurnal and the nocturnal forms of microfilariae look
alike. The microfilariae are ingested by the mosquito vector,
where they complete their development before they are transmitted back to man. Symptoms develop after one year. It was
estimated that a person sleeping indoors in an endemic area
may be bitten by 1,850 infective mosquitos carrying 5,904 infective larvae, and exposed to 115,000 mosquito bites per year.[1]

## CLINICAL FEATURES

The disease is characterized by an initial inflammatory phase,
followed by the obstructive phase:

A.  INFLAMMATORY PHASE: The early phase of the disease
    is characterized by fever (104°F.) and chills often mis-
    taken for malaria. In a day or two, lymphangitis develops
    with tender prominent cord-like red streaks, mostly on the
    upper limbs, associated with regional lymphadenopathy,
    mistaken for streptococcal infection. However, this fever
    may recur periodically for months. Lymphadenitis alone
    might occur with or without fever. Highly tender and en-
    larged testes (orchitis - bilateral or unilateral), with or
    without funiculitis and epididymitis, is a relatively fre-
    quent acute manifestation. On occasion, the adult parasite
    may die and lead to abscess formation in the deep-seated
    fascial planes, particularly in the arm, forearm or in the
    thigh region. Acute synovitis and tenosynovitis may also
    occur due to filariasis.

B.  OBSTRUCTIVE PHASE (Elephantiasis): Obstruction of the
    lymphatics, mainly due to chronic lymphangitis, leads to
    elephantiasis. As the name implies, it is characterized by
    massive non-pitting edema of the leg, arm, mamma or the
    scrotum associated with hydrocele (Fig. 115). The affected
    part of the body enlarges to a massive size and the texture
    of the skin becomes coarse and resembles the skin of an
    elephant. In the East Godavari district of India (Kakinada,
    where I worked as a house officer), elephantiasis was such
    a common household disease that it was rare for anyone to
    raise his eyebrows at this grotesque spectacle. Accumu-
    lation of the lymph (chyle) results in chylothorax, chylus
    ascites or chylocele of the scrotum. Extravasation of the
    lymph may lead to chyluria (lymph in the urine). Filaria-
    sis is the most common cause of chyluria. Chyluria may
    occur as a result of the thoracic duct obstruction.

## DIAGNOSIS

1)  Blood smears: The diagnosis is established by the demon-
    stration of microfilariae in the night blood. The best time
    to collect the blood sample for microfilariae is from 10 p.m.
    to 2 a.m. A thick drop of blood from a finger stick may be
    placed on a glass slide under a cover slip, with its margins
    previously sealed with vaseline and examined under a
    microscope. One may easily see the commotion caused by
    microfilariae disbursing the red blood corpuscles. Expert
    advice is necessary to identify the exact species of the
    filariae. Microfilariae are seldom found during the stage
    of elephantiasis.

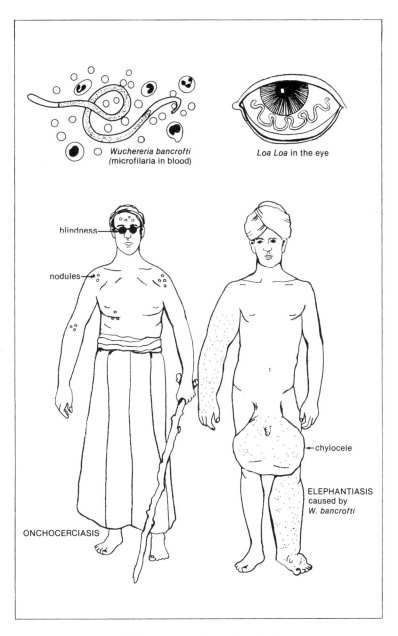

*Wuchereria bancrofti*
(microfilaria in blood)

*Loa Loa* in the eye

blindness

nodules

ONCHOCERCIASIS

chylocele

ELEPHANTIASIS
caused by
*W. bancrofti*

FIG. 115: Human filarial infections.

Knott's method is used for concentrating microfilariae, which consists of diluting 1 ml. of nocturnal blood sample from the patient, diluted with 2% formalin in 9 ml. of water and centrifuging at 2500 r. p. m. for 5 minutes. The microfilariae may be found in a mass in the precipitate. Microfilariae are frequently absent in the very early and chronic phases of elephantiasis.

2) Lymphography may be used to differentiate filarial lymphedema from lymphostatic verrucosis. In chronic and advanced cases of elephantiasis of the leg(s) or arm(s), the lymphatics are obliterated. [2] Lymphography may, by itself, terminate an attack of chyluria in nearly one-half of the patients. [3]

3) Biopsy of the lymph node is not a routine procedure to diagnose filariasis because it can further impede the lymphatic return and worsen the disease process. It is recommended only when the repeated blood smears are negative for microfilariae. Prevalence of eosinophils and lymphocytes, dilated lymphatics and enlarged follicles in a lymph node usually suggests filariasis. When several cut sections of the coils of an adult filarial worm are found in the lymph node biopsy, the diagnosis of filariasis is confirmed.

4) Complement-fixation test using the antigens of Dracunculus medinensis or Dirofilaria (D. ) immitis was found to be non-specific.

5) Skin tests using the antigen derived from the adult D. immitis and an antigen FST (Sawada antigen) were proven to be useful. [4] False-positive results occur with infections of Schistosoma japonicum. Twenty-five per cent of microfilaria carriers may have negative skin tests. The skin tests are useful in cases of elephantiasis when microfilariae are seldom found in the blood.

6) Pandit's reaction: When the blood suspected to contain microfilariae is mixed with serum from a known case of filarial elephantiasis and kept at room temperature for an hour or longer, the embryos become sluggish and become surrounded by adherent leukocytes. This is called Pandit's reaction.

REFERENCES

1. Gubler, D. J. , Bhattacharya, N. C. : A quantitative approach to the study of Bancroftian filariasis. Am. J. Trop. Med. and Hyg. 23:1027, 1974.

2. Cohen, L. B. , et al. : Lymphangiography in filarial lymphedema and elephantiasis. Am. J. Trop. Med. and Hyg. 10:843, 1961.

3. Gandhi, G. M. : Role of lymphography in management of filarial chyluria. Lymphology 9:11, 1976.

4. Sawada, T. , et al. : Intradermal skin test with antigen FST (FSCD1) on individuals in endemic areas. Jap. J. Exp. Med. 38:405, 1968.

## 87: ONCHOCERCIASIS
by H. Thadepalli

Also called blinding filarial disease, onchocerciasis is caused by Onchocerca volvulus, transmitted by Simulium flies (buffalo gnats or black flies).

In the western hemisphere, onchocerciasis is confined to Mexico (Oaxaca and Chipapas states), coffee-growing districts of Guatemala, Venezuela, coastal Columbia, and northwestern Brazil. In the eastern hemisphere, it occurs in several countries of Africa ($15^{\circ}$N. to $13^{\circ}$S. latitude) including Senegal, Sierra Leone, Liberia, Ghana, Dahomey, Nigeria, Chad, Cameroon, Zaire, Tunis, Ethiopia, Uganda, Tanzania, Rhodesia, Malawi, Sudan and Yemen.

## THE PARASITE

Onchocerca volvulus is a thin filarial parasite measuring 35 to 40 cm. (female). The male is short, measuring 2 to 4 cm. The larvae measure 300 $\mu$ in length. Man is its true host. The jinja fly, aptly named as Simulium (S.) damnosum, acts as the vector. The chimpanzee is the suspected reservoir. The American species, S. ochraceum, more frequently bites on the upper part of the body, and the African species, S. damnosum, bites on the lower parts of the body.

## CLINICAL FEATURES

Onchocerciasis occurs in both sexes, in all races, and in all age groups. When the jinja fly bites, the adult worms enter the body. There is an intense sense of itching. At the site of inoculation the adult parasite then forms several subcutaneous nodules[1] varying from the size of a pea to that of a pigeon's egg, and appearing on the head, elbows, knees, axillae and intercostal spaces (see Fig. 115, page 603). In Africa, the nodules are more prevalent around the pelvic girdle, but in the Americas they are more prevalent around the shoulder girdle. These nodules contain the adult worms. The uninvolved skin frequently contains microfilariae. In Kenya and Uganda, chronic onchocerciasis causes "hanging groins", i.e., skin folds of the groin projecting down, simulating inguinal hernias. In America, onchocerciasis causes xeroderma, or dry skin like that of a lizard.

Ocular lesions are the most devastating of all produced by this parasite. Nearly 52,000 people are blind because of this disease. Eye lesions are common when the nodules are found on the head, and infrequent when they are confined to the lower half of the body. Conjunctivitis, punctate keratitis, and sclerosing keratitis extending from the lower part of the limbus to the pupillary region can occur. It can also cause secondary glaucoma, hypopyon ulcer, choroidoretinal lesions, choroid and optic atrophy.

## DIAGNOSTIC TESTS

1) Eosinophilia of 30% to 35% is frequent.

2) Skin biopsy:

   (a) Thin sections of superficial skin from the uninvolved areas of the body may be obtained with a razor blade, mounted in saline under a cover glass and examined under the microscope. The filariae of O. volvulus do not have sheaths, and the tail is slightly curved. Reliance should not be based on a single skin biopsy. Alternatively,

   (b) One may snip off a piece of skin near the nodule and place it in saline solution for 15 minutes at 37ºC.; centrifuge and pipette the bottom layer for microfilariae. Microfilariae of Onchocerca volvulus have diurnal periodicity and are found frequently from 10 a.m. to 2 p.m. A powerful electric light bulb may be placed close to the skin to attract the worms close to the skin, prior to performing the skin biopsy, because these worms are thermotactic. Local anesthetics and freezing are contraindicated prior to biopsy.

3) Scarification: Make several superficial incisions into the skin, prepare a smear of expressed blood and lymph and stain with Giemsa's stain.

4) Conjunctival biopsy: The conjunctival biopsy may be positive even when the skin biopsy is negative.

5) Aspiration or biopsy of the skin nodules may reveal the adult parasite. †

6) Mazzotti test: Administer diethylcarbamazine, 50 mg., by mouth. In positive cases, pruritic skin reaction develops in 24 hours.

7) Urine examination may show the microfilariae in some cases.

8) Slit-lamp examination of the cornea and the anterior chamber may show the migrating microfilariae.

Blood smears are of no value in the diagnosis of <u>Onchocerciasis</u>.

## REFERENCE

1.  Buck, A. A. (Ed. ): Onchocerciasis. Symptomatology, Pathology, Diagnosis. W. H. O. , Geneva, 80 pp. , 1974.

88: LOIASIS
by H. Thadepalli

Loiasis (Calabar or fugitive swelling disease) is caused by the
filarial worm Loa loa, transmitted by "deer" flies (Chrysops).
Loiasis is confined to equatorial Africa.

The adult female of Loa loa measures 7 cm. and the male is
3 to 3.5 cm. The larvae measure 2.5 to 3 mm. Loa loa is a
diurnal parasite; it disappears from the blood during the night –
an adaptation to its vector Chrysops, a daytime feeder. Only
the females of the Chrysops fly bite. The forest monkeys
serve as reservoirs.[1]

Loiasis is characterized by the occurrence of transient swellings called Calabar or fugitive swellings of the size of a hen's
egg. They occur abruptly, are preceded by pain, and disappear within two to three days presumably due to allergic
reaction to the worm. The adult worms may be observed
moving at the rate of one centimeter per minute in areas
where there is loose connective tissue, such as the breast, the
frenum of the tongue, the eyelids, conjunctiva, penis and scrotum. In these areas, the worm can often be seen, for a short
while, moving beneath the skin and disappearing deep into the
tissues. The adult worms moving across in the conjunctiva
can cause a considerable degree of irritation and itching and
the worm itself disappears in 15 seconds to 10 minutes, followed by lacrimation, edema and a painful swelling. Loa loa
does not cause blindness.

DIAGNOSIS

1) Eosinophilia: Twenty to thirty per cent is common in loiasis.

2) Skin test: The test, done with Dirofilaria antigen, may give
positive results.

3) Blood smears, both thick and thin, should be made during
the day (10 a.m. to 2 p.m.) and examined for the microfilariae. The techniques are the same as for W. bancrofti
(see page 602).

REFERENCE

1. Kershaw, W.E.: The epidemiology of infection with Loa
loa. Tr. Roy. Soc. Trop. Med. Hyg. 49:143, 1955.

## 89: DRACONTIASIS
by H. Thadepalli

Dracontiasis is caused by the guinea worm called Dracunculus medinensis. In India, it occurs in areas where the step wells are common (Fig. 116). It is also found in tropical Africa, Arabia, Iran, Russian Turkestan, Pakistan and Afghanistan.

### THE PARASITE

The worm is thread-like and the female is almost one meter long. It is viviparous. The pregnant female migrates from the retroperitoneal space to the lower extremity and creates a blister and a hot burning sensation. When the victim washes his feet in water to cool this sensation, the blister bursts and the uterus of the parasite prolapses, discharging thousands of larvae. The larvae are engulfed by a fresh water crustacean called Cyclops. Infection is acquired by drinking water containing infected cyclops. The cyclops is then digested and the larvae migrate to the retroperitoneal space and remain until they reach the adult size.

### CLINICAL FEATURES

Local irritation of the skin, with blister formation, usually occurs in the leg, where the parasite burrows to discharge its larvae. Generalized allergic reactions may occur at this time. An adult worm, by an act of misadventure, can migrate into the vertebral or joint spaces and causes spinal extra-dural abscess or suppurative arthritis. [1]

### DIAGNOSIS

1) The ulcer on the leg should be washed repeatedly with cold water. A milky drop of discharged embryos or the prolapsed uterus may then be seen. Obtain a drop of this fluid and examine under the microscope for coiled larvae (see Fig. 116).
2) Eosinophilia is frequent.
3) X-ray screening, at times, may show a long calcified worm.
4) The skin tests are unreliable for the diagnosis.

### REFERENCE

1. Reddy, C. R. R. M., Sivaramappa, M.: Guinea worm arthritis of the knee joint. Br. Med. J. 1:155, 1968.

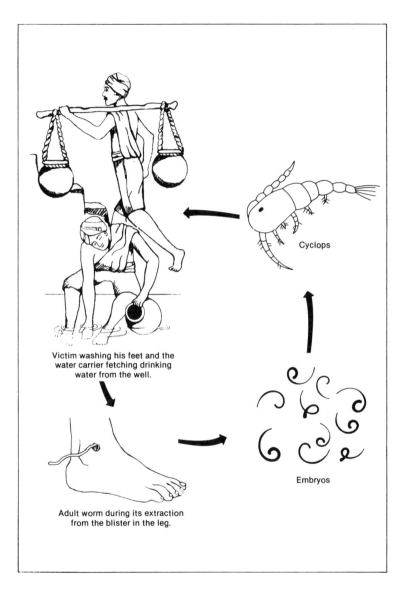

Cyclops

Victim washing his feet and the
water carrier fetching drinking
water from the well.

Embryos

Adult worm during its extraction
from the blister in the leg.

FIG. 116: Life cycle of <u>Dracunculus medinensis</u>.

## 90: TRICHINOSIS
by H. Thadepalli

Trichinosis is characterized by generalized muscle pains ("rheumatism"), periorbital edema and high fever (103⁰ to 105⁰F. ) associated with eosinophilia (30% to 50%). It is caused by the invasion of the skeletal muscles by millions of larvae of Trichinella (T. ) spiralis, an intestinal nematode. Trichinosis can be acquired by eating undercooked pork or bear meat.

Subclinical trichinosis is endemic to the western hemisphere and the United Kingdom. Trichinosis is a reportable disease in the United States. Infection through ingestion of bear meat occurs among the Alaskan Eskimo. Trichinosis is rare in Portugal, Finland, Australia and India.

## THE PARASITE

Infected pork or bear meat may contain nearly a thousand larvae per gram of muscle. When ingested, the larvae enter the duodenum and jejunum, where they live to develop into the adult male (size 1.4 x 1.6 mm. ) and the female (3 to 4 mm. ). The female is viviparous and begins to larviposit the embryos (size 100 x 6$\mu$), which, in turn, enter the bloodstream to settle in the skeletal muscles. This cycle occurs not only in hogs but also in man. In man, the life cycle of the parasite ends here; but in animals, the life cycle is further perpetuated when man or an animal ingests the infected meat.

The adult female dies in sixteen weeks, the male in two weeks, and most of the larvae, die in six months (some live for ten to thirty-one years). The larvae in the muscle arrange with long axis parallel to the fiber and calcify in six to eighteen months.

## THE DISEASE

It may affect an individual or a household five to seven days after the ingestion of the infected pork.

1) Intestinal invasion or early phase is characterized by nausea, vomiting, abdominal pain and diarrhea.

2) Larva migration phase or the invasive phase is the most alarming stage of the disease, characterized by high intermittent fever (103⁰ to 105⁰F. ) lasting one to two weeks.

A skin rash may appear on the twelfth to fourteenth day, which is characterized by generalized scarlatinal form of eruption or urticaria. Subungual splinter hemorrhages are characteristic of this stage of trichinosis. Periorbital edema is a relatively constant feature of trichinosis. The patient may complain of severe aches and pains all over the body (due to myositis). Neurotoxic symptoms, such as confusion and agitation, can occur, but stupor and coma are rare. The spleen is seldom enlarged.

3) Stage of encystation soon ensues; however, this stage may be totally asymptomatic.

## DIAGNOSIS

1) Stool examination: This is of no diagnostic help.

2) Blood: Leukocytosis (20,000 to 50,000/cu. mm. ) with eosinophilia (15% to 50%) is common. The serum enzymes, SGOT, SGPT and the CPK are elevated. The ESR (erythrocytic sedimentation rate) may be normal.

3) Muscle biopsy: This is required to confirm the diagnosis. The preferred sites for biopsy are the tendinous insertion of the deltoid or gastrocnemius muscles. The piece of this specimen may be compressed between two glass slides and examined for the larvae. A portion of the muscle should also be submitted for routine histopathologic examination.

4) Skin tests: When 0.1 ml. of 1:10,000 dilution Bachman antigen (prepared from the Trichinella larvae) is injected intradermally, it causes an erythematous patch within 15 to 20 minutes. Equally significant, but delayed, positive reaction can occur after 24 to 48 hours. This skin test response can be positive for 10 to 20 years after the onset of infection. It is a good practice to inject normal saline on the other arm for control.

5) Bentonite flocculation test: This becomes positive within a month after the infection and remains so for two years.

6) Fluorescent antibody test: This turns positive in seven days.

7) Indirect hemagglutination test, and

8) Complement-fixation test: Usually give variable results. Positive tests are diagnostic, but negative tests are of no diagnostic value.

9) Counterimmunoelectrophoresis: The patient's serum is tested against antigens from mature larvae in the muscle. It seems to offer a promise as the rapid diagnostic test.

## DIFFERENTIAL DIAGNOSIS

Trichinosis can be mistaken for influenza, meningitis, nephritis, typhoid, and typhus fevers, and can pose as fever of undetermined origin. Eosinophilia will distinguish trichinosis from these diseases. Eosinophilia usually suggests parasitic infestation. If one has eosinophilia and periorbital edema, muscle biopsy should be considered to establish the diagnosis of trichinosis.

## TREATMENT

Nearly 95% of the cases are cured spontaneously. Most larvae die in six months. Thiabendazole may be required to cure the infection. Corticosteroids are sometimes required to allay muscle aches during the invasive phase. During the invasive phase 5% - 10% of cases are fatal. Absence of eosinophilia, or a sudden drop of eosinophils to 1%, during the invasive phase of trichinosis, generally warrants poor prognosis.

## 91: VISCERAL LARVA MIGRANS
### by H. Thadepalli

Visceral larva migrans (VLM) is caused by the migration of the larva of the nematodes from the dog, cat, rat or pig; the larvae are unable to complete their lives in man. It is predominantly a disease of the toddler. Most cases are reported from the U.S.A.

### THE PARASITE

The following can cause VLM:

| Parasite | Natural Host | Frequency |
|---|---|---|
| Toxocara canis | Dog | Most common |
| Ascaris canis | Dog | Common |
| Dirofilaria | Dog | Common |
| Toxocara cati | Cat | Common |
| Ascaris suum | Pig | Common |
| Capillaria hepatica | Rat to cat | Rare |

Toxocara (T.) canis is the most common cause of VLM, called toxocariasis. Puppies acquired the infection in utero. Their feces, at three weeks, may be heavily loaded with eggs of Toxocara. Children acquire the infection by geophagy. The larvae then migrate into the circulation and infect almost every organ in the body (Fig. 117). The parasite does not reach maturity in man.

### CLINICAL FEATURES

Subclinical eosinophilia is perhaps the most common feature of toxocariasis, usually brought to light by an unrelated infection. Cough, wheezing, rales, malaise, pallor, anorexia, failure to gain weight, body aches and joint aches are some of the presenting features. Eosinophilia (20% to 80%), with leukocytosis (15,000 to 10,000/cu. mm.) occurring in a child with or without patchy pneumonia, enlarged liver and history of pica, strongly suggests the diagnosis of VLM.

### DIAGNOSIS

The diagnosis of VLM is made on clinical grounds alone. Liver or muscle biopsy and fecal examination are rarely rewarding. If one is lucky, the liver biopsy may show eosinophilic granulomatous hyperplasia. An intradermal saline extract of the

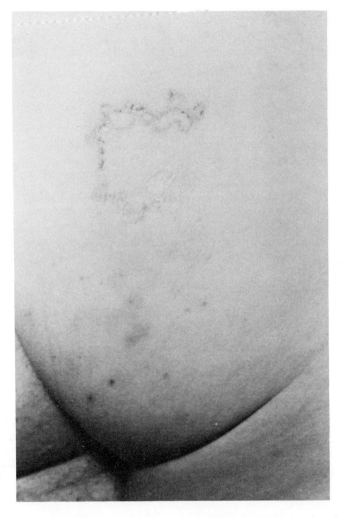

FIG. 117: Larva migrans. Note the serpiginous track left by the larvae under the skin of the gluteal region.

adult parasite, T. canis, is positive in nearly 50% of the cases. Indirect hemagglutination and bentonite flocculation tests are useful, but cross reactions can occur in patients with Ascaris lumbricoides infestation. The chest roentgenogram is often normal in VLM.

## DIFFERENTIAL

VLM is frequently mistaken for other eosinophilic syndromes, like:

1) Tropical eosinophilia (it usually has chest x-ray changes)
2) Eosinophilic leukemia (rare in children)
3) Loffler's syndrome (chest x-ray changes are present)
4) Asthma (responds to steroids)
5) Whooping cough (diagnosed by culture)
6) Strongyloides (by jejunal biopsy)
7) Periarteritis nodosa (biopsy of the artery)

## TREATMENT

Treatment is rarely necessary. Thiabendazole is effective. Methylprednisone may be used if the joint and muscle pains are worse. The entire disease process is self-limiting and ends in 12 to 18 months without any adverse effects.

## 92: TROPICAL EOSINOPHILIA
by H. Thadepalli

The following are the clinical features of tropical eosinophilia:[1]

1) Paroxysms of non-productive cough, with shortness of breath, worsening during the night, occasionally associated with hemoptysis.

2) The chest may be clear on auscultation or associated with several sonorous rales and expiratory wheezes heard on both sides of the chest, rarely at the apices of the lungs.

3) It affects mostly men between the ages of 20 and 30 years.

4) The chest roentgenogram may show mottling or fluffy infiltrates scattered more densely at the periphery and the base than at the apex of the lung, with or without mediastinal lymphadenopathy. Often the chest roentgenogram is negative to start with. Pleural effusions and lobar pneumonia are rare.

5) The leukocyte count is usually increased to 12,000 to 14,000/ cu. mm. The differential eosinophil cell count may increase to 20% to 90%, often around 30% to 40% with corresponding increase in the eosinophil cell precursors in the marrow.

6) Sedimentation rate is increased to 40 to 60 mm. /hour.

7) Splenomegaly is rare.

8) Serum IgE levels are elevated in most patients with tropical eosinophilia. [2]

Tropical eosinophilia is endemic to South India, Pakistan, Sri Lanka, northwest and central Africa, Tanzania, China, Philippines, Samoa, Malaysia and the West Indies. The exact cause of this disease is unknown; although it is generally believed to be due to filarial infection, it is probably a disease of multiple etiologies.

Some of my classmates in the medical school in Guntur, South India suffered from tropical eosinophilia. They were thoroughly investigated for parasitic infection to no avail. They initially failed to respond to diethylcarbamazine (Hetrazan), a drug that was effective against tropical eosinophilia in Singapore and Hong Kong. They responded when Hetrazan therapy was repeated three or four times. <u>Dirofilaria immitis</u>, <u>Brugia pahangi</u>, <u>Brugia malayi</u> and <u>Toxocara canis</u> are some of the filarial parasites that can cause <u>tropical</u> eosinophilia syndrome.

## DIAGNOSIS

Tropical eosinophilia should be differentiated from:

1) <u>Miliary tuberculosis</u>: The eosinophil count in miliary tuberculosis is seldom over 10%.

2) <u>Eosinophilia leukemia</u>: The peripheral white cell counts in leukemia are above 50,000/cu. mm. In tropical eosinophilia, the counts are rarely above 25,000/cu. mm. and seldom above 50,000/cu. mm. A medical student, prior to the discovery of tropical eosinophilia as a clinical entity, was once condemned in a sanatorium for suspected tuberculosis based on the mottling appearance seen in the chest roentgenogram. When he was found to have increased leukocyte count close to 50,000/cu. mm., he was transferred to a general hospital, where he was given tender loving care because of the dreadful diagnosis of leukemia. But, to everyone's surprise, he survived the anticipated six months' prognosis (those days) for acute eosinophilic leukemia; also, his chest x-rays cleared. This led the search for more cases, which resulted in the description of tropical eosinophilia. This young man, 20 years later, was to become the Dean of a medical school.

3) <u>Bronchial asthma</u>

4) <u>Acute bronchitis</u>

5) Other <u>allergic reactions</u>: Unlike the allergic disorders, the eosinophilia in tropical eosinophilia persists in spite of corticosteroid therapy.

6) <u>Viral</u> and <u>Mycoplasma</u> infections

7) <u>Loffler's syndrome</u> secondary to <u>Ascaris lumbricoides</u> and <u>Trichinella spiralis</u>: Infestation is temporary and often the <u>lung fields</u> are clear on the chest roentgenogram.

8) <u>Hodgkin's disease</u>, and

9) <u>Periarteritis nodosa</u> may cause a syndrome similar to that of tropical eosinophilia. They may be differentiated by lymph node biopsy or arterial biopsy. Further, neither of these two diseases improves on Hetrazan therapy.

10) <u>Trichinosis</u> causes eosinophilia (see page 612).

11) <u>Drug allergy</u>: The following drugs may cause pulmonary infiltrates and eosinophilia (PIE) syndrome -

| | |
|---|---|
| aspirin | methotrexate |
| azathioprine | penicillin |
| chlorpropamide | nitrofurantoin |
| isoniazid | sulfonamides |
| mephenesin | tolbutamide |

<u>PIE syndrome is not a diagnosis</u>, and it is not a disease. As its name implies, it is a syndrome or a symptom complex. There are several other favorite, but often meaningless, abbreviations that have crept into American medicine, which include:

ABA (allergic bronchopulmonary - aspergillosis), CPE (cryptogenic pulmonary eosinophilia), and BEAP (bronchiectasis, eosinophilia, asthma and pneumonitis syndrome). They all cause PIE syndrome and at times, their clinical features are indistinguishable from tropical eosinophilia if it occurs under subtropical zones.

Tropical eosinophilia carries an excellent prognosis. Death due to tropical eosinophilia is rare. The autopsy data, collected thus far, are from the accident or trauma victims suffering from tropical eosinophilia. Recurrences are frequent, but rare after a two-year remission.

## REFERENCES

1. Frimodt-Moller, C. , Barton, R. M.: A pseudotuberculosis condition associated with eosinophilia. Indian Med. Gaz. 75:607, 1940.

2. Prakash, N.: Increased circulating IgE in tropical eosinophilia. J. Allergy and Clin. Immunol. 53:189, 1974.

## 93: SCHISTOSOMIASIS
by H. Thadepalli

Schistosomiasis is a disease of the venous system caused by
the trematode called Schistosoma (S. ). Nearly 180 to 200 million people in 71 countries are infected by this parasite. [1] The
three major species of clinical importance are: S. hematobium,
S. mansoni and S. japonicum.   Between 1960 and 1973 (14
years), 3,643 cases of   S. mansoni and S. hematobium were
reported in New York.[2] but none were due to S. japonicum.
Fig. 118 summarizes the characteristic features of this disease.

### THE PARASITE

It is a dioecious (exists as male and female) trematode. The
male measures 1 to 1.5 cm. in length. The mature male em-
braces the thinner, but longer, female in its infold, called
gynecophoric canal. When pregnant, the female separates itself from the male and travels to the terminal venules, where
it plants the spiny eggs as it recedes. These eggs elicit reac-
tionary endophlebitis and perivascular fibrosis. Their eggs
contain live miracidia. When in contact with water, the miracidia are liberated, and in turn invade the fresh water snail (see
Fig. 118), wherein they mature to the stage of cercaria. The
cercariae are the infective forms; they penetrate the skin into
the circulatory system, where they mature to adults. The male
and the female later join in copula and lodge in the venous chan-
nels of the genitourinary system and the large intestine.

### SCHISTOSOMA HEMATOBIUM (vesical schistosomiasis)

Schistosoma hematobium prefers to reside in the venules of
the urinary bladder and, less frequently, the large intestine.
S. hematobium is prevalent in Egypt, Natal, South Africa, Sudan, Uganda, Congo, Rhodesia, Ethiopia, Liberia, Sierra Leone,
Morocco, Algeria, Tunisia, Arabia, Turkey, Iran, Iraq, and
the Ratnagiri district of the Maharashtra state in India.

### CLINICAL FEATURES

Urinary frequency, with or without burning sensation along the
urethra, is a common and an early symptom of this infestation.
Hematuria usually occurs at the end of the act of micturition.
At times, the hematuria can be copious and last throughout.
Dysentery can occur, either due to S. hematobium alone, or
due to the associated S. mansoni infection. On roentgenographic

FIG. 118: Differentiating features of Schistosomiasis.

| | S. HEMATOBIUM | S. MANSONI | S. JAPONICUM |
|---|---|---|---|
| Name of the Disease | Vesical Schistosomiasis | Intestinal Schistosomiasis | Asiatic Schistosomiasis (Katayama disease) |
| Geography | Egypt and several other countries in Africa, Maharashtra (India) | Several countries in Africa, Caribbean, especially Puerto Rico and St. Lucia. South America, particularly Brazil | Japan, China, Formosa and Philippines |
| Clinical Features | Cercarial dermatitis for 2 to 3 days. Hematuria and urinary tract symptoms. Main cause of cancer of urinary bladder in Egypt. X-ray: contracted and calcified bladder, pyelonephrosis | Dermatitis Signs of portal hypertension. Massive splenomegaly. Dysentery. Rectal polyps Appendicitis-like symptoms | Pruritus Hepatosplenomegaly Emaciation, Ascites and Edema. Dysentery |

| | | | |
|---|---|---|---|
| Pulmonary hypertension (Ayerza's disease) | Often present x-ray appearances of cor pulmonale | Common | Occasional |
| Diagnosis | Eggs in urine and feces. Bladder wall biopsy. Sigmoidoscopy and Rectal biopsy | Only in feces. Liver biopsy. Sigmoidoscopy and Rectal biopsy Crypt-aspiration | Eggs in feces. Rectal biopsy. Crypt aspiration. Liver biopsy |
| Egg | 130u | 120-170u | 100x 65u |
| Snail host | Bulinus | Biomphalaria | Oncomelania |

examination, bladder stones and calcification of the urinary bladder wall, bilateral hydro-ureters and hydronephrosis may be found. The spermatic cord may be involved in a bead-like fashion, called "bilharzial rosary". Appendicitis and carcinoma of the urinary bladder may follow as its delayed sequelae.

### SCHISTOSOMA MANSONI (intestinal schistosomiasis)

Schistosoma mansoni, an African disease to start with, was imported to the West Indies and South America along with the import of African slaves. It is endemic to the Nile Delta, Congo River basin and coastal Africa. It is also found in the Middle East and the Caribbean Islands, viz., Dominican Republic, Puerto Rico and St. Lucia. Nearly 29 million people are affected by this parasite. Most patients in the U.S. are Puerto Ricans or Yemenite farm workers.[2,4]

S. mansoni superficially resembles S. hematobium (see Figs. 118, 120). The disease manifests by two clinical types, i. e., dysenteric type and the hepatosplenic type.

Irritative dermatitis, the earliest manifestation of this disease, caused by the penetration of the skin by cercariae, may last for two to three days. Two to three months later, dysentery associated with intense tenesmus may develop. Polypoidal growths can occur in the rectum and be mistaken for piles.

Splenomegaly, with cirrhosis of the liver, may follow within a few months after initial exposure. Those with advanced cirrhosis have few intestinal symptoms; they pass scanty or no eggs in the stool, although they may be abundant in the liver substance. Some develop both dysenteric and hepatolienal forms of the disease simultaneously. The spleen may enlarge and reach down to the umbilicus. The liver, itself, may be enlarged by three to four fingerbreadths below the costal margin. Intermittent fevers are common with hepatolienal forms. Superinfections can occur with Enterobacteriaceae, such as Salmonella and Klebsiella.[5]

### PULMONARY SCHISTOSOMIASIS (Egyptian Ayerza's disease)

Nearly 50% of the cases of S. hematobium and S. mansoni infections develop pulmonary hypertension due to arteritis caused by their eggs. Pulmonary hypertension then leads to right ventricular hypertrophy, and cardiac failure secondary to cor pulmonale. The eggs are rarely found in the sputum.

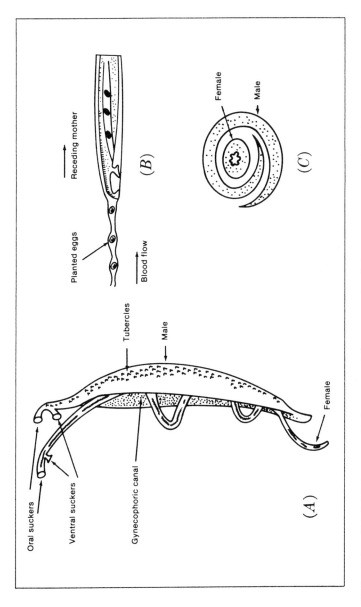

FIG. 119: (A) Schistosoma (S.) mansoni (in copula). (B) The egg-laying female in the blood vessel. (C) Cross section of S. mansoni (in copula).

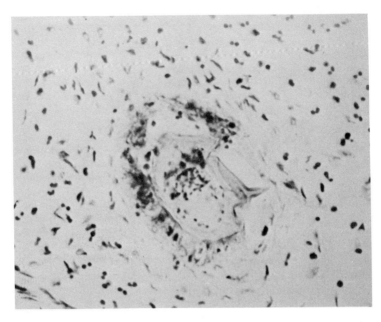

FIG. 120: Ovum of Schistosoma mansoni in tissue showing a peripheral spine and surrounded by a chronic inflammatory infiltrate.

## SCHISTOSOMA JAPONICUM (Katayama disease)

Katayama disease, aptly called Asiatic schistosomiasis, is prevalent along the shores of the Tone and Fuji rivers of Japan; the Yangtze river basin in China; it is also found in Formosa, Philippine Islands (Mindanao); around the Lake Lindu in Celebes, Malaysia; Thailand; Laos and Cambodia. Nearly 45 million people are affected by this disease.

The clinical manifestations of S. japonicum are similar to those of S. mansoni. Pruritus may result from cercarial penetration of the skin, causing dermatitis, called "Kabure" in Japan. This is the first stage or the stage of invasion, which is followed by the second stage or the stage of deposition, characterized by emaciation, dysentery and hepatosplenomegaly, with or without abdominal pain. The third, or the final stage, or the stage of fibrosis, ascites and edema occurs due to hepatolienal fibrosis. Cerebral symptoms, like hemiplegia, and Jacksonian fits, are frequent with S. japonicum infestation.

## LABORATORY DIAGNOSIS

Demonstration of the characteristic eggs in the urine or stool
is of paramount importance to the diagnosis. It is here that
even a single swallow (egg) will make the summer possible.
Several smears should be examined for the eggs. The eggs can
be seen under the low power of the microscope.

Cystoscopy and proctoscopy, coupled with the biopsy of the
vesical or rectal mucosa, are positive in nearly 90% of the untreated cases. Adult worms in copula may be found in the tissue sections. Differentiation of the species is easy and is based
upon the location of the spine (see Fig. 118).

Eosinophilia, up to 50% to 70%, is common in the invasive stage
of the disease. Anemia may result from splenomegaly. Alkaline phosphatase and SGOT may be elevated.

Indirect tests, such as complement-fixation test and the intradermal tests, are non-specific. Similarly, the miracidial
immobilization with the patient's serum; cercarian-Hullen reaction, i. e. , coat formation over the cercaria by the patient's
serum, is also non-specific.

## REFERENCES

1.  WHO expert committee on Bilharziasis. WHO Technical
    Report, Series 299, 1965.

2.  Imperato, P. J. , et al. : Parasitic infections in New York
    City. N. Y. State J. of Med. 77:50, 1977.

3.  Youssef, A. F. , Fayad, M. M. , Shafeek, M. A. : Bilharzia-
    sis of the cervix uteri. J. Obstet. Gynecol. of Brit. Com-
    monwealth 77:847, 1970.

4.  Warren, K. S. , et al. : Schistosomiasis mansoni in Yemeni in
    California: Duration of infection, presence of disease,
    therapeutic management. Am. J. Trop. Med. and Hyg. 23:
    902, 1974.

5.  Neves, J. , et al. : Prolonged septicemic salmonellosis:
    treatment of intercurrent schistosomiasis with niridazole.
    Trans. Roy. Soc. Trop. Med. & Hyg. 63:79, 1969.

## 94: CLONORCHIASIS
### by H. Thadepalli

Clonorchiasis, also called Chinese liver fluke disease, is caused by Clonorchis sinensis, a trematode that inhabits the biliary passages of man.

It is endemic to China, Japan, Korea, Taiwan and Vietnam. It should be considered in the differential diagnosis when the patient is an immigrant from any of these countries. Chinese born in the United States or Canada do not acquire this disease, because of the absence of the snail host needed for this parasite. Nearly 16% of the Chinese surveyed in Montreal, Canada had this infection and between ages 30 and 40, nearly 25% had ova of C. sinensis in the stool.[1]

The adult parasite measures about 20 x 4 mm. and its eggs are about 29 x 16 $\mu$ in size. The eggs of C. sinensis are brown, ovoid and operculated; the operculum resting on the "shouldered" portion of the egg. It has a knob or a boss on the unoperculated end (see Fig. 113, page 592). The adult stays in the biliary tract and the eggs are found in the duodenum and the stool. The snail and the fresh-water fish are its intermediate hosts. The disease is acquired by eating undercooked or raw fish.

### CLINICAL FEATURES

Fever, leukocytosis with eosinophilia, and epigastric pain are the early features of this disease, later followed by diarrhea. Eventually, the liver enlarges. In advanced cases, cirrhosis of the liver with ascites and anasarca might occur. Intense jaundice is an infrequent complication of clonorchiasis.

### DIAGNOSIS

The diagnosis is made by the demonstration of eggs in the feces, bile, or duodenal aspirate (see Fig. 113, page 592). The eggs of C. sinensis, Metagonimus yokogawai, Heterophyes heterophyes and Diphyllobothrium latum so strongly resemble each other that expert advice is needed to tell them apart.

### REFERENCE

1. Seah, S. K. K.: Intestinal parasites in Chinese immigrants in a Canadian city. J. Trop. Med. and Hyg. 76:291, 1973.

95: PARAGONIMUS WESTERMANI (Endemic Hemoptysis)
by H. Thadepalli

Paragonimus (P. ) westermani is a lung fluke of man. It is found in India (states of Assam, Bengal, Kerala and Tamilnadu), Sri Lanka, Bangladesh and other far eastern countries, and Africa. It is also found in Central and South America. P. westermani, the adult parasite, is around 10 x 5 mm. in size and its eggs are of 100 x 50 $\mu$ in size, morphologically resembling the eggs of C. sinensis, Heterophyes heterophyes, and Metagonimus yokogawai. The eggs are expectorated in the sputum or swallowed and passed in the feces. The development of the parasite takes place first in the snail and later in the fresh-water crustaceans. The infection is acquired through eating raw or insufficiently cooked (salted or wine-soaked) crabs. The parasite penetrates through the wall of the alimentary canal and the diaphragm into the parenchyma of the lungs.

## CLINICAL FEATURES

Paragonimiasis is a disease of the young. Most patients are under 25 years of age. [1] Hemoptysis is an outstanding feature of this disease, often confused with tuberculosis. The clinical and radiological appearances of these two diseases are similar. A patient may have both paragonimiasis and pulmonary tuberculosis at the same time. Eosinophilia (30% to 50%) is common. Other intestinal parasitic diseases may also coexist. Extrapulmonary manifestations of paragonimiasis include pleural effusions, empyema, paravertebral abscess and Jacksonian seizures. The chest x-ray may be suggestive of bronchopneumonia, bronchiectasis, lung abscess or necrotizing pneumonia. Calcified spots or pleural thickening may be seen.

## DIAGNOSIS

1) Eosinophils and Charcot-Leyden crystals may be seen in the sputum.

2) Eggs may be seen in the pleural fluid.

3) Sputum examination for eggs: Mix sputum and 3% sodium hydroxide in equal amounts, centrifuge at high speed, decant the supernatant and examine the sediment for the eggs and larvae.

## REFERENCE

1. Nwokolo, C.: Outbreak of paragonimiasis in Eastern Nigeria. Lancet 1:32, 1972.

96:  TAPEWORM INFECTIONS
by H.  Thadepalli


The majority of tapeworm infections in man are caused by five
types:

1) Diphyllobothrium latum, the fish tapeworm
2) Taenia solium, the pork tapeworm
3) Taenia saginata, the beef tapeworm
4) Echinococcus granulosus, the dog tapeworm
5) Hymenolepis nana, the man tapeworm

Table 41 summarizes the differentiating features of tapeworm
infestation in man.

## THE  PARASITE

Diphyllobothrium (D. ) latum is a somewhat pinkish tapeworm
that is 10 meters with 3,000 segments of proglottids.  The egg
of D. latum is of size 60 to 70$\mu$ x 40 to 50 $\mu$ , operculated with a
minute boss at the anopercular end.  The eggs are not infective
to man.  When they reach water, they hatch and liberate larvae
(coracidium) to be ingested by Cyclops, which is later ingested
by small fish, who are then devoured by larger fish, who, in turn,
are captured by man.  It is a disease transmitted predominantly
by eating raw or undercooked fresh-water fish.  The larvae develop to maturity in man and lodge themselves in the jejunum.

D. latum infections are common in Finland, Switzerland, Ru-
mania and Scandinavian countries.  In the United States and
Canada, it occurs around the Great Lakes.  It is reported
in the Alaskan Eskimo.  Those Jewish housewives who habitually
sample gefilte fish before preparation are particularly prone
to developing this infection.

## DIPHYLLOBOTHRIASIS

Pernicious anemia is the outstanding feature of this disease.
In most people, it is asymptomatic, but in others it may cause
anorexia, abdominal pain, nausea, diarrhea and weight loss.
It causes the so-called Bothriocephalus anemia, a megaloblastic anemia resembling pernicious anemia.  However, eosinophilia, which occurs in this disease, is rare with true
pernicious anemia, a distinguishing feature.  Leukocytosis,
when present, is an additional distinguishing feature.  D. latum
infection should, therefore, be considered in the differential

diagnosis of all megaloblastic anemias. Both serum $B_{12}$ and folic acid levels may be low with this disease. D. latum causes anemia, either by mere competition with man for $B_{12}$ and folic acid or by a susceptible host hypersensitivity to lysolecithin, a component of the parasite. [1] A live worm is therefore not always essential to cause the disease.

The diagnosis is established by the demonstration of the characteristic operculated ova in the stool. They resemble the ova of the lung fluke Paragonimus westermani, found in the Orient; Diplogonoporus grandis, found in Japan; and Clonorchis sinensis, found in China (see Fig. 113, page 592). A saline purge may result in the recovery of the proglottids of the worm. The parasitologists identify the species by the arrangement of the reproductive system in the proglottid.

## TAENIA SOLIUM

Taenia (T.) solium, the pork tapeworm, is acquired by eating undercooked pork. It is rare among the Mohammadens and the Jews, who do not eat pork. However, they may acquire the infection by ingestion of the eggs from contaminated raw vegetables or soil. T. solium is found all over the world. The adult tapeworm is 2 to 7 meters long, and the eggs are almost spherical with a diameter of 30 to $40\mu$. The eggs of T. solium and T. saginata are indistinguishable (see Fig. 121). A proglottid is required to tell them apart. T. saginata has nearly 15 lateral uterine branches, and T. solium has nearly 9 such branches (see Fig. 121). The ova are ingested by the hog, where the Cysticercus cellulosae are formed in the muscles, and, when ingested by man, the adult parasite develops in the intestine. The Cysticercus cellulosae stage in man may develop either by auto-ingestion (fecal-oral contamination) or intestinal reverse peristalsis. Live proglottids may migrate down the intestine and actively work their way out from the anus, even when one is not at stool, often to the bewilderment of the host, and at times under very embarrassing circumstances.

## CLINICAL FEATURES AND DIAGNOSIS

The cysticercus lesions may present as multiple subcutaneous nodules. Cerebral cysticercosis can cause focal seizures or other signs of intracerebral space-occupying lesions. Subcutaneous nodules, therefore, should be biopsied in all instances associated with signs of brain tumor. Cysticerci in the soft tissue, subcutaneous and intraocular areas may be no larger than 1 cm. in diameter. The intraventricular, intracerebral

TABLE 41: DIFFERENTIATING FEATURES OF TAPEWORM INFESTATION IN MAN

| Feature | Diphyllobothrium latum | Taenia solium | Taenia saginata | Echinococcus granulosus | Hymenolepis nana |
|---|---|---|---|---|---|
| Adult worm found in | Man | May or may not be found in man | Man | Dog Seldom found in man | Man |
| Approximate size of the adult worm | 8 to 12 m. | 2 to 7 m. | 5 to 10 m. | 3 to 6 mm. | 25 to 40 mm. |
| Intermediate host | Fish | Pig | Cattle | Sheep and man | None |
| Route of in infection | Tasting or eating raw or under-cooked fish | "Measly pork" | Under-cooked "rare" beef | Feces of dog | Man to man transmission |

| | | | | | |
|---|---|---|---|---|---|
| Outstanding clinical features | Eosinophilia and/or megaloblastic anemia | Cysticercus cellulosae cysts presenting as nodules; passing proglottids | No cysticercus lesions in man; passing proglottids | Hepatomegaly or "coin lesion" in the lung | Eosinophilia or other gastrointestinal symptoms |
| Diagnosis (Fig. 121) | Operculated eggs in the stool; no hooklets | The cysts of these three worms look alike. They are round. All have six hooks. | | | Oval in shape, otherwise resemble the cyst of Taenia; has 6 hooks |
| Proglottid (see Fig. 121) | Rarely passed in the stool; disintergrates in large bowel | 5 to 7 lateral uterine branches | 10 to 14 lateral uterine branches | Not found in the stool of man | Much smaller than Taenia |

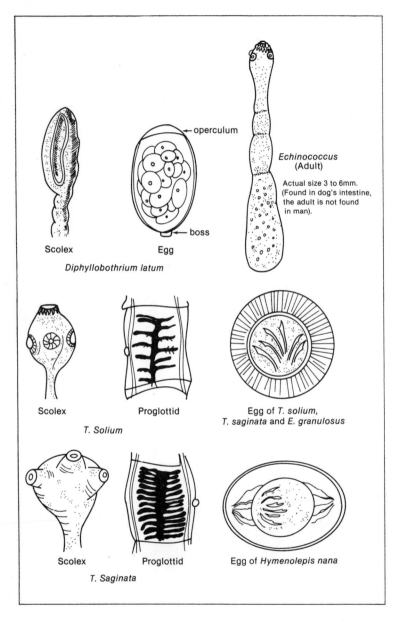

FIG. 121: Identification features for the cystode infestations in man.

cysticerci, may, by osmosis, increase to the size of 5 cm. or more. Therefore, the size of an intracranial lesion should not deter the diagnosis of cysticercosis. Eosinophilia is not a feature of cerebral cysticercosis. Cysticercus cellulosae may be found in the muscles, vitreous of the eye, lungs, liver and kidney.

Another mode of presentation, as mentioned earlier, is that the patient complains, "I am passing something from my rectum. Sometimes they keep falling out when I am walking". This is due to the passing of proglottids. Such symptoms occur with adult worm(s) infestation. The patients that harbor the adult worm may or may not have gastrointestinal symptoms. Patients with the adult tapeworm may have eosinophilia (10% to 15%).

## DIAGNOSIS

1) Biopsy of the subcutaneous nodules (cysticercus lesions) is diagnostic. Examination of the ruptured cyst may reveal the "hooklets", six in number, of the C. cellulosae.

2) Soft tissue x-rays of limbs and the girdles, sometimes even a chest x-ray, may show calcified cysticercus lesions, which look like "rice grain" or "puffed rice". (Fig. 122)

3) A mature proglottid, when passed, may be held between two slides and examined for the lateral uterine branches. T. solium has about 9 (7 to 13) branches (see Fig. 121).

4) Precipitin tests are not helpful.

5) Indirect hemagglutination test in one series has helped in diagnosing 85% of the cases. The antigen was prepared from lyophilized pig cysticerci. [2]

## TAENIA SAGINATA

Taenia (T.) saginata, the beef tapeworm, does not cause cysticercosis in man. The adult parasite inhabits the small bowel. The cysticercus stage occurs in the cattle. The infection is acquired by eating undercooked beef.

The adult T. saginata measures 5 to 10 meters. Unlike T. solium, T. saginata is devoid of hooks on its head, and its proglottid has 15 to 20 lateral uterine branches (twice as many as T. solium). The eggs of T. solium and T. saginata look alike (see Fig. 121). It causes upper gastrointestinal symptoms. Passing the proglottids

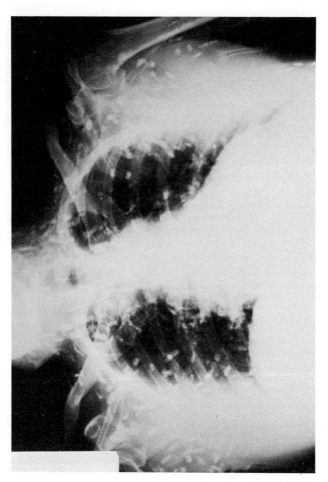

FIG. 122: Disseminated cysticercosis. A 60-year-old man from Mexico admitted for seizures and hemiplegia. Chest roentgenogram revealed multiple radiopaque plaques due to calcified cysts. Autopsy revealed Cysticercus meningitis and massive infiltration of brain.

per os is a common presenting symptom. Diagnosis is made
by actually counting the lateral branches on a defecated proglottid (see Fig. 121).

## HYDATID DISEASE

Hydatid disease is caused by Echinococcus (E. ) granulosus,
a parasite of dogs. Sheep and man do not harbor the adult parasite. The disease in man is caused by its larval (hydatid) phase.
The adult parasite, E. granulosus, is the smallest of all cystodes
infecting man, measuring 3 to 6 mm. It is found in the intes-
tines of dogs, cats and wolves. Human infection results from
the ingestion of the eggs from the feces of the domestic animals,
dogs and cats. The larvae disseminate to the various parts of
the body and subsequently develop into the hydatid cysts over
a period of 15 to 20 years. Fig. 123 depicts the overall incidence of hydatid disease in various organs, as I have illustrated,
based on a large series of patients studied by Reddy et al [4]
from Guntur, India. Sheep acquire this disease by grazing
on fields contaminated with the feces of dogs. In some parts
of the world, 90% of the sheep and 50% of the dogs have hydatid
disease. The dogs acquire this disease by feeding on the un-
cooked meat of the infected sheep. Hydatid disease, therefore,
is prevalent among the sheep-rearing communities. Among
professional sheepherders, for instance, the Basque community in California, hydatid disease is 1,000 times more prevalent. [3] The ova of E. granulosus measures 30 to 38$\mu$, and it
is indistinguishable from the eggs of other Taenia species.

## CLINICAL FEATURES

After the initial exposure, one may remain asymptomatic for
over two decades. Men are more frequently affected than women. A majority of patients are in their third decade of life.
Nearly 40% to 50% may present with abdominal swelling secondary to involvement of the liver, the most frequently affected
organ. Other abdominal symptoms include upper right quadrant
pain, colic and sometimes signs of obstructive jaundice.

Pulmonary symptoms are the next most frequent, found in nearly
20% of the patients. Cough with expectoration is common. Hemoptysis may occur in nearly 3%. See Fig. 123 for other organ sites involved. The right lobe of the liver and the right lung
are more frequently involved. An occasional patient may cough
out, or urinate, the contents of a ruptured hydatid cyst.

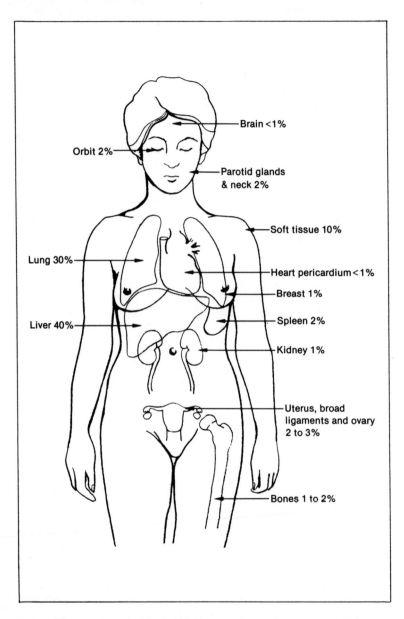

FIG. 123: Incidence of hydatid disease in various organs (adapted from Reddy, D. B. , et al. [4]).

In Guntur, India (see Fig. 123 from the same geographical site), in 1957, a severely malnourished woman was clinically thought to have obstructive jaundice secondary to "post-necrotic scarring", or carcinoma of the liver. One week after she had a normal chest x-ray, she was noted to have seizures, which were thought to be secondary to hepatic encephalopathy. However, a liver biopsy proved unremarkable, and hydatid disease was not clinically suspected. The patient subsequently died, and at the autopsy, which I witnessed, the liver was found to be intensely green and riddled with nearly 40 to 50 hydatid cysts of all sizes. The whole liver weighed nearly 20 pounds and, when removed, looked like a bunch of unripe fruit from a palm tree. These cysts, when the capsules were opened, were found with the germinal epithelium as thin and white as the inside of a tender coconut. Hydatids were also found in the spleen, psoas muscle, both kidneys and the brain.

Although there is no medical treatment for hydatid disease, and surgical resection of all the cysts found in this patient would have been impractical, this case points out that hydatid disease should be considered in the differential diagnosis of carcinoma of the liver. Attempts to obtain liver biopsies from such cases can be fatal.

## DIAGNOSIS

1) Hydatid cysts: The absolute evidence for hydatid disease is the demonstration of hooklets, scolices or laminated membrane in the sputum, urine or any aspirated fluid.

2) Eosinophilia: Ten to fifteen per cent may occur in some cases. The majority of patients reveal no eosinophilia.

3) Casoni test: The Casoni's test is a skin test. The antigen is made from E. granulosus or E. multilocularis. Inject 0.05 ml. of it intradermally on the volar aspect of the forearm and an equal volume of the control antigen (Coca's buffer with thimerosal) on the right. A wheal of ⩾1.2 square centimeters after 15 minutes of the test is considered positive, provided it is at least twice the size of the control. [5] Contrary to popular belief, this test is false-negative in 25% of the proven cases of hydatid disease. False-positive results are rare. In general, a positive skin test is useful, but a negative skin test does not rule out hydatid disease.

4) Chest roentgenogram: Hydatid cyst should be considered in the differential diagnosis of all "coin lesions" in the lung. They may be of any size and located in any portion of the lung, although they are more frequent over the right lower lung field. A positive Casoni's test and a "coin lesion" in the lung suggest that the latter is due to a hydatid cyst. Nevertheless, thoracotomy may be required for final diagnosis.

5) Scans: The rose-bengal liver scan or a Tc-99 liver-spleen scan or the Ga-67 scans may reveal defects of the liver and/ or the spleen. The scans are reliable in 80% to 90% of the cases.[6] False-positive results may occur in 5% to 10%.

6) Angiography: Angiography of the celiac artery territory, including the liver, may be done to exclude malignancy and also for the exact localization of the hydatid cyst.[7]

7) Hemagglutination reaction: This reaction, using formalinized red cells, is considered most useful in the diagnosis of hydatid disease. It appears that hepatic hydatid disease is more immunogenic, therefore, more frequently positive than the pulmonary hydatid disease.[8]

## HYMENOLEPIASIS

Hymenolepiasis is caused by the dwarf tapeworm called Hymenolepis (H.) nana, or H. diminuta. The adult of H. nana measures 25 to 40 mm. It is transmitted from man to man without an intermediate host. The adult worm is usually found lodging itself in the intervillous spaces of the small bowel.

Hymenolepiasis, in most instances, is asymptomatic. Heavy infestation may cause nausea, abdominal pain and diarrhea with or without eosinophilia.

Diagnosis is made by the demonstration of the characteristic cysts in the stool (see Fig. 121).

## REFERENCES

1. Totterman, G.: On the pathogenesis of pernicious tapeworm anaemia. Ann. Clin. Res. 8 (Suppl. 18), 1976.

2. Proctor, E. M., Powell, S. J., Elsdon-Dew, R.: The serological diagnosis of cysticercosis. Ann. Trop. Med. Parasit. 60:146, 1966.

3.  Araujo, F. P. , et al. : Hydatid disease transmission in California: A study of the Basque connection. Amer. J. Epidemiol. 102:291, 1975.

4.  Reddy, D. B. , Suvarnakumar, T. G. , Raju, G. C. : Hydatid disease in Kurnool. J. Indian Med. Assoc. 63:5, 1974.

5.  Kagan, I. G. , et al. : Evaluation of intradermal and serologic tests for the diagnosis of hydatid disease. Am. J. Trop. Med. Hyg. 15:172, 1966.

6.  Serrano Sanchez, P. A. , et al. : Valor diagnostico de la gammagrafia en el quieste hydatidico de higado. Cirurgia Espanola 27:493, 1973.

7.  Diard, F. , et al. : Angiographie des kystes hydatiques due foic. J. Radiol. Electrol. 54:655, 1973.

8.  Tribouley, J. , et al. : Application de la reaction d'hemagglutination passive au serodiagnostic de l'hydatidose. Medicine et Maladies Infectieuses 4:43, 1974.

# SECTION K: RICKETTSIA

## 97: RICKETTSIAL FEVERS
### by H. Thadepalli

Rickettsia (R.) are gram-negative bacilli-like organisms of
0.5 μ diameter, much larger than viruses but smaller than bacteria. They are not filterable (except R. burnetii). These ob-
ligately intranucleolar or intracytoplasmic bodies stain well
with Romanowsky dyes (water adjusted to pH 7.4). Rickettsia
are transmitted by the insect vectors; the louse, the flea, the
tick and the mite.

The clinical picture of the louse-borne typhus is different from
that of the tick-borne, the mite-borne and Q fever.

The following are discussed in this chapter:

A. Louse-borne typhus (epidemic typhus) caused by R. prowazekii

B. Brill-Zinsser's disease (endemic typhus)

C. Murine typhus - rat flea typhus caused by R. prowazekii
   var. mooseri (R. mooseri)

The clinical pictures of A, B and C are similar.

D. Rocky Mountain spotted fever (tick-borne typhus) caused
   by R. rickettsii

E. Tsutsugamushi fever (mite typhus or scrub typhus) caused
   by R. tsutsugamushi

F. Q fever (query fever) air-borne infection transmitted by
   the tick, caused by R. burnetii (Coxiella burnetii)

G. Rickettsialpox, caused by R. akari and transmitted by the
   mouse mite

Table 42 summarizes the epidemiology, clinical features and
diagnostic tests of various rickettsial fevers discussed in this
chapter.

TABLE 42: RICKETTSIAL FEVERS

| Disease | Geography | Vector | Species | Mode of Transmission | Vertebral Host | Distribution of the Rash and Eschar | Reactions to Proteus | | |
|---|---|---|---|---|---|---|---|---|---|
| | | | | | | | OX19 | OX2 | OXK |
| Epidemic louse-borne typhus or Brill-Zinsser disease | World-wide | Louse (also air-borne) | R. prowazekii | Mouse → louse → man → louse → man | Man | Trunk and extremities, axillae; face, palms and soles are spared; no eschar; no rash in Brill-Zinsser disease. | ++ ++ | + | 0 |
| Murine typhus | World-wide | Rat flea | R. mooseri | Rat → rat, flea ⟨ man, rat | Rat | As above | ++ ++ | + | 0 |
| Rocky Mountain spotted fever | Western hemisphere | Tick | R. rickettsii | Tick → tick → dog, Tick ⟨ man, tick | Rodents | As above, but the face is involved; no eschar | + | + | 0 |
| Rickettsial-pox | U.S.A.; U.S.S.R. | Mite | R. akari | Mite → mouse → mite, Mite ⟨ man, mouse | Mice | As above, but an eschar is present | 0 | 0 | + |
| Tsutsugamushi fever | Asia, Australia and Pacific Islands | Larvae of mite | R. tsutsugamushi | Mite → mouse → mite, Mite ⟨ mouse, man | Rat | Generalized rash; eschar present and regional adenitis also present | 0 | 0 | ++ ++ |
| Q fever | World-wide | Tick but no vector is necessary | R. burnetii | Tick → mammal → tick → cattle → airborne → man | Cattle; goats | No rash; no ulcer; pneumonic (not always) | 0 | 0 | 0 |

## PRIMARY LOUSE-BORNE TYPHUS (epidemic typhus)

Louse-borne typhus is caused by R. prowazekii, a coccobacillary diplobacillus-like organism. It stains red by Gimenez method of staining. Louse-borne typhus is a disease of wars, famines and overcrowding. It is transmitted by the body louse Pediculus humanus var. corporis or the head louse var. capitis, but not by the pubic louse, var. pubis. The louse, after a blood meal, leaves the rickettsiae-loaded excreta at the site of the bite. The organisms enter through the raw surface, or by inadvertent killing of the insect. As in the case of ticks (see Rocky Mountain spotted fever, page 646), the louse-borne infections are not transovarially transmitted. Typhus can also spread by droplet infection if the blood is spilled during venipuncture.

### CLINICAL FEATURES

The incubation period is seven to twenty-one days. Fever is the first sign, rising up to 102° to 104°F. within three days, where it remains with little diurnal fluctuation. Intractable headache is a prominent feature associated with myalgias, and sometimes, muscle twitchings (subsultus tendinum). The face is dull and apathetic, or has a flushed, drunken look (facies typhosa). Conjunctivitis is a common feature of louse-borne typhus.

Within four to seven days, the rash starts on the arms, the trunk, and the axillae, then spreads in two days to the entire body, except for the face, palms and soles. The lesions are macular and become dark brown and maculopapular. Unlike, chickenpox, it does not arise in crops of lesions. When a sphygmomanometer is applied, the redness and petechiae become more pronounced.

Epistaxis is common. The pulse rate increases to 110 to 140/minute. Deafness and tinnitus are prominent features of epidemic typhus (80%). Cough with tachypnea occurs in nearly two-thirds of the patients.

Rarely, petechial hemorrhages, disseminated intravascular coagulation, and occasionally intravascular thrombosis secondary to endangiitis can cause gangrene of the skin, extremities, nose or the tip of the penis.

Splenomegaly: The spleen is readily palpable in greater than 50% of the patients.

Mental status: The word typhus means a cloudy state of consciousness. Mania, stupor and coma, however, are rare.

DIAGNOSIS

Chest roentgenogram may show consolidation or pleurisy.

1) Weil-Felix reaction: It is a non-specific agglutination reaction of the patient's serum against a strain of Proteus
   vulgaris OX2 obtained from the urine of a typhus patient
   called Weil-Felix. OX19 and OXK are variants of Proteus OX2.

   Weil-Felix reaction is positive in 90% of the cases of epidemic
   typhus. OX19 may rise to 1:160 or more within eight to twelve
   days; OX2 is variable but the OXK reaction is never positive
   in louse-borne epidemic typhus. Cross reactions can occur
   with relapsing fevers and in those with urinary tract infection
   due to Proteus vulgaris. Occasionally, relapsing fever and
   typhus fever can coexist.

2) Guinea pig inoculation: Obtain heparinized blood or an emul-
   sified blood clot soon after onset of the disease. Inoculate
   intraperitoneally into the male guinea pigs and observe for
   fever, scrotal swelling, hemorrhage, etc. (Neill-Mooser
   reaction). One blind passage may be necessary. Later, the
   animal is sacrificed, and smears are obtained from the
   spleen, scrotal tissue and peritoneum, stained by Giemsa
   or Machiavello's stain, to show intracytoplasmic rickettsial
   bodies. It is positive in two to three weeks. False-positive
   reactions can occur with Salmonella paratyphi and Spirillum
   minus.

3) Complement-fixation test (CFT): Paired blood samples are
   required to do this test; the first sample is taken early during the onset of the disease and the second, two to three
   weeks later. A positive CFT requires demonstration of a
   four-fold or higher increase in the antibody titer between
   the two sera. The test results can be reported within forty-
   eight hours after the receipt of the second specimen.

Epidemic typhus fevers should be differentiated from other
rickettsial fevers (see Table 42), measles, malaria, relapsing
fevers, smallpox, meningococcemia, typhoid fever and toxoplasmosis.

When therapy is delayed, epidemic typhus is associated with 10% to 40% mortality. Mortality is directly proportional to age; benign in childhood (except infancy), 50% at the age of 50 and nearly 100% above the age of 60.

## BRILL-ZINSSER DISEASE

Brill-Zinsser disease is merely a relapse or recurrence of louse-borne typhus; also caused by R. prowazekii. Its clinical course is shorter, lasting for seven to eleven days, and is irregular. It can relapse ten to twenty years after an attack of louse-borne fever. Rash is absent.

## FLEA (murine) TYPHUS

The disease is transmitted by the rat flea, Xenopsylla cheopis, which can also transmit plague. The clinical course of murine typhus is similar to louse-borne typhus, except the fever is often less than 102°F. and headache is an inconstand feature. Weil-Felix reaction for flea and louse-borne typhus fevers are similar.

## ROCKY MOUNTAIN SPOTTED FEVER

This is a disease of the new world. The name, Rocky Mountain spotted fever (RMSF) today carries more historical than geographical meaning. It is no longer confined to the Rocky Mountains. In fact, it is more prevalent in the Appalachian Mountain states than in the Rockies.[1] In the Western U.S., it is transmitted during a blood meal by the tick, Dermacentor (D.) andersoni. In the Eastern U.S., it is transmitted by D. variabilis. These ticks are commonly known as the dog tick, wood tick and the lone star tick. These ticks can also transmit relapsing fevers. The animal reservoirs in the West are the wild goats, sheep, black bear and coyote, and in the East, the meadow mouse and other rodents. The infection among the ticks is transovarially transmitted. It is prevalent during the spring and summer seasons, when outdoor camping is at its height. Nearly 890 cases were reported in the United States during 1976.

## CLINICAL FEATURES

The clinical course of RMSF is more fulminating in the Western U.S., and it runs a benign course in the Eastern U.S.

Fever, exposure to ticks and rash is the diagnostic triad for RMSF.

The incubation period is two to seven days. A history of tick bite is present in nearly 80% of the cases. Most of the patients are less than 15 years old; the age when they are frequently exposed to the vector, the dog tick.

Focal areas: RMSF occurs in certain focal areas. History of a recent visit of the patient to these areas is a useful clue to diagnosis.

Fever: Nearly all (99%) have abrupt or gradual onset of fever with chills. The body temperature may go as high as 105° to 106°F. and decrease by several degrees in the morning. Fever persists throughout the illness, and terminates at the end by lysis.

Headache is very pronounced in 92% of the patients. Myalgias occur, especially of the calf and thigh. These muscles are extremely tender to palpation (78%).

Rash: It often begins within three to five days after the onset of fever, first on the wrists and ankles and later spreading to the trunk, including the palms and soles (92%). Warmth accentuates the rash. These lesions may coalesce and form large blemishes (54%). Sphygmomanometer cuff may accentuate the spots. The rash is often more pronounced over the dependent parts of the body.

Hypotension, oliguria and albuminuria are common. There is no eschar in cases of RMSF. Jaundice is rare. Hepatosplenomegaly is not a constant feature, found in less than one-fourth of the cases.

Malaise (95%) and confusion, restlessness and irritability are common, but stupor (28%) and coma (6%) are infrequent.

Platelet count is usually decreased.

Clinical signs of pneumonia can occur in nearly one-third of the cases.

Leukocytosis (11,000 to 13,000/cu. mm.) is frequent.

Stupor, coma and shock are infrequent, but when present, denote poor prognosis. [2]

In rare instances, disseminated intravascular coagulation can occur.

## DIAGNOSIS

Diagnosis is made by:

1) History of tick bite: In all cases of fever with rash, one should ask if the patient or his dog has been to areas known to have tick infestation. A history of tick bite is given by most patients with RMSF. In cases with the triad of fever, rash and history of tick bite, prompt therapy should be started with chloramphenicol or doxycycline.[3]

2) Weil-Felix reaction is an inconstant, non-diagnostic test for RMSF. However, a four fold rise of titer or a titer of more than 1:160 is suggestive of any rickettsial infection, not necessarily RMSF. This information can be obtained within twenty-four hours after the blood sample is drawn.

3) Culture: Blood cultures can be inoculated into the egg or guinea pig. Neill-Mooser reaction is positive in RMSF. Giemsa or Machiavello stain of the spleen or tunica vaginalis may reveal intranuclear bodies within two to three weeks.

4) Complement-fixation test (CFT) should be performed against all spotted fever groups of organisms. CFT is not as sensitive as the immunofluorescence test. [4]

   A four fold rise in CFT is diagnostic of RMSF. Often, CFT titers and Weil-Felix reaction may not be positive for four to six days after the onset of infection. Early therapy also interferes with this test.

Other useful diagnostic tests include detection of antibodies to R. rickettsii:

5) Microimmunofluorescence

6) Microagglutination, and

7) Hemagglutination

8) Skin biopsy of a surface lesion may reveal endangiitis histology. Machiavello's technique of these lesions may reveal red-stained intranuclear bodies.

9) Immunofluorescence technique of the skin specimens, obtained by biopsy on the fourth and eighth day of illness from RMSF, may confirm the diagnosis earlier than serologic reaction. [5]

Serum immunofluorescence antibodies may persist for ten
to fifteen years after the infection.

10) Monocyte culture technique in the Macaca mulatta: RMSF
can be detected as early as the fourth day of illness by this
method. [6]

DIFFERENTIAL: This is the same as epidemic typhus. Colorado tick fever (CTF) is frequently mistaken for RMSF. Febrile remission and another bout of fever are common with CTF,
which is caused by a virus. Despite its name, CTF is not confined to the Colorado state; it is found in various other parts of
the Western U.S., as well. Fluorescent antibody staining and
culture of the virus will establish the diagnosis.

PROGNOSIS: The overall mortality of RMSF is 7%. In Montana,
the mortality is still high (70% to 90%). RMSF, when it occurs
above the age of 40, carries relatively poor prognosis.

## Q FEVER

Derrick of Queensland, Australia, hesitated to name this disease, and called it "query" fever. Now there is no query about
its cause. It is caused by Rickettsia (Coxiella) burnetii. It will
continue to be called Q (query) fever until the confusion in the
nomenclature of the causative agent is settled between Cox's
fever and Burnet's fever.

Rickettsia (Coxiella) burnetii is a pleomorphic diplobacillus of
size $0.25 \times 0.25\mu$ to $0.25 \times 1.25\ \mu$, carried by the ticks Dermacentor andersoni and Ornithodoros turicata. It is world-wide in
distribution. It is a disease of cattle and sheep farm workers
during the lambing time. The excreta of sheep, goats and cattle,
and fresh-killed meat and raw milk are contagious. In Ohio,
(1966), 41% of the cattle, and 52 of 90 samples of milk examined,
contained this organism. In Los Angeles, where dairying is
done within the city, 90% of the cattle are seropositive; even
the dogs near the herds were infected. Nearly 30% of the population in Los Angeles are seropositive. Drinking raw milk is
a recent fad among the naturalistic-minded youngsters in this
city. The raw milk drinkers are ten times more frequently affected by Q fever than those who drink pasteurized milk. [7]

R. burnetii differs from other Rickettsia in that it is filterable,
does not cross react with Proteus, produces no skin rash, is non-
toxic to large animals, is transmitted by inhalation and, hence,

is considered distinct from other Rickettsia; therefore, called Coxiella burnetii. Q fever is mostly transmitted by inhalation and occasionally by blood transfusion.[8]

## CLINICAL FEATURES

Q fever is a three-phase disease:[9]

1) The incubation period
2) The febrile phase, and
3) The postfebrile phase

1) The incubation period: This may last for two to six weeks. It is inversely proportional to the dose of the contagion. This may be totally asymptomatic.

2) The febrile phase:

(a) Fever is usually acute. It may last for five to fifty-seven days. In most cases, it lasts for one to two weeks. Afterwards, there is a rapid ascent of fever (102° to 104° F.) sometimes broken by remissions. Nearly a third of the patients have biphasic fever, i. e. , when the initial fever touches normal, the second phase of fever begins, which can last once again for one to two weeks. The duration of fever is usually proportional to the age of the patient. Those above 40 years tend to have fevers for longer duration than younger patients.

(b) There is no rash in cases of Q fever.

(c) Headache can be severe.

(d) There may be relative bradycardia.

(e) Loss of weight, 10 to 15 pounds, can occur.

(f) Both liver and spleen may be enlarged, jaundice is occasional (5% to 10%).

(g) Pneumonia: Pneumonitis, when it occurs, resembles atypical pneumonia. Q fevers in Queensland are rarely associated with pneumonia. In most other countries, pneumonia is a prominent symptom (50% to 60%).

3) Postfebrile illness:

    (a) During this period, the organism multiplies in the placenta or the heart valves.

    (b) Abortion, therefore, can occur due to placental invasion.

    (c) Endocarditis can occur as a complication of Q fever because of proliferation of the organisms on the aortic valve. Clubbing of fingers, heart murmurs, intermittent fever, anemia and increased erythrocytic sedimentation rate, and increased immunoglobulin are some of its features. Routine blood cultures are always sterile in Q fever. The Q fever endocarditis, in spite of antibiotic therapy, is often fatal. Surgical resection of aortic valves slightly improves this otherwise grim prognosis.

## DIAGNOSIS

Q fever is diagnosed by the following features:

1) History of exposure to livestock

2) Chest roentgenogram: Nearly 50% show infiltrates or consolidation (not so in Queensland, Australia).

3) Weil-Felix reaction: OX2, OX19 and OXK are all negative.

4) Agglutination test: This may be positive for several months.

5) Hemagglutination test: This is highly sensitive and remains positive for several months.

6) Guinea pig test: The ticks are initially fed on the patient and later transferred on to mice and guinea pigs which develop the infection within ten to twenty-one days. Q fever is highly contagious; it is not safe to cultivate this organism.

7) Complement-fixation antibody: R. (Coxiella) burnetii antibody is produced in two different phases; phase I and phase II. In man, phase I antibodies may not be produced at all. Early in the disease process, phase II antibodies are produced. When phase I antibodies are found in man, it is diagnostic of chronic Q fever. Nearly 9% of the patients have CFT titers during the first, 65% during the second and 100% during the third week of fever. [10]

## TSUTSUGAMUSHI FEVER (scrub typhus)

Japan, Pakistan and northeastern Australia encompass the scrub typhus grid of the world. In this jet age, the scrub typhus acquired from this area can be reported from anywhere in the world. [11] Scrub typhus is caused by R. tsutsugamushi, transmitted by the larvae of the mite called Microtrombidium (Trombicula) akamushi, which has a taste for mammalian blood. They frequent the banks of large rivers and the backyards of the big cities, infesting the long grass. The rat acts as their reservoir. R. tsutsugamushi can be stained in tissues with Giemsa. It takes on an intense blue color with Castenada stain.

### CLINICAL FEATURES

1) Eschar: Nearly 50% or more will have an eschar which starts as a papulovesicle.

2) Regional lymphadenopathy: This is common, mostly in the groin and occasionally in the neck, when it may resemble the "bull neck" in diphtheria (see page 509).

3) Rash: This arises in five to eight days after exposure; is usually macular or maculopapular.

4) Fever: An abrupt rise of fever, sometimes as high as $104^{O}$ to $105^{O}$F. may remain so for fourteen days if untreated.

5) Headache: It is intense and intractable, arising on the fourth to tenth day of illness.

6) Deafness and tinnitus: This can occur in nearly 20%.

7) Conjunctival infection: This is common.

8) Hepatosplenomegaly: This, with moderate enlargement of the spleen, occurs with nearly 50% of the cases.

### DIAGNOSIS

1) The eschar with regional lymphadenopathy, the rash and history of exposure to mite-infested endemic areas, if present, may give the tip-off for the diagnosis.

2) Weil-Felix reaction: OX2 and OX19 are negative, but OXK is strongly positive. A titer of 1:160 is diagnostic. The titer usually increases during the second week of illness.

3) Mouse inoculation: Draw 5 to 10 ml. of blood from the patient; let it clot. Grind the clot up in sodium chloride; centrifuge at low speed and obtain 0.3 ml. of the supernatant fluid and inoculate intraperitoneally into mice. Within ten to sixteen days, Rickettsiae can be seen in the peripheral smears.

4) Immunofluorescence is specific and dependable.

5) Complement-fixation test

PROGNOSIS: Death occurs in 25% to 30% if untreated. Pregnant women may abort. The mortality in pregnancy is formidable.

## RICKETTSIALPOX

Rickettsialpox is caused by R. akari, transmitted by a mite (Allodermanyssus sanguineus) from the mouse (Mus musculus). The mite prefers the mouse, but if the mouse is not around, it bites the man. It is reported from the eastern coastal cities of the United States, most from the city of New York.

### CLINICAL FEATURES

1) Eschar: It is present in 95% of the cases. It may reach the size of 1 to 1.5 cm. , but no rickettsial organisms will be found in the eschar. It becomes papular and sloughs in three days. Scab formation can occur within three weeks.

2) Lymphadenopathy of the region of the eschar: This is common.

3) Fever: This may not begin for four to five days. When the fever (104°F. ) occurs, it is associated with chills and sweats, sometimes three or four times a day.

4) Rash: Maculopapular rash with central vesicles occurs in all areas of the body, except palms and soles. The oropharyngeal mucosa is not involved.

5) Myalgia: Myalgia and headaches are frequent, mostly occurring between the seventh and tenth day of illness.

The entire clinical picture may subside within ten days.

## DIAGNOSIS

Diagnosis is established by:

1) Weil-Felix reaction is negative for all strains of Proteus.
2) Clot culture, and
3) Culture of the vesicle: can be inoculated into mice or guinea pigs. R. akari can be cultured in the egg medium.
4) Complement-fixation test

DIFFERENTIAL: Rickettsialpox is generally benign. It should be differentiated from chickenpox. In chickenpox, the fever does not precede the rash as it does in rickettsialpox.

## REFERENCES

1. Riley, H. D. J.: "Rocky Mountain" spotted fever. Hosp. Pract. 112:51, 1977.

2. Hattwick, M. A., O'Brien, R. J., Hanson, R. F.: Rocky Mountain spotted fever: Epidemiology of an increasing problem. Ann. Int. Med. 84:732, 1976.

3. Perine, P. L., et al.: Single dose doxycycline treatment of louse-borne relapsing fever and epidemic typhus. Lancet 2:742, 1974.

4. Philip, R. N., et al.: A comparison of serologic methods for diagnosis of Rocky Mountain spotted fever. Am. J. Epidemiol. 105:56, 1977.

5. Woodward, T. E., et al.: Prompt confirmation of Rocky Mountain spotted fever. Identification of Rickettsiae in skin tissue. J. Inf. Dis. 134:297, 1976.

6. DeShazo, R. D., et al.: Early diagnosis of Rocky Mountain spotted fever. J. A. M. A. 235:1353, 1976.

7. Bell, J. A., Beck, M. D., Heubren, R. J.: Epidemiologic studies of Q fever in Southern California. J. A. M. A. 142:868, 1950.

8. California Morbidity. Q Fever: A New Mode of Transmission. Dept. of Public Health, State of California, December 4, 1976.

9. Derrick, E. H.: The course of infection with Coxiella burnetii. Med. J. Aust. 1:1051, 1973.

10. Ormsbee, R. A.: Q Fever Rickettsia. In Viral and Rickettsial Infections of Man, 4th Edition. F. L. Hornsfall, Tamm, I. , Pitman Publ. Corp. , London, 1965.

11. Imported Scrub Typhus: Connecticut. Morbidity and Mortality Report. Department of Health, Education and Welfare, Atlanta, March 16, 1974.

## 90. CHICKENPOX - HERPES ZOSTER
### by Larry J. Baraff

Varicella and herpes zoster are caused by the same herpes virus, a DNA virus referred to as varicella zoster (V-Z). Varicella occurs upon first exposure, and herpes zoster upon reactivation of a latent infection.

## CLINICAL FEATURES

The incubation period of varicella is from twelve to twenty-one days. Prodromal symptoms are minimal or absent and consist only of fever and malaise. The exanthem begins on the scalp and trunk, then spreads to the extremities. Lesions begin as erythematous papules, become vesicular, then pustular and finally form crusts. Characteristically, the vesicles are <5 mm in diameter, superficial in the dermis, thin-walled and unilocular. Lesions are usually present in varying stages of development. New lesions rarely appear after the seventh day of illness. Constitutional symptoms include fever to 39.5°C., headache, myalgia and malaise. The illness is more severe in adults. Occasionally lesions are bullous; this may be secondary to bacterial superinfection with phage group II Staphylococcus aureus.

Varicella is highly communicable; usually all susceptible household contacts are infected. Fifty per cent of children are infected prior to school entry. Maternal antibody usually prevents infection in the neonatal period. Patients should be considered communicable until the last vesicle is crusted.

## COMPLICATIONS

Secondary bacterial infection is the most frequent complication of varicella. S. aureus and group A streptococci are the usual associated pathogens. Central nervous system complications include encephalitis, aseptic meningitis, myelitis and cerebellitis with ataxia. The latter is the most common neurologic complication in children. Varicella encephalitis results in approximately thirty deaths annually in the United States. Hematologic complications include thrombocytopenic purpura and purpura fulminans.

Approximately 15% to 20% of adults with varicella have radiologic evidence of pneumonitis. Only one-fourth of these manifest cough or dyspnea. Popcorn-like calcifications of the lung
fields have been reported to be a residua of varicella pneumonitis. Rarely, orchitis, arthritis, myocarditis and acute
glomerulonephritis are associated with varicella. Reye's syndrome of coma, associated with fatty changes of the liver, hypoglycemia, and mitochondria destruction in hepatocytes and
skeletal muscle, is also associated with varicella.

Immunosuppressed or compromised persons (i. e. , those with
thymic deficiencies, hematologic malignancies, or those receiving immunosuppressive agents, including pharmacologic
doses of corticosteroids), may develop a severe form of disease termed progressive varicella. This illness is characterized by high fever to 40.5°C. , and systemic disease involving
the liver, central nervous system and lungs. The rash is more
extensive, and new crops of vesicles may appear for weeks;
lesions may be large and/or hemorrhagic (Figs. 124-127). The
fatality rate in children with leukemia receiving chemotherapy
has been reported to be 7%.

## DIFFERENTIAL DIAGNOSIS

Varicella can usually be easily distinguished from variola major. The latter is characterized by a prodromal period of several days with high fever and prostration, and by lesions which
appear first on the extremities, are deeper in the dermis, are
multilocular, and which are all in the same stage of development. Variola minor may be difficult to distinguish from varicella. Rickettsialpox, insect bites, pustular impetigo and generalized herpes simplex should be considered in the differential diagnosis of atypical cases of varicella.

## HERPES ZOSTER

Zoster probably represents a recrudescence of a latent V-Z
virus infection. It is generally believed that the dorsal root
ganglia is the site of a latent virus infection, and that defects
in cell-mediated immunity result in a reactivation of this infection. Such conditions include Hodgkin's disease, immunosuppressive drugs and old age. However, the majority of patients do not have a demonstrable malignancy.

Zoster usually involves one to three dermatomes. An attack
begins with neuralgic pain in the innervated area; papules,
which progress to vesicles and pustules, develop and dry up

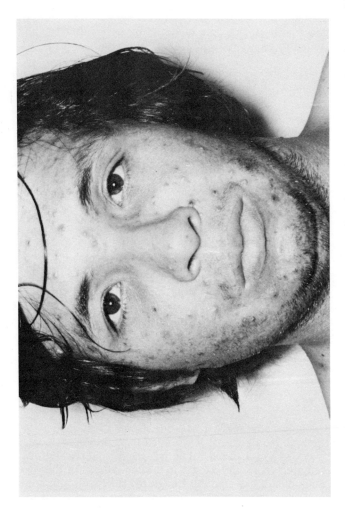

FIG. 124: Chickenpox. The skin lesions are generalized and can be seen in various stages of their development on the face, trunk and the extremities (also see Figs. 125, 126).

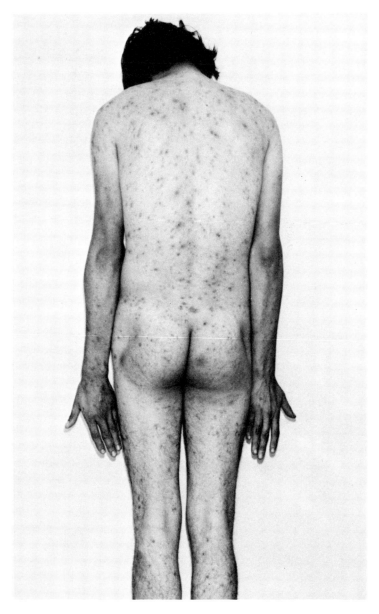

FIG. 125: Chickenpox (same patient as in Fig. 124).

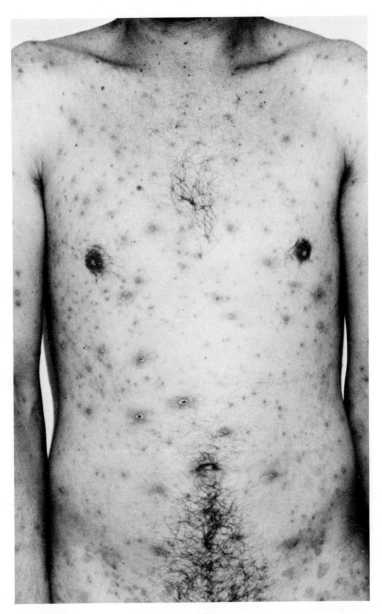

FIG. 126: Chickenpox (same patient as in Figs. 124, 125).

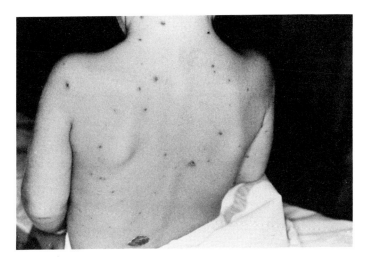

FIG. 127: Hemorrhagic chickenpox. Note the large hemorrhagic area on the lower part of the back. (Courtesy of Paul Kelly, M.D.)

over a course of seven to fourteen days. Regional lymph nodes
are invariably involved. On rare occasions, it may involve the
medulla. In one case, herpes zoster resulted in classical lateral
medullary syndrome (Fig. 128). With involvement of the ophthalmic division of the trigeminal nerve, herpes ophthalmicus
may ensue. Geniculate ganglia involvement produces the Ramsay
Hunt syndrome of paralysis of the facial nerve and vesicles in
the external ear canal. CSF examination usually reveals a mild
pleocytosis. Second attacks of zoster are rare and occur less
than 1% of the time.

Disseminated zoster is defined by the appearance of more than
ten vesicles outside the area of the infected dermatomes. Underlying malignancy is much more common in such individuals
and should be searched for in all cases (see Fig. 132, page 725).

## LABORATORY DIAGNOSIS

V-Z can usually be isolated from vesicles of patients with varicella or zoster. It can be easily cultured in human embryonic
lung fibroblasts. It has also been propagated in primary human
amnion, HeLa cells, African green monkey kidney and other
cell culture systems. To date, only man can be infected with
this virus.

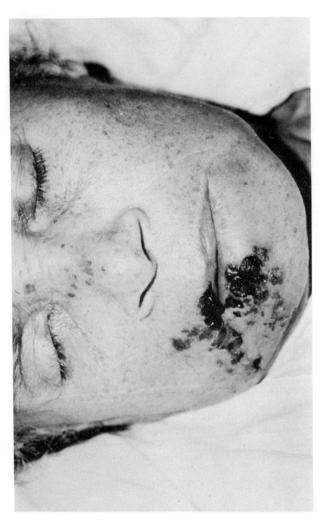

FIG. 128:   Herpes zoster, involving the mental branch of mandibular division and nasociliary branch of ophthalmic division of the trigeminal nerve. This patient was admitted with clinical features of lateral and medullary (Wallenberg) syndrome.

The serologic test usually employed to test for antibody in recent infections is the complement-fixation test. This usually reverts to negative within one year of infection. Other serologic tests rarely employed are neutralization, indirect hemagglutination and indirect fluorescence microscopy. Infection with varicella zoster virus produces eosinophilic intranuclear inclusions, and demonstration of such inclusions in cells scraped from the base of vesicles serves to distinguish varicella from variola.

## ZOSTER IMMUNE GLOBULIN

ZIG is prepared by cold ethanol fractionation of plasma from patients convalescing from zoster. It may be used to prevent or modify varicella in exposed, susceptible, immunocompromised individuals. It is recommended for use within three days of exposure in susceptible children < 15 years of age who are immunocompromised by malignant disease, immunodeficiency disorders, or who are receiving immunosuppressant chemotherapy. In addition, neonates that are born with no lesions, whose mothers developed varicella in the four days prior to delivery, should receive prophylaxis with ZIG to prevent congenital varicella, which has a 20% mortality.

## REFERENCES

1. Hope-Simpson, R. E.: The nature of herpes zoster: a long term study and a new hypothesis. Proc. R. Soc. Med. 58: 9, 1965.

2. Johnson, R., Milbourne, P. E.: Central nervous system manifestations of chickenpox. Can. Med. Assoc. J. 102:831, 1970.

3. Triebwasser, J. H., et al.: Varicella pneumonia in adults; report of seven cases and a review of the literature. Medicine 46:409, 1967.

4. Gerston, A. A., Steinburg, S., Bunell, P. A.: Zoster immune globulin: a further assessment. New Eng. J. Med. 290:243, 1974.

## 99: MEASLES
### by Larry J. Baraff

Measles is a highly communicable viral disease with a char
acteristic prodrome and maculopapular rash. It is caused by
a myxovirus related to the agent responsible for canine dis-
temper. Man is the only known reservoir and transmission is
by respiratory droplets.

## CLINICAL FEATURES

The incubation period is ten to twelve days. The prodrome precedes the rash by two to four days and consists of fever to 40.5°
C. , hacking cough, coryza, conjunctivitis, photophobia, headache, myalgia, irritability and lethargy. Posterior cervical
adenopathy is common. Two days prior to the appearance of
the rash, the pathognomonic Koplik's spots appear. These are
small red macules, with a central bluish-white speck, which
occur on the mucous membrane of the mouth opposite the molars,
on the inner aspect of the lips and on the nasal and vaginal mucosa. Koplik's spots are usually no longer present after the
second day of the exanthem. The rash begins on the face and
neck, then spreads downward and progressively involves the
chest, trunk and extremities. It is an erythematous maculopapular eruption which is discrete and blanches early, but after two to four days becomes confluent, develops a coppery appearance and no longer blanches.

Examination of the lung fields may reveal scattered rales which
usually represent a viral pneumonitis. Immunocompromised
and malnourished patients may develop a more severe Hecht's
giant cell pneumonia. In few cases, severe bleeding into the skin,
mucous membranes and other organs, associated with a decreased platelet count and prolonged bleeding time, results in
the syndrome called black measles. The mortality of this syndrome is high.

Bacterial complications are usually due to group A streptococci, Haemophilus influenzae and Staphylococcus aureus. Otitis
media and pneumonia are most common and should be suspected when fever persists beyond the third day of rash, and
when a leukocytosis develops. Encephalitis occurs in one in
every thousand patients. Approximately sixty per cent of encephalitis patients recover completely, twenty per cent die, and
twenty per cent recover with sequelae. Fifty per cent of measles
patients have an abnormal EEG during the acute phase of the illness.

Other complications include corneal ulceration, purulent cervical lymphadenitis and appendicitis. A positive tuberculin skin test may convert to negative during measles.

A late complication of measles, usually occurring three to ten years after the initial infection, is subacute sclerosing panencephalitis (SSPE). This is a progressive degenerative disease of the central nervous system characterized by progressive dementia, spasticity and coma. Death usually ensues in one year. CSF examination reveals elevated gamma globulin and high measles antibody titers. At least one case has been reported following live attentuated measles virus vaccination.

Prior to the use of the live attenuated measles vaccine, an inactivated vaccine was used. Five per cent of persons immunized with the vaccine develop an atypical measles syndrome when exposed to natural measles. This syndrome consists of a rash which begins on the distal extremities and moves towards the head, pneumonia, edema of the lips and feet, fever and prostration. The rash may be maculopapular, vesicular, urticarial, petechial or purpuric. This syndrome rarely occurs in recipients of the live attenuated measles vaccine.

## DIFFERENTIAL DIAGNOSIS

In rubella, the prodrome is milder, fever less marked, the rash more discrete and of shorter duration; posterior auricular adenopathy is more prominent. In roseola, the rash appears following three to four days of high fever, during which time the patient appears surprisingly well. The rash of scarlet fever is "sandpapery," begins in flexion areas, and is associated with perioral pallor and group A streptococcal tonsillitis or, less commonly, skin infection. Erythema infectiosum (fifth disease) begins with a characteristic slapped-cheek appearance, followed by a red maculopapular eruption on the extensor surfaces of the extremities, which develops a characteristic "lacework" pattern. Constitutional symptoms are mild or absent.

## LABORATORY DIAGNOSIS

Measles virus can be isolated from blood, urine and nasopharyngeal secretions during the prodrome and first 48 hours of the rash. Primary tissue cultures of monkey or human kidney and human amnion are preferred for viral isolation. Multinucleate giant cells are characteristic of infection and can be found in respiratory epithelium, lungs and the brain in cases of encephalitis. Serum neutralizing, hemagglutination inhibiting (HAI) and complement-fixing (CF) antibodies to measles virus are usually detectable within one to four days of the rash. The HAI test is the most sensitive and titers persist indefinitely. CF antibody titers decline to undetectable levels within two years. The virus can be identified in tissue, including the brain of subacute sclerosing panencephalitis cases, by immunofluorescent techniques.

## REFERENCES

1. Koplick, H. : The diagnosis of the invasion of measles from a study of the exanthema as it appears on the buccal mucous membrane. Arch. Pediat. 13:918, 1896.

2. Enders, J. F. , Peebles, T. C. : Propagation in tissue cultures of cytopathogenic agents from patients with measles. Proc. Soc. Exp. Biol. Med. 86:277, 1954.

3. Chen, T. T. , et al. : Subacute sclerosing panencephalitis: propagation of measles virus from brain biopsy in tissue culture. Science 163:1193, 1969.

## 100: MUMPS
### by Larry J. Baraff

Mumps is an acute infectious disease which characteristically produces swelling of one or more of the salivary glands, caused by a paramyxovirus. Other frequently involved glands include the pancreas, ovaries, testes, thyroid and breasts. Approximately 10% of patients will develop meningoencephalitis. It is estimated that one in four infections are asymptomatic; 95% of adults with no history of the disease have serologic evidence of immunity.

### CLINICAL FEATURES

The incubation period is seven to twenty-one days and patients are generally considered infectious for seven days after the onset of symptoms. The parotid gland is most often involved. Characteristically swelling does not extend below the mandible, and the uncinate lobe is palpable under the ear lobe. The submandibular gland may also be involved. Headache, photophobia, lethargy, convulsions and nuchal rigidity are suggestive of meningoencephalitis. Abdominal pain suggests oophoritis or pancreatitis. Diabetes mellitus has been reported to occur after mumps. Orchitis occurs in approximately one-third of postpubertal males; and is bilateral in one-third of the cases. Orchitis occurs without parotitis in 5% of the cases. Sterility is a rare sequela. Unilateral nerve deafness occurs in about 5% of the cases and usually resolves within one year. Aseptic meningitis occurring in the late winter and spring is usually due to mumps. Lumbar puncture will reveal > 500 WBC/mm$^3$ in 40% of patients; this response is not infrequently polymorphonuclear. Complete recovery from meningoencephalitis is the rule; hydrocephalus and death have been reported.

### DIFFERENTIAL DIAGNOSIS

Cervical lymphadenopathy is usually below the mandible; preauricular adenopathy is usually discrete and associated with conjunctivitis. Acute suppurative parotitis is more severe; the gland is red, hot and exquisitely painful. Pus can be expressed from Stenson's duct and the patients are more toxic. Actinomycosis of the mandible is more chronic and results in a firm swelling. Other causes of chronic parotid swelling include tumors, malnutrition, Sjogren's syndrome and sickle cell disease. Other viral infections, including parainfluenza I & III and cytomegalovirus, can produce parotitis, which is indistinguishable from mumps.

## LABORATORY DIAGNOSIS

Mumps virus can be cultured in tissue culture and embryonated eggs. The virus can be isolated from the oropharynx and urine for up to two weeks after infection. Serologic techniques include complement-fixation (CF), hemagglutination-inhibition (HAI) and the neutralization test. The serum amylase determination is a useful indication of inflammation of the pancreas or salivary glands. Mumps skin test antigen is commercially available but cannot be relied upon to determine immunity to mumps.

## REFERENCES

1. Azimi, P. H. , Cramblett, H. G. , Haynes, R. E. : Mumps meningoencephalitis in children. J. A. M. A. 207:509, 1969.

2. Philip, R. N. , Reinhard, K. B. , Lackman, D. B. : Observation on a mumps epidemic in a "virgin" population. Am. J. Hyg. 69:91, 1959.

3. Vuori, M. , Lahikainen, E. A. , Peltonen, T. : A study of 298 servicemen suffering from mumps. Acta. Otolaryngol. 55:231, 1962.

101: RUBELLA
by Larry J. Baraff

Rubella is a usually benign viral exanthem caused by an RNA virus, classified as a togavirus. Until the use of the live attenuated rubella vaccine, the majority of cases occurred in young children. When women are infected during the first and second trimesters of pregnancy, the congenital rubella syndrome may ensue.

## CLINICAL FEATURES

The incubation period of rubella is fourteen to twenty-one days. A prodrome of mild coryza, lymphadenopathy and fever to 38.5° precedes the onset of rash by one to two days. Lymphadenopathy is usually posterior cervical, postauricular and occipital. The rash first appears on the face and neck, then spreads to involve the trunk and extremities. It is a discrete pink to red maculopapular rash which usually lasts approximately three days, does not desquamate and is probably absent in at least 50% of infections. Arthralgia and frank arthritis are frequent complications of rubella in postpubertal females. The arthritis usually begins within five days of the exanthem, and persists from one to two weeks. It involves the proximal interphalangeal and metacarpophalangeal joints, the knees, ankles and wrists. An association of the rubella virus and juvenile rheumatoid arthritis has been suggested.

Complications are infrequent. Encephalitis is reported in one in every five thousand cases. Thrombocytopenic purpura is estimated to occur in one of every three thousand cases. Fatalities are rare.

## DIFFERENTIAL DIAGNOSIS

Scarlet fever, due to Group A streptococci, characteristically has a higher fever (40°C.), leukocytosis, exudative tonsillitis and anterior cervical adenopathy; the rash is a very fine sandpaper-like erythematous papular eruption which is accentuated in the axilla and antecubital fossae. Perioral pallor is characteristic. Measles is preceded by a more pronounced prodrome and the rash is more confluent and lasts longer. Koplik's spots are usually present. The rash of infectious mononucleosis is similar to that of rubella, but the presence of heterophile antibodies and atypical lymphocytes is diagnostic. Many enteroviral infections, due to Coxsackie and ECHO viruses, may result in a clinical syndrome indistinguishable from rubella.

## CONGENITAL RUBELLA

The congenital rubella syndrome occurs in infants of mothers infected in the first two trimesters, usually the first four months of pregnancy. The heart, central nervous system, eyes, ears, hematopoietic and reticuloendothelial systems are most frequently involved. The most frequent cardiac abnormalities are patent ductus arteriosus, and pulmonary artery and valvular stenosis. Deafness is sensorineural and permanent. Ophthalmologic defects are nuclear cataracts, microphthalmia and congenital glaucoma. Neurologic defects occur in 80% of affected infants. The mortality of this syndrome is 20%; most deaths occur in the first six months of life.

## LABORATORY DIAGNOSIS

Rubella virus can be propagated in cell lines from rabbits and African green monkey kidneys. It is detected by its interference with the cytopathic effect produced by challenge enterovirus. Serodiagnosis is usually made with a hemagglutination inhibition assay (HI). A complement-fixation test is also available, but is less sensitive and becomes positive later in the illness.

## REFERENCES

1. Green, R. H. , et al. : Studies of the natural history and prevention of rubella. Am. J. Dis. Child. 110:348, 1965.

2. Horstmann, D. M. , et al. : Maternal rubella and the rubella syndrome in infants. Am. J. Dis. Child. 110:408, 1965.

3. Johnson, R. G. , Hall, A. P. : Rubella arthritis. New Eng. J. of Med. 258:743, 1958.

102: POLIOMYELITIS
by Larry J. Baraff


Poliomyelitis is an acute infectious disease of the central nervous system which infrequently results in paralysis, caused by one of three serologically distinct RNA viruses (poliovirus types I, II and III) which are included in the enterovirus group. Both of the other members of the group, Coxsackie and ECHO viruses, have been infrequently associated with paralytic and non-paralytic disease, clinically distinguishable from poliomyelitis. Polio viruses are resistant to the usual concentrations of chlorine used for water purification. Man is the only known natural reservoir for the virus, and infection is thought to be either by the oropharyngeal-fecal circuit, or, in areas of improved hygiene, by oropharyngeal-oropharyngeal transmission. Poliomyelitis is world-wide in distribution, but its incidence has diminished markedly since the introduction of polio vaccines. The illness is more prevalent in summer, notably in temperate climates.

## CLINICAL FEATURES

During epidemics of poliomyelitis certain organs are identified as high risk due to unknown host factors. The illness is most frequent in childhood; 80% of cases occur in those under ten years of age. Prepubertal boys are affected twice as frequently as girls; however, pregnant women are at high risk. Though less frequent in older individuals, the severity of the clinical illness increases with age. Tonsillectomy predisposes to bulbar poliomyelitis, and suggests the virus gains access to bulbar nuclei directly via severed nerve fibers, or that decreased levels of oropharyngeal IgA may predispose to symptomatic infection. Corticosteroids have been demonstrated to increase the severity of experimental poliomyelitis.

The majority of cases of poliovirus infection do not result in paralysis and probably go unrecognized. The ratio of asymptomatic infection to clinically recognized disease is estimated to be 1000:1. When a susceptible individual is infected, one of four types of responses occurs; in decreasing order of frequency these are (1) asymptomatic infection, (2) abortive poliomyelitis, (3) non-paralytic poliomyelitis, and (4) paralytic poliomyelitis.

ABORTIVE POLIOMYELITIS: This syndrome is indistinguishable from many acute communicable diseases and can be diagnosed only by virologic or epidemiologic evidence, i.e., during outbreaks of recognizable poliomyelitis. It characteristically is a brief, febrile illness, with fever rarely exceeding 39°C. Associated symptoms include headache, nausea, vomiting, malaise, sore throat, abdominal pain and constipation. There are no meningeal signs.

NON-PARALYTIC POLIOMYELITIS: In this form, the headache, nausea and vomiting are more intense. There may be a symptom-free interval after which augmented symptoms again present; this is the so-called dromedary phenomenon. In addition, meningeal signs are usually present. These include soreness and stiffness of the posterior muscles of the neck, back and trunk, and Kernig's and Brudzinski's signs. CSF chemistries and cell counts usually demonstrate a moderate, predominantly mononuclear pleocytosis with a minimally elevated protein, similar to the aseptic meningitis syndromes associated with other viral agents.

PARALYTIC POLIOMYELITIS: This form is similar to non-paralytic poliomyelitis, but in addition, weakness or paralysis of one or more muscle groups is present. Paralysis is flaccid and usually asymmetrical, and is due to destruction of anterior horn cells or medullary motor nuclei, which results in degeneration of whole motor units with a decrease in muscle mass. There are four subclassifications:

1) Spinal: Weakness is present in the muscles innervated by anterior horn cells, including the diaphragm and the extremities. Spinal poliomyelitis is the most frequent type and the lower extremities are most commonly affected.

2) Bulbar: Weakness is present in the muscles innervated by one or more cranial nerves. Pharyngeal, facial and palatal involvement is most common; oculomotor nerves are less frequently affected and smell, vision, hearing and mastication are almost always spared. Death results from involvement of cardiorespiratory centers.

3) Bulbospinal: This consists of a combination of the two preceding forms.

4) Encephalitic: This is characterized by changes in mental status including irritability, disorientation and drowsiness, and can be diagnosed only be epidemiologic clues in the absence of viral isolation or paralysis.

The mortality rate for all types of paralytic polio is between 5% and 15%; that for the bulbar type is 20% to 60%.

## DIFFERENTIAL DIAGNOSIS

The Guillain-Barre syndrome is characterized by an ascending symmetrical paralysis with less fever, headache and meningeal signs. Paraesthesia and sensory changes are frequently present and examination of the CSF usually reveals the characteristic cyto-albumin dissociation. Residual involvement is unusual. Peripheral neuritis is apparent by the sensory loss, distal weakness and history of exposure to heavy metals, avitaminosis, or injections. In encephalitis, paralysis is usually spastic and mental status changes are prominent. Botulism may resemble poliomyelitis but meningismus and pleocytosis are absent. Tick bite paralysis also is without meningeal signs and resolves rapidly with removal of the tick. The periostitis of congenital syphilis results in a pseudoparalysis, but x-rays of long bones are diagnostic. Epidural abscess and spinal cord tumors are usually associated with sensory changes. Less common differential diagnoses include myasthenia gravis, familial periodic paralysis, scurvy, multiple sclerosis and acute porphyria.

## TREATMENT AND PREVENTION

There is no specific therapy for poliomyelitis. Treatment is tailored to the involved muscle groups. Physiotherapy is used for extremities, careful feeding or tube feeding for pharyngeal paralysis, frequent catheterization for bladder paralysis and assisted ventilation for respiratory paralysis. Complications, including secondary bronchopneumonia, hypertension and gastrointestinal bleeding are treated in the usual manner. Hyperimmune human globulin is of no value. Prevention of this illness may be accomplished with either live attenuated oral polio vaccine or the inactivated vaccine. Both are efficacious (see Immunizations, page 692).

## REFERENCES

1. Top, E. H. , Vaughn, H. F. : Epidemiology of poliomyelitis in Detroit in 1939. Am. J. of Public Health 31:777, 1941.

2. Ferris, B. G. , Jr. , et al. : Life threatening poliomyelitis: Boston, 1955. New Eng. J. Med. 262:371, 1960.

3. Poliomyelitis-like disease; a combined Scottish study. Br. Med. J. 2:597, 1961.

## 103: RABIES
by Larry J. Baraff

### PATHOPHYSIOLOGY

Rabies is an acute viral meningoencephalitis usually resulting from the inoculation of the rabies virus, present in the saliva of the biting animal, into the muscle or subcutaneous tissues of the victim. Infection may also result from mucous membrane inoculation. The virus passes, via spinal nerves and dorsal root ganglia, to the cord, then to the brain. Centrifugal axoplasmal spread follows and the virus is distributed to many organs, including the salivary glands, lung, myocardium, kidney, cornea and parafollicular nerve endings.

### CLINICAL COURSE

The incubation period is usually twenty to sixty days, but may be as short as seven days or as long as one year. The initial symptoms of the rabies prodrome are non-specific and include headache, anorexia and fever. Paresthesias in the area of inoculation are present in 50% of patients. Two to seven days following the onset of the prodrome, the acute neurologic phase ensues. Aerophobia, hydrophobia, auditory or visual hallucinations, confusion, lethargy and decreased deep tendon reflexes usually initiate this phase of the illness. Rapid deterioration is characteristic, and seizures, deepening coma, and frequent periods of apnea, progressing to complete respiratory arrest, will result in death if intensive supportive therapy is not instituted. An ascending paralysis similar to the Guillain-Barre syndrome occurs in 10 to 20% of cases, and a total flaccid paralysis is usually seen in patients who are supported by mechanical ventilation.

Pulmonary, cardiac and neurologic complications are seen in patients whose survival is prolonged by intensive supportive care. Pulmonary complications include ventilation-perfusion abnormalities, bronchopneumonia and pneumothorax, usually secondary to mechanical ventilation. Myocarditis is reported to occur in 20% of rabies patients. Bradycardia, hypotension and cardiac arrhythmias are the cause of death in most cases. Neurologic complications include impairment of thermoregulation, manifested by hyper- and hypothermia, the inappropriate antidiuretic hormone syndrome, diabetes insipidus and disorders of autonomic function which play a role in the development of hypotension and bradycardia. Rabies should be included in the diagnosis of all febrile encephalopathic patients. Many rabies patients are initially felt to have functional neuropsychiatric complaints.

## LABORATORY DIAGNOSIS

The diagnosis of rabies is dependent upon the demonstration of the rabies antigen, by viral isolation in mice or cell cultures, electron microscopy or immunofluorescent rabies antibody (FRA) staining; the development of significant antibody titers is also diagnostic. Rabies virus can be isolated from saliva, brain biopsy, and occasionally urine and rectal swabs. FRA staining may be used to demonstrate the virus in corneal touch preparations (40% of cases), brain biopsies, and more recently, in parafollicular neurons of skin biopsy specimens obtained from the neck or face. This latter technique appears to be reliable and is positive from the onset of symptoms. Serologic tests include neutralization, indirect fluorescent antibody (IFA) and fluorescent foci inhibition tests (FFIT). In patients who have not received vaccine or serum, any titer is diagnostic. In those who have received either of these, titers $\geqslant 1:5,000$ are presumptive.

## RABIES PROPHYLAXIS

Dog bites are responsible for the majority of human rabies cases world-wide. In the United States, because of extensive domestic animal immunization, there has not been an instance of human rabies associated with a dog bite since 1966; however, at least six U. S. cases were linked to dog bites which occurred outside the country in this same period. Feral animals most often found to be rabid are skunks, insectivorous bats, raccoons and foxes. The wolf and mongoose are significant reservoirs in other countries.

Pre-exposure prophylaxis is indicated for individuals at high risk of exposure to rabies such as veterinarians, animal handlers and certain laboratory workers. No cases of human rabies have occurred in individuals with rabies antibodies in their serum at the time of exposure. The recommended pre-exposure prophylaxis schedule is duck embryo vaccine (DEV), two 1.0 ml. subcutaneous injections one month apart, followed by a third dose six months later; or three 1.0 ml. injections at weekly intervals, and a fourth dose three months later.

Post-exposure prophylaxis should be provided for individuals bitten by an animal known or suspected to be rabid. For specifics of therapy, see the section on Immunizations, page 692.

## REFERENCES

1. Bryceson, A. D. M. , et al. : Demonstration during life of rabies antigen in humans. J. Infect. Dis. 131:71, 1975.

2. Hattwick, M. A. W. : Human rabies. Publ. Health Rev. 3:229, 1974.

3. Dupont, J. R. , Earle, K. M. : Human rabies encephalitis: A study of forty-nine fatal cases with a review of the literature. Neurol. 15:1023, 1965.

4. Bhatt, D. R. , et al. : Human rabies: Diagnosis, complications and management. Am. J. Dis. Child. 127:862, 1974.

104: GUILLAIN-BARRE LANDRY STROHL SYNDROME
by Larry J. Baraff

The Guillain-Barre syndrome is an acute infectious polyneu-
ronitis of unknown etiology, characterized by an ascending
muscular paralysis and cyto-albumin dissociation in the cerebrospinal fluid. Sensory deficits are usually absent.

## CLINICAL FEATURES

This syndrome affects children and adults and occurs during
all seasons. It frequently follows an acute infection or vaccination. The principle symptoms are those of peripheral and
cranial nerve involvement. Pain is unusual, but paresthesia
is common. Symmetrical weakness associated with absent
deep tendon reflexes, which first appears in the legs, and then
ascends to involve the thorax, upper extremities and muscles
of respiration, is most frequent. The cranial nerves are usually spared, but facial diplegia may occur. The abdominal reflexes are usually preserved. In most cases, there is muscular tenderness to deep pressure. Muscular atrophy is unusual
due to the acute onset of the illness. Fever is uncommon. In
most cases, complete recovery ensues after weeks or months,
but may take up to two years. Death results from complications.

## COMPLICATIONS

Respiratory paralysis may be gradual in onset. Vital capacity
should be measured daily, and respiratory assistance given,
when it falls 30% below normal or when hypoxia or hypercapnia
ensues. Pneumonia complicates hypoventilation and assisted
ventilation. Instability of the autonomic nervous system resulting in hyper- and hypotension and cardiac arrhythmias is rare.

## DIFFERENTIAL DIAGNOSIS

The symmetrical and ascending nature of the paralysis, and
the CSF findings differentiate the Guillain-Barre syndrome
from poliomyelitis. Acute myelitis is marked by sensory-motor
deficits below a given spinal level. Diphtheritic polyneuritis is
apparent because of the other aspects of the illness. Cranial
nerves are usually involved first and the paralysis is descending. Porphyric polyneuropathy may, on occasion, be ascending
and affect only motor fibers. The CSF protein is usually normal and psychosis and convulsions are occasionally present.
Polyarthritis nodosa with polyneuropathy may rarely present

as an acute idiopathic polyneuritis and be diagnosed only by
muscle biopsy. Tick paralysis can be excluded by a careful
search for an engorged, usually gravid, female tick.

## LABORATORY FINDINGS

The cerebrospinal fluid pressure is usually normal and the
cell count normal, but the protein elevated in the majority
of cases. Ten per cent of patients may have a pleocytosis of
from ten to one hundred cells. Not infrequently, a second lumbar puncture is needed four to seven days after the first to reveal the CSF abnormality.

## ASSOCIATED ILLNESSES

As stated earlier, this syndrome frequently follows viral infections and vaccinations. Diseases with which the Guillain-
Barre syndrome has been linked include mumps, varicella,
influenza, rubella, measles, mycoplasma infections, infectious mononucleosis and enteroviral infections. It has followed
vaccination for poliomyelitis, influenza and smallpox. The
relationship of these preceding factors and the syndrome is
yet to be clearly elucidated, but many feel it may be secondary
to a hypersensitivity syndrome.

## REFERENCES

1.  McFarland, H. R. , Heller, G. L. : Guillain-Barre complex:
    A statement of diagnostic criteria and analysis of 100 cases.
    Arch Neurology 14:196, 1966.

2.  Haymaker, W. , Kernohan, J. : The Landry Guillain-Barre
    syndrome. Medicine, 28:59, 1949.

## 105:  INFECTIOUS MONONUCLEOSIS
### by Larry J. Baraff

Infectious mononucleosis is an acute infection of the lymphatic system caused by the DNA herpes group Epstein-Barr (E. B.) virus, which usually occurs in young adults and is character- ized by the clinical triad of fever, sore throat and lymphadeno- pathy. This virus has also been strongly linked to Burkitt's lymphoma, from which it was first isolated, and to nasopharyn- geal carcinoma in the Far East.

## CLINICAL FEATURES

The incubation period of mononucleosis is thirty to fifty days and averages six weeks. The route of transmission is presumed to be oral-oral in adolescents and oral-fecal in young children. Prodromal symptoms include fatigue, anorexia, headache, chilliness and a distaste for cigarettes. In young adults, the representative clinical features are sore throat, fever and lymphadenopathy. One-third of the cases manifest a tonsillar exudate which is usually grayish-white, confluent and malo- dorous. Dysphagia may be marked. Petechiae may be seen on the hard palate in the first week of the illness. Fever fluctuates from $38^{\circ}$ to $40.5^{\circ}C$. Posterior cervical adenopathy is usually present. The spleen can be palpated in one-half of the patients. A morbilliform rash is present in 5% to 10% of the patients; if ampicillin is taken, then a rash will occur in more than 90% of the patients.

Infection in young adults is characteristic of developed coun- tries. In the United States, only one-fourth to one-half of col- lege freshman are immune and it is estimated that 10% to 15% of susceptible college students are infected annually. E. B. virus infection in young children is less characteristic. It may be asymptomatic or result in marked hepatosplenomegaly, gen- eralized adenopathy, neutropenia and atypical rashes. Diag- nosis is more difficult, as heterophil antibodies are rarely present in young children.

## COMPLICATIONS

More than 90% of cases are benign. Hepatitis occurs in 10% of the cases as manifested by liver tenderness and elevated en- zymes; one-half of these patients are jaundiced. A viral-like pneumonitis occurs in 2% to 5% of the patients. Neurologic complications, including the Guillain-Barre syndrome, encephalitis and aseptic meningitis, occur in 1% of the patients. Rare complications include agranulocytosis, hemolytic anemia, thrombocytopenia, myocarditis, glomerulonephritis and orchitis. Ten per cent of the patients have a throat culture positive for group A Streptococcus. Significant tonsillar hypertrophy may result in airway obstruction. Splenic rupture is a rare complication and has been associated with firm palpation.

## DIFFERENTIAL DIAGNOSIS

Three diseases need to be differentiated from infectious mononucleosis: group A streptococcal tonsillitis, cytomegalovirus and toxoplasmosis infections. Streptococcal tonsillitis can be differentiated clinically by the presence of a yellow follicular exudate, tender anterior cervical adenopathy, soft palate petechiae and the absence of splenomegaly. The heterophil test is negative, the throat culture positive, and the leukocytosis is predominantly polymorphonuclear. In cytomegalovirus (CMV) mononucleosis, exudative tonsillitis is rare; hepatomegaly is more common, occurring in 50% of the patients, and heterophil test is negative. CMV can be isolated from urine and CMV antibody titer rises are diagnostic. In toxoplasmosis, sore throat and tonsillitis are rarely present and lymphocytosis is unusual. Serologic tests are diagnostic. Rarely serum-sickness may mimic mononucleosis. In protracted cases of mononucleosis-like illness, it is imperative to rule out chronic lymphatic malignancies such as Hodgkin's disease.

## LABORATORY DIAGNOSIS

The E. B. virus cannot be propagated in tissue culture. It can be demonstrated in cultured lymphocytes by immunofluorescence techniques and electron microscopy. It can usually be demonstrated as a leukocyte transforming factor in the throats of mononucleosis patients and may persist in oral secretion for longer than one year.

Serologic confirmation of infection is usually obtained by the demonstration of heterophil antibodies, which can be demonstrated in 90% of young adults. Sera should be pre-absorbed with guinea pig kidney prior to incubation with horse red cells. Beef cell hemolysin titers may also be used but are less sensitive. A heterophil antibody titer of $\geqslant 1:28$ is usually diagnostic. Specific E. B. virus serologies, such as viral capsid antibody, antibody to early antigen, and IgM anti-E. B. virus, should be employed only when heterophil tests are negative.

Hematologic findings are characteristic but not specific. The majority of patients will demonstrate an increase in lymphocytes and monocytes to over 50% of all leukocytes. Ten per cent or more of these cells will be atypical, i. e. , have abnormal nuclei with a dense chromatin network and excess foamy vacuolated cytoplasm.

## REFERENCES

1. Henle, W. , et al. : Epstein-Barr virus and infectious mononucleosis. New Eng. J. Med. 288:263, 1964.

2. Henle, G. , Henle, W. , Diehl, V. : Relation of Burkitt's tumor associated herpes-type virus to infectious mononucleosis. Proc. Natl. Acad. Sci. U.S.A. 59:94, 1968.

3. Evans, A. S. : Complications of infectious mononucleosis: Recognition and management. Hosp. Med. 3:24, 1967.

4. Sawyer, R. N. , et al. : Prospective studies of a group of Yale University freshmen. I. Occurrence of infectious mononucleosis. J. Infect. Dis. 123:263, 1971.

5. Henle, G. , Henle, W. : Observations on childhood infections with Epstein-Barr virus. J. Infect. Dis. 121:303, 1970.

## 106: YELLOW FEVER
by H. Thadepalli

Yellow fever is sparsely distributed in equatorial Africa and Central and South America, caused by an arbovirus (RNA virus) of size 30 ± 5 m$\mu$, transmitted either from man to man or from a non-human primate to man by the mosquito Aedes aegypti. The mosquito itself may not become infectious for two to three weeks after the ingestion of the virus.

### CLINICAL FEATURES

Yellow fever should be suspected in anyone returning from an endemic zone and becoming ill within three to five days, which is the incubation period of this disease. The pulse rate is disproportionately low as compared with the body temperature. This relative bradycardia is called Faget's sign. Headache, body aches and backache may be very pronounced. The liver is often palpable, but the spleen is not. In some instances, the patients are asymptomatic. In others, the initial fever is followed by remission within five to seven days, when the patient feels better. This "period of calm" may continue or relapse into another bout of fever. The pulse rate may rise during this second attack. A quickening pulse rate with a falling temperature is generally regarded as an ominous sign.

Obvious jaundice is rare in yellow fever. Patients with yellow fever may have very little icterus. The conjunctivae are of light yellow color and so is the skin. Obvious jaundice should suggest viral hepatitis rather than yellow fever.

Proteinuria is a constant feature of yellow fever, sometimes patients have cylindruria.

Coagulation abnormalities are common. Occasionally, yellow fever is complicated by disseminated intravascular coagulation. Hemorrhages, petechiae and bleeding from the gastrointestinal tract may then occur.

### DIAGNOSIS

1) Blood cultures: Viraemia may be present during the first three days. Not only should blood cultures be drawn, but a sample of serum separated and saved for titers and also for future reference.

2) Animal inoculation: Blood samples may be inoculated into the Rhesus monkey or intracerebrally into mice. Development of specific antibody to yellow fever in the serum can be demonstrated by the mouse protection test.

3) Liver biopsy: This should not be taken lightly. In yellow fever, coagulation studies should always be obtained before liver biopsy. Profuse internal hemorrhage is a known complication of this procedure. Coagulative midzonal degeneration of the hepatic cells is characteristic of this disease. Postnecrotic scarring seldom occurs.

DIFFERENTIAL: The following should be considered in the differential diagnosis:

1) Influenza
2) Leptospirosis
3) Relapsing fever
4) Typhoid
5) Dengue and malaria

## THERAPY

Hyperimmune serum is the only known therapeutic amelioration in cases of yellow fever. The current yellow fever vaccine, with attenuated yellow fever virus, is a very effective prophylaxis.

## 107: VIRAL HEPATITIS
### by Larry J. Baraff

Hepatitis refers to an inflammatory process involving the liver, which may be either acute or chronic and may be caused by several infectious agents, toxins and drugs, hypersensitivity or immune mechanisms, and metabolic diseases. Infectious agents which have been associated with hepatitis include enteroviruses, the Epstein-Barr virus, cytomegalovirus, yellow fever virus, Leptospira, type A and B hepatitis viruses and Listeria monocytogenes. This discussion will be primarily confined to hepatitis caused by the type A and B hepatitis viruses (HAV and HBV). Neither of these viral agents has been propagated in tissue culture systems; however, both have been demonstrated serologically and by electron microscopy in patients with hepatitis. Together they account for the majority of clinical hepatitis. In 1977 in the United States, hepatitis was the fourth most frequent notifiable disease after gonorrhea, varicella, and rubeola. More than 55,000 cases were reported of which approximately 30,000 were type A, 16,000 type B and 9,000 type unspecified. Man and certain primates are the only known natural reservoirs for these hepatitis viruses which are world-wide in distribution.

### CLINICAL FEATURES

The clinical features of hepatitis due to type A or B virus are similar, and in individual cases, the few distinctions do not allow reliable differentiation. The initial or prodromal symptoms include lassitude, loss of appetite, malaise, myalgia, nausea and vomiting, headache, feverishness and epigastric abdominal pain. These symptoms usually persist for three to ten days, after which the urine becomes brownish in appearance. Jaundice follows in icteric cases. In anicteric illness, the symptoms are less severe. Itching and an evanescent rash may occur in a minority of patients with hepatitis A. Characteristically, the onset of hepatitis A is relatively sudden, with symptoms developing over a 24- to 48-hour interval. In contrast, in the majority of cases of hepatitis B, the onset is gradual. Joint manifestations and hypersensitivity type rashes are characteristic of hepatitis B. Occasionally, the arthritis associated with hepatitis B may be so prominent in the prodromal period as to suggest rheumatoid arthritis.

The most prominent signs in hepatitis are jaundice, hepatomegaly and hepatitic tenderness. Spider angiomata and palmar erythema do occur and may not indicate chronic liver disease.

Manifestations distinct from those associated with viral hepatitis have also been associated with hepatitis B virus infections. These include polyarthritis, glomerulonephritis, and cryoglobulinemia, all presumed to be secondary to antigen-antibody complex formation.

## EPIDEMIOLOGY

Hepatitis A has been previously called infectious hepatitis. Its incubation period is short, usually from 15 to 45 days. It is more common in younger age groups, especially school age children, and person to person spread by the fecal-oral route is the usual mechanism of transmission. A few epidemiologic investigations suggest the possibility of respiratory spread. Common vehicle epidemics due to contaminated food and drinking water also occur. Ingestion of raw or incompletely cooked mollusks, especially clams, is the most important non-contact mode of transmission. Transmission by blood products or contaminated instruments can occur in the late incubation period.

Patients with hepatitis A are most infectious when experiencing prodromal symptoms. Patients are unlikely to transmit the agent at the time the diagnosis is made. Immunity seems to be life long. The mortality rate is reported to be one in every thousand overt cases.

Hepatitis B has been previously called serum hepatitis or post-transfusion hepatitis. Since the advent of sensitive serologic tests for viral antigens associated with this infection, and routine screening of blood donors, this type of hepatitis rarely follows blood transfusions. The incubation period ranges from 30 to 180 days, and infection usually occurs in infants (perinatal or vertical transmission) or in adults (horizontal transmission). The infectious agent has been demonstrated in blood, saliva, urine, semen, synovial fluid, cerebrospinal fluid and breast milk. It is absent in bile or feces. Transmission by blood now occurs in three circumstances: (1) maternal-fetal blood mixing, usually perinatally; (2) accidental blood transfer, i. e. contaminated needle puncture and in dialysis units; (3) transfusion of blood products, especially commercial clotting concentrates.

Infection with hepatitis B virus may result in acute or chronic infection. Acute infection may be subclinical or clinical. Patients

with acute infection may be infectious for three months following resolution of symptoms. A small percentage of patients
(10%-15%) remain chronically antigenemic following acute infection. Chronic antigenemia is more likely to follow vertical
transmission. If acute hepatitis B occurs in the third trimester
of pregnancy, or in the two months following delivery, approximately 70% of infants will be infected. Vertical transmission
from chronically antigenemic mothers to their offspring is less
frequent and varies from 10% to 50%.

Individuals who are chronically antigenemic, following an asymptomatic infection or acute hepatitis, usually can be divided into three groups: (1) asymptomatic with normal liver function
tests and liver biopsies; (2) asymptomatic with slight elevations of transaminases; and (3) more severe abnormalities on
liver biopsy, which may progress to cirrhosis (chronic active
hepatitis). At the present, it is best to consider all chronically
antigenemic persons as possibly infectious.

In hospitals, hepatitis B is a problem in specialized areas including hemodialysis units, oncology units and institutions for
the mentally retarded. Sexual contact is an efficient means of
transmission of type B hepatitis and probably is responsible
for the majority of cases in the general population. Approximately 25% of sexual partners may develop hepatitis following exposure to acute type B hepatitis in their mate.

Eighty-five per cent of patients with acute type B hepatitis make
a full recovery, approximately 15% become chronically antigenemic. The mortality rate associated with acute infection is
1%.

## LABORATORY DIAGNOSIS

Hepatitis A is caused by a 27nm. RNA virus (HAV), which can
be demonstrated in serum and fecal samples by immune electron microscopy. Serum antibody against HAV has been demonstrated by radioimmunoassay, immune adherence hemagglutination and complement-fixation. These techniques are
research laboratory methods, and at present, diagnosis is usually based upon clinical and epidemiological data in the absence
of a laboratory diagnosis of type B hepatitis.

Hepatitis B is caused by a 42nm. DNA virus called the Dane
particle. It is composed of a 27nm. inner core (HBcAg) containing double stranded DNA and DNA polymerase and an outer surface antigen (HBsAg). The protein coat or HBsAg is frequently

manufactured in amounts greatly in excess of that required to cover nucleoprotein cores, and forms small spherical particles and tubular forms which predominate in the circulation of patients with hepatitis B. HBsAg appears in the circulation late in the incubation period and usually persists from one to three months following recovery. Antibody to HBsAg (anti-HBsAg) develops two to six months following cessation of antigenemia in about three-fourths of the patients. HBcAg can be detected in some patients during the incubation period and early acute illness. Antibody to HBcAg (anti-HBcAg) develops early in the acute illness and persists in recovery, and it may be useful in diagnosis when the HBsAg tests are falsely negative. Another recently described antigen-antibody system, the "e" system, has been associated with hepatitis B. The presence of eAg appears to be of value in identifying HBV carriers likely to develop active forms of chronic liver disease, and to be infectious to their contacts. In contrast, the presence of anti-e may indicate non-infectivity despite the presence of HBsAg.

The most useful single test for the diagnosis of hepatitis B is radioimmunoassay for HBsAg. This antigen was previously called the hepatitis-associated antigen (HAA) or Australia antigen. Counter immunoelectrophoresis, immune adherence hemagglutination and passive hemagglutination are usually less sensitive and more difficult to perform. Assays for anti-HBs, eAg, HBcAg, anti-HBc and anti-e are still research tools.

Routine laboratory tests useful in the diagnosis of hepatitis are transaminases (SGOT, SGPT), bilirubin, serum alkaline phosphatase, and prothrombin time. Usually the degree of elevation of the transaminases exceeds that of the alkaline phosphatase, indicating the hepatocellular, rather than obstructive, nature of the illness. The degree of prolongation of the prothrombin time correlates directly with the severity of the clinical illness and is a useful aid in determining the need for hospitalization.

### PROPHYLAXIS

Pre-exposure prophylaxis for hepatitis A is indicated for travelers who go to developing countries and bypass ordinary routes, and for persons in close contact with recently imported nonhuman primates. Immune serum globulin (ISG) in a dose of 0.05 ml/kg is recommended. Post-exposure prophylaxis for hepatitis A is recommended for household contacts and institutional contacts of patients with acute hepatitis A within two weeks of exposure. The dose of ISG in these cases is 0.02 ml/kg. Such prophylaxis is usually not indicated for school, hospital or work contacts.

Recently a high titer immune globulin preparation, hepatitis B immune globulin (HBIG), has become available for passive prophylaxis of hepatitis B. With few exceptions, there is no epidemiologically convincing evidence that HBIG is superior to ISG containing low titers of anti-HBs (manufactured after 1072) for hepatitis B prophylaxis. However, the use of HBIG is recommended in the following circumstances: (1) following a single acute exposure to blood known to contain HBsAg by needle puncture, or ocular or mucous membrane inoculation; (2) to sexual partners of patients with acute hepatitis B; (3) to infants born to mothers with acute hepatitis B in third trimester of pregnancy or the ensuing two months. In all cases, HBIG should be administered within seven days of exposure. The dose for adults is 0.05 - 0.07 ml/kg and for infants 0.13 ml/kg. HBIG should not be given to HBsAg positive individuals. It is not indicated for anti-HBsAg positive patients.

<h2 style="text-align:center">NON-A, NON-B HEPATITIS</h2>

Several investigators have now reported the occurrence of three well separated bouts of hepatitis in a single patient. Usually, such patients are intravenous drug users. With serologic tests, it is now possible to demonstrate that at least one of these episodes is not due to any of the currently recognized causes of infectious hepatitis. In addition, there are now several reports of transfusion-associated hepatitis not associated with serologic evidence of hepatitis B. A small proportion of these cases are due to CMV; however, it is likely that we shall soon identify other viral agents responsible for transfusion-associated hepatitis.

<h2 style="text-align:center">REFERENCES</h2>

1. Krugman, S., Freedman, H., Lattimer, C.: Viral hepatitis, type A. Identification by specific complement fixation and immune adherence tests. New Eng. J. Med. 292:1141-43, 1975.

2. Villarejos, V. M., et al.: Role of saliva, urine and feces in the transmission of type B hepatitis. New Eng. J. Med. 291:1375-78, 1974.

3. Feinstone, S. M., et al.: Transfusion associated hepatitis not due to viral hepatitis type A or B. New Eng. J. Med. 292:767-70, 1975.

4. Immune globulins for protection against viral hepatitis. Morbidity and Mortality Weekly Report 26:425-42, 1977.

5. World Health Organization: Advances in viral hepatitis. Report of the Expert Committee on Viral Hepatitis (WHO Tech Rep No. 602) Geneva, 1977, pp. 1-62.

6. Mosley, J. W. : The epidemiology of viral hepatitis: An overview. Am. J. Med. Sci. 270:253, 1975.

7. Schweitzer, I. L.: Infection in neonates and infants with the hepatitis B virus. Prog. Med. Virol. 20:27-48, 1975.

## 108: VIRAL DIARRHEA
### by H. Thadepalli

The first manifestation of viral gastroenteritis is vomiting, followed by watery diarrhea (five to twenty stools per day), abdominal cramps and low-grade fever. This diarrhea may be aggravated by food and relieved by fasting. The diarrhea itself lasts longer than vomiting, but the entire episode settles down in one to two days, followed by rapid recovery. Occasionally, in children and debilitated aged patients, the disease may be fulminating with rapid dehydration, collapse and death. Viral gastroenteritis is mainly a disease of children. It occurs during the summer in the tropics, and during the winter in the subtropics. Most attacks begin with abrupt vomiting or diarrhea or both, followed by abdominal colic and profuse watery stools.

The leukocyte count and the sedimentation rate are normal, but when dehydration occurs, the leukocyte count and the hematocrit may rise.

Viral gastroenteritis is caused by varieties of agents: Reovirus-like agent, arbor virus-like agent, ECHO virus, rota virus, adenovirus and several other viral particles were demonstrated in the stools,[2,4] duodenal aspirates and in the biopsy of the small intestine. Viral diarrhea is a disease of the small bowel.[1] It rarely involves the large bowel; hence, fecal leukocytes are rare in viral gastroenteritis.

### DIFFERENTIAL

The diagnosis of an isolated case of viral diarrhea is confusing. It may be confused with travelers' diarrhea (perhaps this disease is also produced by viruses), and other bacterial diarrheas. Sigmoidoscopy in viral enteritis might show edematous, but not inflamed mucosa, and rarely minute ulcerations. Specific immune bodies may be detected from the patient's serum. It is important to note that the presence of a recognized bacterial pathogen in the stool does not exclude the viral etiology. Viruses and bacteria have been isolated together in cases of diarrhea.[3] Bloody stools and mucus stools are infrequent in viral diarrhea. Vomiting and mild watery diarrhea, without blood or mucus and without leukocytes, suggests small bowel disease, possibly viral enteritis.

## REFERENCES

1.  Schreiber, D. S. , Blacklow, N. R. , Triev, J. S. : The mucosal lesion of the proximal small intestine in acute infectious non-bacterial gastroenteritis. New Eng. J. Med. 288:1318, 1973.

2.  Middleton, P. J. , et al. : Orbivirus acute gastroenteritis of infancy. Lancet 1:1241, 1974.

3.  Echeverria, P. , Blacklow, N. R. , Smith, D. H. : Role of heat-labile toxigenic Escherichia coli and reovirus-like agents in diarrhea in Boston children. Lancet 2:1113, 1975.

4.  Cameron, D. J. S. , et al. : New virus associated with diarrhoea in neonates. Med. J. Aust. 1:85, 1976.

## 109: IMMUNIZATION
by Larry J. Baraff

Immunizations are one of the major health care efforts responsible for the dramatic decline in the morbidity and mortality associated with infectious diseases world-wide. Despite their proven efficacy, it is estimated that between 20%-40% of U.S. children, and certainly more in many other countries, are inadequately immunized against the common infectious diseases. Updating of adult immunizations is unfortunately usually limited to tetanus toxoid post-injury and vaccinations for international travel. All physicians should be aware of the principles of immunizations, the recommendations for childhood and adult vaccination, and for vaccinations for international travel.

### ACTIVE IMMUNIZATION

The administration of an immunogen which results in the production of antibody by the host is termed active immunization. Active immunization is usually initiated prior to exposure to the communicable disease which it is intended to prevent. It provides protection, not only for the individual, but when widely practiced within a population, for the unimmunized, by decreasing their exposure to the infectious agent; this is termed "herd immunity." Antigens employed for active immunization include both live attenuated and inactivated viruses, killed bacteria, and bacterial toxins altered so as to be immunogenic but non-toxic, i. e. toxoids. Inactivated viral vaccines may be composed of whole virus, or selected viral antigens, i. e. split vaccines (e. g. , influenza vaccines). Bacterial vaccines may also contain only a portion of the disease-producing bacterium to minimize adverse reactions (e. g. , meningococcal vaccines). In all instances, the primary goal of active immunization is to expose the individual to a modified form of the disease-producing organism or toxin which will provide immunity with few or no adverse effects. Protection is usually quantitated by the titer of specific antibodies present in the sera. The role of cell-mediated immunity in the protection afforded by several vaccines is currently being actively investigated.

Live attenuated viral vaccines differ from inactivated vaccines and toxoids, because in most cases only a single dose is necessary to provoke protective levels of antibody, and immunity is long-lasting with no need for boosters. Three doses of trivalent oral polio vaccine are used to immunize because of possible interference of one poliovirus with the immunogenicity of

another, and because of the potential neutralizing effect of passively acquired maternal antibody. Inactivated antigens seldom
are immunogenic in a single dose; a primary series is required
to invoke immunity, and boosters are necessary to maintain
suitable protection.

IMMUNIZATION SCHEDULES: Routine childhood immunizations are generally given as soon as they will invoke immunity
(Table 43). Because of the lack of passively acquired protection to pertussis, and the gravity of this illness in early
infancy, immunization with DTP vaccine is usually instituted
at the age of two months. Simultaneous administration of T-OPV
is now recommended. Other vaccines are withheld until after
the first birthday to minimize the interference with immunization associated with maternal antibodies. Measles, mumps,
and rubella vaccine are usually given in the second year of life
and may be given as a combined vaccine at the age of fifteen
months. The seroconversion rates with these vaccines is approximately 90%. Factors which may be responsible for vaccine failure include passive acquisition of maternal antibodies,
improper handling of vaccine, undetermined host factors, and
in the past, the simultaneous administration of measles immune
globulin with measles vaccine.

## TABLE 43: RECOMMENDED ROUTINE IMMUNIZATIONS

| Vaccine | Primary | Childhood Boosters | Adult Booster Intervals |
|---------|---------|--------------------|-------------------------|
| DTP | 2, 4, 6 mos. | 18 mos. & 5 yrs. | N. A. |
| Td | | | 10 yrs. |
| T-OPV | 2, 4, 6 mos. | 18 mos. & 5 yrs. | Travel |
| MMR | 15 mos. | None | None |
| Smallpox | No longer recommended | | Travel |

DTP   : Diphtheria Tetanus Pertussis Vaccine
Td     : Diphtheria Tetanus Vaccine - Adult Type
T-OPV: Trivalent Oral Polio Vaccine
MMR   : Measles Mumps Rubella Vaccine
N. A.   : Not Advised

The recommended schedules are only guidelines, and if it is
necessary to alter the suggested intervals, this can usually be
accomplished with little or no loss of efficacy. It is not necessary to start a primary immunization series over again when
it has been interrupted for some reason.

The routine use of smallpox vaccine has now been discontinued
for all persons except those at high risk because of their occupation, i. e. laboratory workers who are associated with variola virus, health workers in infectious disease centers that
are designated to care for smallpox patients, and those who
plan to travel to countries that require vaccination. At this time
(June 1979) smallpox has been eradicated world-wide.

With the exception of the Tetanus-Diphtheria Vaccine (Adult
type), adult immunizations are only recommended for those
at special risk because of occupation or travel. The adult Td
vaccine has one-third of the diphtheria toxoid of the pediatric
preparation and should be given every ten years. Except when
known allergenicity to diphtheria toxoid is present, pure tetanus toxoid should not be used. If an individual has had the primary DTP series, plus boosters every ten years, there is no
need for additional tetanus wound prophylaxis, except in the
case of dirty wounds, when an additional Td should be given
if it is more than five years since the last tetanus toxoid. The
recommendations for active and passive tetanus wound prophylaxis are presented in Table 44. A reliable knowledge of
the patient's immunization history is necessary to determine
the tetanus prophylaxis to be given. When this is not available,
the patient should be managed as though he had no previous immunizations.

NON-ROUTINE ACTIVE IMMUNIZATIONS: In addition to the
routinely administered active immunizing agents, there are at
least fifteen other antigens available for special use (Table 45).
Smallpox, cholera, yellow fever and typhoid vaccines are recommended for international travel to selected areas where exposure to these diseases is possible. Smallpox and yellow fever vaccines provide solid immunity for three and ten years
respectively; both are live attenuated viral vaccines. The protection offered by the killed cholera and typhoid bacterial vaccines is less effective and is short-lived (six months); thus they
are of limited value. The Bacillus Calmette-Guerin vaccine for
tuberculosis is prepared from an attenuated strain of Mycobacterium tuberculosis var. bovis. It is widely used in countries
where tuberculosis is prevalent to prevent dissemination of

TABLE 44:  GUIDE TO TETANUS PROPHYLAXIS
IN WOUND MANAGEMENT

| History of Tetanus Immunizations (Doses) | Clean, Minor Wound | | All Other Wounds | |
|---|---|---|---|---|
| | Td* | TIG | Td | TIG |
| Uncertain | Yes | No | Yes | Yes |
| 0 - 1 | Yes | No | Yes | Yes |
| 2 | Yes | No | Yes | No |
| 3 | ⩾10 yrs** | No | ⩾5 yrs** | No |

Td  : Tetanus Diphtheria Toxoids - Adult Type
TIG: Tetanus Immune Globulin
* DTP if ⩽ 6 yrs of age
** Td to be given if interval since last immunization greater
than indicated

disease, and has been shown to be 80% effective over a 15-year
period. Its use may result in disseminated disease in immunocompromised individuals. The U. S. Public Health Service ad-
vises against the widespread use of BCG in this country. The
chief objection to its use is that it invalidates the tuberculin skin
test as a diagnostic and epidemiologic tool.

Influenza is the only infectious disease that still causes world-
wide epidemics that result in significant excess mortality. Those
at both extremes of life (i. e. the very young and very old), and
those with cardiopulmonary, renal and metabolic disease are
most prone to serious complications associated with influenza.
Because of periodic major shifts in the antigenic structure of
the influenza virus, and the short-lived protection associated
with the vaccine, it is usually recommended that vaccination
be done annually. The antigenic nature of the vaccine is determined by the specific influenza virus associated with human disease in the current and previous years. During the massive
"swine flu" vaccination program of 1976, it was noted that there
was an increased incidence of the Guillain-Barre syndrome,
which was subsequently related to vaccine administration and
caused the termination of this immunization program. The incidence of this syndrome was estimated to be 1/100,000 vaccinees. The exact relationship of this syndrome and vaccine
administration has not yet been determined.

## TABLE 45:  VACCINES AND ANTISERA FOR HUMAN USE

| DISEASE | ACTIVE | | | PASSIVE | |
|---|---|---|---|---|---|
| | Live, Attenuated | Inactivated | Toxoid | Human | Equine |
| Adenovirus | | S | | | |
| Botulism | | | | | S |
| Cholera | | T | E | | |
| Clostridial Myonecrosis | | | | | L |
| Cytomegalovirus | E | | | | |
| Diphtheria | | | R | | S |
| Equine Encephalitis Eastern Western | | S S | | | |
| Gonococcal | | E | | | |
| Haemophilus influenzae, Type B | | E | | | |
| Hepatitis A | | | | T/S* | |
| Hepatitis B | | | | S | |
| Influenza | E | R | | | |
| Measles | R | S | | S* | |
| Meningococcus A & C | | S | | | |

Table 45 (Cont'd)

| DISEASE | ACTIVE | | | PASSIVE | |
|---------|--------|--|--|---------|--|
| | Live, Attenuated | Inactivated | Toxoid | Human | Equine |
| Mumps | R | | | L | |
| Myco-plasma | | E | | | |
| Para-tyhpoid A & B | | S | | | |
| Pertussis | | R | | L | |
| Plague | | S | | | |
| Pneumo-coccus | | S | | | |
| Polio | R | S | | L | |
| Rabies | | S | | S | |
| Rocky Mountain Spotted Fever | | S | | | |
| Rubella | R | | | | |
| Smallpox (Vaccinia) | T | | | S | |
| Snakebite | | | | | S |
| Spiderbite | | | | | S |
| Tetanus | | | R | S | |
| Tubercu-losis | S | | | | |
| Typhoid | | T | | | |

Table 45 (Cont'd)

| DISEASE | ACTIVE | | | PASSIVE | |
|---|---|---|---|---|---|
| | Live, Attenuated | Inactivated | Toxoid | Human | Equine |
| Typhus | | S | | | |
| Varicella-Zoster | E | | | S | |
| Yellow Fever | T | | | | |

E: Experimental
L: Limited Value
R: Routine
S: Special Use
T: Travel
* Immune Serum Globulin, no specific high titer antiserum

Other active immunizing agents available for special use include inactivated viral vaccines for eastern and western equine encephalitis, rabies and adenovirus, killed bacterial vaccines for meningococcal types A and C, plague, a dodecavalent pneumococcal vaccine and killed rickettsial vaccines for typhus and Rocky Mountain spotted fever. Vaccines are being developed for cytomegalovirus diseases, syphilis, varicella-zoster, gonorrhea, Haemophilus influenzae type B, hepatitis A and B and malaria.

COMPLICATIONS AND CONTRAINDICATIONS OF ACTIVE IMMUNIZATION: Hypersensitivity reactions, including anaphylactic shock, may occur with any biological substance. They are most likely to occur in an individual allergic to products used in vaccine preparation. Live viral vaccines are much freer of these production-related allergens than killed vaccines. This is especially true of vaccines produced in tissue culture (polio vaccine). Rabies and influenza vaccines may cause severe reactions in recipients allergic to eggs. Other vaccines are quite reactogenic, in part because of the nature of the immunizing antigen; these include cholera, plague and typhus. As previously mentioned in the instance of influenza vaccine, occasionally neurologic complications follow vaccination. Rabies vaccines have been associated with numerous CNS complications, including transverse myelitis, encephalitis and the Guillain-Barre syndrome; influenza vaccine with the Guillain-Barre syndrome, measles vaccine with encephalitis and subacute sclerosing pan-encephalitis, and pertussis vaccine with encephalopathies. In most cases, the risk of these complications is minimal; however, recipients should be warned of them prior to administration. Rarely, poliomyelitis has followed administration of oral polio vaccine (approximately 1/7,000,000 vaccinees). Encephalitis has been reported to occur within 30 days following measles vaccination in 1/1,000,000 recipients as compared with 1/1,000 cases of measles. Neurologic complications following the duck embryo rabies vaccine occur in approximately 1/225, 000 vaccinees.

Live attenuated viral vaccines should not be used in immuno-compromised individuals, whether primary or induced by drugs or radiation. This includes patients with lymphomas, leukemias and other malignancies, and those treated with immuno-suppressive therapy, including steroids. If an alternate killed virus vaccine (polio or measles) is available, this should be used. Though there is no evidence that any live viral vaccine is teratogenic,these agents should not be administered during pregnancy. Though rubella infection during pregnancy may result in the congenital rubella syndrome, no cases of this syndrome have yet been reported in women who received the rubella vaccine and who went to term. The number of cases recorded to date is sufficient to state that the risk of the congenital rubella syndrome in an infant born to a susceptible mother who received the live attenuated rubella vaccine in the first trimester of pregnancy is less than five per cent. Therefore, therapeutic abortion is not recommended in the event of this occurrence. In extenuating circumstances, live viral vaccines may be given during pregnancy with precaution: smallpox vaccine may be given, if necessary, with vaccinia immune globulin to modify viral replication.

The existence of an acute febrile illness usually delays immunization; however, febrile illness is not a contraindication to immunization. If immunization is necessary, viral syndromes or the common infectious diseases should not delay vaccination. Likewise, all available data suggest that the simultaneous administration of multiple vaccines have little effect on reactogenicity or antibody response. As many as twelve antigens have been given simultaneously with no decrease in antibody response. In most cases, if vaccines are not recommended to be given concomitantly, it is best to space live viral vaccinations at least one month apart. Whenever it is not possible to observe the one-month interval, it is best to give live virus vaccines on the same day at different sites.

## PASSIVE IMMUNIZATION

Passive immunization is the parenteral administration of antibody against an infectious agent. It is necessarily of brief duration, i.e., the half-life of IgG is 23 days. As more active immunizing vaccines are developed, the importance of passive
immunization has declined. Passive immunization is used (1)
when no active immunizing agent exists; (2) post-exposure, when
there is not time for an antibody response to active immunization; (3) in combination with active immunization when immediate and prolonged protection is necessary (rabies).

In the past, all passive immunization was accomplished with
animal sera (usually equine). Now specific, high titer, homologous, immune globulin preparations of human origin are prepared by cold ethanol fractionation, and reduce the risk of anaphylactic and serum sickness reactions and hepatitis B. Such
preparations are available for rabies, varicella-zoster, hepatitis B, pertussis, vaccinia and tetanus. These preparations
cannot be given intravenously, as they may activate complement and cause fatal anaphylactic reactions. Heterologous sera
of equine origin are still used to treat diphtheria, botulism,
snake bite and spider bites (Latrodectus) (see Table 45). Other
antisera are of limited value. When heterologous sera are used,
adverse reactions are likely to occur. The two major types of
adverse reactions are anaphylaxis and serum sickness. Anaphylactic reactions occur minutes to hours after administration of sera and consist of shock, respiratory distress, and
urticaria. Serum sickness usually occurs five to ten days after
injection of sera and is characterized by rash, fever, arthralgias and vasculitis. The risk of serum sickness increases
with age; from 5% to 25% of patients will develop some degree
of serum sickness after administration of heterologous sera.
Treatment of these hypersensitivity reactions includes epinephrine, antihistamines, corticosteroids and supportive measures.

## POST-EXPOSURE RABIES PROPHYLAXIS

There are approximately 500,000 animal bites annually in the
United States. Very few of these present a risk of rabies. Currently there is only one accepted regimen of post-exposure
rabies prophylaxis, which entails the use of human rabies immune globulin and duck embryo vaccine (Table 46). Prior to
utilization of this regimen, it is necessary to determine if a
given exposure presents a risk of rabies. Domestic animal
rabies is now extremely unusual in the United States. Only
unprovoked domestic animal bites should be considered a

TABLE 46: POST-EXPOSURE RABIES PROPHYLAXIS GUIDE

| ANIMAL AND ITS CONDITION | | TREATMENT | |
|---|---|---|---|
| Species | Condition | Bite | Non-bite |
| **Wild** Skunk | Escaped | S+V[1] | S+V |
| Fox | Killed and Brain FRA Neg | none | none |
| Raccoon Bat | Killed and Brain FRA Pos | S+V | S+V |
| **Domestic** Dog Cat | Provoked - Healthy | none | none |
| | Unprovoked - captured | none[2] | none[2] |
| | Unprovoked - escaped | S+V | S+V |
| Other | Consider Individually | | |

[1]S+V: Human Rabies Immune Globulin: 20 IU/kg. IM Duck Embryo Vaccine, 23 one cc. S.C. doses: two doses daily for seven days, then one dose daily for seven days, followed by boosters ten and twenty days later. Serum rabies titer should be checked at end of therapy to confirm presence of protective antibody.

[2]If severe bites of head, animal should be sacrificed and brain examined for presence of rabies antigen. For other unprovoked bites, animal should be observed for ten days, and if unusual behavior develops, it should be sacrificed and brain examined. If FRA positive, S+V should be started immediately.

possible rabies exposure. If the animal can be observed for ten days and exhibits no unusual behavior, rabies prophylaxis is not necessary; if the animal has escaped, prophylaxis may be indicated. At present, New York and Philadelphia are considered domestic animal rabies-free, and bites in these geographical areas are considered possible rabies exposures only under the most unusual circumstances.

Foxes, bats, raccoons and skunks are the wild animals that present the greatest risk of rabies. In the event of bites by these animals, post-exposure prophylaxis should be undertaken immediately, unless the animal is captured, sacrificed, and its brain is negative for rabies virus by the fluorescent rabies antibody (FRA) technique. Rabies is almost non existent in rodents and lagomorphs (i. e. rats, mice, rabbits, squirrels), and bites of these animals can usually be considered to present no risk of rabies. Treatment of all other wild animal bites should be individualized, depending upon the circumstances of the bites and the prevalence of rabies in the geographic area.

## REFERENCES

1. Report of the Committee on Infectious Diseases. American Academy of Pediatrics, Evanston, Illinois, 1974.

2. Collected Recommendations of the Public Health Service Advisory Committee on Immunization Practices. Morbidity and Mortality Weekly Report 21: Dec. , 1972.

SECTION M: MISCELLANEOUS CATEGORIES

110: GRAM-NEGATIVE ROD BACTEREMIA
AND SEPTIC SHOCK
by H. Thadepalli

Nearly 71,000 to 142,000 cases of gram-negative rod bacteremia occur in the United States and nearly 25% die as a
direct result of this infection each year.[1]  Introduction of
"broad spectrum" antibiotics coincided with this increased
incidence of gram-negative rod bacteremia.

## CLINICAL FEATURES

First described in detail by Waisbren,[2] classically, the syndrome consists of an elderly patient who appears otherwise
well, has a fever of 105°F. , and has no recordable blood pressure due to gram-negative bacteremia. Most patients we see
today vary greatly in their presentation from this classic
description.

1) Fever and chills: Fever is almost universal in gram-negative rod (GNR) bacteremia, although it may be minimal
   in some patients, more so if they are on steroids. Frequently,
   fever may be the only sign of GNR bacteremia. On rare
   occasions, hypothermia may be the presenting feature of
   gram-negative sepsis.

2) Hypotension: This occurs within 40 to 60 hours after the
   onset of fever. Significant lowering of blood pressure occurs in 40% of patients with GNR bacteremia. Septic shock
   in the hospital is as frequent as cardiogenic shock and more
   frequent than posthemorrhage shock.[3] Shock should be considered as an integral part of sepsis and treated as such.

3) Pulmonary manifestations, such as hyperpnea and tachypnea or respiratory alkalosis in the absence of pulmonary
   abnormalities, may be the initial manifestations of bacteremia. Later, the chest roentgenogram may show infiltrates

703

resembling bacterial pneumonia. These are more frequent
in cases of GNR sepsis arising from below the diaphragm.
Metabolic acidosis secondary to tissue anoxia may be found
later. In some patients, unexplained tachypnea may be the
subtle manifestation of GNR bacteremia.

4) Oliguria or anuria without a cause, especially among the
elderly, may indicate GNR bacteremia. Often it is secondary to "septic shock", a form of pre-renal azotemia. Bacteremia is not always essential. Abscesses alone can cause
glomerular failure,[4] a reversible process if recognized
and promptly treated.

5) Coagulation abnormalities: Thrombocytopenia is the most
frequent (50% to 60%) of all hematologic manifestations in
GNR bacteremia. Disseminated intravascular coagulation
(DIC) may occur frequently. DIC rarely occurs in patients who are not in shock (except meningococcal septicemia). DIC may cause extensive hemorrhages and, therefore, a shocklike state.

6) Mental changes: Unusual drowsiness, apathy, listlessness,
incoherence in thought and action and, infrequently, even
delirium and coma may supervene. Some patients may remain surprisingly alert to the end. Unexplained mental
changes in an elderly nursing home case or hospitalized patient should lead to the suspicion of septicemia (bacteremia).

7) Evidences for predisposing causes: A thoughtful history
and physical often may yield clues to the possible source
of sepsis (see Table 47).

8) Microbiology: The type of offending agent depends on the
source of underlying infections. It also depends on whether
or not the patient was on antimicrobial agents before. Sub-
inhibitory serum levels of antibiotics may lead to periodic
bacteremia, called "break-through" bacteremia. See Table
48 for the list of the etiologic agents in gram-negative bacteremia. Prior antimicrobial therapy may cause a shift
from the relatively benign to the malignant flora. More
often than not, the causative agent may be susceptible to
the antibiotic the patient is already on.

Most of the GNR that affect these patients are their own
organisms, with the exception of Pseudomonas, which is
a true nosocomial infection. Staphylococcus aureus, the
scourge of the fifties, has vacated its place, occupied today

## TABLE 47: PREDISPOSING CAUSES FOR SEPTIC SHOCK*

| SITE OF ORIGIN | PREDISPOSING CAUSE | MOST LIKELY CAUSATIVE AGENT(S) |
|---|---|---|
| Genitourinary[5] | Instrumentation of infected urinary tract, obstruction due to stones, tumor or stric- ture, catheterization | E. coli <u>Klebsiella</u> Erterobacter Serratia Proteus S. aureus <u>Pseudomonas</u> |
| Gastrointestinal | Surgery, trauma, abscess, appendicitis, diverticulitis, perforation, peritonitis | As above and anaerobes, especially Bacteroides |
| Biliary Tract | Cholelithiasis, cholecystitis, surgery of the biliary tract | E. coli <u>Klebsiella</u> Salmonella Enterococcus |
| Liver | Cirrhosis and liver abscess, tumor, trauma | Anaerobic cocci are common in liver abscess; both aerobes and anaerobes in cirrhosis |
| Reproductive System | Septic abortion, pelvic inflammation, pelvic abscess, surgery, fetal monitoring, pro- longed labor | Anaerobic organisms are more fre- quent than aerobes Enterococcus |

(Cont'd)

## TABLE 47 (CONT'D)

| SITE OF ORIGIN | PREDISPOSING CAUSE | MOST LIKELY CAUSATIVE AGENT(S) |
|---|---|---|
| Respiratory Tract | | |
| Upper | Tracheostomy<br>Bronchoscopy | Pseudomonas<br>Klebsiella, Serratia |
| Lower | Pneumonia<br>Lung abscess<br>Empyema | Pneumococcus, S. aureus<br>Bacteroides<br>Clostridia |
| Meninges | Meningitis | Pneumococcus<br>N. meningitidis<br>H. influenzae (in children only) |
| Intravascular | Intravenous catheters, pacemakers, prosthetic valves | S. aureus<br>Klebsiella, Serratia<br>Pseudomonas<br>Streptococcus, yeast |
| Skin and Soft Tissue | Abscess, cellulitis | S. aureus, Streptococcus, Clostridia<br>Anaerobic cocci |
| | Burns<br>Decubitus ulcers[6] with or without underlying osteomyelitis | Pseudomonas<br>Proteus, Bacteroides, anaerobic cocci |

| Malignancy | Leukemia, cancer, multiple myeloma, perirectal abscess | S. aureus<br>Pseudomonas<br>Klebsiella<br>E. coli<br>Yeast<br>Aspergillus<br>Anaerobes |
|---|---|---|
| Ear | Otitis media | Streptococcus, H. influenzae, S. aureus |
| Nose | Sinusitis | α Streptococcus, anaerobes |
| Throat | Retropharyngeal abscess<br>Stomatitis<br>Tonsillitis | Streptococcus<br>S. aureus<br>Pneumococcus |
| Undetermined Origin | Nosocomial from I.V. fluids, tablets and other environs | Klebsiella, Pseudomonas, Candida and other fungi |

*This is by no means a complete list, and the prevalence of a given organism need not necessarily be in the order given and may vary from one hospital to another.

by a host of gram-negative organisms. See Table 48 for the relative frequency of the etiologic agents in GNR bacteremia.

TABLE 48: ETIOLOGIC AGENTS IN
GRAM-NEGATIVE BACTEREMIA

| ORGANISM* | TOTAL | PER CENT |
|-----------|-------|----------|
| Escherichia coli | 183 | 43. 6 |
| Klebsiella | 51 | 12. 2 |
| Pseudomonas | 43 | 10. 3 |
| Bacteroidaceae | 37 | 9. 0 |
| Enterobacter | 35 | 8. 4 |
| Proteus | 23 | 5. 5 |
| Serratia | 20 | 4. 8 |
| Haemophilus | 12 | |
| Citrobacter | 4 | |
| Providencia | 4 | |
| Salmonella | 3 | |
| Veillonella | 2 | 6. 7 |
| Shigella | 1 | |
| Pasteurella | 1 | |
| Acinetobacter | 1 | |
| | 420 | |

* Above results were derived from 16,242 blood specimens submitted for culture. [5]

Escherichia coli is by far the most frequent cause of gram-negative bacteremia, followed by Klebsiella.

It is not essential that the "septic shock" should be produced always by GNR. Gram-positive organisms, even viruses and fungi, may also produce similar illness. I have seen patients with miliary tuberculosis, without other associated bacterial infections, present with this syndrome.

9) Ecthyma gangrenosum, the punched-out, scattered, gangrenous lesions, can occur with septicemia due to Pseudomonas aeruginosa (Fig. 129).

### DIAGNOSIS

The diagnosis of GNR bacteremia should be made when the previously mentioned clinical features are encountered, either by themselves or in combination. Therapy should be promptly

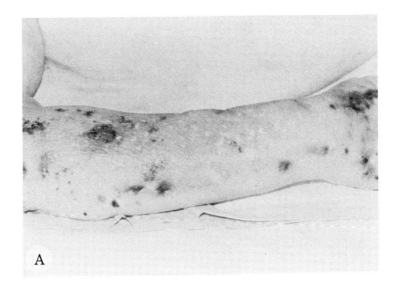

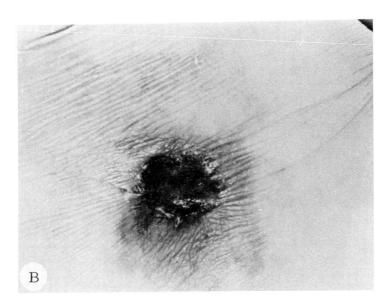

FIG. 129: (A) Ecthyma gangrenosum in a patient with Pseudomonas septicemia (B) Close-up of such a lesion.

instituted in this otherwise fatal disease. The following diagnostic procedures can be used to confirm the clinical suspicion:

1) Blood cultures: A positive blood culture is imperative to
   prove the diagnosis, but it should be remembered that cultures may be negative in cases otherwise typical of "septic shock", because endotoxemia alone can produce a clinical syndrome indistinguishable from GNR bacteremia. Remember the "rules of three" - if three separate blood cultures are drawn and more than three days have elapsed
   since the last culture, it is less likely that bacteremia can
   be documented.[5] Refer to Chapter 36 on Infective Endocarditis for details on the techniques for blood culture.

2) Nitroblue tetrazolium test (NBT): In normal people, a certain percentage of the polymorphonuclear leukocytes reduce
   the colorless nitroblue tetrazolium to formazan, which appears as a dark blue globule within the cell's cytoplasm.[7]
   When infection occurs, there is an increase in the number
   of positive cells. The NBT test can be negative in one-half
   of the cases, despite the presence of bacteremia.[8] Several
   other reports[9] also indicate that the NBT test can be misleading. Basic hematologic data, such as increased total
   white cell and polymorphonuclear cell counts with a shift to
   the left, presence of toxic granulation, Dohle bodies and
   vacuolization of the neutrophils, can in fact, yield far more
   dependable results than the NBT test.[7] The NBT test was
   found to be positive in non-infectious disorders as well.[10,11]
   Conflicting data on NBT tests suggest that it is of little diagnostic value.

3) Limulus lysate test: The limulus test is based on the reaction of lysates derived from blood cells (amoebocytes)
   of the horseshoe crab (limulus) with endotoxin, and can detect as little as $0.0005 \mu g/ml$. of endotoxin.[12] It is controversial, however, whether the limulus lysate test of the
   blood can accurately predict the presence of endotoxin and
   gram-negative rod bacteremia. In three separate studies
   evaluating the limulus test as a diagnostic tool for gram-
   negative sepsis, one group found that it was not only specific[13]
   for the diagnosis of gram-negative sepsis, but also a good
   indicator of prognosis - a positive test indicated poor prognosis. Other investigators doubted the value of this test[14,15,16]
   because there were too many false-positive and false-
   negative results. It was later confirmed that the limulus test
   per se had no clinical usefulness in the detection of endotoxemia or gram-negative septicemia.[17]

However, the limulus test appears to be of diagnostic value to detect gram-negative meningitis in children due to H. influenzae and Neisseria meningitidis.[18] It was found to be useful as a rapid bedside diagnostic test to detect gram-negative meningitis within one hour after performing the lumbar puncture[19] (see Chapter 30 on Meningitis). When the urine was tested with limulus lysate, it was found to be useful in the detection of urinary tract infection due to gram-negative bacilli.[20] It was claimed to be specific because all urine samples containing $> 10^5$ GNR/ml. gave positive results. Excellent correlation was noted between positive limulus test of the synovial fluid and arthritis due to GNR.[21] The value of the limulus test in the detection of urinary tract infections and synovitis due to GNR has not been fully verified.

Certain antibiotics, like polymyxin B and semi-synthetic penicillins can exhibit the limulus lysate assay for endotoxin.[22]

The limulus lysate test is of limited value as a diagnostic tool for GNR bacteremia. It is extremely useful in the diagnosis of gram-negative meningitis in children when the Gram's stain preparations of CSF are negative.

## TREATMENT

The most important rule is that the clinician should first consider the source of sepsis and suspect certain potential pathogens, before choosing therapy to "cover" them. Irrational selection of antibiotics in fixed doses and combinations is discouraged. An "intelligent and educated guess", based on the source of infection, the flora indigenous to the hospital and the antimicrobial susceptibility patterns of the local hospital flora, should be the considerations for selecting the antibiotic regimen. One should also consider if the chosen antibiotic is safe and effective at the site of infection in a given patient. Following is a brief outline of certain steps to be considered during the evaluation of the septic patient:

1) Remove all intra-caths, indwelling Foley's catheters, and any other foreign body likely to be the source for sepsis.

2) Identify the source of infection.

3) "Guess" the most likely causative agent based on previously obtained culture results (if available) and also by the site of infection. Consider the following:

   (a) Consider the likely pathogen (Table 47) based on the source of sepsis.
   (b) Previous antibiotic therapy may change the flora.
   (c) If the patient with a Foley's catheter had Klebsiella in a recent urine culture, it is likely that Klebsiella would be the cause for sepsis.
   (d) Undrained abscess may cause persistent bacteremic infection in spite of appropriate therapy.

4) Consider the nature of the "host". If the patient has leukemia or other forms of malignancy, one may expect infection due to practically "anything".

5) Antibiotic therapy: Selection of the antibiotic should be based on the following considerations:

   (a) It should be generally known to be effective against the suspected bacteria in that hospital. For instance, if the Pseudomonas strains are resistant to a compound "X", an alternative antibiotic should be chosen when infection due to this organism is suspected.

   (b) Therapy should be promptly instituted pending culture results and antimicrobial susceptibility patterns.

   (c) To be effective, antibiotic should be available in sufficient concentration at the site of infection. Penicillins and cephalosporins are preferred for urinary tract infections. Intravenous aminoglycosides are generally ineffective against gram-negative meningitis when intrathecal therapy is required.

   (d) Aggressive, early use of antibiotics is crucial to achieve success, especially in leukopenic patients with fever.

   (e) A single effective antibiotic is preferable to a double or triple antibiotic regimen. Some would question the wisdom of and the need for, using more than two antibiotics at a time. Combined chemotherapy, contrary to what may seem to be "synergistic", may in a real patient at best yield only "additive" if not "indifferent" chemotherapeutic effect. In other than leukopenic patients, routine usage of multiple antibiotics is unnecessary.

(f) To monitor the efficacy of any antibiotic, serum antibiotic levels should be monitored and the in vitro susceptibility data examined. This data is valuable in the management of the patient and in adjusting the antibiotic dosage.

6) If there are any abscesses, they should be drained.

7) Symptomatic therapy to raise the blood pressure to monitor the "shock state" is also important. The role of steroids is a matter of great controversy.

## REFERENCES

1. Wolff, S. M. , Bennett, J. V. : Gram-negative rod bacteremia (Editorial). New Eng. J. Med. 291:733, 1974.

2. Waisbren, B. A. : Bacteremia due to gram-negative bacilli other than the Salmonella. A clinical and therapeutic study. Arch. Intern. Med. 88:467, 1951.

3. McCabe, W. R. : Gram-negative bacteremia. Disease a Month, (Ed. ), H. F. Dowling. Year Book Med. Pub. , Chicago, December, 1973.

4. Beaufils, M. , et al. : Acute renal failure of glomerular origin during visceral abscesses. New Eng. J. Med. 295:185, 1976.

5. Young, L. S. , et al. : Gram-negative rod bacteremia. Microbiologic, immunologic and therapeutic considerations. Ann. Int. Med. 86:456, 1977.

6. Galpin, J. E. , et al. : Sepsis associated with decubitus ulcers. Am. J. Med. 61:346, 1976.

7. Matula, G. , Paterson, P. Y. : Spontaneous in vitro reduction of nitroblue tetrazolium by neutrophils of adult patients with bacterial infection. New Eng. J. Med. 285:311, 1971.

8. Steigbigel, R. T. , Johnson, P. K. , Remington, J. S. : The nitroblue tetrazolium reduction test versus conventional hematology in the diagnosis of bacterial infection. New Eng. J. Med. 290:235, 1974.

9. Soonattrakul, W. , Anderson, B. R. : Diagnostic accuracy of the nitroblue tetrazolium test. Arch. Int. Med. 132: 529, 1973.

10. Lauter, C. B. , et al. : The nitroblue tetrazolium test and acute myocardial infarction. Ann. Int. Med. 79:59, 1973.

11. Chang, J. C. , Appleby, J. , Bennett, J. M. : Nitroblue tetrazolium test in Hodgkin's disease and other malignant lymphomas. Arch. Int. Med. 133:401, 1974.

12. Levin, J. , Tomasulo, P. A. , Oser, R. S. : Detection of endotoxin in human blood and demonstration of an inhibition. J. Lab. Clin. Med. 75:903, 1970.

13. Levin, J. , et al. : Gram-negative sepsis: Detection of endotoxemia with the limulus test. Ann. Int. Med. 76:1, 1972.

14. Martinez, G. L. A. , Quintiliani, R. , Tilton, R. C. : Clinical experience on the detection of endotoxaemia with the limulus test. J. Inf. Dis. 127:102, 1973.

15. Stumacher, R. J. , Kovnat, M. J. , McCabe, W. R. : Limitation of the usefulness of the limulus lysate assay for endotoxin. New Eng. J. Med. 288:1261, 1973.

16. Feldman, S. , Pearson, T. A. : The limulus test and gram-negative bacillary sepsis. Arch. J. Dis. Child. 128:172, 1974.

17. Elin, R. J. , et al. : Lack of clinical usefulness of the limulus test in the diagnosis of endotoxaemia. New Eng. J. Med. 293:521, 1975.

18. Nachum, R. , Lipsfy, A. , Siegel, S. E. : Rapid detection of bacterial meningitis by the limulus lysate test. New Eng. J. Med. 289:931, 1973.

19. Ross, S. , et al. : Limulus lysate test for gram-negative bacterial meningitis - Bedside application. J. A. M. A. 233: 1366, 1975.

20. Jorgensen, J. H. , Jones, P. M. : Comparative evaluation of limulus assays and the direct gram stain for detection of significant bacteriuria. Am. J. Clin. Path. 63:142, 1975.

21. Tuazon, C. U. , et al. : Detection of endotoxin in cerebrospinal and joint fluids by limulus assay. Arch. Int. Med. 137:55, 1977.

22. McCullough, K. Z. , Scolnick, S. A. : Effect of semisynthetic penicillins on the limulus lysate test. Antimicrob. Agents. Chemother. 9:856, 1976.

## 111: DISSEMINATED INTRAVASCULAR COAGULATION (DIC)
by H. Thadepalli

"Consumption Coagulopathy"

DIC is an acquired progressive hypercoagulable state due to augmentation of hemostatic mechanisms, triggered by a procoagulant stimulus leading to deposition of stable fibrin clots throughout the microcirculation. It is then followed by plasminolytic clot digestion and by the release of the fibrin split products into the circulation. Hemorrhage and tissue necrosis are the two outstanding clinical features of this disease. Paradoxical as it is, the anticoagulant, heparin, is the treatment of choice. Generally, DIC, is not a disease; but it is a complication of another disease.

### CLINICAL FEATURES

Fever, tachycardia and tachypnea are the most frequent signs. Bleeding tendencies are present and may be manifested by petechiae, purpura or blotchy hemorrhagic patches over the skin. Gangrenous lesions of the skin; fingers and toes; or ears, nose or lips, can occur along with the hemorrhagic lesions (Fig. 130). Slight icterus may be present, but pronounced jaundice due to DIC is rare. Vaginal bleeding, hematemesis, melena or passing fresh blood in the stool may occur with or without external signs of bleeding. Other clinical signs are those of the underlying disease, but are not specific for DIC. Vaginal bleeding may follow an obstetric or gynecologic disease. It may occasionally occur spontaneously in acute viral infections, such as hemorrhagic chickenpox and smallpox. The patient may have hemoptysis and signs of pulmonary edema. Of 120 consecutive cases of DIC in one study,[1] 76% had shock and 73% had hemorrhagic lesions. Depressed mental state is common. On occasion, coma and seizures can occur due to lesions of the nervous system. Hypotension may lead to oliguria and azotemia.

### DIAGNOSIS

1) Peripheral blood smear: The peripheral blood smear may show fragmented erythrocytes, due to forced filtration of the red cells through fibrin strands (Fig. 131).

2) Hemolysis: Microangiopathic hemolytic anemia is common. Indirect bilirubin may be increased. The LDH levels and the haptoglobin levels may be increased.

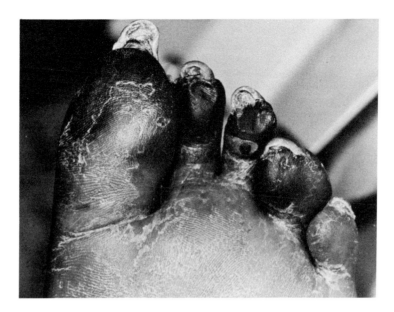

FIG. 130: Gangrene of the toes in a patient with gram-negative sepsis and disseminated intravascular coagulation (DIC).

3) The platelet count is decreased (generally less than 2,500/
cu. mm. ). In cases of infection due to gram-negative bacilli, the platelet count decreases before a demonstrable decrease can be shown in the plasma clotting factors. In infections due to gram-positive cocci, viruses and Rickettsia,
both platelet count and clotting factors are decreased simultaneously (Table 49). [2] The platelet survival time is also
decreased in DIC. When DIC is suspected and the platelet
count is within normal limits, it should be repeated four
hours later, because a precipitous drop may be observed
later.

4) Prothrombin time, partial thromboplastin time and thrombin generation time are prolonged, due to depletion of factors I, V, VII, IX and XI.

5) Fibrinogen: The fibrinogen levels are either normal or decreased. At the end stage of the disease when shock is imminent or already present, the fibrinogen level may be as
low as 100 mg. %.

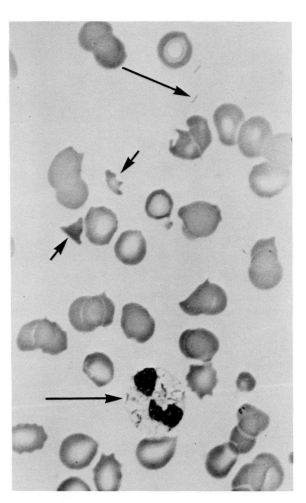

FIG. 131: Peripheral blood smear showing fragmented red blood corpuscles (short arrows) and several intraleukocytic and free gram-negative bacilli (long arrows) in a fatal case of disseminated intravascular coagulation and renal microangiopathic (hemolytic-uremic) syndrome. Patient was bitten by a dog three days prior to admission. The blood cultures grew Bacteroides. (Courtesy of Harry M. Bauer, M.D., Clinical Associate Professor of Pathology, University of Southern California, Los Angeles).

TABLE 49: INFECTIOUS AGENTS THAT MAY CAUSE DIC

A. BACTERIA:

    1) Streptococcus (Groups A & B)
    2) Staphylococcus aureus
    3) Pneumococcus
    4) Neisseria (N.) meningitidis
       (Waterhouse-Friderichsen syndrome)
    5) Clostridium perfringens (welchii)
    6) Escherichia coli
    7) Pseudomonas aeruginosa
    8) Mycobacterium tuberculosis
    9) Other gram-positive and gram-negative organisms

B. VIRUS:

    1) Herpes simplex
    2) Varicella zoster
    3) Smallpox
    4) Hemorrhagic fevers
    5) Cytomegalovirus

C. RICKETTSIA:

    1) Rocky Mountain spotted fever

D. FUNGUS:

    1) Aspergillus
    2) Histoplasma

E. PARASITIC:

    1) Malaria
    2) Kala-azar
    3) Trypanosomiasis

F. MISCELLANEOUS

    1) Purpura fulminans

G. NON-INFECTIOUS CAUSES THAT MIMIC INFECTIOUS DISEASES:

    1) Snake bite*
    2) Heat stroke

* Rattlesnake bite can cause DIC. [4] Snake venom is now being tested in the treatment of DIC.

6) Fibrin split products (FSP): FSP are usually present in DIC. Several tests are being used for detecting FSP:

    (a) Staphylococcal clumping test using lyophilized bacteria is easy to do, but commercial reagents have variable potency and reliability. [3]

    (b) Tanned erythrocyte hemagglutination inhibition test is time-consuming and technically difficult.

    (c) Agglutination of latex particles, coated with specific antibody to fibrinogen degradation products, is a simple and reliable method for the detection of fibrinogen degradation products in DIC.

    (d) Ethanol gelation test, and

    (e) Serial dilution of protamine sulfate test (SDPS test): Fibrin split products clot in the presence of ethanol or protamine sulfate. Positive gelation occurs in DIC but not in primary fibrinolysis. A negative ethanol gelation test, or SDPS, does not rule out DIC.

### DIFFERENTIAL DIAGNOSIS

Table 50 shows the differentiating features of DIC from other conditions:

1) Primary fibrinolysis may occur due to metastatic prostatic carcinoma.

2) Liver disease: Heparin corrects most of the clotting abnormalities in DIC but not in liver disease. The effect of heparin, used to observe this differentiation, if necessary, can be quickly corrected by protamine sulfate.

3) Obstetric problems: Heparin and epsilon amino caproic acid (EACA) will usually raise the fibrinogen levels to greater than 100 mg. %.

4) DIC should also be differentiated from thrombotic thrombocytopenic purpura (TTP). In TTP, neurological manifestations are common (92%).

5) DIC should be differentiated from hemolytic uremic syndrome, which usually occurs during the first year of life. It is rarely a disease of the adult. The blood smear appearance in a rare case of hemolytic uremic syndrome that

TABLE 50: COAGULATION TEST PROFILES OF DIC WITH INFECTION AND WITH
PRIMARY AND SECONDARY FIBRINOLYSIS

| Coagulation Test (Normal Value) | DIC Due to Infection | Amniotic Fluid Embolism | Primary Fibrinolysis Due to Metastatic Prostatic Carcinoma |
|---|---|---|---|
| Platelet count 150,000 - 350,000/cu. mm. | Low 2,500 | Low 13,000 | Normal 195,000 |
| Activated partial thromboplastin time: < 45 sec. | Prolonged 101 sec. | Prolonged 88 sec. | Normal to slightly prolonged 46 sec. |
| Prothrombin time 13 sec. | Prolonged 28 sec. | Prolonged 51 sec. | Normal to slightly prolonged 22 sec. |
| Fibrinogen 150 - 350 mg. % | Normal to very low 316 mg. % | Very low 25 mg. % | Very low 21 mg. % |
| Ethanol gelation/SDPS (Negative/Negative) | Positive/Positive | Positive/Positive | Negative/Negative |
| Bedside clot observation Stable | Stable | Stable | Lysed |
| Euglobulin clot lysis > 6 hr. | > 2 | > 2 | < 2 |

occurred in an adult following Bacteroides septicemia secondary to dog bite is shown in Fig. 131.

6) "Pseudo-DIC" is caused by repeated heparin administration used to prevent clotting of blood in the indwelling catheters.

## REFERENCES

1.  Larcan, A. , et al. : Les coagulopathies aigues de consommation: 120 observations. La Nouvelle Presse Medicale 2: 2771, 1976.

2.  Pierce, L. E. : Disseminated intravascular coagulation. Amer. Family Phys. 7:118, 1973.

3.  Carvalho, A. C. A. , Ellman, L. L. , Colman, R. W. : A comparison of the staphylococcal clumping test and agglutination test for detection of fibrinogen degradation products. Amer. J. Clin. Path. 62:107, 1974.

4.  Raby, C. , Franc, B. , Mugneret, P. : Coagulopathie de consommation aigue apres morgure de crotalidae. La Nouvelle Presse Medicale 2:2949, 1973.

112:  INFECTIONS IN THE COMPROMISED HOST
by H. Thadepalli


Improved survival in patients with leukemia, Hodgkin's disease, and carcinoma has increased the incidence of opportunistic infections. Various mechanisms have been implicated for the causation of sepsis in such patients. Myeloperoxidase deficiency, G-6-PD deficiency, Chediak-Higashi syndrome, lazy leukocyte syndrome, Wiscott-Aldrich syndrome and complement C-3 deficiency, etc. are some such examples.

## DIABETES MELLITUS

Diabetes mellitus is a common compromising disease state. Not all diabetics are prone to infection, but those who are older than 45 years with undiagnosed diabetes are the most prone. Nearly 80% of them present with infection. Nearly 50% of insulin-dependent patients tend to develop serious infections within five years. The most common offending pathogen is Staphylococcus aureus, presenting either in the form of a boil or carbuncle, pneumonia, or even septicemia. Escherichia (E.) coli and Mycobacterium tuberculosis are the next most frequent offending pathogens. It is not proven that diabetics have an increased incidence of tuberculosis, but very severe infections of tuberculosis do occur among diabetics.

Escherichia coli is the most common cause of gas gangrene in diabetes mellitus. Sometimes, the gaseous cellulitis can be very extensive and spread to the scrotum, pelvis and abdominal cavity. It can cause gaseous cellulitis of the urinary tract (see Fig. 58).

Mental disturbances, stupor, coma and seizures in cases of diabetes mellitus should make one suspect the possibility of cryptococcal meningitis, even if the patient is afebrile.

## LEUKEMIA

Infection is the most common cause of undiagnosed fever in leukemia. When the total neutrophil cell count falls to 500 or less, leukemics are at risk to develop infections. In acute leukemia, when the leucocyte count falls below 1,000, 50% develop infections. Below 100 leucocytes/cu. mm., nearly all of them develop infections, of which nearly 28% can be fatal. When the leucocyte count is maintained at 2,000 cells/cu. mm. or above, only 2% develop infections.[1]

Anorectal infections are frequent in acute leukemia. Twenty-five per cent of all patients with acute leukemia develop rectal abscess. [2] Nearly 60% of monocytic leukemia patients have a tendency to develop perianal infections. I saw two such patients who were admitted to the surgical wards for drainage of rectal abscess. They were later diagnosed to have monocytic leukemia. Perianal infections occur more frequently in monocytic leukemia than myelomonocytic, myelogenous or lymphoblastic leukemia. They occur with greatest frequency when the cell count is less than 500/cu. mm. Staphylococcus aureus used to be the most frequent offender, followed by Pseudomonas. Pseudomonas aeruginosa is the most frequent isolate in such patients today. The majority of these infections can be managed with the currently available antibiotics, but they are occasionally terminal.

Until 1940, Candida infections were noted in less than 3% of the patients, but after the introduction of broad-spectrum antibiotics, the incidence has increased to 30%. Aspergillus fumigatus septicemia is now being increasingly reported as a final fatal infectious complication in immunologically compromised patients. In most instances, it is diagnosed at autopsy.[3]

Cytomegalovirus infection is perhaps the most common viral infection associated with leukemia today.

### RENAL TRANSPLANT

Staphylococcus aureus infections are the most common; however, if the patient was treated with anti-staphylococcal agents, gram-negative infections due to E. coli and Pseudomonas dominate. Pneumocystis carinii infections are also common in the renal transplant patients. Other frequently associated infections in transplant recipients include herpes simplex infections and Cytomegalovirus infections. These infections do not appear to be related to the presence of immunoglobulins in the serum. Paradoxically, it appears that if infection precedes the rejection of the transplant, it is fatal in nearly 60% of the patients; in contrast, there were no deaths when infection followed the rejection. Some of these infections will be discussed later.

### HODGKIN'S DISEASE

Hodgkin's disease patients are prone to develop a complex disarray of infections due to T-cell dysfunction and defective phagocytosis. Characteristically, intracellular infections, such as tuberculosis, Listeria, toxoplasmosis and herpes zoster (Fig. 132) are more common with Hodgkin's disease.

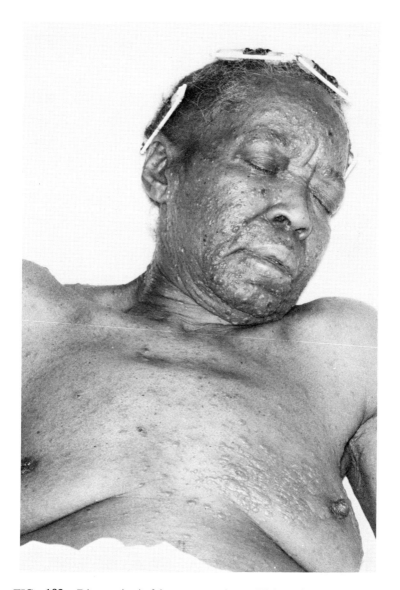

FIG. 132: Disseminated herpes zoster. This patinet had splenectomy done for staging of Hodgkin's disease. She
was admitted for zoster lesion on the chest and later
developed disseminated zoster.

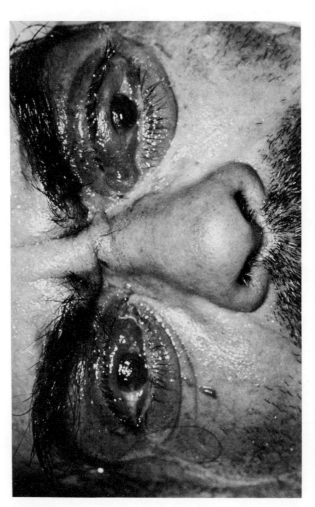

FIG. 133: A case of thyroid storm with <u>Bacteroides fragilis</u> septicemia. He was admitted with fever and conjunctival edema. He was taking penicillin eye drops. Thyroid was not palpable. Several hours later, he developed fever (105°F.) without chills and shock. He was suspected to have gram-negative sepsis, which he indeed had, but the underlying cause, thyrotoxicosis, was initially missed.

Splenectomy is often done for staging the Hodgkin's disease patients, who may also be prone to infections of varying types Recognizing the possible sources of serious infections in Hodgkin's disease patients, one wonders if three more commandments should be added to the usual ten commendments for patients with Hodgkin's disease:

Thou shalt feed no pigeons lest thou might cough up Cryptococcus or mellow with Cryptococcal meningitis.

Rear not the cats, lest thou be taxed with Toxoplasma.

Thou shalt not pet any dogs, for they are impure to thee with toxocariasis.

SICKLE CELL DISEASE: See page 521

## MALNUTRITION

Intracellular infections, like miliary tuberculosis, herpes simplex and zoster infections are more common in patients suffering from malnutrition then in the normal population. They is not due to iron deficiency, because there is ample evidence that iron deficiency may, in fact, protect one from developing infection. [4] It does not appear to be due to hypoproteinemia, either.

## INFECTIONS OF THE CENTRAL NERVOUS SYSTEM

Of 104 consecutive cases studied at Sloan Kettering Institute in New York, [5] Cryptococcus was the most common pathogen found in central nervous system infections, affecting nearly one-fourth of the patients. It does not necessarily mean that this would be true for all cancer patients all over the world. Each hospital must develop its own epidemiologic patterns to recognize the chances of incidence. Among bacterial infections, the most common is Listeria monocytogenes. Both Cryptococcus and Listeria more frequently affect the lymphoma patients than other cancer patients. In countries where antibiotics are not widely used, pneumococcus and Staphylococcus aureus might be the most predominant. In all instances of suspected cases of compromised host, the cerebrospinal fluid should be examined with India ink for Cryptococcus. It should also be gram-stained for Listeria.

## PNEUMONIA

Infections associated with malignancy of the genitourinary and gastrointestinal tract may result in pneumonia in nearly 50% of the patients and septicemia in the remaining 50%. In malignancies above the diaphragm, pneumonia is the most common infection in 80% and septicemia in 20%. The most common causes of such pneumonias are Staphylococcus aureus, Escherichia coli, Pseudomonas aeruginosa and anaerobic infections, including Bacteroides.

Bizarre and totally unexpected clinical situations can occur because of sepsis in a compromised host. Often they present because of sepsis, thus favoring the detection of the underlying disease. Fig. 133 illustrates one such example.

## REFERENCES

1. Bodey, G. P.: Infections in cancer patients. Cancer Treatment Reviews 2:89, 1975.

2. Schimff, S. C., Wiernik, P. H., Block, J. B.: Rectal abscess in cancer patients. Lancet 2:844, 1972.

3. Young, R. C., et al.: Fungaemia with compromised host resistance. Ann. Int. Med. 80:605, 1974.

4. Weinberg, E. D.: Iron and susceptibility to infectious disease. Science 184:952, 1974.

5. Singer, C., Kaplan, M. H., Armstrong, D.: Bacteremia and fungaemia complicating neoplastic disease. Am. J. Med. 62:731, 1977.

## 113: FEVER OF UNDETERMINED ORIGIN (FUO)
by H. Thadepalli

Most self-limiting fevers of short duration remain either undiagnosed, or, at best, blamed on a "virus", which perhaps
is more sinned against than sinning. Be that as it may, the
fevers that last for weeks and months are more worrisome to
the clinician; and the troubled patient is the subject of multiple
consultations, until the fever either subsides or its cause is
determined. Incomplete history and physical examination are
the major causes for the so-called FUO. Faulty data collection
further compounds the faulty initial impressions. Nearly 10%
to 20% of fevers still remain undiagnosed, in spite of a match-
less and keen systematic approach characteristic of Sherlock
Holmes.

CRITERIA FOR FUO:[1]

1) Illness of more than three weeks' duration
2) Fever higher than 101°F. on several occasions
3) Diagnosis uncertain after one week of study in the
   hospital

The above criteria are by no means rigid. Some hospitals may
need more than a week to do initial routine tests that can be done
in one day at another hospital. It has been our experience with
the indigent patients that even temperatures less than 101°F.
need to be investigated, for most of them have low-grade fevers
even when they have serious infections.

FUO is not a diagnostic entity; it simply means that the physician
has not yet diagnosed the fever. FUOs are not fevers due to
some rare and unusual causes; they are mostly misdiagnosed
but common infections, often prematurely treated; or sometimes
a common disease occurring in an uncommon geographical
location. For instance, tuberculosis, malaria, typhoid fever,
pyelonephritis, and liver and biliary tract infections are by
no means uncommon, yet they form the bulk of the cases of
FUO.

During the past seven years, I was consulted on nearly 2,300
patients suspected of having infections, of which the first 200
that fit the criteria for FUO (we allowed ten days for investigations in the hospital) are shown in Table 51.

## TABLE 51: SOME OF THE COMMON CAUSES OF FUO

|  | NUMBER OF PATIENTS |
|---|---|
| **A. INFECTIONS:** | |
| 1) Iatrogenic and nosocomial infections | 23 |
| 2) Subdiaphragmatic and liver abscess, cholecystitis, hepatic and biliary cirrhosis | 14 |
| 3) Partial bowel obstruction (also ureteric or biliary tract obstruction) | 11 |
| 4) Pelvic infections (chronic PID, T-O abscess, endometritis) | 11 |
| 5) Intra-abdominal abscess (retroperitoneal, pancreas, prostate, internal hernia) | 9 |
| 6) Tuberculosis (miliary, abdominal and genitourinary) | 7 |
| 7) Dental infection and sinusitis | 7 |
| 8) Amoebisis presenting as dyspepsia | 6 |
| 9) Decubitus ulcers, perirectal abscess | 6 |
| 10) Septicemia of unexplained origin | 6 |
| 11) Infections due to foreign bodies such as hip pins, prosthetic valves, pacemakers, shunts | 5 |
| 12) Vertebral osteomyelitis in addicts | 4 |
| 13) Actinomycosis | 3 |
| 14) Intestinal parasites other than amoebae (ascariasis, bilharziasis) | 3 |
| 15) Malaria | 2 |
| 16) Endocarditis | 2 |
| 17) Cryptococcus, Nocardia | 2 |
| 18) Histoplasmosis | 1 |
| 19) Splenic abscess | 1 |
|  | 123 |
| **B. MALIGNANCY:** | |
| 1) Hodgkin's disease | 2 |
| 2) Leukemia (acute lymphatic, acute monocytic) | 2 |
| 3) Hypernephroma (one with and other without infection) | 2 |
| 4) Carcinoma of the pancreas | 1 |
| 5) Bronchogenic carcinoma with metastasis (alveolar cell carcinoma) | 5 |
|  | 12 |

| TABLE 51 (CONT'D) | NUMBER OF CASES |
|---|---|

**C. AUTO-IMMUNE DISEASES:**

| | |
|---|---|
| Lupus erythematosus | 2 |
| | 2 |

**D. MISCELLANEOUS:**

| | | |
|---|---|---|
| 1) | Drug fevers (INH, dilantin, sulfonamides, penicillin, cephalothin) | 17 |
| 2) | Erythema multiforme (Stevens-Johnson syndrome) | 17 |
| 3) | Factitious fever | 2 |
| 4) | Thyrotoxicosis | 2 |
| 5) | Periodic disease (Mediterranean fever) | 1 |
| | | 39 |

**E. PROVEN VIRUS INFECTIONS:**

| | | |
|---|---|---|
| 1) | Herpes (simplex, zoster) | 2 |
| 2) | Hepatitis (HAA positive) | 3 |
| 3) | Cytomegalovirus | 1 |
| | | 6 |

| F. NO PROVEN ETIOLOGY | 18 |
|---|---|

| GRAND TOTAL | 200 |
|---|---|

### INFECTIONS

1) IATROGENIC AND NOSOCOMIAL INFECTIONS: Hospital-acquired infections are the major cause of the so-called FUO today. For the most part, they are due to thrombophlebitis; abscesses at the sites of insertion of venous and Foley catheters; contamination from certain procedures, such as insertion of chest tubes, and pleural biopsies; acquired infections from hyperalimentation, endotracheal tubes; and infections precipitated by intra-uterine fetal monitoring devices. Most iatrogenic fevers begin while the original fever is subsiding. In many instances, persuasion to discontinue these devices, whenever possible, was all that was required to cure the so-called FUO!

2) SUBDIAPHRAGMATIC INFECTIONS, INFECTIONS OF THE LIVER AND BILIARY SYSTEM: Pyogenic abscess, subdiaphragmatic abscess, cholecystitis (acute or chronic, with or without cholelithiasis):

   (a) Cholangitis: Ascending cholangitis, either secondary to hemorrhoids or due to bile duct (intrahepatic or extrahepatic) obstruction can give rise to fever and leukocytosis. Progressive increase in the bilirubin and the leukocyte count is the tip-off for the diagnosis. Blood cultures are required to exclude the possibility of gram-negative sepsis, often associated with the condition.

3) PARTIAL BOWEL OBSTRUCTION: High incidence of bowel obstruction in our series is merely a reflection of our interest in the surgical infections. Abdominal pain and fever, with or without positive blood cultures, are the outstanding features of this disease. History of prior abdominal (elective gastrointestinal and gall bladder or gynecologic) surgery is often present. Vomiting may not start during the early stages. One should not wait for vomiting to develop to diagnose bowel obstruction. Partial bowel obstruction is often clinically indistinguishable from an abdominal abscess. Exploratory laparotomy may be required to establish the diagnosis. Partial bowel obstruction is listed here because it is often associated with fever and bacteremia. Scintiscans (Ga-67) in the postoperative period may be misleading, as well.

4) PELVIC INFECTIONS: Chronic pelvic inflammatory disease, pelvic abscess, tubo-ovarian abscess, and endometritis should be considered.

   The eleven cases of pelvic infection, noted previously, had failed earlier on routine penicillin therapy. Diagnosis was established by culdocentesis (see page 323).

5) INTRA-ABDOMINAL ABSCESS: Retroperitoneal abscess (see page 461), pancreatic abscess (see page 83), and prostatic abscess (see page 332) are some of the hard-to-diagnose infections listed here.

6) TUBERCULOSIS: Tuberculosis is often the commonest cause of FUO; but it was not so in my experience. In our hospital more than 100 patients were proven to have tuberculosis during this period. In cases where no AFB were seen in sputum smears, we have routinely performed transtracheal aspiration (TTA) within the first three to five days of admission. If we had not used TTA for the diagnosis of tuberculosis in the sputum smear-negative patients, tuberculosis would have been the leading cause for FUO in our study (see Tuberculosis, Chapter 23 for details).

7) DENTAL INFECTION AND SINUSITIS: Periodontal abscess and chronic sinusitis should be considered in the differential diagnosis of FUO. When they are suspected, dental films should be obtained.

8) AMOEBIC COLITIS: Dyspepsia and fever with or without dysentery (walking dysentery) should lead to the suspicion of chronic amoebic colitis.

9) DECUBITUS ULCERS: It is perplexing to note how even the best clinicians can miss such an obvious lesion as a glaring decubitus ulcer or an unseatingly painful perirectal abscess. On one occasion, seven physicians successfully diagnosed a lung abscess but failed to note its source, an incompletely drained perirectal abscess. When questioned, the patient said that "an internist would not be interested in the rectal abscess" because, "It is the surgeon's territory"! Another patient was suspected to have an intra-abdominal abscess because of positive blood cultures for three organisms at a time, i.e., Bacteroides fragilis, Clostridium ramosum, and Proteus mirabilis - most of us missed a large decubitus ulcer, which was the real source for sepsis.

10) SEPTICEMIAS OF UNEXPLAINED ORIGIN: Persistent septicemia can occur without a heart murmur or a specifically local focus for sepsis. Even extensive investigations may not reveal the source for sepsis. They respond to appropriate therapy.

11) INFECTIONS DUE TO FOREIGN BODY: These include infections of the prosthetic valve, orthopedic devices, pacemaker and other prosthetic devices. One patient with FUO had a metallic foreign body in the soft tissue of the fourth interdigital area, discharging foul-smelling pus through an interdigital sinus. He was admitted for fever. His blood

cultures grew <u>Staphylococcus aureus,</u> but the source of sepsis was not obvious until the patient was re-examined thoroughly from head to toe. This diagnosis was missed during two separate episodes of fever for which he was hospitalized previously.

12) VERTEBRAL OSTEOMYELITIS: Vertebral osteomyelitis should be suspected when an intravenous drug abuser complains of a low back pain. Tuberculosis is still the most common cause for vertebral osteomyelitis. But, in the United States, staphylococcal or gram-negative rod osteomyelitis in the addict is common. Since the clinical symptoms precede the radiologic evidence of osteomyelitis by several weeks, it is often missed. Gallium 67 scan may show increased uptake at the site of osteomyelitis long before there are any visible abnormalities in the Tc-99 scan or on routine roentgenograms.

13) ACTINOMYCOSIS: Actinomycotic infections can be missed by improper culture techniques or confused with other bacterial infections.

14) INTESTINAL PARASITES: Intestinal parasites are often neglected in the differential diagnosis of FUO. Stool should be examined for ova and cysts in all cases of FUO. If intestinal symptoms are present, duodenal aspirates and jejunal biopsies should be obtained.

15) MALARIA: Malaria is often missed because it is not thought of. One woman who was admitted for post-abortion sepsis was treated with antibiotics for nearly 17 days. She had dilatation and curettage, and at least four different antibiotic regimens tried at different times. The fever subsided with each of the therapeutic or surgical procedures and when it spiked again another therapeutic trial was given with a different antibiotic. Finally, she was suspected to have pyometra. While hysterectomy was being contemplated, malarial parasites were discovered by a hematology technician. This is an example of FUO due to a common disease occurring in an uncommon geographical location.

A five-year-old boy from Mexico was being investigated for splenomegaly with low-grade fever. He had several scans and all the other tests, but the blood smears were not examined. Ten days later, the thin blood smears were positive for malarial parasites.

16) ENDOCARDITIS: Nearly sixty patients were diagnosed to have endocarditis during this five-year period in our hospital. We had missed the diagnosis of endocarditis in two patients investigated for FUO, in spite of repeated cultures; hypertonic media were of no help in these two cases. The diagnosis was established at autopsy.

17) CRYPTOCOCCUS AND NOCARDIA: One patient with myelomonocytic leukemia was investigated for FUO and treated with several antibiotics for suspected gram-negative infection. When his mental status deteriorated, a lumbar puncture was performed; he was then found to have cryptococcal meningitis.

One elderly patient with emphysema was in an accident, and developed a massive hemothorax which later became infected. Gram's stains of this fluid showed acid-fast bacilli. He was treated with antituberculosis chemotherapy. Subsequent cultures yielded Nocardia. He responded to clindamycin alone.

18) HISTOPLASMOSIS (see page 209): An elderly gentleman was seen for FUO and weight loss. Physical examination revealed a nodule on the lip which, on biopsy, showed Histoplasma. He was originally from Arkansas, where he raised chickens until he was 16 years old, when he moved to California. He was found to have Addison's disease, presumably secondary to Histoplasma.

19) SPLENIC ABSCESS: (See page 523).

### MALIGNANCY

1) HODGKIN'S DISEASE: A heroin addict was admitted with fever and chills. He had several negative blood cultures. Chest x-ray, on admission, revealed a needle in the right lower lobe which he had aspirated two or three months prior to admission. It was removed under direct bronchoscopic visualization, following which he promptly defervesced. He was readmitted two weeks later with fever and chills. At this time, the physical examination revealed

cervical adenopathy which, on biopsy, confirmed the diagnosis. He spent nearly six weeks in the hospital before the correct diagnosis was made.

2) ACUTE LYMPHOCYTIC AND MONOCYTIC LEUKEMIA: Infection is the most common cause for fever in leukemia. Occasionally, acute leukemia or lymphoma can present with fevers.

3) HYPERNEPHROMA: One patient who was seen for hematuria had normal renal arteriograms. He was then referred to us because of the preoperative roentgenogram of the chest, which revealed miliary lesions. This case was discussed at three separate teaching conferences held for infectious disease, pulmonary and gastroenterology divisions, and was thought to be miliary tuberculosis. The liver biopsy showed granuloma with central necrosis, and the lung biopsy also showed giant cells with necrosis, thought to be due to miliary tuberculosis. He lived for three weeks on rifampin, INH and streptomycin. At autopsy, he was found to have hypernephroma with miliary metastasis to the lung.

4) PANCREAS: Another patient also had a similar syndrome. Hypernephroma was thought of. He died of pancreatic carcinoma.

5) LUNG: Radiographically insignificant factors can cause distant metastasis. An elderly lady suspected to have carcinoma of the liver had several negative liver biopsies. At autopsy, a 5 to 7 mm. lesion was noted in the bronchus. Another patient was in and out of the hospital for nearly three months before a nodule developed on the sternum which, on biopsy, was confirmed as squamous cell carcinoma.

### AUTO-IMMUNE DISEASES

1) LUPUS ERYTHEMATOSUS: Lupus erythematosus should always be considered in the differential diagnosis of FUO. One woman admitted for pleural effusion had several negative L. E. preparations, but the antinuclear antibody test was strongly positive.

### MISCELLANEOUS

1) DRUG FEVERS: Drug fever is a common problem. It occurs five to seven days after the administration of a penicillin or cephalosporin antibiotic. The drug fever is

often periodic, sometimes associated with chills, and with or without eosinophilia. Drug fevers are sometimes hard to separate from the nosocomial infections caused by bacteria. Certain drugs can cause Stevens-Johnson syndrome with fever often mistaken for infectious diseases.

2) ERYTHEMA MULTIFORME (Stevens-Johnson syndrome): The most difficult challenge that I had during the early days of my practice of infectious disease was Stevens-Johnson syndrome (SJS). SJS presents like an infectious disease and therefore an infectious disease specialist is called. SJS can be mistaken for bacterial pneumonia or secondary syphilis and several other diseases (see page 426 for details).

3) FACTITIOUS FEVER: Two addicts trying to escape a court trial hospitalized themselves with fevers. They had several investigations for fever, which were negative. The real nature of the fever became obvious when the nurse insisted on staying in the room with the patient while the temperature was being taken.

Recording simultaneously the urine temperature along with oral and rectal temperatures is helpful in the diagnosis of factitious fever due to manipulation of the thermometer. The urinary temperatures are normally within 1 to 1.5°C. of simultaneous oral temperatures and within 2°C. of rectal temperatures over a wide range of body temperatures. [2] A greater discrepancy should suggest factitious fever.

4) THYROTOXICOSIS: Thyrotoxicosis is often forgotten as a hypercatabolic state which may cause increase in the body temperature. Fever should be considered as a heralding sign for thyroid storm. One patient, an alcoholic who was seen for fever and edematous conjunctiva was thought to have gram-negative sepsis with allergic reaction of the conjunctiva to penicillin. Indeed, he had septicemia due to Bacteroides fragilis, which was eradicated with intravenous carbenicillin, but he continued to have high fevers (104° to 105°F.) when thyrotoxicosis was suspected and subsequently proved (see Fig. 133).

5) PERIODIC DISEASE: See page

VIRUS INFECTIONS

The virus that so often gets the blame was proven to be the cause of FUO in only six instances. One patient, a woman, had slow endometritis and later amnionitis from CMV.

Hepatitis can present with fever, joint pains and rash mistaken for rubella. One patient who was thought to have gonococcal arthritis had several cultures that were negative, and failed to respond to antibiotic therapy. This patient was later proven to have hepatitis by HAA titers and liver biopsy.

## INVESTIGATIONS TO BE DONE IN CASES OF FUO

1. Take a good history: It should include travel and occupational history and history of anyone sick in the same household. If a child was sick, inquire about the health status of parents and grandparents. There are so many subtle questions that one may ask to gather relevant data. History-taking is an art. Tact is required for asking the right questions in the right manner to get all the answers.

2. Re-examine the patient thoroughly from head to toe. Do not assume anything.

3. Examine the chart and the notes written by the physicians, and, more importantly, the notes made by the nurses and paramedical personnel.

4. Build a data base from 1, 2 and 3 and plan a strategy for further investigations if necessary.

5. Blood cultures: In cases of FUO, certain procedures may have to be repeated. Blood culture is one of them. The antibiotic therapy may have to be discontinued, if tolerated, for at least 24 hours prior to drawing blood cultures. Hypertonic media to detect cell wall deficient organisms are of doubtful value [3] (see Chapter 36 for details on blood cultures).

6. Go where the money is: This is popularly known in the U.S.A. as Willie Sutton's law. Mr. Sutton, a bank robber, apparently was asked by the judge why he always robbed the banks. He never robbed houses or railroads as other robbers did in those days. Mr. Sutton simply answered, "That is where the money is!" The same rule applies to the diagnostic investigations. Tissue diagnosis is preferred. When a lymph node is enlarged, if necessary, it would seem to be the most logical site to biopsy. When miliary tuberculosis of the lung is suspected, and the sputa and the transtracheal aspirate are smear-negative, then lung biopsy would be the next most logical step. In cases of anemia, one does a bone marrow aspiration; likewise, in cases of

pneumonia, one should consider transtracheal or transthoracic needle aspiration. If the liver is enlarged, liver
biopsy is useful. Biopsy of skin nodules and lesions in the
mucous membrane is sometimes useful.

7. Bone marrow and bone biopsy: Bone marrow, in contrast
to bone biopsy, is the least rewarding procedure to establish the diagnosis of FUO. The expected yield from bone
marrow in cases of miliary tuberculosis, for example, is
low. Bone biopsy may perhaps have better yield.

8. Serologic tests: Unfortunately, serologic tests are not available for all bacterial infections. One of the routinely re-
quested tests in cases of FUO is the "febrile-agglutinins
test", which consists of detecting agglutinins of typhoid O
and H and paratyphoid A and B, Brucella abortus and Proteus OX19, OXK and OX2 for Rickettsia. More often than
not, the test should be repeated for verification and for evidence of increase in the titer. Increasing titers are diagnostic. In one study of 812 cases of FUO in Delhi, India,[4]
nearly 13% had positive titers for typhoid and paratyphoid;
7% for typhus; 6% for brucellosis and 5% for Q fever. By
serologic procedures alone, 70% of these cases of FUO remained undiagnosed. Other serologic procedures include
VDRL, C-reactive protein, and ASO titer for steptococcal
infections, mononucleosis slide test and heterophil antibody titers for evidence of infectious mononucleosis, rheumatoid arthritis (latex) test and latex fixation titer, antinuclear antibody test, cold agglutinins, hemagglutination
and complement-fixation for amoebiasis, thyroid ($T_3$, $T_4$)
tests and hepatitis-associated antigen. Serologic tests for
fungal infections are discussed separately (see page 192).

9. Ultrasound: If the source of the infection is known, then
one may request ultrasound examination. It is a useful test
to detect the size of the gallbladder and the presence of gall-
stones when the patient is severely jaundiced. Ultrasonic
examination of the abdomen or pelvis can be used for the
detection of abscess (see page 69).

10. Scans: It is a good practice to consult the specialist in nuclear medicine for help before requesting the scans. "Routine total body scanning" with all available radionuclides
is unwise. Abscesses and malignancies are the two things
that can be detected by the gallium-67 scan (see Chapter 118
for details on diagnostic tests in nuclear medicine).

11. Investigate for malignancy: Intravenous pyelography, upper and lower gastrointestinal examination with barium and sputum cytology, if indicated, should be performed. Pancreatic carcinoma is the most difficult of all malignancies to diagnose with the currently available tests. Exfoliative cytology of the duodenum was used with some success.

12. Viral cultures: These are useful, provided a specific virus or a group of viruses are suspected (see Chapter 115 for virus cultures).

## REFERENCES

1. Petersdorf, R. G. , Beeson, P. B. : Fever of unexplained origin: Report of 100 cases. Medicine 40:1, 1961.

2. Murray, H. W. , et al. : Urinary temperature: A clue to early diagnosis of factitious fever. New Eng. J. Med. 296: 23, 1977.

3. Gleckman, R. , Esposito, A. , Madoff, S. : Fever of unknown origin: Attempts to isolate L-forms and other aberrant bacterial forms. J. Clin. Microbiol. 5:225, 1977.

4. Mohan, K. , et al. : Investigations of cases of pyrexia of uncertain origin in Delhi with particular reference to brucellosis. The J. Conv. Dis. 6:329, 1974.

## 114: OTHER CONDITIONS THAT MIMIC INFECTIOUS DISEASES
### by David D. Ulmer

Many of the manifestations of infection arise from the host response to circulating organic molecules, released either from the infectious agent or from destruction of host cells. However, the range of potential host responses to alien substances is limited; hence, exposure to non-infectious foreign materials often produces signs and symptoms mimicking illness caused by microbial pathogens. For example, fever and arthralgias commonly accompany infection but also are frequently observed side effects of drugs used to treat infection, posing a common clinical dilemma. Less often, but of more serious concern, are drug reactions which present as prolonged and baffling infectious-like illnesses and which both vex the physician and dishearten the patient. An exhaustive review of toxic responses which have been confused with infection is beyond the scope of the present volume; however, it is intended that this chapter provide a few examples of drugs, plant and animal toxins, metals, and chemical substances of occupational risk, each of which induces an infection-like response in one or several major organ systems of the host and, in this manner, call attention to the constant necessity for considering toxins in the differential diagnosis of infectious disease (Table 52).

### GENERAL COMMENTS

### PHARMACOLOGIC AGENTS

Adverse responses to pharmacologic agents, including antimicrobials, are now recognized as a major cause of morbidity and, during the past few decades, the increasing use of multiple, highly potent agents has led to a corresponding growth in the number of infectious-like illnesses which may be attributed to drug therapy. Of note, a portion of this morbidity, particularly that owing to antibiotics, appears to be avoidable. For example, a recent study at Duke University Medical Center revealed that more than one-third of all hospitalized patients received antibiotics and, in nearly two-thirds of such cases, their administration either was not indicated or was inappropriate in terms of drug or dosage. [1] Such studies serve to emphasize the need for continued attention to teaching and monitoring prudent use of drugs.

## TABLE 52: EXAMPLES OF TOXINS WHICH MIMIC INFECTIONS

### CLASS: DRUGS

| Toxic Agent | Usual Source of Exposure | Infection Mimicked | Principal Manifestations | Diagnostic Source or Test | Remarks |
|---|---|---|---|---|---|
| Methicillin | Therapeutic | Pyelonephritis | Fever; rash; proteinuria | Renal biopsy | Immune reaction |
| Clindamycin | Therapeutic | Ulcerative colitis | Diarrhea; abdominal pain; fever; leukocytosis | Large bowel biopsy | Also observed with lincomycin, ampicillin, tetracycline, chloramphenicol |
| Erythromycin | Therapeutic | Hepatitis | Jaundice | Liver biopsy | Also observed with triacety-oleandomycin, oxacillin, nitrofurantoin |
| Cephalosporins | Therapeutic | Endocarditis | Fever; arthralgias; myalgias; rash | Subsides with drug cessation | Observed with high dosage, I.V. use, prolonged use |

| Hydrochloro-thiazide | Therapeutic | Pneumonia | Recurrent fever and pulmonary infiltrates | Chest x-ray | Sensitivity reaction |
|---|---|---|---|---|---|
| CLASS: PLANT TOXINS | | | | | |
| Phallotoxins | Poisonous mushrooms | Gastroenteritis | Nausea; vomiting; abdominal pain; diarrhea | Examine mushrooms | Thiotic acid of possible therapeutic benefit |
| Amatoxins | (Amanita phalloides) | Hepatitis | Hepatorenal syndrome | Same | — |
| "Hypoyglycins" | Unripe akee (a fruit) | Gastroenteritis / Encephalitis | "Jamaican vomiting sickness" - convulsions; coma; hypoglycemia | History; low blood sugar, increased urinary fatty acids | — |
| Atropine Scopolamine | Tea, cigarettes of "Jimson weed" (Datura stramonium) | Encephalitis | Restlessness; ataxia; blurred vision; hallucinations | History of Datura use | — |

(Cont'd)

TABLE 52: (CONT'D)

CLASS: FISH TOXINS

| Toxic Agent | Usual Source of Exposure | Infection Mimicked | Principal Manifestations | Diagnostic Source or Test | Remarks |
|---|---|---|---|---|---|
| Ciguatoxin | Ciguatera; red snapper, grouper, etc. | Polio; infectious polyneuritis | Paresthesias; muscular weakness; cranial nerve palsies; respiratory paralysis | History of ingestion | Heat-stable toxin acquired in food chain |
| Scrombotoxin | Scrombroid fish, e.g., tuna, mackerel | Gastroenteritis | Nausea; vomiting; diarrhea; flushing; dizziness; urticaria | History of ingestion | Histamine-like toxin formed by bacteria in fish muscle |
| Tetrodotoxin | Puffer fish, e.g., ocean sunfish | Poliomyelitis | Muscle weakness; respiratory paralysis | History of ingestion | High mortality |

| | | | | | |
|---|---|---|---|---|---|
| "Red-Tide" toxin | Shellfish exposed to toxic dinoflagellates | Poliomyelitis Gastroenteritis | Muscle paralysis; nausea; vomiting; diarrhea | History of ingestion | Occasionally fatal owing to respiratory paralysis |

CLASS: TRACE METALS

| | | | | | |
|---|---|---|---|---|---|
| Zinc | Welding | Influenza | "Metal fume fever"; chills; cough; nausea; vomiting | History of fume exposure | Benign and self-limited |
| Cadmium | Inhalation of fumes | Pneumonia | Headache; fever; chills; chest pain; dyspnea | History of fume exposure | Secondary pulmonary infection and toxic hepatitis |
| | Chronic ingestion | Osteomyelitis Pyelonephritis | "Ouch-ouch" disease; bone pain with pseudofracture; chronic renal disease | Increased blood and urine cadmium | Affects older, multiparous women |
| Arsenic | Acute ingestion, e.g., pesticides | Gastroenteritis | Nausea; vomiting; diarrhea; abdominal pain | Increased blood and urine arsenic | 70-180 mg. arsenic trioxide is fatal |

(Cont'd)

TABLE 52: (CONT'D)

### CLASS: FISH TOXINS

| Toxic Agent | Usual Source of Exposure | Infection Mimicked | Principal Manifesta- tions | Diagnostic Source or Test | Remarks |
|---|---|---|---|---|---|
| | Chronic ingestion | Infectious polyneuritis and encephalitis | Headache; lethar- gy; confusion; peripheral neu- ritis; skin rash | Increased blood and urine arsenic | BAL for treatment |
| Nickel | Nickel carbonyl fumes | Pneumonitis | Fever; cough; dyspnea; headache | History of exposure to fumes | Fatalities from pulmonary hemorrhage and atelectasis |
| Mercury | Ingestion of soluble salt | Gastroen- teritis  Colitis | Nausea; vomiting; pharyngitis; stomatitis; bloody diarrhea; tenesmus | Mercury levels in blood or urine | Neurological signs predominate with chronic poisoning |

### CLASS: OCCUPATIONAL TOXINS

| Toxic Agent | Usual Source of Exposure | Infection Mimicked | Principal Manifesta- tions | Diagnostic Source or Test | Remarks |
|---|---|---|---|---|---|
| Fluorocarbon polymers | Pyrolysis fumes | Bronchitis Broncho- pneumonia | Fever; chills; cough; myalgias; dyspnea | History of exposure to fumes | "Meat wrappers" illness is similar |

| | | | | | |
|---|---|---|---|---|---|
| Oxides of Nitrogen | Freshly filled silos | Broncho-pneumonia | "Silo-fillers" disease; cough; fever; dyspnea | History of inhalation of fumes | Can cause fatal pulmonary fibrosis |
| Uncertain | Moldy hay fumes | Interstitial pneumonia | "Farmers lung" disease; fever; chills; dyspnea; cyanosis | Granulomas; obliterative bronchitis by lung biopsy | Hypersensitivity pneumonitis; also seen with sugar cane, cotton, mushroom - compost workers, and pigeon breeders |

The most common syndromes of drug toxicity which must be differentiated from infection are those which result either from sensitization and allergic reactions or from idiosyncratic responses. However, considerable diversity in the nature of adverse reactions may be encountered with certain drugs. For example, diphenylhydantoin may induce a spectrum of toxic responses which mimic infections including serum sickness, hepatitis, cholangitis, polyarthropathies, pseudolymphomas, thyroiditis, and an infectious mononucleosis-like syndrome. [2,3] An illness suggesting botulism ranks amongst the more bizarre reactions to diphenylhydantoin and has been described in two patients. [4]

## ANIMAL AND PLANT TOXINS

Poisonous or venomous animals are found in every phylum except the birds and include about 250 species of snakes, 700 species of arthropods, and more than 1000 species of marine animals. In general, illnesses which follow the bites and stings of land animals are readily identified as toxic responses; hence, they are seldom confused with infection. Rarely, the initial bite of the black widow spider may not be recognized as such and the subsequent intense abdominal pain be mistaken for peritonitis. Tick-bite paralysis, which manifests as a severe neurotoxic syndrome, may also elude diagnosis in the early stages.

In contrast to illnesses caused by bites and stings of land animals, poisoning from toxic marine species is frequently confused with an infectious process. Vertebrate fish may contain toxins in the muscles, viscera, skin or mucus (ichthyosarcotoxic fish), gonads (ichthyotoxic fish), or blood (ichthyohemotoxic fish). Although gastrointestinal symptoms are often the presenting signs of such poisoning, neurotoxicity is the most serious manifestation (vide infra).

Knowledge of toxic, as opposed to edible plant life, gleaned by trial and error, presumably constitutes a portion of the earliest survival information regularly passed from generation to generation. Since primitive times, man has been plagued by problems of mistaken identification of the choice of plants for food, or suffered illness from plants employed in ritual ceremonies, owing to their content of pharmacological agents. Vestiges of these problems remain today in the form of illnesses such as those caused by poisonous mushrooms or the use of "jimson weed" (vide infra).

## METAL INTOXICATIONS

More than two dozen elements, including trace metals ordinarily present in the body only in minute concentrations, have essential biological functions and are required for normal growth, development and the maintenance of health. [5] However, all elements are potentially toxic if presented to an organism in high concentrations. Metal intoxications produce a variety of acute and chronic illnesses which may simulate infectious disease. As with other forms of poisoning due to external agents, a careful history revealing metal exposure is the key to timely diagnosis.

## OTHER TOXINS

In addition to drugs, plant or animal toxins, and metals, human reactions to a wide variety of environmental substances are commonly observed and serve to remind the clinician that fever, pneumonitis, gastroenteritis, arthritis, or anemia often are of non-infectious origin. Several examples will be cited in the section on respiratory syndromes.

## MAJOR MANIFESTATIONS OF TOXICITY

## GASTROINTESTINAL SYNDROMES

ANTIBIOTICS: Mild nausea, vomiting and diarrhea are common side effects of many drugs. However, more serious illness such as pseudomembranous colitis, presenting with profuse watery diarrhea, severe abdominal pain, fever, and leukocytosis, occurs in as many as 10% of patients who receive clindamycin. [6] The syndrome most frequently follows administration of oral clindamycin but also occurs after parenteral therapy. [7] Diagnosis is based upon recognition of yellow-white plaques at proctoscopy or colonoscopy that, upon biopsy, show a bland pseudomembrane. Early recognition of the syndrome and cessation of clindamycin therapy generally result in prompt recovery, although topical or parenteral steroids are occasionally required. In addition to clindamycin, the syndrome has been observed with lincomycin, ampicillin, tetracycline and chloramphenicol. However, the basic mechanism of this idiosyncrasy remains undefined.

As the primary site for drug metabolism, the liver is especially vulnerable to toxic damage produced by drugs or their breakdown products. For example, it has long been recognized that adverse reactions to certain antibiotics may produce clinical illness which resembles viral hepatitis or cholecystitis. Reversible cholestatic jaundice is observed with use of triacetyloleandomycin, erythromycin estolate, oxacillin and nitrofurantoin.

More severe cellular damage and, sometimes, progressive
liver failure may follow therapy with sulfonamides or parenteral tetracyclines, especially in pregnant patients with reduced
renal function. Novobiocin can also produce a hepatocellular
type of jaundice. Massive hepatic necrosis is a rare, but devastating, complication of antituberculous therapy with isoniazid.

MUSHROOM POISONING: Illnesses resulting from ingestion of
poisonous mushrooms, (principally Amanita phalloides, also
known as "death cap" or "destroying angel") are dramatic, if
infrequent, events and readily confused with acute infectious
processes. Nearly 30% of persons who ingest Amanita are fatally
stricken. After a latent period of eight to twenty-four hours, the
toxin causes a profound watery diarrhea, abdominal pain, nausea and vomiting, sometimes culminating in rapid death owing
to the cholera-like manifestations. Even if the patient survives
the acute gastrointestinal phase of the illness, however, improvement is short-lived; a fatal hepatorenal phase of the disease follows in three to five days, eventually leading to a
hepatic failure and death.

Two types of unusual sulfur-containing cyclopeptides have been
identified as the major lethal toxins in Amanita[8]: "phallotoxins,"
which act upon the endoplasmic reticulum of liver cells, and the
more potent "amatoxins", which exert cytopathogenic effects
upon the cell nucleus, including binding to, and inhibition of,
RNA polymerase. Other potent, biologically active substances
have also been isolated from poisonous mushrooms, including
muscurine from A. muscaria, but are less toxic than the cyclopeptides.

Until the last decade, no specific therapy for Amanita poisoning has been available; however, the mitochondrial heme protein, cytochrome c, has been found to exert a protective action in experimental animals [9] and, in recent years, thiotic
acid has been employed with good response reported in European victims of mushroom poisoning. [10]

JAMAICAN VOMITING SICKNESS (Akee Poisoning): Jamaican
vomiting sickness provides another example of severe disease
resulting from ingestion of a plant toxin, and is occasionally
confused with infection. The illness has been known to occur
endemically in Jamaica for more than 100 years, principally
afflicts children, and is manifested by the sudden onset of
severe vomiting, usually followed by convulsions, coma and

death [11]. Profound hypoglycemia occurs in most cases, and autopsy reveals marked depletion of liver glycogen with a characteristic type of diffuse fatty infiltration of liver, kidney and other organs.

The disease has been shown to result from the action of toxins, designated hypoglycins, found in the arilli and seeds of unripe akee, a local fruit. The hypoglycins are unusual amino acids which, after ingestion, are metabolized to methylene cyclopropylacetic acid, an agent which strongly inhibits transport into mitochondria and oxidation of long chain fatty acids. This results in depression of gluconeogenesis, hypoglycemia, and a marked increase in excretion of short and medium chain fatty acids into the urine. [12] Speculation that vomiting sickness might represent a Jamaican variant of Reye's syndrome is not supported by comparison of urinary excretion of metabolites in the two diseases.

METAL INTOXICATIONS: Acute or chronic ingestion of metals may produce gastrointestinal symptoms easily confused with infection. Thus, acute poisoning owing to ingestion of metallic copper resembles other forms of food poisoning. If severe, the early manifestations of nausea, vomiting and diarrhea may be followed by hematemesis, melena, hypotension and coma. Centrilobular hepatic necrosis may produce jaundice. The manifestations of metal intoxication are seldom confined solely to the gastrointestinal tract of course. Thus, copper poisoning may also result from the rapid absorption of copper sulfate through the skin, as may occur in the therapy of burns, or directly into the blood, owing to the use of copper-lined dialysis equipment; an acute hemolytic anemia results from either circumstance.

Acute human poisoning with cobalt is manifested by nausea, vomiting, diarrhea, tinnitus and loss of hearing. In contrast, chronic administration of cobalt induces polycythemia and, by blocking iodine uptake, produces goiter, especially in children. During the 1960s, cobalt, added to beer as an antifoaming agent, produced several localized epidemics of an extraordinary cardiomyopathy, often accompanied by pericardial effusion, frequently with fatal outcome. The mechanism of this illness remains uncertain, but the myocardiopathy epidemic ceased upon removal of cobalt from the beer. Inhalation of aerosols of finely powdered cobalt has been implicated in the development of progressive interstitial lung disease, although the data are not yet conclusive.

Poisoning by a number of other metals, usually by acute ingestion of their soluble salts, produces a clinical syndrome of gastroenteritis which may, initially, be confused with food poisoning. Associated signs and symptoms may prove helpful in arriving at an accurate diagnosis. Thus, the mercuric ion is highly corrosive, and acute poisoning with mercuric chloride causes severe local inflammation of the mouth and throat. Since mercury is also excreted into the colon, enteritis may be accompanied by bloody diarrhea and tenesmus. Renal tubular damage may lead to anuria and uremia. Chronic mercury poisoning causes a less severe gastrointestinal syndrome; neurologic changes, including tremors, vertigo, irritability, moodiness and depression predominate.

Silver poisoning, usually from silver nitrate, also causes nausea, vomiting, and diarrhea, accompanied by deep staining of the tissues of the mouth and throat. The salt is caustic and causes local burning pain. Chronic silver poisoning, usually from nose drops, produces a characteristic bluish discoloration of skin (argyria).

The gastroenteritis of thallium ingestion is accompanied by leg pains, progressing to weakness and paralysis of the legs. Visual and mental disturbances may also be observed. Loss of hair within a few weeks is a strong diagnostic clue if the etiology of the poisoning has remained uncertain.

Nausea, vomiting, diarrhea, and abdominal pain from fluorine intoxication, in the form of insect poison, is often complicated by tetany, owing to formation of calcium fluoride. Death may result from cardiovascular collapse.

## PULMONARY SYNDROMES

METAL FUME FEVER: Metal fume fever (welder's fever; zinc chills) is a rather common, benign and self-limited illness of short duration. It afflicts welders and other metal tradesmen within a few hours of exposure to, and inhalation of, fumes of various metals, most commonly zinc. The syndrome is characterized by fever, chills, salivation, dry cough, nausea, vomiting, headache, chest discomfort and pronounced leukocytosis. Symptoms and signs usually subside within 24 hours.

CADMIUM INTOXICATION: Cadmium poisoning may occur either through inhalation of metal fumes or by ingestion.[13] Inhalation of cadmium fumes, freshly evolved by heating, welding, or burning of cadmium-containing metals, is almost entirely of occupational origin and is among the most dangerous of health hazards faced by metal workers. Symptoms of severe bronchitis, dyspnea and chest pain do not appear until many hours after exposure and may be accompanied by dryness and irritation of the throat, headache, dizziness, fever and chills. The illness is often mistaken by welders for the familiar metal-fume fever (vide supra) and causes them to delay seeking prompt medical care. In 12 to 36 hours, chest pain and dyspnea may become severe and be accompanied by x-ray changes of patchy pulmonary infiltrates or pulmonary edema. Toxic hepatitis or secondary pulmonary infection may complicate the picture, and death may occur during the first week. However, with good care, most patients survive and ordinarily recover without evidence of permanent damage.

Chronic poisoning owing to cadmium inhalation follows prolonged exposure to small amounts of cadmium dusts. Lung damage gradually results in progressive dyspnea and the slow development of emphysema but without cough. Kidney damage accompanies the lung pathology and, often, is more prominent. Cadmium accumulates in the renal tubular epithelium and, initially, results in excretion of low molecular weight proteins followed, in many cases, by progression to a complete Fanconi's syndrome. There may be associated bony demineralization, bone pain, and gastrointestinal disturbances. Removal of workers from the source of cadmium exposure may permit the lung and kidney lesions to stabilize.

A somewhat different, non-occupational form of chronic cadmium poisoning has been recognized in Japan as the cause, at least in part, of Itai-Itai Byo or "Ouch-Ouch" disease. This painful, often fatal illness mainly afflicts multiparous women 50 to 60 years of age and is characterized by demineralization of bone (osteomalacia) and nephropathy. Affected individuals manifest extreme bony pain and develop pseudofractures, waddling gait and finally inability to walk. They also exhibit proteinuria, aminoaciduria, glucosuria and hypercalcemia. The incidence of hypertension appears to be increased in victims. Urinary and tissue cadmium are increased. The disease has been traced to contamination of river water by waste products of cadmium mines, and crops, watered by the river, show increased cadmium concentrations. While malnutrition and other factors may play a role, it seems likely that prolonged ingestion of metal-contaminated water and food are primary factors in producing the clinical illness. [14]

OTHER METALS: Although a number of nickel compounds are toxic to humans, nickel carbonyl, formed from nickel and carbon monoxide, is the most dangerous and induces a severe alveolar inflammatory response and liver necrosis. After excessive industrial exposure to nickel fumes, symptoms of dyspnea, headache, and vomiting appear within a few hours. During the subsequent one to two days, the victim develops chest tightness, fever, productive cough and shortness of breath. In severe cases, progressive respiratory distress, owing to hemorrhage and atelectasis, may lead to death within a week. Sodium diethyldithiocarbamate or dimercaprol have been recommended for treatment.

Silicon exposure does not produce an acute toxic syndrome, but inhalation of fine particles of free crystalline silica ($SiO_2$) produces a pulmonary inflammatory response and granuloma formation, leading to chronic fibrosis (silicosis).

OTHER CHEMICAL AGENTS: An influenza-like syndrome characterized by cough, fever, chills, myalgias and shortness of breath has been described in textile mill workers exposed to fumes of a fluorocarbon polymer.[15] Investigation revealed, however, that only cigarette smokers in the plant were afflicted. It was postulated that cigarettes became contaminated with polymer carried on the fingers of the smokers and inhalation of the pyrolysis products of the burning cigarettes induced the illness. In an analogous fashion, respiratory symptoms and illness have been described in meat wrappers who were exposed to polyvinylchloride pyrolysis fumes while working with hot wire cutting machines.[16]

Such "infectious-like" occupational illnesses are not restricted to workers in industrial plants and factories, of course. Farmbelt laborers have long been known to fall victim to such respiratory afflictions as "silo-filler's disease", an acute and sometimes fatal fibrosing bronchiolitis, owing to inhalation of oxides of nitrogen evolved in freshly filled silos. "Farmer's lung," an acute interstitial pneumonitis secondary to mold hypersensitivity, may also mimic an infection and is akin to the acute respiratory syndromes in sugarcane or cotton processing workers. Doubtless, many such host responses remain to be identified, but serve to emphasize the necessity for careful elicitation of historical information and for positive identification of microorganisms when considering an infectious etiology for pulmonary illness.

## NEUROLOGICAL SYNDROMES
DRUGS: An extrapyramidal syndrome which superficially resembles tetanus is a rather frequent complication of therapy
with the phenothiazine group of drugs. Muscle spasms about
the face and neck, which may prevent swallowing, are very
frightening to the patient and family members but respond
promptly to administration of diphenhydramine or anti-Parkin-
sonism drugs.

PLANTS: The medicinal use of herbal preparations dates from
antiquity but, in recent years, there has been a marked increase in the use of potent herbal products in cigarettes, other
smoking mixtures, tea, and in capsular form as hallucinogens,
euphoriants, aphrodisiacs and as substitutes for marijuana.
Many such preparations contain substantial amounts of psycho-
active substances, which induce behavioral disorders that require clinical attention. [17] Certain ones may be confused with
infectious processes. For example, consumption of kavahava
tea, prepared from the roots of the kava plant, is alleged to
have euphoric and relaxing effects. However, overindulgence
may produce a chronic "high", anorexia, diarrhea, neurologic
changes, dermatosis and a yellow discoloration of the skin.
Dihydromethysticin in the tea appears responsible for the central relaxant effect. Myristicin, a monamine oxidase inhibitor,
is the active agent in nutmeg tea, and may cause dizziness,
vertigo, headache, sweating, dryness in the mouth and throat,
and hallucinations. "Jimson weed", tea made of Datura stra-
monium, produces flushing, ataxia, restlessness, blurred vision, pronounced thirst and hallucinations. Certain herbal
cigarettes also contain jimson weed and may produce an identical clinical picture. The plant and leaves of Datura contain
high concentrations of atropine and scopolamine, which account
for the toxic symptoms.

MARINE ORGANISMS: Ingestion of toxic marine species often
results in both gastrointestinal and neurologic syndromes; the
latter are usually more serious.

Ichthyosarcotoxism is the most common of fish poisonings that
are of risk to man. That due to ciguatera (red snapper, amber-
jack, grouper, barracuda) presents as abdominal cramps, nausea, vomiting and watery diarrhea, appearing within a few
hours after ingestion of the toxic fish. Numbness, paresthesias,
myalgias, and arthralgias may follow, and neurotoxicity occasionally progresses to cranial nerve palsies and respiratory
paralysis. Ciguatoxic fish are predominantly bottom dwellers
and are believed to acquire the toxin via their food chain. Ciguatoxin is a relatively heat-stable substance, hence not destroyed

by cooking. The toxin, as yet poorly characterized, inhibits cholinesterase, but the mechanism of its effects on humans is more complex and not yet well understood. Treatment is entirely supportive.

Symptoms of poisoning with scrombroid fish (tuna, mackerel, bonito and skipjack) resemble those of a histamine reaction with flushing, dizziness, headache, burning of the throat, abdominal cramps, nausea, vomiting and diarrhea. Urticaria and pruritis are frequent. Symptoms appear within minutes to a few hours after ingestion of the meal in which toxin has formed by the action of bacteria on fish muscle, usually owing to the improper refrigeration of the freshly caught fish. Scrombrotoxin, like ciguatoxin, is not well defined but may contain histamine as well as other heat-stable substances. The illness generally lasts only a few hours and mortality is unusual. No specific treatment is available.

Poisoning from ingestion of puffer fish, including ocean sunfish and porcupine fish, produces the most serious of the vertebrate fish-induced illnesses and may be accompanied by a mortality as high as 50-60%. In Japan, more than 100 persons die each year from ingestion of the poisonous species. [18] The puffer poison, tetrodotoxin, exerts potent curare-like effects on the neuromuscular system. In victims, initial lethargy and ataxia are followed by rapid and progressive weakness of voluntary muscles of the limbs and, later, respiratory paralysis. The site of neuromuscular block is apparently at the nerve axon and muscle membrane rather than at end-plate receptors, but a direct central nervous system action also seems likely.

Shellfish constitute another rather common source of human poisoning. Severe neurotoxicity, leading to muscle weakness and paralysis, usually appears within 30 minutes of ingestion of bivalve mollusks (especially mussels, clams, oysters and scallops) contaminated with the heat-stable neurotoxins of the dinoflagellates, Gonyanlax catenella or Go. tamarensis. Nausea, vomiting and diarrhea may accompany the neuromuscular symptoms. In severe cases of poisoning, death, owing to respiratory paralysis, may follow within 12 hours. Gastric lavage and cathartics may speed removal of toxin from the intestine but, otherwise, treatment is supportive. Outbreaks of poisoning may occur whenever the toxic species of dinoflagellates rapidly increase in number as water temperature warms during the summer months. The proliferation of dinoflagellates may impart a red or reddish-brown color to the water ("red-tide"), but non-toxic species may also generate a red tide and shellfish may become poisonous from toxic organisms in the absence of visible proliferation.

Gymodinium breve, still another toxic dinoflagellate, frequently causes red tides off both Florida coasts and leads to a milder form of neurotoxic shellfish poisoning characterized by nausea, vomiting, diarrhea, ataxia and paresthesias, but without paralysis. Aerosolization of the dinoflagellate in the surf may also induce, in shore-dwellers, a self-limited upper respiratory syndrome with conjunctivitis, rhinorrhea and cough.[19]

ARSENIC INTOXICATION: Accidental arsenic poisoning may result from industrial exposure, medication containing arsenic (e.g., Fowler's solution), or from many environmental sources, most notably arsenical pesticides.[20] White arsenic has also been a popular homicidal agent for many centuries and is still used by some classicists of the art. The cardinal manifestations of arsenical intoxication are dependent upon the form of arsenic employed and the time-dose relationship.

The fatal dose of arsenic trioxide for man is 70 to 180 mg., although toxicity may result from much smaller quantities. Ingestion of solid arsenic may produce, in 30 minutes to several hours, burning and dryness of the mouth and throat, dysphagia, colicky abdominal pain, vomiting, profuse diarrhea and sometimes hematuria. Shock due to diarrhea and dehydration may develop rapidly. If the patient survives the initial symptoms, recovery may be complicated by encephalitis, myelitis or nephritis. Therapy includes fluid replacement, gastric lavage with one per cent sodium thiosulfate in warm milk or water, and dimercaprol, 2 to 3 mg. per kg. every four hours until symptoms abate.

Chronic intoxication with solid arsenicals produces a clinical state highlighted by polyneuritis and motor palsies. As with lead intoxication, which acts at similar biochemical sites, weakness is most likely to affect the long extensors of the fingers and toes. However, arsenical neuritis is said to be more symmetrical, widespread and painful than that seen with lead. Personality changes, headache, drowsiness, memory loss and confusion may be part of the neurologic syndrome, and a clinical similarity to Wernicke's syndrome and Korsakoff's psychosis has been noted. In addition to the prominent neurological changes, chronic arsenical intoxication may be accompanied by hoarseness, cough, laryngitis, conjunctivitis and abdominal pain. A diffuse, dry, brawny, non-pruritic desquamation of the skin with hyperkeratosis, especially of palms and soles, regularly occurs. Transverse white striae of the fingernails (Mee's lines) are a useful diagnostic sign. Laboratory abnormalities include leukopenia, eosinophilia and evidence of hepatitis. Most signs and symptoms of toxicity are reversible upon removal of the source of exposure and treatment with dimercaprol. However, recovery from the neurologic changes usually requires many months.

Arsine gas is the most dangerous form of arsenic exposure, and poisoning may occur whenever hydrogen is generated in the presence of the element, usually from the action of acid on metals containing small amounts of arsenic. Toxicity results from hemolysis of red cells, which may be massive and rapidly fatal or, with chronic low grade exposure to arsine, slow hemolysis may produce anemia of varying severity. Removal of the victim from the source of exposure results in prompt recovery.

## RHEUMATIC SYNDROMES

Acute arthritis and other rheumatoid syndromes are frequent manifestations of adverse drug reactions and have been observed even more commonly in recent years with the growth in number of patients receiving anti-hypertensive agents. The lung may also serve as the "shock organ" for "rheumatoid" drug reactions; for example, severe, recurrent pneumonitis may result from sensitivity to hydrochlorothiazide. [21]

Administration of cephalothin or cephapirin in high doses (2 grams) by rapid intravenous infusion several times daily, as might be employed in treating bacterial endocarditis, after two to four weeks, uniformly induces a serum sickness syndrome characterized by fever, malaise, weakness, arthralgia, myalgia, lymphadenopathy and pruritic skin rash. [22] However, the frequency of such reactions is low with smaller, more conventional dosage, alternate methods of administration, and shorter times of therapy. These observations emphasize the importance of selecting the proper antibiotic, minimal effective dosage, and shorter length of treatment, if excessive sensitivity is to be avoided. Even in patients with renal failure, the risks (e.g., central nervous system toxicity manifested by convulsions) of high dose therapy with penicillin and its analogues are reduced significantly by efforts to monitor serum drug concentrations and correct dosage relative to creatinine clearance. [23] Safety in the administration of antibiotics, like other potent drugs, should improve with the growing availability of techniques for rapid and accurate measurements of serum drug concentrations and clearance rates.

## NEPHROTOXICITY

Interstitial nephritis leading to renal failure is a well recognized complication of therapy with penicillin derivatives, particularly methicillin. [24] The disease presents with fever, rash, proteinuria and eosinophilia, beginning several days after initiation of antibiotic therapy; renal biopsy reveals a predominantly mononuclear interstitial infiltrate with focal tubular degeneration; vessels and glomeruli are essentially normal. Antitubular basement membrane antibodies, directed against a methicillin-derived dimethoxyphenypenicilloyl-tubular-basement-membrane "hapten protein conjugate", may be responsible for the immunopathogensis of this disease. [25]

## DIAGNOSIS

A high index of suspicion and a careful history are the keys to toxicological diagnosis. In particular, attention should be focused upon the use of medication, including home remedies and tonics: upon any variations in the usual diet, be they from use of new or different foods at home or from eating out; upon the recent or long term usage of pesticides, herbicides and rodenticides in the home or garden; and upon possible occupational exposure to chemicals, fumes, dusts or solvents.

If recent or acute exposure to a toxin is suspected, an effort should be made to obtain, for inspection and analysis, specimens of the food, drug, or other material. Biological materials may deteriorate quickly at ambient temperatures and samples should be placed in clean plastic containers and frozen for later examination. Emergency management of the patient should include collection of vomitus, gastric contents obtained by lavage, blood or urine, as appropriate.

Many chemicals, including hypnotics and street drugs, can now be rapidly identified by procedures such as thin layer chromatography, or gas chromatography-mass spectroscopy. These procedures are most useful when the general class of compounds to be screened is known or may be surmised. Metals in blood, urine, nails or hair can be quantified by emission, atomic absorption, or atomic fluorescence spectroscopic procedures. However, it is important that samples for analysis be stored in polyethylene containers which have been previously acid cleaned and rinsed with deionized water. Often 10-15 ml. of blood and 100-200 ml. of urine are sufficient for metal analysis but, ideally, aliquots of 4-hour urine collections, upon which creatinine is also determined, should be submitted for

analysis. Many plant and animal toxins, particularly neurotoxins, can be identified only by tedious bioassay, if at all, and
it is usually of much greater importance to examine the possible
source of the toxin and consider epidemiological features of
the exposure in an effort to determine the likelihood of poisoning.

Finally, all practicing physicians should be familiar with a
source book on poisons, [26-29] the telephone number of a functioning poison information center which provides 24-hour service, and the location of the nearest local, state and federal
laboratories which perform special chemical diagnostic examinations.

## REFERENCES

1. Castle, M. , et al.: Antibiotic use at Duke University Medical Center. J. A. M. A. 237:2819-2822, 1977.

2. Zidar, B. L. , et al.: Diphenylhydantoin-induced serum sickness with fibrin-platelet thrombi in lymph node microvas-
culature. Am. J. Med. 58:704-708, 1975.

3. Editorial: Adverse effects of hydantoins. Med. J. Aust. 2:
346, 1971.

4. Wand, M. , Mather, J. A.: Diphenylhydantoin intoxication
mimicking botulism. New Eng. J. Med. 286:88, 1972.

5. Ulmer, D. D.: Trace elements. New Eng. J. Med. 297:318-
321, 1977.

6. Wells, R. F.: Clindamycin-associated colitis. Editorial.
Ann. Int. Med. 81:547-548, 1974.

7. Tedesco, F. J. , Barton, R. W. , Alpers, D. H.: Clindamycin-associated colitis. A prospective study. Ann. Int. Med.
81:429-433, 1974.

8. Weiland, T.: Poisonous principles of mushrooms of the
genus Amanita. Science 159:946-952, 1968.

9. Floersheim, G. L.: Curative potencies against $\alpha$-amanitin
poisoning by Cytochrome c. Science 177:808-809, 1972.

10. Quoted by Culliton, B. J.: The destroying angel: A story of a search for an antidote. Science 185:600-601, 1974.

11. Hill, K. R.: The vomiting sickness of Jamaica. A review. West Indian Med. J. 1:243, 1952.

12. Tanaka, K. , Kean, E. A. , Johnson, B.: Jamaican vomiting sickness. New Eng. J. Med. 295:461-467, 1976.

13. Vallee, B. L. , Ulmer, D. D.: Biochemical effects of mercury, cadmium and lead. Ann. Rev. of Biochem. 41:91-120, 1972.

14. Emerson, B. T.: "Ouch-Ouch" Disease: The osteomalacia of cadmium nephropathy. Ann. Int. Med. 73:854-855, 1970.

15. Wegman, D. H. , Peters, J. M.: Polymer fume fever and cigarette smoking. Ann. Int. Med. 81:55-57, 1974.

16. Falk, H. , Portnoy, B.: Respiratory tract illness in meat wrappers. J. A. M. A. 235:915-917, 1976.

17. Siegel, R. K.: Herbal intoxication. J. A. M. A. 236:473-477, 1966.

18. Kao, C. Y.: Tetrodotoxin, saxitoxin and their significance in the study of excitation phenomena. Pharmacol. Rev. 18:997-1049, 1966.

19. Hughes, J. M. , Merson, M. H.: Fish and shellfish poisoning. New Eng. J. Med. 295:1117-1120, 1976.

20. Vallee, B. L. , Ulmer, D. D. , Wacker, W. E. C.: Arsenic toxicology and biochemistry. AMA Arch. Indust. Health 21:132-151, 1960.

21. Beaudry, C. , Laplante, L.: Severe allergic pneumonitis from hydrochlorothiazide. Ann. Int. Med. 78:251-253, 1973.

22. Sanders, W. E. , Johnson, J. E. , Taggart, J. G.: Adverse reactions to cephalothin and cephapirin. New Eng. J. Med. 290:424-429, 1974.

23. Bryan, C. S. , Stone, W. J.: "Comparably massive" penicillin G therapy in renal failure. Ann. Int. Med. 82:189-195, 1975.

24. Simenhoff, M. L. , Guild, W. R. , Dammin, G. J.: Acute diffuse interstitial nephritis: Review of the literature and case report. Am. J. Med. 44:618-625, 1968.

25. Border, W. A. , et al. : Antitubular basement-membrane antibodies in methicillin-associated interstitial nephritis. New Eng. J. Med. 291:381-384, 1974.

26. Gleason, M. N. , et al. : Clinical Toxicity of Commercial Products, 3rd Edition. Williams and Wilkins Co. , Baltimore, 1969.

27. Arena, J. M.: Poisoning. Charles C Thomas, Springfield, 1970.

28. Hamilton, A. , Hardy, H. L.: Industrial Toxicology, 3rd Edition. Publishing Sciences Group, Inc. , Acton, 1974.

29. Dreisbach, R. H.: Handbook of Poisoning, 9th Edition. Lange Med. Publ. , Los Altos, 1977.

SECTION N: DIAGNOSTIC PROCEDURES

115: VIRAL DIAGNOSTICS (Collection of Specimens
and General Laboratory Techniques)
by Larry J. Baraff

There are three methods by which one may attempt to diagnose
a viral infection:

1) Microscopic examination of tissues for direct or indirect
   evidence of viral material;

2) Isolation and identification of the virus;

3) Demonstration of a rise in titer of specific antibody during
   the course of the illness.

One or more of these methods may be used in any illness to
confirm a viral etiology. Because of the fragile nature of viral
material and the possibility of bacterial contamination, it is
imperative that specimens be handled properly prior to their
processing. Tissues will undergo autolysis or bacterial put-
refaction, making microscopic examination impossible, unless
they are properly handled. In general, small pieces (five by
five mm. ) should be frozen to -20°C. and shipped, packed in
dry ice. Material for viral isolation, including swabs, tissues
and biological fluids, must also be handled with care. These
should be refrigerated immediately and kept cold during shipment up to the time they are inoculated into the appropriate
test host systems. They should be stored at -70°C. Serum specimens should be stored at -20°C.

## MICROSCOPIC METHODS

These include ordinary light microscopy, fluorescent microscopy and electron microscopy. These methods detect the presence of virus in tissues directly by immunologic mechanisms
or by the presence of pathognomonic changes. In general, his-
tiopathologic methods are of limited value in virology. Routine
light microscopy, by demonstrating the presence of inclusion
bodies or certain types of syncytial cells, may point to a viral
etiology. For example, the diagnosis of rabies may be made
by the examination of brain tissues for the presence of Negri

bodies. However, even in experienced hands, no Negri bodies may be seen in culture-positive rabies tissues. The cytomegalovirus was named for the typical inclusion-bearing giant cells which are present in the urine and tissues of patients infected with this agent, and microscopic examination of the scrapings from the base of a vesicle may be useful in differentiating varicella from variola.

Light microscopy, though of historical value, has limited application today. It has been largely replaced by immunofluorescence microscopy. This method utilizes specific high titer antibody directed against the viral antigen. Antibody may be prelabeled with fluorescent dye; or a two-step procedure may be utilized in which the tissue is first incubated with a specific, high titer antibody containing sera, and then incubated with fluorescent labeled antibody directed against the antibody used to conjugate with the viral antigen. For identification of rabies virus, the fluorescent antibody technique gives results that correlate well with those of mouse inoculation tests. This technique can be used to demonstrate the presence of most viral agents in tissues.

Similar antibody techniques are being developed which utilize other markers. Antibody may be conjugated with an enzyme which, when incubated with a specific substrate, results in color change visible on light microscopy. An example of this technique is the use of horseradish peroxidase conjugated to specific high titer antibody. Such techniques eliminate the need for the specialized equipment that fluorescent microscopy requires.

## ISOLATION OF VIRUSES

With the availability of tissue culture systems, viral isolation has been greatly simplified. However, this is an extremely time-consuming and expensive process. Consequently, for most diagnostic purposes, serodiagnosis is generally preferred to virus recovery. When viral isolation techniques are used, the following principles must be remembered:

1) Specimens must be collected from the appropriate sites as early as possible in the illness to assure the presence of virus.

2) Specimens must be properly handled en route to, and in, the laboratory to maintain viral viability.

3) Material must be inoculated into appropriate (susceptible) laboratory test systems.

In most common viral infections, the materials collected include nasal, throat, and rectal swabs and urine specimens. In selected illness, i.e. ARBO encephalitides and hemorrhagic fevers, virus may be isolated from blood specimens. In instances of viral (aseptic) meningitis, virus may be isolated from cerebrospinal fluid. Virus may also be isolated from infected tissue obtained by biopsy or at post-mortem examination. Vesicular fluid and scrapings from the base of vesicles may be utilized for viral isolation in the case of these exanthems. When swabs are used, they must be placed in the appropriate holding media to maintain viral viability. Such holding media should be proteinaceous and buffered to a neutral pH. Examples of commonly used media include veal infusion broth (V. I. B. ) and Hank's balanced salt solution with added V. I. B.

The host system employed for viral identification may include tissue culture, chick embryo or specific animals, including the suckling mouse, guinea pig or hamster. Tissue culture systems are generally derived from human embryonic tissues, human carcinomas and animal organs. Evidence of viral infection in tissue culture systems is demonstrated by cytopathic effect or hemadsorption. Evidence of infection in chicken embryos may manifest as the development of hemagglutinins, enfeeblement or death of the embryo, or the presence of plaques on the allantoic membrane. The source of material for viral isolation, host system employed, route of inoculation in the case of animal systems, and evidence of infections varies with the etiologic viral agent. For example, specimens for adenoviral isolation are usually obtained from throat or rectal swabs and identified in primary diploid human embryonic fibroblasts by the presence of a specific cytopathic effect. Influenza viruses are obtained from nasopharyngeal swabs, and may be identified in chick embryos by the development of hemagglutinins or in tissue culture (primary monkey kidney) by hemadsorption. Coxsackie viruses are isolated from rectal swabs and cerebrospinal fluid in suckling mice which demonstrate weakness, tremors, paralysis and death after intracerebral inoculation.

Tissue cultures have come to be the most important system for the isolation of viruses. Their usefulness for this procedure is being continually broadened through expansion of the spectrum of susceptible cell types.

## SEROLOGIC METHODS

Most viral infections are identified by a rise in specific anti-body titer during the course of illness. In general, paired sera obtained at least two, and preferably three, weeks apart are necessary to diagnose a viral infection. The presence of a high titer in convalescent serum may be suggestive of a specific etiologic diagnosis. Serologic techniques commonly used include complement-fixation, agglutination, hemagglutination inhibition, and in vitro neutralization techniques. More recent serologic techniques that shall be widely used in the future are the ELISA method (enzyme-linked immune serum assay) and the indirect fluorescent (IFA) test. The preferable serologic test varies with the type of viral infection. Complement-fixation is currently the most widely used technique. The choice of antigen is crucial in all serologic tests.

## REFERENCE

1.  Lennett, E. H. , Schmidt, N. A. (eds. ) : Diagnostic Procedures for Viral and Rickettsial Infections. American Public Health Association, 4th edition, 1969.

116:  ULTRASOUND: In the Diagnosis and Management
of Infectious Disease
by Caroline Yeager

## BASIC PRINCIPLES

In order to understand how diagnostic ultrasound images are
generated, what information can be obtained from these images
and what the limitations of such images are, it is necessary
first to consider the physical principles that govern sound waves.
The propagation of a sound wave depends on the vibration of
the molecules of the material through which it passes. That is,
the ·molecule must move from point A to point B and back to
point A again. Solid materials vibrate, but because of their
rigid structural bonds, they dampen the vibrations of the sonic
beam. Liquid materials vibrate very well and, because of their
looser molecular bonds, require less energy to do so. Gases
have such loose bonds that vibration is poor, especially at the
high frequencies used in diagnostic ultrasound, so that propagation of a sound wave is ineffective for diagnostic purposes.

Sound waves travel at a uniform speed through a single medium. When high frequency sound waves reach an interface between two medias, they are either reflected, refracted or
transmitted. The amount of the beam that is reflected depends
on the difference in the sonic properties of the materials forming the interface. This reflection is called an echo and is recorded as information on the ultrasound image. The sound that
is not reflected is transmitted through the interface. Thus, the
ultrasound image is composed of reflected sound waves, or
echos.

Fluid-filled structures, such as the gallbladder or an abscess,
have few internal surfaces for reflection and are characteristically echo-free. The reflections from their posterior walls
show the strong reflection of a fluid-solid interface. Because
fluids vibrate well, with little absorption of the sonic beam,
there is increased transmission of the beam through a fluid-
filled structure when compared to a solid structure.

Solid structures do not transmit sound as well, having absorbed
the beam energy and, depending on the homogeneity of the solid
structure, have few to many internal reflecting surfaces that
give an organ "texture" on the ultrasound image, which varies
from a light to a dark gray tone.

These same properties that allow us to create a diagnostic image with sound waves also impose limitations on its use. Because bone absorbs so much of the beam energy, the lack of significant penetration through bone precludes adequate imaging through bone at the present time. For example, during renal scanning, the ribs frequently obscure the upper third of the kidney in its longitudinal plane. The iliopsoas muscles are scanned easily from the dorsal aspect to the level of the iliac crest. Below the iliac crest, they must be scanned from the ventral aspect. In addition, gas does not allow transmission of the sonic beam with present technology. Thus, bowel gas and the lungs will prevent the imaging of structures where gas is interposed between the structure and the ultrasound transducer. Degassing agents have been used with varying success to overcome the problem of epigastric bowel gas. Scanning the abdomen below the umbilicus requires a distended bladder to displace colon and small bowel gas. The limitations of ambient air interposed between the transducer and the skin have been overcome with coupling agents, such as mineral oil or gel preparations. However, interruptions of skin continuity, such as scars, incisions or bandages still cause disruption of the useful sonic beam.

The ultrasound examination is performed after adequate patient preparation to minimize the limitations that have been described above. The patient's anatomy is reconstructed in a series of transverse, longitudinal and oblique sections, which are made in a logical sequence with adjustments in the angle and direction of the section, so that the anatomic reconstruction is tailored to the individual patient. Accurate identification of variant and pathological anatomy often depends on the painstaking demonstration of anatomical relationships on serial sections, rather than a gestalt of three dimensional structures in two dimensions.

With the recent development of gray-scale and real-time display, the ability to produce detailed images has made the ultrasound an increasingly important tool in the diagnosis and management of infectious diseases. The examination can be done with minimal patient preparation, discomfort, or morbidity. Ultrasound examination can be performed on even the most toxic patient with very little patient cooperation, if any. From the clinician's point of view, ultrasound is a rapid, non-invasive method for outlining the nature of a suspected lesion. Is there a mass present? If so, is it cystic, solid, vascular or related to a specific organ? Ultrasound can also determine the location and the extent of an abscess and even, on occasion, discover a previously unsuspected source for fever, thus obviating the need for the usual invasive diagnostic techniques. For the critically ill patients, portable scanning units are ideal.

## ECHOENCEPHALOGRAPHY (A-Mode)

At the present time, echoencephalography is limited to a simple determination of the position of the intracranial midline in the posterior two-thirds of the cranial vault. [1] Thus, as an initial screening modality, the examination is quick, harmless and may demonstrate a lateralizing sign in the initial evaluation of patients presenting with symptoms of intracranial infection, alerting the clinician to the possibility of a focal abnormality, such as abscess, hematoma or tumor rather than a generalized encephalitis. Since bone limits the penetrability of the sonic beam, anatomic imaging of the intracranial contents is best performed using CT scanning, radioisotope imaging or angiography.

## ECHOCARDIOGRAPHY (M-Mode)

Ultrasound scanners equipped with M-Mode (motion) display can make reproducible measurements of the size of the ventricular and left atrial cavities, septal and ventricular wall thicknesses, and can assess the functional motion of the mitral and aortic (and occasionally the tricuspid and pulmonic) valves. Unlike abdominal B-Mode scanning, which produces recognizable two dimensional "slices" of internal organs, M-Mode display relies on the linear-time display of the relative positions of the various intracardiac structures.

Infectious endocarditis is an entity that requires rapid, accurate diagnosis and continued clinical monitoring during therapy. Unfortunately, bacterial vegetations are usually small. By visualizing the functioning valve surfaces in motion, one can demonstrate these bacterial vegetations only if they are greater than 3 mm. in size. [2] On the other hand, the large, exophytic vegetations of Candida and Actinobacillus are more easily demonstrated on ultrasound, the echo pattern being rather characteristic for those entities. [3] The non-invasive demonstration of valvular vegetations may allow for more careful planning of such procedures as angiography, so that the morbidity from embolization is decreased and hastens surgical valvular replacement where needed.

In the presence of echocardiographically demonstrated endocarditis, the patient should be followed for such serious

complications as valvular ulceration, perforation rupture or
acute left ventricular failure. Flutter of the anterior leaflet of the mitral valve is seen in aortic insufficiency. When
this finding is associated with an otherwise normal aortic
valve, an infectious etiology should be suspected. In addition,
if there is an early closure of the mitral valve, it suggests
a severe aortic insufficiency, a finding that should alert
the clinician for rapid surgical intervention. [4] Paradoxically,
the abnormal thickening and shaggy non-uniform echoes of aortic valve vegetations have shown an increase during medical
therapy, possibly due to fibrosis of the valves as a result of
healing, rather than an increase in the growth of the vegetations. [5] Some patients may show resolution of the abnormal
pattern and return to a normal valve pattern after the course
of therapy is completed. [6]

The demonstration of pericardial effusion is best made by ultrasound (Figs. 134, 135). The method is simple, accurate,
harmless and may be performed at the bedside of a critically
ill patient. Collections of more than 35 ml. may be demonstrated with adequate technique. [5] The reproducibility of the
findings allows a simple and safe method of following the course
of pericardial effusions. On occasion, the demonstration of a
less than clear pericardial effusion may suggest the possibility
of a purulent effusion.

Pericardiocentesis can be performed using ultrasound visualization. The draining needle is introduced through the central
canal of a biopsy transducer. The needle or catheter tip and
epicardium are continually visualized during the procedure,
thus decreasing the potential morbidity and allowing the direction of the needle to the site of the fluid for drainage. [5]

### CHEST AND MEDIASTINUM (A-and M-Mode)

Evaluation for pleural effusion is most efficiently accomplished
radiographically, using plain film and horizontal beam technique.
With the use of a biopsy transducer, the draining needle or
catheter and its relationship to the pleural surface can be
visualized during thoracentesis, decreasing the morbidity of
this procedure and the risk of associated pleural puncture. [5]

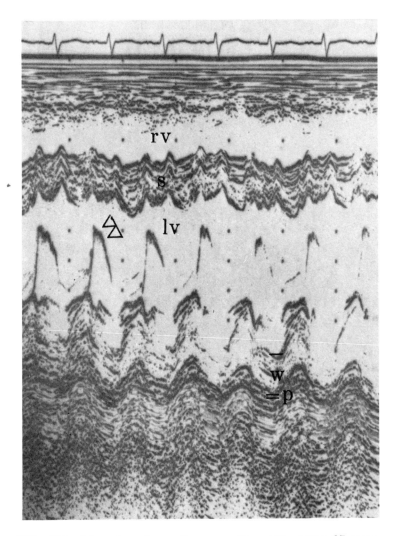

FIG. 134: M-mode echocardiogram. The patient is a 37-year-
old Black male with staphylococcal endocarditis secondary to heroin abuse. The flutter of the anterior
leaflet of the mitral valve is seen in aortic insufficiency (double arrowheads). The left ventricular posterior wall (-w-) is in apposition to the pericardium
(p). (Interventricular septum=s; right ventricle=rv;
left ventricle=lv).

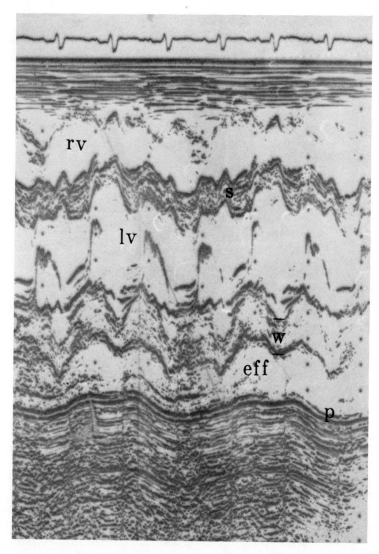

FIG. 135: Same patient as in Fig. 134. Ten days later, a moderate to large pericardial effusion (eff) is seen interposed between the left ventricular posterior wall and the pericardium (rv = right ventricular cavity; s = interventricular septum; lv = left ventricular cavity).

Evaluation of the mediastinum in adults is limited by the interposition of the bony sternum or air-filled lung between the transducer and the area to be studied. In children, this limitation
is minimal. Nevertheless, many mediastinal masses lend themselves to evaluation by ultrasound. By using a combination of
A-and M-Mode examination, the general characteristics of some
mediastinal masses can be determined prior to such invasive
procedures as mediastinoscopy. A-Mode evaluation of the presence and pattern of internal reflections can determine whether
a mass is solid or cystic. Abscesses, true cysts and vascular
structures have a "cystic" ultrasound appearance. M-Mode
evaluation can determine if the characteristic pulsatile motion
of a vascular structure is present. True cysts tend to have a
more characteristic location and spherical, smooth-walled appearance. Obviously, the non-invasive determination of the nature of the lesion may help in the selection of more specific
diagnostic procedures.[7]

## ABDOMINOPELVIC SONOGRAPHY (B-Mode)

Improvements in B-Mode scanning have resulted in more clearly
recognizable images of the abdomen and pelvis. For sono-
graphic purposes, the "abdomen" can be divided into the abdomen,
retroperitoneal space and pelvis. Abdominal sonography includes
evaluation of the diaphragm, intra-abdominal organs above the
level of the umbilicus and retroperitoneal organs anterior to the
spine. Usually, the patient is scanned in the supine position,
using longitudinal and transverse sections. Retroperitoneal
sonography encompasses examination of the retroperitoneal
structures lateral to the spine. This portion of abdominal scanning is performed with the patient prone; longitudinal and transverse sections being made from the dorsal aspect of the patient. In this position, the patient may be examined from the
lower extent of the pleural reflection to the iliac crest. The
remainder of the retroperitoneal examination, i.e., below the
level of the iliac crest, is performed from the ventral aspect,
using the technique of pelvic sonography. Retroperitoneal scanning from the dorsal aspect eliminates the intrusion of bowel
gas, and it requires no patient preparation. Occasionally, placing support, such as a pillow, under the patient's abdomen in
the prone position may aid in more adequate visualization of
the retroperitoneal structures superior to the iliac crest. Pelvic sonography is performed from the ventral aspect of the patient's abdomen with the patient supine. It is essential that the
patient's urinary bladder be fully distended in order to displace

intervening small bowel and colon gas so that a "sonic window" is created for examination of the intrapelvic contents and retroperitoneal structures lying inferior to the iliac crest.

Appropriate examination of the intra-abdominal and retroperitoneal contents depends on the adequate visualization and identification of solid parenchymal organs, vascular structures and bony anatomical landmarks. Gray-scale identification of the solid parenchymal organs of intra-abdominal, intrapelvic and retroperitoneal portions of the abdomen depends on adequate demonstration of the appropriate "texture" for that organ, as well as the relationship of that organ to the adjacent surrounding vascular structures.

In very general terms, inflammatory processes, such as the edema of inflammation, decrease the echo texture of the parenchymal portion of a solid organ and enlarge that organ. Degenerative changes, such as calcification and fibrosis, tend to increase the echo texture of the organ and decrease the size of the organ. Fluid collections, whether they are intraparenchymal or not, appear as echo-free spaces that distort the normal anatomical appearance. [8] It is difficult to determine the nature of a fluid collection by ultrasound. Although it is true that an abscess is more likely to have irregular borders and internal debris than a true cyst or early hematoma, the differentiation is often difficult. Occasionally, correlating the clinical course and laboratory findings with the ultrasonographic appearance of a fluid collection may help make this distinction. In addition, some solid masses are so homogeneous that they may lack the necessary internal reflecting surfaces necessary to differentiate a cystic from a solid mass.

In any event, diagnostic ultrasound is invaluable in the detection of intra-abdominal and intraparenchymal inflammatory changes secondary to infectious processes. Occasionally, ultrasound examination may localize an infectious process in an area not previously suspected to be involved. Because of its non-invasive nature, diagnostic ultrasound is quite suitable for following the course of a known intra-abdominal infectious lesion.

A combination of B-Mode and A-Mode scanning is helpful in the evaluation of diaphragmatic motion and contour. On the right, the diaphragm is identified as a perimeter of dense echoes at the superior and posterior periphery of the liver. On the left, the diaphragm is not visualized as well, being obscured frequently by a gas-filled stomach or small bowel. Examination on the left is facilitated by filling the stomach with fluid through a nasogastric tube. Even small motions of the diaphragm can be identified when B-Mode scanning and A-Mode evaluation are used together. Absence of diaphragmatic motion is a frequent indication of the presence of a subdiaphragmatic inflammatory process, such as a subdiaphragmatic abscess. [9] In most instances, especially on the right, careful scanning technique will demonstrate a cystic collection interposed between the liver and the diaphragm. On the left, because of the presence of bowel gas and a relatively echo-free spleen, identification of the abscess itself is less successful. Because the diaphragmatic echoes are usually readily identifiable, differentiation can usually be made between pleural and subdiaphragmatic fluid. Ascites and hemorrhage localized to the subdiaphragmatic space can give an identical ultrasound image. The clinical setting may help to differentiate these etiologies.

The liver image is reconstructed using longitudinal and transverse sections with the patient supine. The liver has a moderate gray-tone texture, slightly less echogenic than the pancreas. The hepatic and portal veins are visualized near their confluens. The biliary system is usually not visualized unless it is dilated. The gallbladder is frequently visualized, especially if the patient is fasting. Evaluation of the hepatic, vascular and ductal structures can differentiate obstructive from non-obstructive jaundice with a high degree of reliability, even in patients with a significantly elevated serum bilirubin. In acute, generalized inflammatory parenchymal disease, the liver may be enlarged with a decrease in the gray-tone texture. No distinctive pattern can be used to make a diagnosis of chronic, toxic or infectious hepatitis. This may be due to the changing appearance of the organ with different stages of the disease. However, as fibrosis replaces atrophic parenchyma in the development of cirrhosis, the general gray-tone pattern of the liver increases, and areas of fibrosis may be identified by focal increases in echogenicity. In this late stage, portal hypertension can be demonstrated if it is present by observing a general dilatation of the portal system, including the splenic vein, and splenomegaly.

Patients with known or suspected infectious or parasitic hepatic disease are usually examined with ultrasound, following the demonstration of a focal area of decreased uptake on a hepatic radioisotope scan. Although ultrasound imaging alone may demonstrate cystic areas of focal involvement in the liver parenchyma, such areas may be overlooked during routine

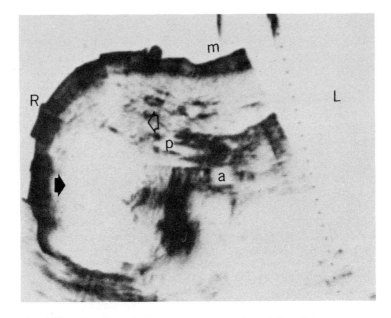

FIG. 136: Abdominal B-scan sonography of the liver. Transverse supine section. The normal liver texture (open arrow) is lost in the posterior portion of the right hepatic lobe (solid arrow), where there is the echo-free appearance of a fluid-filled area. (a = aorta; p = portal vein; m = ventral midline; R = right; L = left.)

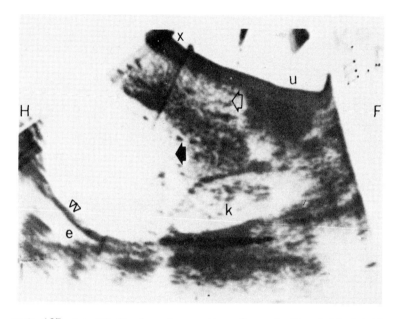

FIG. 137: Longitudinal supine section, 6 cm. to the right of midline (same patient as in Fig. 136). Again, the echo-
free focus in the posterior portion of the right hepatic
lobe is seen (solid arrow). This is a frequent location
for amoebic abscess. There is an accompanying pleural effusion seen as an echo-free space (e) superior
to the diaphragm (double arrowhead). (H = cephalad;
F = caudad; x = xiphoid; u = umbilicus; k = kidney).

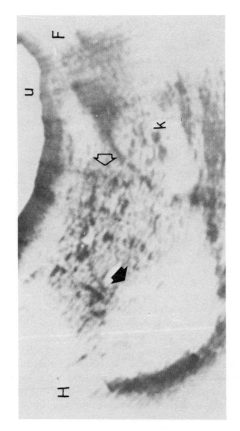

FIG. 138: Abdominal B-scan sonography of the liver. Longitudinal supine section, 6 cm. to the right of midline. Although this is a different patient, the echo-free portion of the posterior right hepatic lobe (solid arrow) can be differentiated from normal liver texture (open arrow). The patient is a 38-year-old Mexican-American male with an amoebic abscess. (H = cephalad; F = caudad; u = umbilicus; k = kidney).

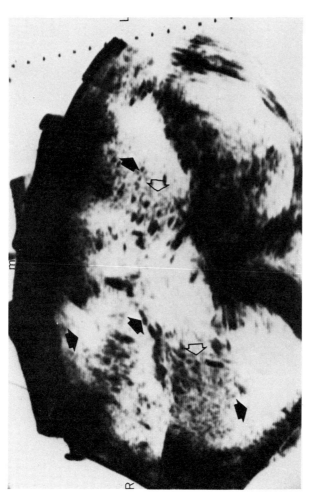

FIG. 139: Abdominal B-scan sonography of the liver. Transverse supine section. Multiple echo-free areas (solid arrows) are seen interspersed among areas of relatively normal liver texture (open arrows). The patient is a 33-year-old Mexican-American female with multiple anaerobic abscesses secondary to ascending cholangitis. (R = right; L = left; m = midline).

examination if radionuclide imaging does not direct scanning to the appropriate portion of the liver. "Blind spots" created by overlying ribs can be compensated for if directed by the existence of a focal abnormality on the radioisotope scan. Although cysts, abscesses or hematomas may have a similar appearance on ultrasound, that is, the echo-free appearance of fluid, a few differential features are recognized (Figs. 136-139). A pyogenic abscess can be seen as single or multiple echo-free areas scattered throughout the liver. Amoebic abscesses tend to occur more frequently in the posterior portion of the right hepatic lobe, possess somewhat irregular walls and may have the complex appearance of numerous internal reflecting surfaces. When hydatid cysts are first examined, they tend to be large.

Echinococcal cysts have a varied appearance, from simple and echo-free, occasionally with septa or necrotic debris, to the demonstration of the diagnostic "ring" of the internal daughter cyst. [10] Echinococcal cysts can also be demonstrated in the pelvis, but the appearance is different. There are more internal echoes. In a female patient, the appearance of the pelvic echinococcal cyst cannot be differentiated from an ovarian cyst. In a male patient, it would be rare to see cysts of another etiology.

Differentiating a pyogenic abscess located within the parenchyma of the liver from a necrotic tumor or cyst will depend more on the clinical picture than the ultrasonographic appearance of the echo-free area. Ultrasonic differentiation of cystic areas in the liver from pancreatic pseudocysts or a renal cystic mass rests upon the ultrasonic demonstration of organ continiity with the cystic structure.

It is interesting to note that liver abscesses appear to regress more rapidly on the ultrasound scan than on radioisotope images, [11] suggesting that form is re-established more promptly than function.

The normal "texture" of the spleen is a good example of an anechoic, or echo-free, solid mass. Because of this relatively echo-free appearance, demonstration of internal focal cystic areas is somewhat limited in the spleen. Echinococcal cysts have been identified in the spleen. Hematomas and abscesses have an echo-free appearance but are usually identified only at very high gain settings. The clinical picture is necessary for differentiation. Diffuse, chronic infectious processes that affect the spleen can result in a generalized increase in the gray-tone texture of the spleen. The demonstration of an abscess or other fluid collection in the retroperitoneum, adjacent to the spleen, relies on the demonstration of a wall separating a normal spleen from the cystic area.

In the evaluation of the pancreas, ultrasound offers a modality more sensitive than radioisotope scanning, an insignificant morbidity when compared to other methods of studying the retroperitoneum, except for the upper GI series, which is less specific than diagnostic ultrasound. However, interposition of bowel gas limits adequate visualization of the pancreas more frequently than other intra-abdominal organs. The examination of the pancreas includes scanning the patient in the prone position, through the left kidney, to look for the tail of the pancreas which lies ventral to that organ. The pancreas is usually identified as a solid structure that lies ventral to the splenic vein and dorsal to the left lobe of the liver. Its echo texture is slightly coarser and darker than the normal hepatic texture. The edematous pancreas is slightly enlarged with a generalized decrease in echo texture (Fig. 140). Pseudocysts or abscesses are seen as echo-free areas with a strong posterior wall reflection[9] (Fig. 141). The presence of internal septations, necrosis or debris appears as scattered internal echoes in an otherwise echo-free or cystic area. At times, pancreatic carcinoma can have an echo-free appearance. However, carcinoma demonstrates the absorption of the sonic beam characteristic of solid masses, and a strong posterior wall reflection should not be present. Measurement of the wall of a pseudocyst is important in determining the type of drainage that is performed in the absence of spontaneous resolution of the pseudocyst. Because ultrasound is a rapid and simple examination, the progress of a pseudocyst can be followed at frequent intervals, often demonstrating the rapid resolution that can be seen in pseudocysts.

Renal sonography is performed with the patient prone, scanning in transverse and oblique longitudinal sections over the area of the renal beds. No patient preparation is required. The renal shape demonstrated conforms to the plane of the section. The parenchyma has a very light gray-tone texture which, at moderately low gain settings, appears to be anechoic. The collecting systems are seen as a crowded collection of dense echoes located centrally within the renal parenchyma. Visualization of the superior third of the kidneys may be obscured by overlying ribs, which absorb the sonic beam, or limited by failure to demonstrate the separation between the left kidney and the spleen. Unless contraindicated, it is advisable to perform

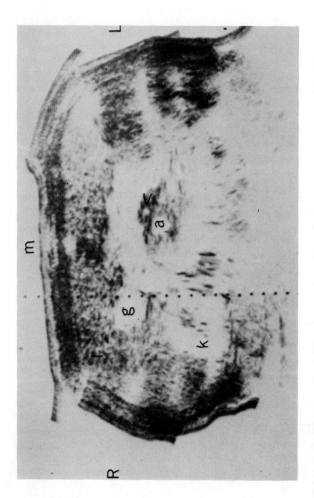

FIG. 140: Abdominal sonography of the pancreas. Transverse supine section, 10 cm. above the umbilicus. The pancreas is enlarged with a generalized decrease in texture compatible with edema in a patient with acute alcoholic pancreatitis. (R = right; L = left; m = midline; a = aorta; < = superior mesenteric artery; k = right kidney; l = liver; g = gallbladder).

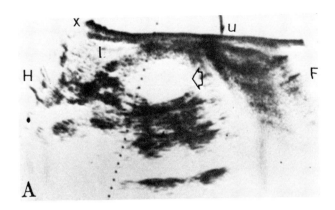

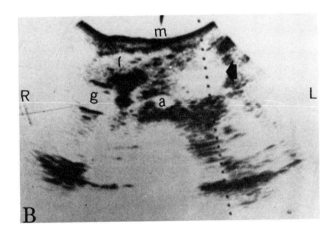

FIG. 141: Abdominal sonography of the pancreas. (A) Longitudinal supine section, 3 cm. to the left of midline. The enlarged, echo-free area (open arrow) can be seen in pseudocyst, abscess, hematoma of fluid-filled stomach. (B) Transverse supine section, 8 cm. superior to the umbilicus. The location of the cystic structure is shown to be the pancreatic tail. Clinical correlation confirms that this is a pancreatic pseudocyst. (R = right; L = left; H = cephalad; F = caudad; u = umbilicus; x = xiphoid; l = liver; g = gallbladder; a = aorta; m = midline).

the excretory urogram prior to renal sonography, so that the ultrasonographer is directed to evaluation of a specific renal finding. Entities such as pyelonephritis, papillary necrosis and glomerulonephritis are best differentiated on excretory urography. The mild calycectasis that can be demonstrated with ultrasonography requires excretory urography for confirmation and to delineate fine differentiation of the calycectatic pattern. In the kidney, diagnostic ultrasound is best used in the evaluation of renal masses previously identified by excretory urography. When directed at a specific site, ultrasound is a very sensitive means of differentiating cystic from solid masses in, or around, the kidney. [12] Use of a biopsy transducer provides non-invasive assistance in cyst puncture, obtaining culture samples and decompressing pyonephrosis and renal carbuncle so that specific antibiotic therapy may be initiated without delay. Especially in the case of renal carbuncle, the use of ultrasound to obtain culture samples has resulted in improved clinical management. [13]

Perirenal fluid collections are more easily visualized with diagnostic ultrasound than with any other modality. Unless there is significant renal displacement on excretory urography, perirenal fluid collections may be easily missed. Visualization of the kidneys with ultrasound not only demonstrates very minimal changes in renal position, but localizes small perirenal fluid collections accurately. This is especially important in patients who are otherwise asymptomatic or whose clinical state has been altered by steroids or immunosuppressive drugs. Perirenal fluid collections, such as abscesses, hematomas, seromas and urinomas all can have a similar ultrasonographic appearance. [11] Abscess may be more strongly suggested by scattered internal echoes within the cystic area if debris is present.

Xanthogranulomatous pyelonephritis is a diagnosis frequently missed preoperatively. Although occasionally excretory urography may demonstrate exuberant peripelvic fat proliferation, usually only a large kidney with poor or no function is seen. Retrograde pyelography and angiography demonstrate variable findings which are non-specific. However, ultrasound can demonstrate the presence of a large kidney which, in xanthogranulomatous pyelonephritis, has a normal parenchymal texture. The absence of solid tumor, pyonephrosis and the demonstration of obstruction all argue in favor of xanthogranulomatous pyelonephritis. [14]

Evaluation of the ureters, unless they are markedly dilated, is uniformly unrewarding with ultrasound. For evaluation of peri-ureteral masses, contrast-enhanced CT scanning is the preferred modality. Evaluation of the distended urinary bladder is easily performed with ultrasound, demonstrating its size, contour, intraluminal masses and extravesicular connections.

Evaluation of retroperitoneal structures, other than the pancreas and kidneys, depends on how the structure relates to the spine and iliac crest. If the structure is anterior to the spine, such as the aorta and the periaortic lymph nodes, evaluation is best performed in the supine position. Periaortic lymph nodes are seen as anechoic masses surrounding, elevating and impressing upon the aorta. Occasionally, retroperitoneal lymph node enlargement can be mistaken for a pancreatic head mass. Correlation of ultrasonographic sections of the retroperitoneum with contrast-enhanced CT body scanning of the lymph nodes may be a better method of making this differentiation.

Ultrasonographic evaluation of the retroperitoneal musculature, especially the iliopsoas muscles, is divided into two portions. The portion of the iliopsoas muscles superior to the iliac crest is best scanned with the patient prone. The portion of the iliopsoas muscles inferior to the iliac crest is best scanned with the patient supine, using the distended urinary bladder as a sonic window. The iliopsoas muscles are generally reasonably echo-free, but solid. Iliopsoas abscesses can be identified as echo-free areas that remain at high gain settings. [15] The demonstration of an iliopsoas abscess should alert the clinician to the possibility of tuberculosis as an etiologic agent with associated intraspinal disease.

Pelvic sonography is a well-developed field. It has long been used in the evaluation of obstetrical and gynecological diseases. Recently, pelvic sonography has been used in efforts to evaluate the prostate in male patients.

Adequate examination of the pelvis by ultrasound relies on distention of the urinary bladder and the absence of recent surgical incisions or bandages overlying the suprapubic portion of the abdomen. The distended urinary bladder not only displaces air-filled small bowel and colon from the pelvis, but acts as a known echo-free standard in the evaluation of cystic masses.

In the evaluation of pelvic inflammatory disease, pelvic sonography is useful for demonstrating changes in the uterine texture and the loss of definition of the pelvic musculature that may differentiate acute from chronic pelvic inflammatory disease [16] (Fig. 142). Gonococcal pelvic inflammatory disease frequently leads to adhesions, creating hydrosalpinx, which has a cystic adnexal appearance that is usually more funnel-shaped or tubular than the spherical-to-irregular appearance of a tubo-ovarian abscess or ovarian cyst. In many of these patients, serial examination may demonstrate the development of changes, indicating chronic or subacute stages of this disease. Pyogenic pelvic inflammatory disease may show more dramatic uterine texture changes, such as cystic areas of uterine necrosis and less severe adnexal changes in its acute form.

Non-gynecological pelvic abscesses can occur in ruptured appendicitis, Crohn's disease or other causes of peritoneal or pelvic infection (Fig. 143). These abscesses usually are demonstrated as an irregular cystic mass or masses in the vesiculorectal or rectouterine recesses of the pelvis and may have septations. The ultrasonic demonstration of the nature of the inflammatory process and its anatomical relationships may be helpful in planning whether drainage or conservative management of the process is the most beneficial form of therapy. In this country, experience with pelvic sonography of the prostate is limited. Nevertheless, demonstration of a cystic area within the prostatic texture argues in favor of prostatic abscess. [17]


## CONCLUSION

Diagnostic ultrasound is a relatively new and rapidly expanding field that provides a means of non-invasive imaging in the diagnosis of infectious diseases and is a simple method of frequent monitoring of those disease processes during therapy. In many instances, it may be the only reasonable method of alerting the clinician to the necessity for modification of the patient's clinical management. By balancing a basic knowledge of the principles and limitations that govern sound waves against the clinical problem to be solved, the clinician will be rewarded with the assistance of a useful tool of increasing importance and versatility.

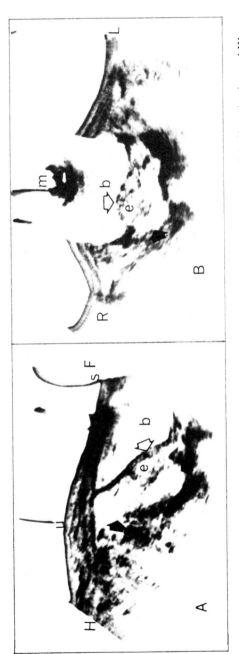

FIG. 142: Pelvic B-scan sonography. (A) Longitudinal supine section, directed to the uterine midline. (B) Transverse supine section, directed to a transverse section of the uterine body. The decreased intra-uterine echoes (e) create an echo-free "halo", indicating endometrial involvement. The multiple echo-free areas (solid arrows) are fluid collections in the adnexa and pelvis. This is a 29-year-old Mexican-American female with pelvic tuberculosis. Nevertheless, the findings are also seen in acute gonococcal pelvic inflammatory disease. (H = cephalad; F = caudad; R = right; L = left; m = midline; u = umbilicus; s = symphysis pubis; b = bladder).

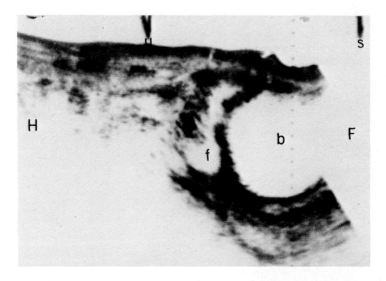

FIG. 143: Pelvic B-scan sonography. Longitudinal midline section. Intraperitoneal fluid is seen as an echo-free
collection in the vesiculorectal recess (f) in this male
patient who developed pelvic and subdiaphragmatic
abscesses post-appendectomy. (H = cephalad; F =
caudad; s = symphysis pubis; u = umbilicus; b = urinary bladder).

## REFERENCES

1. King, D. L.: Diagnostic Ultrasound. C. V. Mosby, St. Louis,
   1974.

2. Dillon, J. C., Feigenbaum, H.: Echocardiographic manifestations of valvular vegetations. Am. Heart J. 86:698,
   1973.

3. Moorthy, K., Prakash, R., Aronow, W. S.: Echocardiographic appearance of aortic valve vegetations in bacterial
   endocarditis due to Actinobacillus actinomycetemcomitans.
   J. Clin. Ultrasound 5:49, 1977.

4. Feigenbaum, H.: Echocardiography. Lea and Febiger,
   Philadelphia, 1972.

5. Goldberg, B. B. , Pollack, H. : Ultrasonic aspiration techniques. J. Clin. Ultrasound 4:141, 1976.

6. Nomier, A. , Watts, E. , Philip, J. R. : Bacterial endocarditis. Echocardiographic evaluation during therapy. J. Clin. Ultrasound 4:23, 1976.

7. Goldberg, B. B. : Mediastinal ultrasonography. J. Clin. Ultrasound 1:114, 1973.

8. Conrad, M. R. , Sanders, R. C. , James, A. E.: The sonolucent "light bulb" sign of fluid collection. J. Clin. Ultrasound 4:409, 1976.

9. Holm, H. H. , et al. : Abdominal Ultrasound. University Park Press, Baltimore, 1976.

10. King, D.: Ultrasonography of echinococcal cysts. J. Clin. Ultrasound 12:64, 1973.

11. Hassani, I. N.: Ultrasonography of the Abdomen. Springer-Verlag, New York, 1976.

12. Leopold, G. , Talner, L. , Asher, W.: An updated approach to the diagnosis of renal cyst. Radiology 109:671, 1973.

13. Pederson, J. F. , Hancke, S. , Kristensen, J. K.: Renal carbuncle: Antibiotic therapy governed by ultrasonically-guided aspiration. J. Urology 109:777, 1973.

14. Morgan, C. L. , et al. : Ultrasound in the diagnosis of xanthogranulomatous pyelonephritis: A case report. J. Clin. Ultrasound 3:301, 1975.

15. Leopold, G. : A review of retroperitoneal ultrasonography. J. Clin. Ultrasound 1:82, 1973.

16. Sample, F.: Pelvic Inflammatory Disease. Ultrasonography in Obstetrics and Gynecology, by Sanders, R. C. , James, A. E.. Appleton-Century-Crofts, New York, 1977.

17. Bartrum, R. J. , Crow, H. C. : Gray-Scale Ultrasound: A Manual for Physicians and Technical Personnel. W. B. Saunders, Philadelphia, 1977.

117: GAS CHROMATOGRAPHY (For Rapid Identification
of Bacterial Infections)
by H. Thadepalli

The diagnosis of bacterial infections involves laborious and
time-consuming culturing techniques. It is often important to
quickly arrive at the diagnosis. Gas chromatography appears
to serve this purpose. Most bacteria, aerobic and anaerobic,
produce a variety of metabolic by-products that can be detected
from the clinical specimens. [1,2] Each may have its own characteristic "fingerprint" pattern.

There are various methods for identification of bacterial infections. It may involve analysis of the metabolic products, or
a whole cell hydrolysate examination of the bacteria. Gas
chromatography is sensitive and specific enough to detect the
characteristic metabolites, even when they are produced in
such small concentrations as a nanogram or picogram level.

## BACTERIAL PNEUMONIA

Bacterial pneumonitis due to Diplococcus pneumoniae, Klebsiella pneumoniae or Herellea vaginicola, or tuberculosis, can
be detected by analysis of their by-products in the serum.[3] The
distinctive peaks obtained for each bacteria were considered
specific and highly reproducible. Gas chromatography is not
in wide application for the diagnosis of bacterial infections.

## ARTHRITIS

Arthritis can be diagnosed by gas chromatographic examination
of synovial fluids. Heptafluorobutyric anhydride derivatives of
these extracts are analysed on the gas chromatograph equipped
with an electron capture detector. [4] It was found that staphylococcal and gonococcal arthritis can be diagnosed by their characteristic patterns produced by this technique. Thus, they can
be readily distinguished from post-traumatic arthritis. These
patterns need to be standardized.

## CANDIDA SEPTICEMIA

The chromatograms of the serum from patients with Candida
albicans septicemia can be distinguished from bacterial septicemia. [5] Some of these peaks are identified by their chemical
nature, and others simply designated as A, B, C or D. The
advantage is that gas chromatograms of the candidemic sera
may become positive long before blood cultures.

## MENINGITIS

The activity of meningitis can be diagnosed by the quantity of lactic acid present in the cerebrospinal fluid. The quantities of lactic acid produced increase directly proportional to the degree of infection in cases of active meningitis; correspondingly, during therapy, there is a steady decline in quantity and a total disappearance on cure. [6] The spinal fluid samples in cases of Candida albicans meningitis, and the serum samples in cases of Candida septicemia, may show certain characteristic fingerprint patterns, diagnostic of Candida infection. Gas chromatography can also be used for the diagnosis of cryptococcal meningitis. [7,8]

## DIAGNOSIS OF ANAEROBIC INFECTIONS

Identification of anaerobic bacteria is done by means of gas-liquid chromatography. [9] In fact, gas chromatography is routinely used for the identification of anaerobic bacteria in the laboratory. For example, a gram-positive, non-spore-forming anaerobic bacillus which produces large quantities of propionic acid would be defined as a Propionibacterium, and a gram-negative bacillus which produces large quantities of butyric acid would be defined as Fusobacterium. We have evaluated more than 100 samples of clinical specimens suspected to have anaerobic infections (Fig. 144). In our experience, in 96% the diagnosis of anaerobic infection was made with certainty within an hour. In a small percentage of samples, when an anaerobe that does not produce volatile fatty acids is involved, gas chromatography may be unrewarding. This procedure can be done in the laboratory within a period of 20 minutes, in contrast to 48 to 72 hours required by routine culture techniques.

Identification of anaerobic gram-negative bacilli is important because most of the conventionally used antibiotics are ineffective against these organisms. We have reported that the presence of isobutyric, butyric and succinic acids indicated the presence of these organisms in the clinical specimens. False-positive and false-negative reactions occur, however, infrequently. [10]

Not all gas chromatographic patterns seen on gas chromatography are due to by-products of the bacteria found in the clinical specimen. Occasionally, the by-products from the host can be a result of the host reaction to the infection.

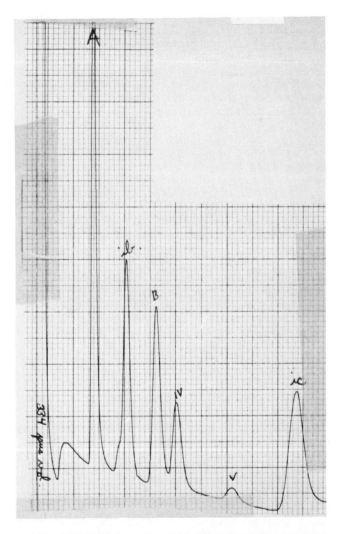

FIG. 144: Gas-liquid chromatography of an ether extract from the clinical specimen of empyema fluid revealing multiple volatile fatty acid peaks. A: acetic acid; ib: isobutyric; B: butyric; iv: isovaleric; v: valeric; and ic: isocaproic acid. Culture of the pus yielded Bacteroides fragilis ss. NGF, Peptococcus magnus, Eubacterium contortum and Streptococcus.

REFERENCES

1. Gorbach, S. L. , et al. : Rapid diagnosis of anaerobic infection by direct gas-liquid chromatography of clinical specimens. J. Clin. Invest. 57:478, 1976.

2. Phillips, K. D. , Tearle, P. V. , Willis, A. T. : Rapid diagnosis of anaerobic infection by gas-liguid chromatography of clinical material. J. Clin. Path. 29:428, 1976.

3. Mitruka, B. M. , Kundargi, R. S. , Jonas, A. M. : Gas chromatography for rapid differentiation of bacterial infections in man. Medical Res. Engineering. March-April, p. 7 1972.

4. Brooks, J. B. , et al. : Gas chromatography as a potential means of diagnosing arthritis. I. Differentiation between staphylococcal, streptococcal, gonococcal and traumatic arthritis. J. Inf. Dis. 129:660, 1974.

5. Miller, G. , et al. : Rapid identification of Candida albicans septicemia in man by gas-liquid chromatography. J. Clin. Invest. 54:1235, 1974.

6. Controni, G. , et al. : Cerebrospinal Fluid Lactate Determination: A New Parameter for the Diagnosis of Acute and Partially Treated Meningitis. Chemotherapy 1. (Eds. ) Williams, J. D. , Geddes, A. M. , Plenum Press, New York, 1975.

7. Davis, C. E. , McPherson, R. A. : Rapid diagnosis of septicemia and meningitis by gas-liquid chromatography. Microbiology. (Ed. ) Schlessinger, D. , American Society Microbiol. , page 55, 1975.

8. Schlossberg, D. , Brooks, J. B. , Shulman, J. A. : Possibility of diagnosis of meningitis by gas chromatography: Cryptococcal meningitis. J. Clin. Microbiol. 3:239, 1976.

9. Holdeman, L. V. , Moore, W. E. C. (Eds. ): Anaerobic Laboratory Manual, 3rd Edition. Virginia Polytechnic Institute and Anaerobic Laboratory, University of Virginia, Blacksburg, 1975.

10. Thadepalli, H. and Gangopadhyay, P. : Rapid Diagnosis of Anaerobic Empyema by Gas Liquid Chromatography Chest (in press) 1979.

118: NUCLEAR MEDICINE (Its Role in Infectious Diseases)
by Toshiyuki Tanaka

Nuclear medicine has advanced to a state where it can contribute effectively to the diagnosis and monitoring of therapy of infectious diseases. Such progress was possible because of instrumentation and rapid development in the field of radiopharmacology. The benign and the relatively non-invasive nature of nuclear medicine procedures, and their ability to ascertain natural events favored their usage in the detection of abscesses, osteomyelitis and such inflammatory processes. Obviously, no one procedure can give all the answers. Intelligent application of a combination of imaging modalities can increase the probability of a correct diagnosis. Consultation with the nuclear physician is important to ascertain the value of scanning in a given patient.

Radionuclear images, unlike x-rays, involve several hours of delay to obtain a scan. This may vary from five to ten minutes, as in the case of a liver scan, to 72 hours for a gallium-67 citrate (Ga-67) scan of the abdomen. The time for the actual scan depends upon the activity found within the body or the organ. A minimum of 300,000 (300K) counts are necessary for an adequate scintigraph of large organs in most cases. A repeat, delayed view may occasionally be helpful to enhance probability of finding a lesion by virtue of better target to non-target ratio. Further, scanning procedures may involve somewhat tiresome procedures, like bowel cleansing for Ga-67 scanning to eliminate obfuscation by overlying gut activity. This is not desirable in desperately ill patients, who, indeed, are the ones who need rapid diagnosis.

## SKELETAL SYSTEM [1]

Bone scanning is a sensitive method for discovering skeletal abnormalities, but it lacks specificity. In hematogenous osteomyelitis, the scan may become positive within 24 hours of the clinical symptoms. Abnormal scan findings may precede roentgenographic changes by 10 to 14 days. The radiopharmaceutical presently in favor is the Tc-99m labeled phosphate compounds. These agents accumulate at the sites of osteoblastic activity and are chemi-adsorbed onto the hydration shell of the hydroxyapatite. The differentiation of osteomyelitis and septic arthritis from cellulitis can be made by a combination of blood pool scanning and delayed bone scans. The blood pool scan is performed immediately after the intravenous injection of the bone agent. If the abnormality on the bone scan, a focal, well-defined lesion, matches precisely with the increased blood pool, the scan is compatible with hematogenous osteomyelitis (see Figs. 82-85, pages 453-456). Septic arthritis shows similar matching immediate and delayed image findings localized to a joint space (Figs. 145, 146). On the other hand, if no skeletal uptake is noted on delayed images, and increased blood pool activity is found immediately after injection, soft tissue inflammation is most likely. [2] Blood pool images of the spine are of less value because of underlying organs which obscure the hyperemic response.

The differentiation between osteomyelitis and infarction can be made by the temporal changes seen on serial images. Osteomyelitis will show an increased uptake at the involved site and either progressively increase or remain the same. Early in the course of an infarct, high resolution scintigraphs may actually reveal areas of decreased uptake, corresponding to the infarcted or devitalized bone, with a surrounding area of increased uptake due to the osteoblastic activity.

Diseases which cause periosteal reaction and hence an abnormal bone scan, but are of non-purulent nature, may be differentiated from osteomyelitis by using Ga-67 citrate, which does not concentrate in sterile reactive bone, but does concentrate in septic processes.

The earliest stages of osteomyelitis may be missed, and repeat scans are justified in those patients in whom the clinical suspicion remains high. Alterations of bone blood flow due to immobilization or lack of usage may show abnormal patterns; hence, a careful analysis is necessary. Confusing images may be seen in patients who are on large doses of antibiotics or anti-inflammatory drugs which reduce the response of bone to injury and hence reduce uptake. These may be resolved, at times, by the judicious use of Ga-67 citrate which concentrates in acute osteomyelitis. Occasionally, a lesion which fails to concentrate the bone imaging agent may be noted as a "cold" area on bone scans done early in the course of osteomyelitis. This may be the result of vascular compromise. Such a lesion may eventually become "hot". Thus, a lesion due to osteomyelitis may appear "cold" or "hot" on the bone scan, depending upon when, during the course of the disease, it is obtained.

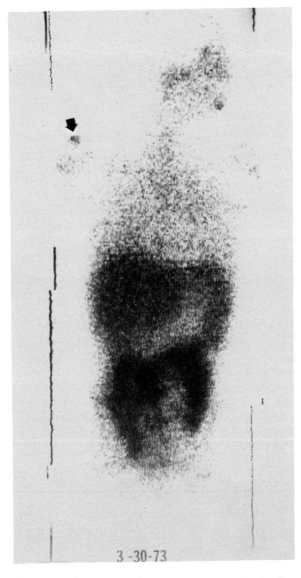

FIG. 145: Acromioclavicular arthritis due to Coc-
cioides immitis. Note the increased uptake of Ga-67 radionuclide at this site
(arrow). Also see Fig. 149 for followup.

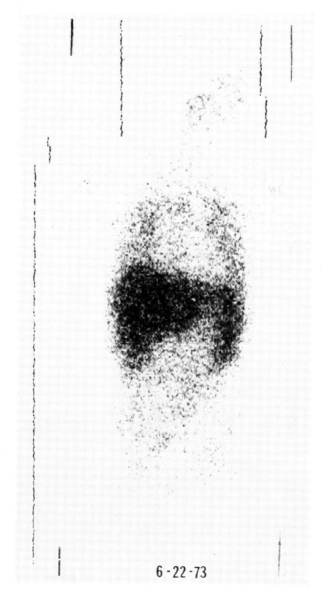

6 - 22 - 73

FIG. 146: Same as Fig. 145 after therapy with amphotericin B. Note the absence of uptake
of Ga-67.

## ABDOMINAL ABSCESS [3]

Gallium-67 citrate is a versatile, non-specific radiopharmaceutical which has affinity for inflammatory and tumor tissue.
The mechanism underlying this affinity is unclear. The empir-
ical observation of the affinity of gallium for the two types of
abnormal tissues has been exploited widely in the search for
an infectious source and neoplastic lesions. In abscess formation, the gallium concentrates in the wall of the abscess, presumably via the leukocyte carriers. Actual bacterial incorpor-
ation of the radionuclide has been demonstrated and it, too, adds
to the localization. In order to enhance the abscess wall uptake, leukocytes have been tagged with gallium and other radionuclides in vitro with no significant improvement in the images.

Patients suspected of amoebic abscess of the liver should initially have a liver scan. Amoebic abscesses of the liver usually appear as large focal areas of decreased activity on the
conventional technetium-99m sulphur colloid scan. They are
often in the right lobe of the liver, located just beneath the
"bare" area where the triangular ligament sweeps off the liver
(see Fig. 105, page 544). A complementary gallium scan will
reveal a ring of activity around the abscess, but the defect itself is generally smaller in radius than on the technetium scan
(see Fig. 106, page 545). While serial technetium scans may
show dramatic shrinkage of the apparent lesion, there may be
only minimal size changes on the gallium study. The reason
for this disparity is thought to be the temporary loss of phagocytic activity in the region surrounding the abscess. The tech-
netium-99m sulphur colloid is actively phagocytized by Kupffer's
cells. The return of normal phagocytic activity results in the
apparent "healing" on the conventional liver scans, as opposed
to both clinical and gallium scan findings. [4] Rarely, the scintigraphic appearance of a necrotic liver metastasis may be identical with that of amoebic abscess. Pyogenic abscess of the liver
will show patterns similar to that of an amoebic abscess. (Figs.
147-149).

At times, the abnormal concentration of gallium in the hepatic
area may be due to acute cholecystitis or empyema of the gallbladder; there is also increased uptake in the pancreatic bed
in many cases of acute pancreatitis. An additional useful procedure in the case of possible liver abscess is to perform a
flow study with Tc-99m sulphur colloid. In abscess, the flow
shows a rim of increased activity appearing late in the arterial
phase and persisting into the venous phase. This is due to the
dual blood supply of the liver. However, the study is limited in

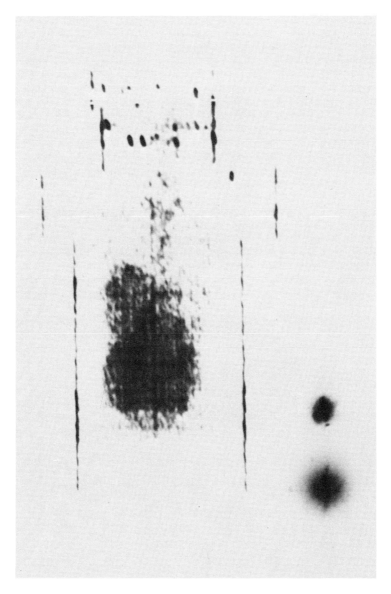

FIG. 147: Ga-67 scan showing increased uptake in the abdomen,
due to generalized peritonitis secondary to rupture of
an infected pseudocyst of the pancreas.

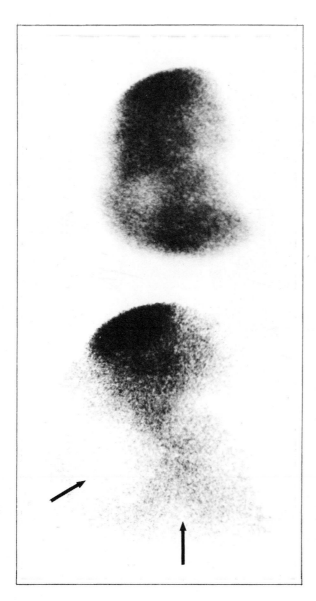

FIG. 148: Liver scan. A case of pyogenic liver abscess secondary to cholangitis, cholelithiasis and biliary obstruction. Note the multiple defects in the liver (arrows) shown on the left. The scan on the right was obtained approximately one month after surgical drainage and antibiotic therapy. The pus, on culture, yielded <u>Streptococcus viridans</u>, Peptostreptococcus and Peptococcus. The patient also had septicemia due to <u>Streptococcus viridans</u>.

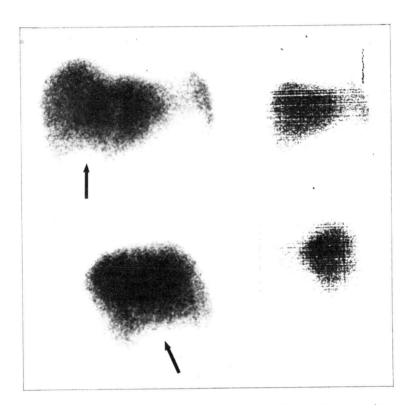

FIG. 149: Liver scan in a case of pyogenic liver abscess. (Anterior view on the top and right lateral view below). Note the defects marked by arrows, noticed before therapy. Two abscesses were drained and treated with antibiotics. Two weeks later, the scan was repeated (right). Note the absence of the previously noted defects.

the presence of a small lesion. Two centimeters is the smallest size of a lesion which can be detected with present instrumentation.

The search for an abscess in the abdomen is complicated by the normal concentration of activity in the gut. Bowel cleansing with laxatives and enemas may eliminate the unwanted activity. If an abnormal accumulation is noted, serial scans may often differentiate the transient and moving gastrointestinal activity from the fixed, persistent activity in the lesion. Simultaneous liver-lung scans have been used in addition to the gallium study to localize subphrenic abscesses. While a "gap" of activity between the two organs is compatible with a sizable subphrenic abscess, there are many pitfalls. If there is atelectasis, parenchymal lung disease at the base, loculated effusion or large pleural effusion, the examination is invalid. A liver scan alone is as useful, and less misleading than the combined lung-liver scan in detecting right-sided subphrenic abscess. On the left side, scanning is not as sensitive.

The true positive gallium scans for abdominal abscess range between 50% and 90% in the literature. False-positives are in the 5% to 10% range, false-negatives, 10% to 20%, and true negatives are around the 90% range.[5] The figures vary considerably from one series to another.

The gallium scan should be the last nuclear medicine procedure to be ordered if other scans are to be performed, since its long effective half-life will affect other studies when performed within a week of the injection, i. e. , there will be high "background noise".

## PULMONARY SYSTEM

Most active inflammatory diseases of the lungs will show increased gallium uptake (Figs. 150, 151) (Also see Figs. 12 and 14, pages 118, 124). Gallium scanning can be helpful in deciding whether a lesion seen on the chest roentgenogram represents an active process, or an old, burned-out process. Active, sputum-positive tuberculosis has positive lung images in nearly all cases (see Fig. 21, page 148). Sputum-negative cases of pulmonary tuberculosis may have normal gallium scans. In cases with suspected pulmonary embolism where there is an infiltrate on the chest x-ray and, consequently, an indeterminate lung scan, a gallium study can differentiate between pulmonary infarction, which has no avidity for gallium (Figs. 152, 153) and pneumonitis, which has avidity for gallium[6] (see Figs. 150, 151). Active sarcoidosis, silicosis, asbestosis and other inflammatory lung diseases will have positive images as well.

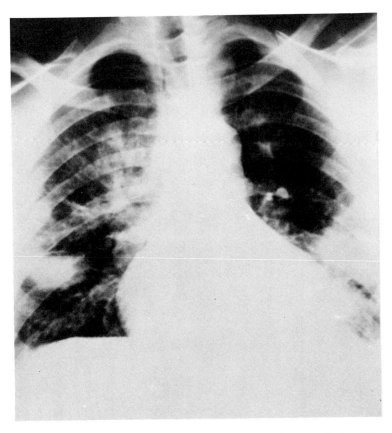

FIG. 150: Staphylococcal endocarditis in a drug addict. The chest roentgenogram shows septic infarcts on both sides of the lung (see Fig. 151 for Ga-67 scan).

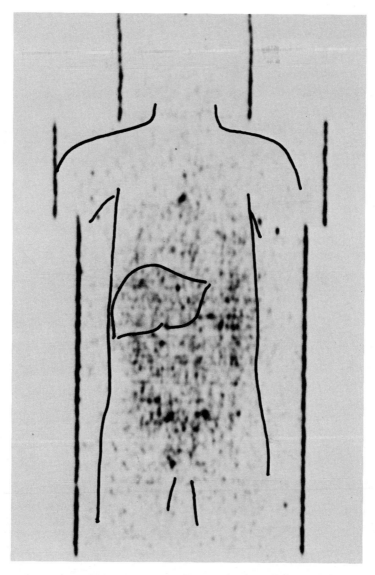

FIG. 151: Ga-67 scan of the patient shown in Fig. 150 depicts
increased uptake of Ga-67 in both lower lobes. S.
aureus was isolated from the blood and transtracheal
aspirate. Compare this with Figs. 150 and 152.

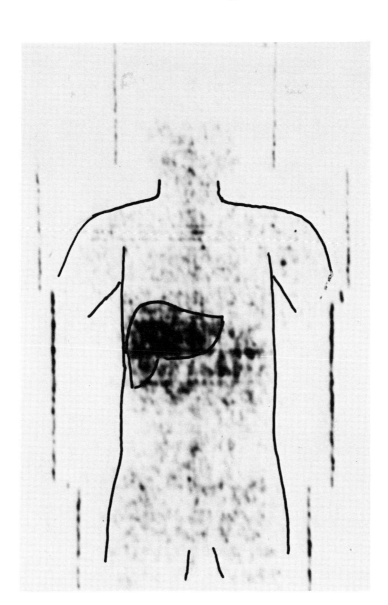

FIG. 152: Ga-67 scan in a case of pulmonary embolism. Note
the absence of any increase in the uptake of gallium
in the chest.

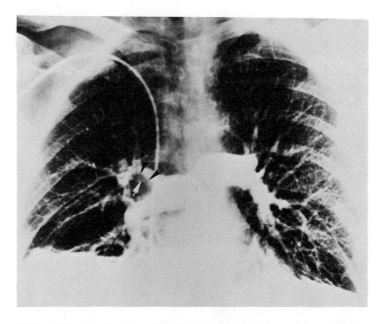

FIG. 153:   Angiogram of the same patient as in Fig. 152 showing radiolucency (arrows) in the right pulmonary
trunk; "cutoff sign" due to an embolus. (Courtesy of
Fred S. Mishkin, M. D. , Charles R. Drew Postgraduate Medical School, Los Angeles, California).

Conventional ventilation/perfusion lung scan has little value in
infectious disease involving the lungs, other than in quantita-
ting functional impairment of ventilation and perfusion. When
infiltrates are seen on the chest films, the scans will invariably be abnormal. Often the abnormalities on the lung perfusion scan are more extensive than expected from the chest
roentgenogram. Further, abnormalities may precede and lin-
ger longer than the chest film changes.

## GENITOURINARY SYSTEM

Renal uptake of gallium has been associated with acute pyelonephritis, perinephric abscesses (Fig. 154), acute tubular necrosis, vasculitis and malignant disease. [7] Approximately 15%
of the injected gallium is excreted via the genitourinary system
during the first 24 hours and minimally thereafter. Hence, renal
concentration after the first day is considered abnormal. The
differentiation among the previously mentioned disease entities

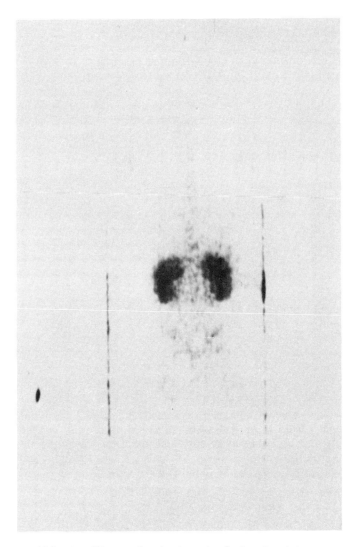

FIG. 154: Ga-67 scan (posterior view) showing intense uptake of the radionuclide in the parenchyma of
both kidneys.

must be clarified clinically and with other examinations. In one series, there was 84% accuracy in the diagnosis of acute pyelonephritis by gallium. Patients who have undergone recent transfusions may have saturation of transferrin, in which case the renal uptake of gallium is observed. Specificity, as in abdominal gallium scan, is lacking in gallium renal imaging. However, the gallium scan can help furnish evidence to distinguish between infection of the kidneys and the lower urinary tract. [8]

Inflammatory disease of the scrotum can be differentiated from torsion, which is potentially an acute surgical case, by scanning. [9] The study requires only an intravenous injection of Tc-99m pertechnetate. Sequential flow study images are obtained immediately after injection, and a static 300K count scintigraph is taken. The time required for the study is less than ten minutes and immediate interpretations can be made. Inflammatory disease will show increased blood flow to the involved side (Fig. 155); no focal area of decreased activity is seen within the involved testicle unless an abscess is present. Torsion will have a central "clear" area with hyperemic rim around the involved testicle (Fig. 156).

## CENTRAL NERVOUS SYSTEM

Brain abscesses are detected with a high degree of reliability by the brain scan. The advent of computerized axial tomography may supersede brain scans in the near future, but abscess detection via the brain scan is extremely sensitive, detecting lesions which may be missed by angiography. [10] The flow study may show bowing of the artery away from the abscess if the lesion is near the vessel. Immediate uptake as a result of the blood-brain barrier breakdown is seen. In some cases, a "doughnut" shaped lesion with a central "lucency" is visualized because of the necrotic tissue in the center. The course of therapy can be followed by serial scans of the resolving abscess. Gallium has also been used and, in one reported series, showed higher sensitivity than technetium brain scan.

Encephalitis is generally undetected on brain scans, but, on occasion, when the blood-brain barrier breaks down, increased uptake may be seen. In acute non-herpetic encephalitis, the brain scans are normal; in herpetic encephalitis, either bitemporal or frontotemporal, uptake may be seen. [11] Toxoplasmosis has also been reported to cause positive brain scans.

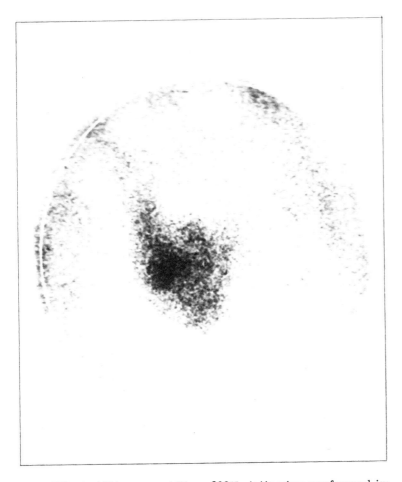

FIG. 155: Epididymo-orchitis - 300K static view performed immediately after the injection of Tc-99m pertechnetate.
There is increased uptake in the right scrotal contents. Etiology unknown.

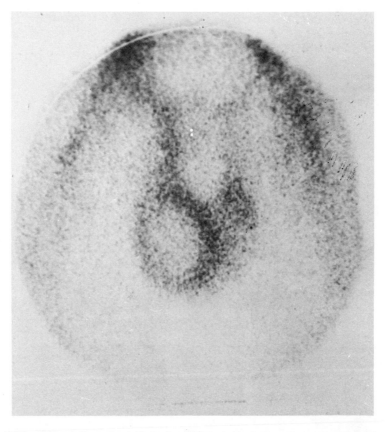

FIG. 156: Subacute torsion - 300K static scan shows a central area of decreased activity in the right scrotal content. There is hyperemic "rim" around the right testicle from the pudendal vessel. This case was surgically proven to have been torsion.

Tubercular meningitis may be diagnosed in suspected patients by oral administration of bromine-82 as ammonium bromide (0.6 uCi/kg), and measuring the cerebrospinal fluid/plasma ratio of Br-82 at 48 hours. A ratio of less than 1.9 is highly specific for tubercular meningitis. The Mantoux reaction may be rendered ineffective in cases where malnutrition and overwhelming tubercular infection exist; hence, the bromine test is of value. Unfortunately, external probe counting has not been successful and the patient must undergo a lumbar puncture. [12]

Rhinocerebral mucormycosis is a result of an opportunistic fungus and has had a rise in frequency as a consequence of immunosuppressive drug usage in transplant patients. It is also found in heroin users. The brain scans in these patients show a large triangular "shadow" in the naso-orbital region of the calvarium. Again, serial scans may assist in the assessment of therapy. [13]

Determination of a normal cerebrospinal fluid pathway, prior to intrathecal administration of drugs for therapy, may be performed by cisternography with a radiopharmaceutical such as Indium-111 DTPA (diethylene triamine pentacetic acid). In fungal meningitis, intrathecal administration of hyperbaric solution of amphotericin B must be preceded by the assurance of patent pathway. [14] The DTPA is a chelating agent, and it will avoid the possible aseptic meningitis formerly caused infrequently by albumin, a stigma which has been attached to radioiodinated serum albumin.

## RADIOBACTERIOLOGIC METHODS [15]

By inoculating appropriate samples onto culture media which contain carbon-14 labeled substrates such as C-14-C-1 glucose, one may detect bacterial respiration of radioactive $CO_2$ before bacterial growth is detectable by visual means. Such an approach can readily be automated and provides a sensitive and specific indicator of bacterial growth.

Radioactive techniques, because of their extreme sensitivity and ability to be quantitated, may be applied to many in vitro assay techniques. For example, anti-streptolysin-O determinations can be made simply and accurately. [16] Such methods have broad applicability, but have not been widely used.

## FUTURE DEVELOPMENTS

The future appears to be in the development of radiopharma-
ceuticals that offer more specificity. The goal is to develop
radiolabeled antibodies, the most specific agents in biochemistry. The production of purified antigen is the preliminary
step. The carcinoembryonic antigen tagged with iodine-131 has
been in use for several years as a laboratory procedure. Myoglobin antigen has been labeled for the detection of myocardial
infarct. [17] Antistaphylococcal antibody has been labeled, rather
crudely, and initial trials in a rabbit model have had promise. [18]
Further purification of antigen is necessary before adequate
images can be obtained. Once this major problem is overcome,
the sought-for specificity in the scan diagnosis may be attain-
able.

## CONCLUSION

The role of nuclear medicine in infectious diseases is an active and expanding one. Many radionuclide techniques provide
sensitive means of detecting abnormalities. Lack of specificity is a major drawback, but correlation with clinical findings
and other diagnostic procedures will generally result in valid
final diagnoses. The nuclear medicine contribution to laboratory bacteriology is not widely used, but can provide sensitive
means of early detection of bacterial growth. The development
of radiolabeled antigen is expected to enhance greatly the role
of nuclear scanning in infectious disease.

## REFERENCES

1.  Handmaker, H. , Leonards, R. : The bone scan in inflam-
    matory osseous disease. Sem. Nucl. Med. 6:95, 1976.

2.  Gilday, D. L. , Paul, D. J. , Patterson, J. : Diagnosis of
    osteomyelitis in children by combined blood pool and bone
    imaging. Radiology 117:331, 1975.

3.  Selby, J. B. : Radiologic examination of subphrenic disease
    processes. CRC Crit. Rev. Diagnostic Imaging 9:229, 1977.

4.  Maze, M. , Wood, J. : Uptake of $^{67}$Ga in space-occupying
    lesions in the liver. J. Nucl. Med. 16:443, 1975.

5.  Harvey, W. C. , Podoloff, D. A. , Kopp, D. T. : Gallium-67
    in 68 consecutive infection searches. J. Nucl. Med. 16:2,
    1975.

6. Mishkin, F. S. , et al. : Gallium lung imaging as an aid in the differential diagnosis between pulmonary infarction and pneumonitis. J. Nucl. Med. 16:551, 1975.

7. Kumar, B. , Coleman, R. E. : Significance of delayed Ga-67 localization in the kidneys. J. Nucl. Med. 17:872, 1976.

8. Hurwitz, S. R. , et al. : Ga-67 imaging to localize urinary tract infection. Brit. J. Radiol. 49:156, 1976.

9. Mishkin, F. S. : Differential diagnostic features of the radionuclide scrotal image. Am. J. Roentgenol. 128:127, 1977.

10. Crocker, E. F. , et al. : Technetium brain scanning in the diagnosis and management of cerebral abscess. Am. J. Med. 56:192, 1974.

11. Pexman, J. H. W. , McFreely, W. E. , Salmon, M. V. : The angiographic and brain scan findings in acute non-herpetic encephalitis. Brit. J. Radiol. 472:862, 1974.

12. Da Costa, H. , Barker, A. , Loken, M. : Distribution of orally administered bromine-82 in tubercular meningitis. J. Nucl. Med. 18:123, 1977.

13. Zwas, S. T. , Czerniak, P. : Head and brain scan findings in rhinocerebral mucormycosis. J. Nucl. Med. 16:925, 1975.

14. Alazraki, N. P. , et al. : Use of a hyperbaric solution for administration of intrathecal amphotericin B. New Eng. J. Med. 290:641, 1974.

15. DeBlanc, H. J. , Jr. , et al. : Automated radiometric detection of bacteria in 2,967 blood cultures. Appl. Microbiol. 22:846, 1971.

16. Deland, F. H. , Wagner, H. N. , Jr. : A new, accurate and simple technique for the assay of anti-streptolysin-O antibodies. J. Clin. Invest. 46:1049, 1967.

17. Parkey, R. W. , et al. : Localization of a specific I-131 antibody to myoglobin in myocardial tissue and factors which influence myoglobin release from cardiac cells. J. Nucl. Med. 18:611, 1977.

18. Huang, J. , et al. : Tc-99m-labeled antibacterial antibody scan for the diagnosis of infective endocarditis (in rabbits). Internatl. J. Nuc. Medicine & Biol. 5:169-174, 1978.

### 119: COMPUTERIZED AXIAL TOMOGRAPHY
by Lalit H. Vora

### INTRODUCTION

Computed tomography (CT), an idea, was tentatively put forward in 1961 by Oldendorf (a clinical neurologist), but conceived and developed independently by Hounsfield. It is a new method of "imaging" in which the patient is scanned by a narrow beam of x-rays. Measurements of the transmission of x-ray photons across a section of a part of the body are taken by an arrangement of crystal detectors, in such a way that a picture can be constructed by a computer and displayed on a cathode-ray tube. This system is approximately 100 times more sensitive [2] than conventional x-ray systems, to such an extent that variations in soft tissues of nearly similar density can be displayed. The most obvious difference from conventional radiography is that CT presents a cross-sectional view of the body.

### TECHNOLOGY

The following basic types of scanners are available:

FIRST GENERATION CT SCANNERS: These units consist of a single-beam x-ray tube operating in rotational and translational movements and one or two detectors. First generation scanners require approximately four minutes to obtain two cross sections of the body.

SECOND GENERATION SCANNERS: These employ larger numbers of detectors and a modified x-ray fan beam. Like the first generation units, they operate in rotational and translational motion, but they can obtain one or two cross sections in 20 seconds. These units often minimize artifacts due to respiratory motion.

THIRD GENERATION SCANNERS: In these scanners, in contrast to first and second generation machines, the motion of the x-ray tube and detector is purely rotational, without translating motion of earlier generations. Multiple detectors and true fan beams are used. Scan times of two to nine seconds will hopefully preclude artifacts due to respiratory motion.

FOURTH GENERATION SCANNERS: These units would be capable of scanning in fractions of a second without any motion of the x-ray tube or detector. Artifacts or blurring due to cardiac motion will be the challenge of the fourth generation devices.

## CONTRAST ENHANCEMENT

Intravenous administration of iodinated contrast medium has been proved to enhance the images of intracranial neoplasms, vascular malformations, abscesses and cerebral infarcts. Examination is carried out after rapid (one to five minutes) intravenous infusion of the equivalent of 200 ml. of 30% aqueous contrast material. CT is started at the end of the infusion; another 100 ml. is allowed to infuse slowly during the examination to maintain constant blood levels.

## DEMONSTRATION OF INTRACRANIAL INFECTIONS BY CT

It is shown to be a highly accurate, non-invasive technique of examining the brain. Diagnosis and management of various disease processes, such as meningitis, cerebritis, cerebral abscess, ventriculitis and epidural, subdural and subgaleal infection have become much easier than ever before.

MENINGITIS: CT findings may be normal in early meningitis and in successfully treated cases. In inadequately treated cases, fulminant cases and in cases of the sequelae of meningitis, CT might be helpful to delineate the disease process. Leptomeningeal inflammation may be associated with sterile subdural empyema. Loculation of cerebrospinal fluid, chiefly in the basilar cisterns, may result from pia-arachnoidal adhesions. Adhesions may cause communicating hydrocephalus, while obstructive hydrocephalus can result secondary to aqueductal occlusion.

Meningitis causes congestion in leptomeningeal capillaries, and increased blood volume, along with slow blood flow in these capillaries, which may lead to cortical infarction [3,4] (Fig. 157). Infarction may also occur secondary to vasculitis and septic thrombosis.

CEREBRITIS: Initially, a CT scan may be normal, but subsequently, a scan may show mottled areas of enhancement associated with a mass effect. [3] Neuropathologically, septic cerebritis consists of vascular congestion, petechial hemorrhages, cerebral softening and edema.

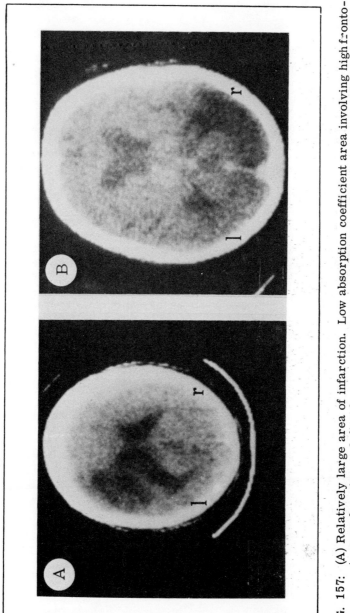

FIG. 157: (A) Relatively large area of infarction. Low absorption coefficient area involving high frontotemporal region on left side, consistent with an infarction. (B) Also shows relatively large area of infarction involving right parieto-occipital region.

CEREBRAL ABSCESS: The area of cerebral softening in cerebritis may undergo liquefaction, resulting in an abscess. In the
later stage, there may be capsule formation, which usually
consists of granulation tissue, collagen layer and reactive glial
tissue. Demonstration of the abscess capsule by CT is very
important, because it will be helpful in deciding when to drain
and subsequently, when to excise the capsule (Fig. 158). It has
been shown that the surgical results are considerably better
when the abscess capsules are excised. Besides the capsule
visualization, CT would accurately locate the abscess anatomi-
cally and would also identify multiple loculi when present (Figs.
159, 160).

Also important in the management of these cases is information
regarding the degree of mass effect, since cerebral herniation
is a leading cause of death, and the prognosis for recovery is
much worse after pressure cones have occurred preoperatively. [6]
Follow-up CT scans are useful in the evolution of intracranial
abscesses.

EPIDURAL AND SUBDURAL INFECTION: Epidural infection
is usually due to paranasal or mastoid sinus infection, osteomyelitis of the skull, postcraniotomy infection or septic phlebitis of emissary veins. CT would show an extracerebral area
of abnormality with a mass effect. Subdural empyema occurs
predominantly over the cerebral convexities and rarely at the
skull base (Fig. 161).

GRANULOMATOUS BASAL ARACHNOIDITIS: Clinical findings
are often insufficient to diagnose the basal arachnoiditis, and
conventional neuroradiological imaging techniques (angiography,
pneumoencephalography, or radionuclide imaging) often fail to
demonstrate the inflammatory process. CT scans usually can
demonstrate the circle of Willis and the basilar cisterns. CT
scanning may prove to be the most accurate and sensitive radiographic test for basal arachnoiditis (Fig. 162).

VENTRICULITIS: Chronic process may result in ependymitis
and may lead to hydrocephalus secondary to blockage of the
foramen of Monro or the aqueductus sylvius, or secondary to
meningitis, which results from ventriculitis.

TOXOPLASMOSIS (Fig. 163): Cytomegalic inclusion disease
and cysticercosis (Figs. 164, 165), tuberculomas (Fig. 166),
viral infection and fungal infection, etc. , may cause intracranial disease and can be detected by CT. Intracranial calcification can be detected with CT much earlier than conventional
x-ray, and this would be very helpful for early diagnosis.

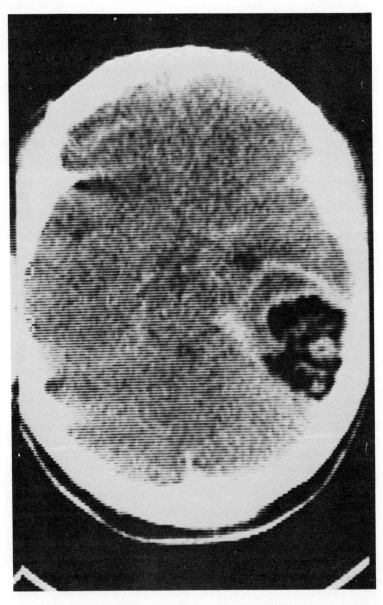

FIG. 158: Scan shows an abscess with early thin capsule formation. Low density of the abscess is suggestive of the
gas formation.

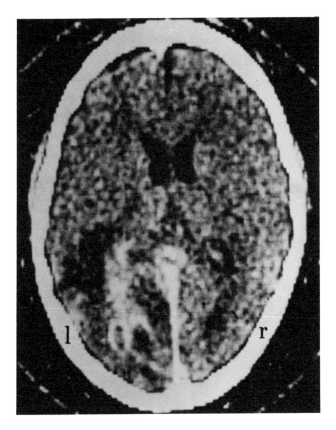

FIG. 159: Nocardia cerebritis with abscess formation.
This 55-year-old male had fever, headaches
and right homonymous hemianopsia. Lumbar
puncture showed 2,500 WBCs with 90% polymorphs in CSF. Scan shows irregular, poorly
defined areas of low absorption and contrast-
enhanced areas of left parieto-occipital region consistent with cerebritis. Just posterior
to these areas, there appear ring shadows
consistent with abscesses. Surgery with needle
aspiration demonstrated Nocardia. (Courtesy
of Drs. J. Bentson and L. O'Connor).

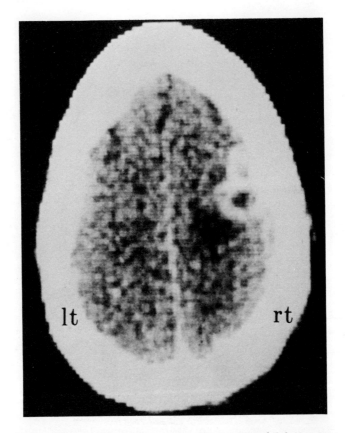

FIG. 160: Cortical abscesses. Scan obtained following
IV injection of contrast agent in this young
heroin addict. Ring appearance of these two
abscesses is due to contrast enhancement
consistent with capsule. The lesions are located at high frontoparietal region on right
side.

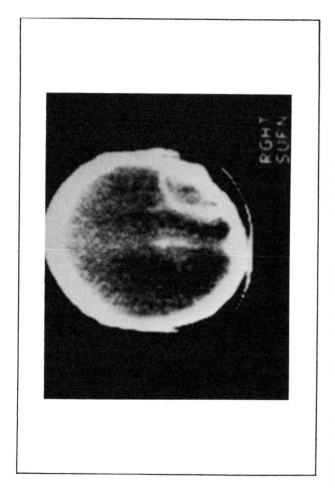

FIG. 161: Epidural abscess. Scan obtained following I.V. injection of contrast agent. It shows thick contrast-enhanced capsule surrounding a low absorption coefficient area. There was localized mass effect on ventricular system.

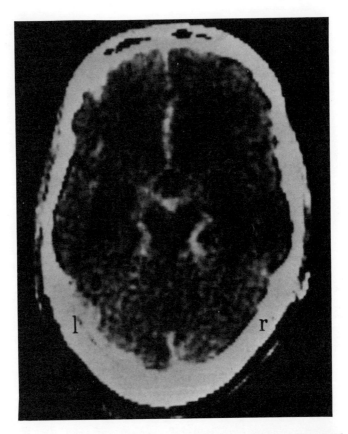

FIG. 162: Coccidioidal meningitis. Scan shows abnormal
staining of basal cisterns, following intravenous injection of contrast agent. Findings are
consistent with basal arachnoiditis. Ventricular system appeared grossly enlarged, indicating communicating hydrocephalus. (Courtesy of Drs. J. Bentson and L. O'Connor).

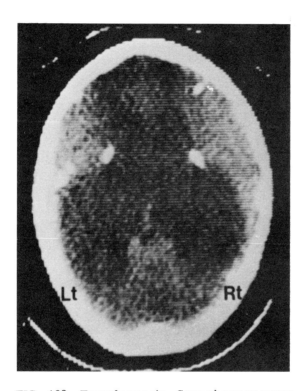

FIG. 163: Toxoplasmosis. Scan shows paraventricular and relative peripheral parenchymal calcifications with marked hydrocephalus of both ventricles.

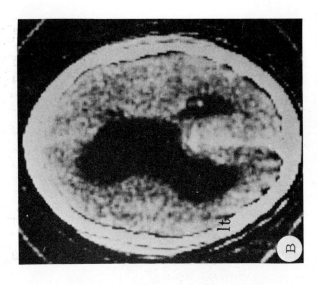

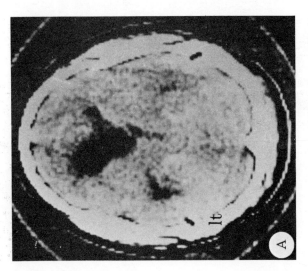

FIG. 164: (A) Upper cut at the level of frontal horns and (B) lower cut at the level of bodies of the lateral ventricles show cysticercosis cyst. Scans show unilateral hydrocephalus of frontal and temporal horns and body of left lateral ventricles. Contrast ventriculogram confirmed the site of obstruction. At surgery, cysticercosis cyst obstructing foramen of Monro was noted. (Courtesy of Drs. J. Bentson and L. O'Connor).

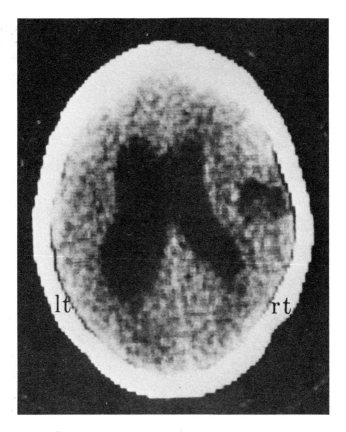

FIG. 165: Cysticercosis cyst. A well-defined low absorption coefficient area at high right frontotemporal region represents a cysticercosis
cyst. (Courtesy of Drs. J. Bentson and L.
O'Connor).

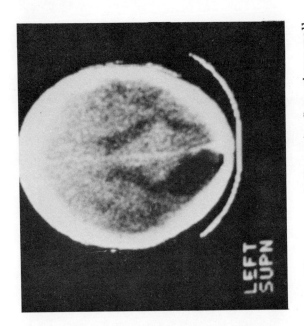

FIG. 167: Porencephalic cyst. Scan shows well-localized, low absorption coefficient (black) area, like CSF density, in close relation to posterior horn of left lateral ventricle.

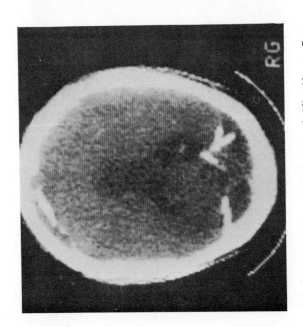

FIG. 166: Old granulomatous calcifications. Scan shows peripheral parenchymal calcifications with previous history of tuberculosis. Diagnosis of old tuberculomas was presumed.

CT CHARACTERISTICS: Plain scan may reveal areas of diminished absorption. With contrast medium injection, the capsule may be demonstrated. The capsule may appear regular or irregular in both thickness and contour.

DIFFERENTIAL DIAGNOSIS OF ABSCESS ON CT SCANS: Clinical and laboratory evidence of active infection is important in making the specific CT diagnosis of abscess. Metastasis, glioblastoma, granuloma, infarction and changes from recent cerebral surgery may show an area of low absorption surrounded by an enhancing rim and perifocal edema. Any of these lesions may sometimes appear identical to a cerebral abscess on CT scans. A porencephalic cyst, on scanning, may show a well localized, low absorption coefficient in close relation to the ventricles (Fig. 167).

PREFERRED ORDER OF RADIOLOGICAL STUDIES:[6] A high quality, plain radiographic skull examination should be obtained first. Paranasal sinuses and mastoids may be supplemented as required. Second, the CT scan, with plain scans followed by high dose contrast enhancement, would be necessary.

## EXTRACRANIAL COMPUTED TOMOGRAPHY

ORBIT: The retrobulbar space, difficult to assess clinically and by other radiological techniques, can now be rapidly evaluated for abnormal tissue without discomfort to the patient. Evaluation of globe, optic nerve and some of the ocular muscles is possible almost routinely (Fig. 168). It seems a higher resolution CT system will give considerably more detail of the lens and sclera and also ocular muscles. In short, orbital evaluation by CT scanning promises a new and, above all, safe method of investigation.

PARANASAL SINUSES AND PHARYNGEAL AREAS: These can be evaluated at a better advantage. Experience in this area is limited. Since lesions are seen in three dimensions at various planes, the localization of a lesion appears easier. Bony destruction and soft tissue abnormalities are well appreciated.

THORAX: The evaluation of pleural disease is unique because the extent of involvement of the pleura can be seen in a circumferential fashion (Fig. 169). Detection of an underlying lung parenchymal lesion in the presence of pleural effusion is very helpful. Extent of chest wall lesion can be studied accurately by CT scanning. Additional nodules, undetected on the chest film, are being detected by CT. A nodule can be better evaluated

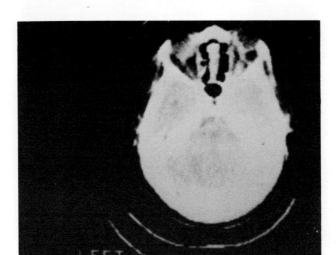

FIG. 168: Optic neuritis. Asymmetric optic nerves, with irregular thickenings of right optic nerve consistent with optic neuritis.

by CT, as it is more sensitive for detection of early calcium deposition, which may be unrecognized by conventional chest x-rays. In this situation, CT can show us a benign nature of a nodule (Fig. 170).

The mediastinum is difficult to assess, because the density of masses in this region is not much different from those of normal structures. Contrast enhancement may be helpful.

ABDOMEN:

Liver: The normal liver appears slightly more dense than other intra-abdominal organs, is homogeneous in density and is variable in size and configuration. Intravenous administration of contrast medium increases the density of both the normal and abnormal tissue, which tends to accentuate this density difference. CT allows the detection of smaller and deeper lesions than does the nuclear scan (Fig. 171). Hepatic abscesses are less dense than the liver and are less sharply marginated than neoplastic lesions. Gallbladder usually can be seen on CT scans of the liver (Fig. 172).

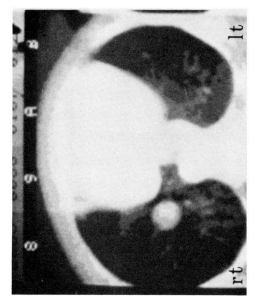

FIG. 170: Granulomatous lung parenchymal lesion. A well-defined, rounded, soft tissue nodule at the right midlung field with central calcification. Visualization of calcification is most likely indicative of benignity. Cardiac silhouette and spines are seen.

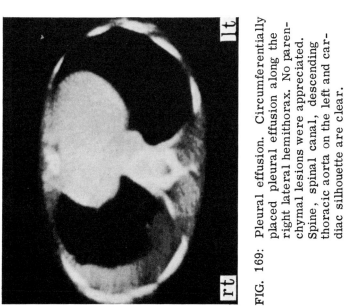

FIG. 169: Pleural effusion. Circumferentially placed pleural effusion along the right lateral hemithorax. No parenchymal lesions were appreciated. Spine, spinal canal, descending thoracic aorta on the left and cardiac silhouette are clear.

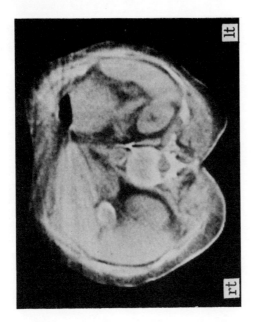

FIG. 172: Porcelain gallbladder. Scan shows a calcified ring near the porta hepatis consistent with porcelain gallbladder. Liver, spleen, kidneys, aorta and air fluid level in the stomach are well visualized.

FIG. 171: Cystic liver lesion. A well-defined, low absorption coefficient area in the left lobe of liver is suggestive of a cystic lesion.

Pancreas: The pancreas, or a portion of it, can be identified
on most scans, because it is separated from other organs by
fat planes. The pancreas is oriented in the abdomen, either
horizontally or obliquely. If it is oriented horizontally, the entire organ can be seen on one or more of the slices. However,
if the pancreas is oriented obliquely, only a portion will be seen
on any one slice.

Recognition of the pancreas can also be aided by its relationship to other organs. The tail is near the hilum of the spleen
and extends anteriorly ventral to the upper pole of the left kidney, where the body passes over the vertebral body and aorta
and immediately in front of the superior mesenteric artery.
The head lies in the loop formed by the second and third portions of the duodenum and is often inseparable from the bowel
by virtue of density alone (Fig. 173).

Detection of pancreatic lesions depends on recognition of alteration in the size or morphologic contour of the gland and
on secondary signs, such as pseudocyst. Distinction between
an inflammatory and a neoplastic mass is usually not possible
on the basis of a CT scan alone (Fig. 174).

Retroperitoneum: The retroperitoneal space is an area that is
difficult to evaluate with routine radiographic techniques. CT
scans appear to be one of the best examinations to detect retroperitoneal disease and its extent. The aorta and inferior vena
cava are sharply defined structures in the normal patient. Their
obliteration, compression or displacement can serve as indicators of disease.

Kidney and genitourinary tract: The kidneys are particularly
well demonstrated on abdominal CT scans, because they are
surrounded by perinephric fat, which demarcates the outer margin of the renal cortex; and they contain renal sinus fat, which
outlines the inner margin of the renal parenchyma. Evaluation
of flank masses and inflammatory processes is very helpful
(Fig. 175). The bladder and prostate have had limited study.

Pelvis: Distended urinary bladder and the rectum are routinely
identified as landmarks by the CT scans. The uterus, prostate
and the seminal vesicles can commonly be seen. Pelvic masses
can then be localized in relation to these anatomical sites.

Musculoskeletal: The muscle bundles and bones are seen very
well in cross section.

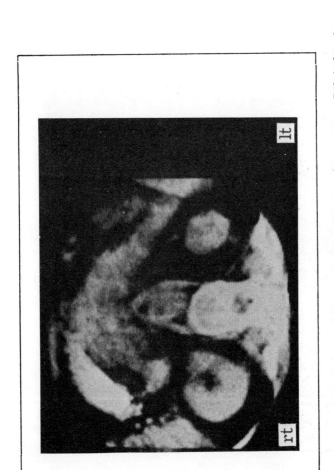

**FIG. 173:** Pancreatitis. Enlarged head and proximal portion of body of pancreas. Diluted water-soluble contrast material is seen in the stomach, delineating upper and right margin of head of the pancreas. Both kidneys, aorta and crus of diaphragms are seen. Tail of the pancreas reaches the hilum of spleen, and it appears unremarkable.

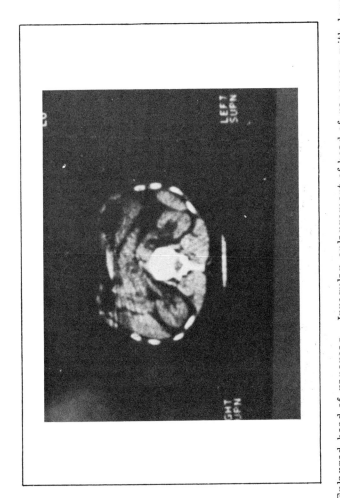

FIG. 174: Enlarged head of pancreas. Irregular enlargement of head of pancreas with loss of planes of surrounding organs. Differentiation of inflammatory process from malignancy is not possible without clinical correlation.

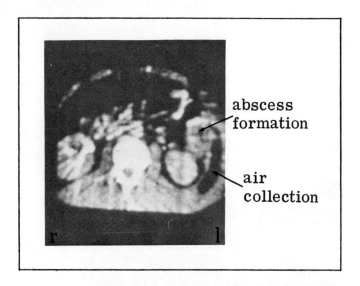

FIG. 175: Diverticulitis with abscess formation. This male patient presented in energency room with pain and tenderness in left flank. He had fever and leukocytosis. Clinically, he was diagnosed to have perinephric abscess. Plain films of abdomen showed suspicious tiny air collections in left flank. He was sent to scan room for emergency CT scanning. Scan showed a well-localized pocket of air collection in left flank with adjacent, irregular soft tissue mass anteriorly. Both kidneys were well-delineated with no abnormalities. At surgery, patient was found to have diverticulitis with localized area of abscess formation.

## CT-GUIDED BIOPSY AND ASPIRATION PROCEDURES (Fig. 176)

CT-assisted biopsy is an extremely useful diagnostic tool. Aspiration of abscesses and inflammatory processes of various body parts is possible, which has proven helpful for the best management and treatment. Utilization of this modality may preclude the morbidity, mortality and expense of laparotomy.

### IMAGE DEGRADATION IN CT SCANNING

The following are practical problems in best CT imaging:
1) Large amount of gas in intestine

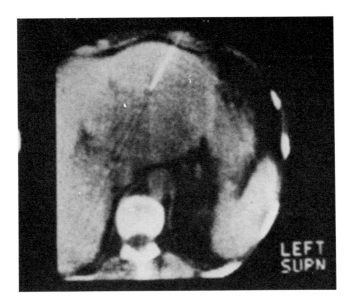

FIG. 176: CT-guided biopsy. A needle was manipulated in the large liver mass (left lobe of liver). Exact site of biopsy is possible by this means.

2) Residual barium
3) Surgical clips
4) Motion: This is probably the largest contributor to the loss of resolution and to the production of streak artifacts.
   - voluntary and involuntary musculature
   - peristaltic
   - respiratory
   - cardiovascular

Hopefully, faster scanning would eliminate some of the above artifacts due to motion. Peristalsis may be controlled by drugs (glucagon).
5) Very thin or debilitated patients: This is because of poor fat planes
6) Ascites might interfere in appreciating density difference.

## CONCLUSION

CT is one of the most significant diagnostic advances in radiology. It has been established as one of the safest and least invasive methods available for diagnosis and follow-up of intracranial diseases. CT of the body adds a new dimension to diagnostic radiology, and has a promising future.

## REFERENCES

1. Backer, H. L., Jr.: Computed tomography and neuroradiology: A fortunate primary union. Amer. J. Radiol. 127: 101, 1976.

2. Hounsfield, G. N.: Computerized transverse axial scanning (tomography). I. Description system. Brit. J. Radiol. 46: 1016, 1973.

3. Zimmerman, R. A., Patel, S., Bilaniuk, L. T.: Demonstration of purulent bacterial intracranial infections by CT. Amer. J. Radiol. 127:155, 1976.

4. Butler, I. J., Johnson, R. T.: Central nervous system infections. Pediatric Clin. N. A. 21:649, 1974.

5. Lott, T., et al.: Evaluation of brain and epidural abscesses by computed tomography. Radiology 122:371, 1977.

6. Paul, F. J., Davis, K. R., Ballantine, H. R.: Computed tomography in cerebral abscesses. Radiology 121:641, 1976.

7. Dieter, R., et al.: Computed tomography of granulomatous basal arachnoiditis. Radiology 120:341, 1976.

8. Momose, K. J., et al.: The use of computed tomography in ophthalmology. Radiology 115:361, 1975.

9. Alfidi, R. J., Haagg, J. R.: Computed tomography of the body. Postgrad. Med. 60:133-136, 1976.

10. Sheedy, P. F., et al.: Computed tomography of the body: Initial clinical trial with the EMI prototype. Amer. J. Radiol. 127:23, 1976.

11. Stephens, D. H., et al.: Initial clinical experience with CT of the body. Rad. Clinics of N. A. XIV(1):149, 1976.